Neurological Disorders: Advances in Neurology

Neurological Disorders: Advances in Neurology

Editor: Billy Acord

AMERICAN
MEDICAL PUBLISHERS
www.americanmedicalpublishers.com

AMERICAN
MEDICAL PUBLISHERS
www.americanmedicalpublishers.com

Cataloging-in-Publication Data

Neurological disorders : advances in neurology / edited by Billy Acord.
p. cm.
Includes bibliographical references and index.
ISBN 978-1-63927-316-4
1. Nervous system--Diseases. 2. Neurology. I. Acord, Billy.
RC347 .N48 2022
616.8--dc23

American Medical Publishers,
41 Flatbush Avenue,
1st Floor, New York,
NY 11217, USA

ISBN 978-1-63927-316-4 (Hardback)

Contents

Preface

This book has been a concerted effort by a group of academicians, researchers and scientists, who have contributed their research works for the realization of the book. This book has materialized in the wake of emerging advancements and innovations in this field. Therefore, the need of the hour was to compile all the required researches and disseminate the knowledge to a broad spectrum of people comprising of students, researchers and specialists of the field.

A neurological disorder is a condition of the nervous system that causes symptoms such as muscle weakness, loss of sensation, paralysis, poor coordination, seizures, altered levels of consciousness, confusion and pain. People with neurological disorders are susceptible to associated disability and suffering. The study, diagnosis and treatment of such disorders, fall within the scope of neurology and clinical neuropsychology. Neurological disorders may be classified based on the primary type of dysfunction involved, the primary location affected, or the primary cause. Brain disorders, spinal cord disorders, autonomic nervous system disorders, peripheral nervous system disorders, movement disorders, etc. are some of the categories in which neurological disorders are classified. Modern neurosurgery is guided by advanced neuroradiological imaging techniques. Open surgery, microsurgery, stereotaxy, endoscopic surgery, stereotactic radiosurgery, endovascular surgical neuroradiology, etc. are some of the techniques of neurosurgery. This book contains some path-breaking studies in diverse neurological disorders. It elucidates concepts and innovative models around prospective developments with respect to the diagnosis and management of such disorders. Students, researchers, experts and all associated with neurology will benefit alike from this book.

At the end of the preface, I would like to thank the authors for their brilliant chapters and the publisher for guiding us all-through the making of the book till its final stage. Also, I would like to thank my family for providing the support and encouragement throughout my academic career and research projects.

Editor

1

Surfen, a proteoglycan binding agent, reduces inflammation but inhibits remyelination in murine models of Multiple Sclerosis

Jordan R. Warford[1], Anna-Claire Lamport[1], Derek R. Clements[1], Alicia Malone[1], Barry E. Kennedy[1], Youra Kim[1], Shashi A. Gujar[1], David W. Hoskin[1,2] and Alexander S. Easton[1*]

Abstract

Proteoglycans are promising therapeutic targets in Multiple Sclerosis (MS), because they regulate many aspects of the immune response. This was studied using surfen, an agent that binds both heparan sulphate proteoglycans (HSPGs) and chondroitin sulphate proteoglycans (CSPGs). Initial cell culture work on bone marrow derived macrophages (BMDMs) found that surfen reduced concentrations of the chemokines CCL2, CCL4 and CCL5, with reduced messenger (m)RNA expression for Tumor Necrosis Factor, IL-6, IL-1β and inducible nitric oxide synthase. These data were further explored using Experimental Autoimmune Encephalomyelitis (EAE) in mice. Surfen reduced clinical signs during EAE when administered from disease onset, and reduced infiltration by CD4 positive T cells and macrophages into the central nervous system. These mice also showed reduced mRNA expression for the chemokines CCL3 and CCL5, with reduced concentrations of CCL2, CCL3 and CCL5. During EAE, surfen treatment induced a persistent increase in Interleukin (IL)-4 concentrations which may enhance T helper 2 responses. During EAE, surfen treatment reduced mRNA expression for HSPGs (NDST1, agrin, syndecan-4, perlecan, serglycin, syndecan-1) and the CSPG versican. By contrast, surfen increased mRNA expression for the CSPG aggrecan, with no effect on neurocan. During EAE, significant positive correlations were found between mRNA expression and clinical score for syndecan-4, serglycin and syndecan-1 and a significant negative correlation for aggrecan. These correlations were absent in surfen treated mice. Repair in the later stages of MS involves remyelination, which was modeled by injecting lysolecithin (lysophosphatidylcholine, LPC) into mouse corpus callosum to create regions of demyelination. When surfen was injected 2 days after LPC, it delayed remyelination of the lesions, but had no effect when injected 7 days after LPC. The delayed remyelination was associated with local increases in CSPG expression. Therefore surfen suppresses inflammation but inhibits remyelination in these models. A mechanism in common may be increased CSPG expression.

Keywords: Surfen, Lysolecithin, Proteoglycan, Experimental autoimmune encephalomyelitis, Multiple sclerosis

* Correspondence: Alexander.Easton@dal.ca
[1]Department of Pathology, Dalhousie University, Sir Charles Tupper Medical Building, 5850 College Street, PO Box 15000, Halifax, NS B3H 4R2, Canada
Full list of author information is available at the end of the article

Introduction

Multiple Sclerosis (MS) is a chronic disabling disease of the Central Nervous System (CNS) that is characterized by plaque formation in the brain and spinal cord parenchyma. These plaques have a prominent inflammatory component in the early stages, associated with myelin stripping from axons (known as demyelination). As the disease progresses, the loss of myelin contributes to atrophy and loss of axons which leads to permanent disability [3]. The pathogenesis of MS is unknown. It may be caused by a persistent failure of myelin formation, either because myelin is biochemically abnormal, or because of damage to myelin forming oligodendrocytes, or be triggered by an auto-antigen that causes autoreactive T cell clones to invade the CNS and trigger demyelination [25]. A puzzling aspect of the disease is the varied ability of plaques to undergo remyelination, which occurs when new myelin sheaths form around previously damaged axons. Many studies have focused on the factors that regulate remyelination, in the hope that restoring the myelin sheath may prevent axonal loss and prevent progression to permanent disability. This progression is untouched by current therapies, which dampen the immune response, but fail to arrest axonal loss. Studies of remyelination have revealed a paradox. While inflammation characterizes the disease, it also plays a role in orchestrating repair and remyelination [7, 18, 21]. Infiltrating macrophages play a role by generating growth factors that stimulate oligodendrocyte precursors to remyelinate axons [13]. However macrophages were also shown to generate chondroitin sulphate proteoglycans (CSPGs) which inhibit maturation of oligodendrocyte precursors, thereby inhibiting remyelination [14].

Proteoglycans (PGs) are macromolecules composed of a protein core covalently linked to glycosaminoglycan (GAG) side chains. GAGs are linear polysaccharides made of repeating disaccharide units and an amino sugar; they comprise heparin, heparan sulphate, hyaluronic acid, chondroitin sulphate, dermatan sulphate and keratan sulphate. The family of heparan sulphate PGs (HSPGs) have heparan sulfate side chains, while chondroitin sulphate PGs (CSPGs) have chondroitin sulphate side chains. The HSPG family includes perlecan, syndecan, serglycin and agrin, while CSPGs include aggrecan, versican, neurocan and brevican. PGs are a major component of the extracellular matrix of the developing CNS where they guide the migration and targeting of neurons to their final anatomic sites [32]. In the adult CNS they are localized in particular sites such as nodes of Ranvier, perineuronal nets and perivascular basement membranes. However their expression in the brain's extracellular matrix (ECM) increases during many diseases in the process of glial scar formation, as resident astrocytes respond to injury. Reactive astrocytes produce increased amounts of CSPGs, which are inhibitory to axon outgrowth in culture, and play a role in inhibiting axonal regeneration following injury in vivo [5]. In MS autopsy material, in early active plaques there was an accumulation of CSPGs (aggrecan, versican, neurocan) as well as dermatan sulphate PGs at the lesion edge associated with reactive astrocytes, with phagocytosis of PGs by macrophages at the lesion centre [23]. In another study, HSPGs normally associated with the perivascular basement membrane were widely distributed in the parenchyma of active plaques [27]. The role of PGs in the pathogenesis of MS is likely to be multifaceted, given the diverse roles attributed to these molecules, but one effect that they have is to inhibit remyelination. Similar to their ability to inhibit axonal growth and regeneration, a cluster of studies point to the capacity of CSPGs to inhibit remyelination through inhibitory effects on oligodendrocyte precursor cells [14, 17]. However, the effect of PGs is likely to be wider still, since PGs act as binding partners for a variety of factors that regulate immune responses, including cytokines, chemokines and growth factors [22]. Moreover, PGs not only bind to other molecules, but when bound they themselves trigger intracellular signaling events that control cellular responses, including in T cells which are major effector cells in MS [28].

To date there have been relatively few studies that target PGs in an attempt to develop new therapies for MS. A recent study used an inhibitor of CSPG synthesis (fluorosamine) in Experimental Autoimmune Encephalomyelitis (EAE) and lysolecithin (lysophosphatidylcholine, LPC)-induced demyelination and found that fluorosamine improves outcomes in both models. CSPGs alone, or astrocyte generated extracellular matrix containing CSPGs normally inhibits process formation by cultured oligodendrocyte precursors, but this inhibition was partially reversed when the astrocytes laying down the matrix were pretreated with fluorosamine [12]. The focus of this study is surfen, a compound known to bind the GAG side chains of PGs with high affinity. Surfen was first described as a component of depot insulin, and binds with greatest avidity to heparin, followed (in order) by dermatan sulphate, heparan sulphate and chondroitin sulphate [20]. It is therefore broader in its targeting of PGs than CSPG synthesis inhibitors like fluorosamine, with greater binding to HSPGs than CSPGs. Following on from our previous work in T cells [28], we began by studying the impact of surfen on cultured bone marrow derived macrophages

(BMDM) in vitro. Since macrophages are major effector cells in MS, we then went on to study the impact of surfen on two in vivo murine models of MS that respectively utilize EAE and LPC-induced demyelination. These models study complimentary aspects of MS. EAE models the early inflammatory changes seen in MS plaques, and allows detailed study of immunologic aspects of disease. LPC-induced demyelination, which permits the study of remyelination in isolation, mimics the later reparative phases of MS associated with a degree of remyelination, and provides insights into mechanisms of repair.

This study therefore investigates the impact of surfen on activated BMDM which model peripheral macrophages that have infiltrated the CNS during MS, and it goes on to explore the therapeutic potential of surfen in EAE, as well as its effects on remyelination in the LPC model. We report that surfen ameliorates inflammatory responses in EAE, but inhibits remyelination after LPC injection into the corpus callosum. Surfen in EAE has many effects on immune responses, including the expression of chemokines and cytokines, which reflect results obtained in BMDM cultures. The effect of surfen on PG expression has been studied in both animal models, leading to the conclusion that its divergent effects result in part from the increased expression of CSPGs. Surfen therefore inhibits remyelination, not just by binding to PGs, but by triggering increased local expression of CSPGs, which are well known to inhibit remyelination [14, 17]. The beneficial impact of surfen in EAE, and increased CSPG expression, also suggest that CSPGs are protective in the early inflammatory stages of MS, and do not just act as inhibitors of remyelination. These multimodal effects illustrate the complexity of using proteoglyan binding agents as therapies for the different phases of MS.

Materials and methods

Reagents and supplies

The peptide fragment containing amino acids 35-55 of Myelin Oligodendrocyte Glycoprotein (MOG_{35-55}) was obtained from Stanford Protein and Nucleic Acid Facility (CA). Acetic acid, ammonium sulphamate ($H_6N_2O_3S$), bovine serum albumin (BSA), brefeldin A from *penicillium*, complete Freund's adjuvant (CFA) containing *mycobacterium tuberculosis* H37RA (10 mg/ml), concanavalin A, dimethyl sulfoxide (DMSO), chondroitinase ABC, cysteine hydrochloric acid (HCL), 3-(4,5-dimethylthiazol-2-yl)-2,5-diphenyltetrazolium bromide (MTT), eriochrome cyanine, Dulbecco's Modified Eagle's Medium (DMEM), 10% buffered formalin, Griess reagent for nitrite, ketoprofen, L-α-Lysophosphatidylcholine (lysolecithin) from egg yolk, phosphate buffered saline (PBS; pH 7.4), pertussis toxin from *Bordetella pertussis*, Roswell Park Memorial Institute 1640 medium (RPMI), heparinase-III, ionomycin, bacterial lipopolysaccharide (LPS) from *E. coli* 0111:B4, papain from papaya latex, phorbol 12-myristate 13-acetate (PMA), sodium azide (NaN_3), sodium citrate, sodium nitrite ($NaNO_2$), sodium phosphate (NaH_2PO_4), SIGMA*FAST*® protease inhibitor cocktail tablets, surfen (bis-2-methyl-4-amino-quinolyl-6-carbamide hydrate), and Triton-X-100 were obtained from Sigma-Aldrich Canada (Oakville, ON). Fetal bovine serum (FBS), 10,000 U/ml penicillin/10,000 µg/mL streptomycin solution, 200 mM L-glutamine, 1 M 4-(2-hydroyethyl)-1-piperazineethanesulfonic acid (HEPES) buffer solution, and 0.4% trypan blue dye solution were obtained from Invitrogen Canada (Oakville, ON). Ethylene diamine tetraacetic acid (EDTA) was purchased from EM 46 Industries Inc. (Hawthorne, NY). Anhydrous ethyl alcohol was obtained from Commercial Alcohols (Brampton, ON). Purified functional grade anti-mouse CD28 (clone 37.51), purified functional grade anti-mouse CD16/32 (clone 93), and 7-amino-actinomycin D (7-AAD) were purchased from eBioscience (San Diego, CA). Neutral red was obtained from Fisher Scientific (Nepean, ON). Bio-Rad Protein Assay Dye Reagent, complementary deoxyribonucleic acid (cDNA) iScript, and Arium Total ribonucleic acid (RNA) extraction kits were obtained from Bio-Rad (Mississauga, ON). All cell culture plastics were obtained from Sarstedt Inc. (Montreal, QC) unless otherwise specified.

Antibodies (Ab)

The following Ab were used for flow cytometry: Phycoerythrin (PE)-conjugated anti-CD25, fluorescein isothiocyanate (FITC)-conjugated anti-CD69, PE-conjugated anti-mouse CD3e (clone eBio500A2), APC-conjugated anti-mouse IFN-γ (clone XMG1.2) were all purchased from eBioscience. Alexa Fluor® 488-anti-mouse CD4 (RM4-5), PE-anti-mouse CD3e (145-2C11), PerCP/Cy5.5-anti-mouse CD8a (53-6.7), APC-anti-mouse CD45 (30-F11), and APC-F4/80 (BM8) were obtained from Biolegend (San Diego, CA). FITC-anti-mouse CD11b (M1/70) was purchased from BD Bioscience (Mississauga, ON).

The following Ab were used for immunofluorescence: an unconjugated primary mouse anti-CSPG polyclonal Ab was obtained from Sigma-Aldrich Canada. An unconjugated rabbit anti-Iba-1 polyclonal Ab was obtained from Wako Chemicals (Wako, TX). Conjugated fluorescent secondary donkey anti-mouse IgG H&L (Alexa Fluor® 555) and donkey anti-rabbit IgG H&L (Alexa Fluor® 488, pre-adsorbed) Abs were obtained from Abcam (Cambridge, UK).

Bone marrow derived macrophages (BMDM)

Cell culture

Mice were killed by cervical dislocation and bone marrow flushed from the tibia and femurs. Red cells were removed by osmotic lysis and the bone marrow cell suspension washed twice with PBS and cultured at a density of 1×10^6 cells/well in 6-well plates in BMDM medium made of 85% RPMI-1640 and 15% L929-conditioned DMEM containing macrophage colony stimulating factor. 6 days later, culture medium and non-adherent cells were removed and fresh BMDM medium added. On day 7 after plating, the purity of BMDMs was 90% based on surface expression of the macrophage marker F4/80 (FACSCalibur, BD Bioscience).

Assay conditions

In all experiments, BMDMs were activated with 100 ng/mL of bacterial lipopolysaccharide (LPS), except for the Griess assay and iNOS expression studies which used 500 ng/mL. For nitric oxide assays, flow cytometry, and multiplexed ELISA, BMDMs were seeded in 24-well plates at 2.5×10^5 cells/well in 1 mL of cRPMI medium. Cells were plated at 1×10^6 cells/well in a 6-well plate for qPCR in 3 mL of cRPMI medium. For 7-AAD viability staining, MTT assays and surfen binding, cells were plated in 96-well plates at 1.5×10^4 cells/well in 100 μL cRPMI medium.

Protein expression

BMDMs were seeded on 24 well plates in RPMI-1640 and left to adhere for 4 h. One set of wells were left untreated, while others were treated with surfen (5 μM) or vehicle (0.1% DMSO) for 24 h. Culture supernatants were then collected and stored at −80 °C prior to use. Another set of cells were washed briefly in PBS and stimulated with LPS (100 ng/ml) for a further 24 h, at which point the supernatants were collected and stored at −80 °C prior to use. Cytokine levels in the supernatants were assessed using a Bio-Plex Pro™ premixed 8-plex mouse cytokine kit (Bio-Rad, Hercules, CA, USA) that measures the level of the cytokines IL-1β, IL-6, IL-10, TNF and the chemokines KC, CCL2, CCL4 and CCL5, as described above (section 4.3). Data was acquired using Bio-Plex Manager software version 6.1 with five-parameter logistic regression curve fitting (Bio-Rad).

Griess assay

After treatment, as outlined in section 1.3, culture supernatants were collected and 100 μL of supernatant combined with 100 μL of Griess reagent in individual wells of a 96-well plate and incubated for 5 min at RT in the dark. Nitric oxide levels for each condition were measured by reading the absorbance at 570 nm using a ELx800 UV universal microplate reader (BioTek Instruments, Winooski, VT) and comparing it with known concentrations of sodium nitrite (Sigma-Aldrich) in PBS using SOFTmax® PRO software (version 4.3; Molecular Devices, Sunnyvale, CA).

mRNA expression

After treatment, as outlined above, cells were washed with PBS, and 345 μL of RLT cell lysis buffer (Qiagen) was added to each well of a 6 well plate. RNA was harvested from the lysis buffer using an RNeasy Mini Kit (Qiagen) following manufacturer instructions. The purity and concentration of each RNA sample was determined using a NanoDrop 2000 device (Thermo Fisher Scientific, MA). The purity of the sample was based on the ratio of absorbance at 280 nm over 260 nm (A_{280}/A_{260} ratio) in which a value between 1.7 and 2.0 is considered acceptable [25]. Using 500 ng of RNA, cDNA was prepared with an iScript Advanced cDNA synthesis kit (Bio-Rad), as outlined in section 4.4. Transcript levels for individual proteins were determined using an SsoAdvanced Universal SYBR Green Supermix® (Bio-Rad) as outlined in section 4.4. For BMDMs the optimal housekeeping gene was determined to be GAPDH.

Viability assays

Viability was assessed by labeling with 7-AAD or MTT. 7-AAD labels non-viable cells by binding to nuclear DNA and is detected by flow cytometry, while the dehydrogenases of viable cells reduce MTT from its yellow tetrazole form to purple formazan, detected by absorbance. In the 7-ADD assay, BMDMs were treated with surfen (1, 2.5, 5, 10, 20 μM) or vehicle (0.1% DMSO) for 24 h. Following treatment, cells were washed with PBS, resuspended in FACS buffer, and labeled with 7- AAD (0.25 μg in 5 μL) for 5 min. Samples were immediately analyzed by flow cytometry. In the MTT assay, following 24 h surfen treatment, 10 μL of MTT solution (5 mg/ml in PBS) was added to each well of a 96-well plate and the BMDMs were incubated for 2 h at 37 °C in a humidified 5% CO_2 incubator. Following incubation, the plates were centrifuged, supernatants discarded, and 100 μL of 100% DMSO was added to each well. Plates were then shaken for 5 min at 550 g on a Microplate Genie (Montreal Biotech, Montreal, QC). The absorbance at 570 nm was read on an Expert 96 microplate reader (Biochrom ASYS, Cambridge, UK).

Surfen binding assay

Unstimulated murine BMDMs were collected and treated with surfen (5, 10, 20 μM) or vehicle (0.1% DMSO) for 2 h. A separate group of BMDMs were pretreated with heparitinase-III (0.001 U/ml) or chondroitinase ABC (10 U/ml) for 2 h and washed once with PBS before surfen or vehicle was added at the stated doses for an additional 2 h. The cells were washed to remove excess surfen, and fluorescence read at an emission wavelength of 488 nm in a spectrophotometer.

Mice

C57BL/6 adult female mice (16-20 g, 6-8 weeks of age) were purchased from Charles River Laboratories Canada (Saint Constant, QC) and housed in the Carleton Animal Care Facility (Dalhousie University). Mice were housed for approximately 2 weeks prior to experiments. Experimental procedures conform to 'Principles of laboratory animal care' (NIH publication 86-23, revised 1985). All applicable international, national and/or institutional guidelines for the care and use of animals were followed, including guidelines from the Canadian Council on Animal Care. All procedures performed in studies involving animals were in accordance with the ethical standards of the institution at which the studies were conducted and were approved by the Dalhousie University Committee on Laboratory Animals.

Experimental autoimmune encephalomyelitis (EAE)

Induction and surfen treatment

Experimental Autoimmune Encephalomyelitis (EAE) was induced as follows. On day 0, mice were briefly anesthetized with isoflurane (3 L/min) and inoculated subcutaneously (sc) bilaterally at the base of the tail, with a 1:1 mix of MOG_{35-55} and CFA (100 μL each side containing 150 μg MOG_{35-55} and 500 μg *mycobacterium tuberculosis* H37RA) combined with intraperitoneal (ip) pertussis toxin (PTX, 500 ng in 100 μL). The PTX injection was repeated on day 2. Antigen control mice received CFA + PTX but not MOG_{35-55}. Mice were scored clinically, based on the assessment of tail and hindlimb paralysis. At day 3, any mice showing lower limb gait disturbances resulting from the immunization procedure were excluded from the study. The scoring scale was 0 - no clinical deficits, 0.5 - partially limp tail, 1 - paralyzed tail, 2 - beginning of walking deficit, 2.5 - one hindlimb paralysed, 3 - both hindlimbs paralysed, 3.5 - hindlimbs paralysed with weak forelimbs, 4 - bilateral hindlimb paralysis and 5 - moribund [24]. At the onset of clinical signs (scores of 0.5 or greater) in mice with EAE, these mice as well as the CFA + PTX group received either vehicle (2.5% DMSO dissolved in PBS [*v*/v], i.p. every other day) or surfen (5 mg/kg, i.p. every other day). Animals were killed on day 21 with a lethal dose of sodium pentobarbital (100 mg/kg, i.p.). CNS tissues were harvested from these animals for subsequent analysis.

Extraction of immune cells and flow cytometry

Suspensions of immune cells were obtained from spinal cord and cerebellum. Fresh tissue was dissected, dissociated using a razor blade, and filtered with 70 μm cell strainers to remove debris. Cells were washed in PBS containing 5 mM EDTA, and treated with potassium lysis buffer for 20 min to induce lysis of contaminating red blood cells. Cells were washed twice, blocked with anti-CD16/32 antibody, and incubated with primary conjugated antibodies. Following incubation, cells were washed and fixed with 4% paraformaldehyde prior to flow cytometry acquisition and analysis. Flow cytometry data were collected with a FACSCalibur flow cytometer and CellQuest Pro software (BD Bioscience) or collected with a BD LSRFortessa™ cell analyzer using BD FACSDiva™ software (BD Bioscience). Post-acquisition data analysis was conducted using FCS 6 Express software (DeNovo Software, Los Angeles, CA).5.3 Protein expression.

Protein extracts from EAE and CFA + PTX spinal cord tissue were obtained by homogenization in 500 μL of PBS containing SIGMA*FAST*® protease inhibitor cocktail tablet (2 mM 4-[2-aminoethyl] benzenesulfonyl fluoride, 14 mM E-64, 130 μM bestatin, 1 μM leupeptin, 0.3 μM aprotinin, and 1 mM EDTA). Tissue was homogenized on ice for 1 min using a Pro 200 handheld homogenizer (Pro Scientific Inc., CT). Homogenates were centrifuged at 10000 × g for 10 min, supernatants collected, and protein concentrations determined using a Bradford protein assay. The supernatants were adjusted to a working concentration of 500 μg/mL using PBS buffer containing protease inhibitor and stored at −80 °C prior to use. A Bio-Plex Pro™ premixed 23-plex mouse cytokine kit (from Bio-Rad) was used to measure eotaxin, G-CSF, GM-CSF, Interferon (IFN)-γ, Interleukin (IL)-1α, IL-1β, IL-2, IL-3, IL-4, IL-5, IL-6, IL-9, IL-10, IL-12 (p40), IL-12 (p70), IL-13. IL-17A, KC, CCL2, CCL3, CCL4, CCL5, and Tumor necrosis factor (TNF). Standards were reconstituted with PBS buffer containing protease inhibitor and a 0.1% BSA [*w*/*v*] carrier. A standard curve was constructed using a 4-fold dilution series of beads with a known fluorescence spectrum unique to each cytokine. Magnetic anti-cytokine Ab conjugated beads (50 μL/well) were added to the wells of a 96-well plate and washed twice with 100 μL of assay buffer. Each sample was measured in duplicate wells, by adding 50 μL of undiluted supernatant to each well. The plate was covered and incubated in the dark at room temperature (RT) on a shaker set at 850 rpm for 30 min followed by 3 washes. Next, biotinylated detection Ab was added to each well and incubated in the dark at RT on a shaker set at 850 rpm for 30 min followed by 3 washes. Lastly, streptavidin-PE (50 μL) was added to the wells and incubated in the dark at RT on a shaker set at 850 rpm for 10 min.

Lastly, beads were washed 3 times, resuspended in assay buffer and analyzed with the Bio-Plex® 200 Suspension Array System (Bio-Rad). Data was acquired using Bio-Plex Manager software version 6.1 with five-parameter logistic regression curve fitting (Bio-Rad).

Messenger RNA (mRNA) expression

Fresh spinal cord tissue was immersed in 10 × the volume of an RNA stabilization reagent (RNAlater, Qiagen, Toronto, ON) for 24 h at 4 °C, and then stored at −20 °C prior to RNA extraction. Tissue was subsequently placed in 2 mL tubes containing 1.5 mm triple-pure zirconium beads (Benchmark Scientific Inc., NJ) and 1 mL of PureZol™ RNA isolation reagent (Bio-Rad). Spinal cord tissues were thoroughly homogenized by placing the bead-filled tubes into a BeadBug microtube homogenizer (Benchmark Scientific, NJ) for 45 s at 4000 rpm. Total RNA was extracted from the homogenized PureZol™ RNA reagent using an Aurum™ Total RNA Fatty and Fibrous Tissue kit (Bio-Rad) following the procedures outlined by the manufacturer. RNA quality was assessed with an Experion RNA StdSens Analysis Kit (Bio-Rad) used in conjunction with an Experion bioanalyzer system. cDNA was prepared with an iScript Advanced cDNA synthesis kit (Bio-Rad). The iScript reaction mix (4 μL) and iScript reverse transcriptase (1 μL) were added to 10 μL of nuclease-free water and 5 μL of input RNA. The reaction was incubated in a Bio-Rad T100™ Thermocycler using the following reaction protocol: 20 min at 46 °C, 1 min at 95 °C, and 5 min at 25 °C. Once synthesized, cDNA was stored at −20 °C for future use. A no-RT control reaction was included in every run to control for genomic DNA carryover by replacing reverse transcriptase volume with nuclease-free water. The transcript level for individual proteins was determined using an SsoAdvanced Universal SYBR Green Supermix® (Bio-Rad). Mouse KiCqStart® SYBR® Green Primers were purchased from Sigma-Aldrich Canada (listed in Additional file 1: Table S1). Each primer set contained a GC content of between 50 and 60%, no secondary structure, melting temperature between 60 °C ± 5 °C, and was between 18 and 24 base pairs long. The optimal annealing temperature for each primer set was determined with a temperature gradient that ranged from 53.0 °C – 65 °C in 2 °C increments using a CFX 96 Touch™ real-time PCR detection system with CFX manager 2.1 software (Bio-Rad). The temperature which produced the lowest quantitation cycle value was chosen as the optimal annealing temperature for that specific primer pair. Next, the linear dynamic range of the samples was established for each primer set by pooling 2 μL of cDNA from each cDNA sample and making a two-fold serial dilution series that ranged from 1/5 to 1/640. Primer efficiency was calculated using the pooled cDNA standard curve and was kept within 90-105% with an R^2 value >0.980. Subsequent cDNA dilutions were specific to each primer set based on efficiency results. Housekeeping genes were determined by calculating a geNorm expression stability m-value. The m-value represents the maximum amount of heterogeneity across experimental groups that can be tolerated by any given housekeeping gene and must be a value ≤ 1 [26]. The optimal housekeeping genes for spinal cord tissue were GAPDH along with HPRT1 to determine relative expression. The gene B2M was also tested but produced an m-value >1 for spinal cord tissue. PCR amplification and fluorescence detection were performed in triplicate using a CFX 96 Touch™ real-time PCR detection system with CFX manager 2.1 software. PCR cycling conditions were 95 °C for 30 s, followed by 40 cycles of 95 °C for 30 s and the experimentally determined annealing temperature (Additional file 1: Table S1) for 20 s. To confirm that the PCR reaction had produced the appropriate products, a melt curve analysis was conducted with temperatures ranging from 65 to 95 °C in 0.5 °C increments for 5 s each. Results are expressed as relative changes from the housekeeping calibrators and calculated using the $2^{-\Delta\Delta Ct}$ method [15].

Lysolecithin (lysophosphatidylcholine, LPC) model

Injection of LPC into the corpus callosum

Mice were anesthetized with isoflurane (3 L/min) and the head fixed in a stereotactic frame (Model 900, Kopf Instruments, CA). A 1 cm midline incision was made over the scalp. Two holes were drilled in the skull, one 1.2 mm anterior and 1.0 mm left of bregma, the other 1.2 mm anterior and 1.0 mm right of bregma. Using a microinjection unit (Model 5000, Kopf Instruments), 1 μL of 1% LPC [*w*/*v*] dissolved in PBS was injected into the corpus callosum on each side to a depth of 3.7 mm using a 2 μL Hamilton Neuros® 7001 metal syringe (Hamilton Company, NV). To prevent backflow, the needle was kept in place for 30 s before being retracted. The incision was sutured with 5-0 prolene, and the mice allowed to recover. 2 or 7 days later, separate cohorts of mice were reanesthetized with isoflurane, and the midline incision reopened. Through the left burr hole, 1 μL of vehicle (2% DMSO dissolved in PBS) was injected using a Hamilton metal syringe to a depth of 3.7 mm. The right burr hole was used to inject 1 μL of 100 μM surfen in a similar manner to a depth of 3.7 mm. The needle was kept in place for 30 s, retracted and the incision resutured. Sham mice received an injection of either PBS or the needle was inserted but no injection was made, to control for mechanical injury. Different cohorts of mice were killed 2, 7, 14, or 21 days after LPC injection with a lethal dose of sodium pentobarbital (100 mg/kg, i.p.).

Myelin staining

Mice were perfuse-fixed through the heart (10 mL PBS followed by 10 mL 10% buffered formalin). The brain was removed and immerse-fixed in formalin for a minimum of 4 days. Paraffin embedded tissue was then sectioned (5 μm). Myelin was stained using eriochrome cyanine with neutral red as counterstain. Briefly, paraffin sections were deparaffinized in 100% xylene, rehydrated in graded ethanols (100%, 95%, 70%), stained with eriochrome cyanine (15 min), washed in tap water (1 min) and differentiated in 0.5% ammonium hydroxide (NH_4OH) for 5 s. The eriochrome solution consisted of 40 mL of 0.2% eriochrome [*w*/*v*] diluted in 0.5% aq. H_2SO_4 [*v*/v] brought to 50 mL with 2% $FeCl_3$ [v/v] dissolved in water. Tissue was counterstained with 1% neutral red [w/v] for 2 min, then washed in tap water. Tissue was dehydrated in graded ethanols (70%, 95%, 100%), cleared in 100% xylene and coverslipped using Cytoseal (Stephen's Scientific, Riverdale, NJ, USA).

Immunofluorescence

Formalin fixed paraffin embedded sections were deparaffinized, and sections underwent antigen retrieval in sodium citrate buffer (11 mM sodium citrate, 0.05% Tween 20, pH 6.0) using a decloaking chamber (Biocare Medical, CA). Protein blocking was carried out in 5% donkey serum (Vector Laboratories, CA) dissolved in Tris buffered saline with Tween 20 (TBST) for 1 h at 37 °C. Primary Abs were diluted in TBST and placed directly on each section and incubated for 18 h at RT in the dark using a Simport StainTray™ (Simport Scientific, Beloeil, QC). Next, sections were washed three times with TBST and fluorescent conjugated secondary Ab diluted in TBST and placed directly on the sections for 2 h at RT in the dark. Lastly, sections were washed three times with TBST to remove excess secondary Ab and immediately coverslipped using Vectashield® mounting medium containing the nuclear counterstain DAPI (4,6-diamidino-2-phenylindole, Vector Laboratories, Burlingame, CA).

Electron microscopy

A cohort of mice were used following administration of LPC on day 0 and further treatment with surfen or vehicle on day 2. After death on day 7, the brains were removed fresh without transcardial perfusion. The corpus callosum from each side was resected and placed in 3.5% glutaraldehyde and post-fixed for at least 7 days. After fixation, the tissue was washed in Sorensen's phosphate buffer (0.2 M Na_2HPO_4, pH 7.4-7.6) for 2 min. The tissue was then treated with 1% osmium tetroxide (1 h, 4 °C), rinsed in buffer solution (2 min) and passed through a graded series of ethanols (70%, 95%, 100%, 15 min each) followed by treatment with propylene oxide (30 min on mixer). Embedding resin was then added to the tissue (2 h on mixer) and resin added to an embedding mold, pre-warmed in a 70 °C oven. The tissue was transferred to the mold and kept at 70 °C overnight before cooling to RT. Ultrathin sections were cut with a diamond knife on an ultra microtome. The resulting grids were stained with uranyl acetate (8 min), washed three times in 30% ethanol (10 s each wash) and then stained with lead citrate (8 min) and washed three times in distilled water (10 s each wash). The grids were dried, mounted and examined with a Hitachi TT7700 transmission electron microscope. Electron photomicrographs were obtained for different lesions, and stored in image files, coded to blind their identity during image analysis.

Image analysis

To evaluate LPC induced lesions in the corpus callosum, slides were scanned with an Aperio AT2 Digital Pathology scanner at 20 × magnification (Leica Biosystems, Wetzlar, Germany). The size of the lesion was determined using Aperio ImageScope software (Leica Biosystems) in which the region of demyelination within the corpus callosum was manually traced with a Wacom Intuos® touch tablet (Wacom Co. Ltd., Kazo, Japan) and the area calculated in mm^2. Representative photomicrographs of sections that displayed immunoreactivity were captured at 100 × magnification with a Zeiss Axio Imager Z2 fluorescent microscope (Zeiss AG, Oberkochen, Germany). Image quantification was performed using ImageJ software (NIH version). Briefly, preprocessing involved background substraction and application of a noise reduction filter. Next, a global threshold was set to define detection levels across all micrographs. Lastly, fluorescent intensities were quantified in terms of pixel counts translated to area by a scale bar. On electron micrographs, myelination was assessed using the ratio of axon circumference to full circumference (including myelin sheath, if present) of the fiber (G-ratio) using ImageTrak software (written by Dr. Peter Stys; www.ucalgary.ca/styslab/imagetrak). A ratio of 1 represents a completely demyelinated axon, whereas a ratio of 0.5 would be an average ratio of a large myelinated axon. Briefly, lesion electron photomicrographs were imported into the ImageTrak and each axon manually traced with a Wacom Intuos® touch tablet. G-ratios were then automatically calculated.

Statistics

Where two groups were compared, Student's t-test and Mann Whitney U test were used to calculate differences between groups with normal and non-Gaussian distributions, respectively. Comparison between three or more groups was performed using a one-way ANOVA with Tukey's post-hoc analysis. EAE curves were analyzed using a two-way ANOVA with Bonferroni's post-hoc analysis. All statistics were computed using GraphPad Prism version 7.0 for Macintosh (GraphPad Software, San Diego, CA). $P < 0.05$ was considered significant.

Results

Impact of surfen on macrophage cell cultures

Surfen may reduce disease in MS by impacting the function of peripheral macrophages, either in the periphery, or once they have migrated into the CNS parenchyma and undergone local activation. To explore this possibility, cell culture studies were carried out on murine bone marrow derived macrophages (BMDM). 5 μM was the highest dose of surfen that did not reduce numbers or viability of BMDM (significant reductions were noted at 10 and 20 μM, Additional file 2: Figure S1). 5 μM surfen also resulted in significant binding to the cells, as assessed by fluorescence, that was partially inhibited by pretreatment with heparitinase-III and chondroitinase ABC, enzymes that degrade the GAG side chains to which surfen binds (Additional file 2: Figure S1). Surfen significantly reduced concentrations of the chemokines CCL2, CCL4 and CCL5 released by lipopolysaccharide (LPS)-stimulated BMDM (Fig. 1a). Various cytokines were also studied. In LPS-stimulated BMDM, surfen significantly reduced mRNA expression for IL-1β, IL-6 and TNF (Fig. 1b). Concentrations of IL-6, TNF and IL-10 produced by LPS-stimulated BMDM were significantly reduced by surfen, while, by contrast, the concentration of IL-1β was significantly increased (Fig. 1c). In LPS-stimulated BMDM, surfen significantly reduced the mRNA expression of inducible nitric oxide synthase (iNOS), and induced a dose dependent reduction in NO production (Fig. 1d). These data show that surfen alters the production of key mediators by peripheral macrophages, which may affect their ability to contribute to CNS diseases such as MS, or the animal models we went on to study.

Surfen ameliorates experimental autoimmune encephalomyelitis (EAE)

Having obtained data from one effector cell of relevance to MS, we went on to study the impact of surfen on EAE, a key model of the inflammatory-immune aspects of the disease. Treatment with surfen from onset of clinical signs during EAE (between 7 and 11 days after induction) resulted in a significant reduction in clinical scores between days 13-21 (Fig. 2a). The mean clinical score for vehicle treated EAE over this period was 2.84 ± 0.05 (mean ± standard error the mean/sem, $n = 9$, averaging the mean for each time point) reducing to 1.96 ± 0.04 (n = 9) in surfen treated mice. A clinical score of ~ 3 represents significant gait impairment with partial hind limb paralysis, while a score of ~ 2 represents mild ataxia. The ordinal scale is limited because the degree of disability is not the same between each interval. Therefore, the number of days spent with a score of ^{3} 2.5 was also calculated, because this reflects substantial gait impairment and paralysis associated with significant spinal cord demyelination [6]. During vehicle treated EAE, mice spent 6.14 ± 0.64 (mean ± sem) days at this level of disability, compared to just 1.87 ± 0.51 days for surfen treated animals (Fig. 2b). There was a significant loss of weight in vehicle treated EAE compared to surfen treated EAE between days 13-19 (Fig. 2c); mean weight over this period in vehicle treated EAE fell to 18.08 ± 0.19 g ($n = 7$) compared to 20.31 ± 0.03 g (n = 7) in the surfen treated group, a reduction in mean weight of 11%. Weights of disease free, CFA + PTX treated control mice remained stable (Fig. 2d) and clinical scores remained at zero in these mice throughout the experimental period. Therefore surfen reduces several disease parameters in the EAE model.

During EAE, surfen reduces CD4 positive T cell and macrophage infiltration into the CNS

Since EAE is driven by infiltrating immune cells, surfen might ameliorate disease by reducing cellular infiltration. T cells and macrophages were identified by flow cytometry in extracts from the spinal cord and cerebellum. Compared to vehicle treated EAE, surfen treatment produced a significant reduction in the percentage of CD4 positive T cells in both spinal cord and cerebellum (Fig. 3a) and of macrophages in spinal cord but not cerebellum (Fig. 3b). In the spinal cord, the percentage of CD8 positive T cells increased during vehicle treated EAE (in CFA + PTX treated controls: 5.02 ± 0.88% ($n = 10$) rising to 14.12 ± 2.12% ($n = 17$) in vehicle treated EAE), but there were no differences between vehicle treated EAE and surfen treated EAE (surfen treated EAE: 12.06 ± 2.34% ($n = 18$)). Representative flow cytometry plots are shown to indicate the gating strategy as well as scatter in surfen treated mice (Fig. 3a,b). In parallel to its effects on the spinal cord, surfen increased the number of cells in peripheral lymph nodes taken from mice with EAE. Surfen also reduced the percentage of proliferating CD4 positive T cells isolated from the lymph nodes and stimulated ex vivo. However surfen had no effect on the percentage of CD4 positive T cells in splenic extracts from mice

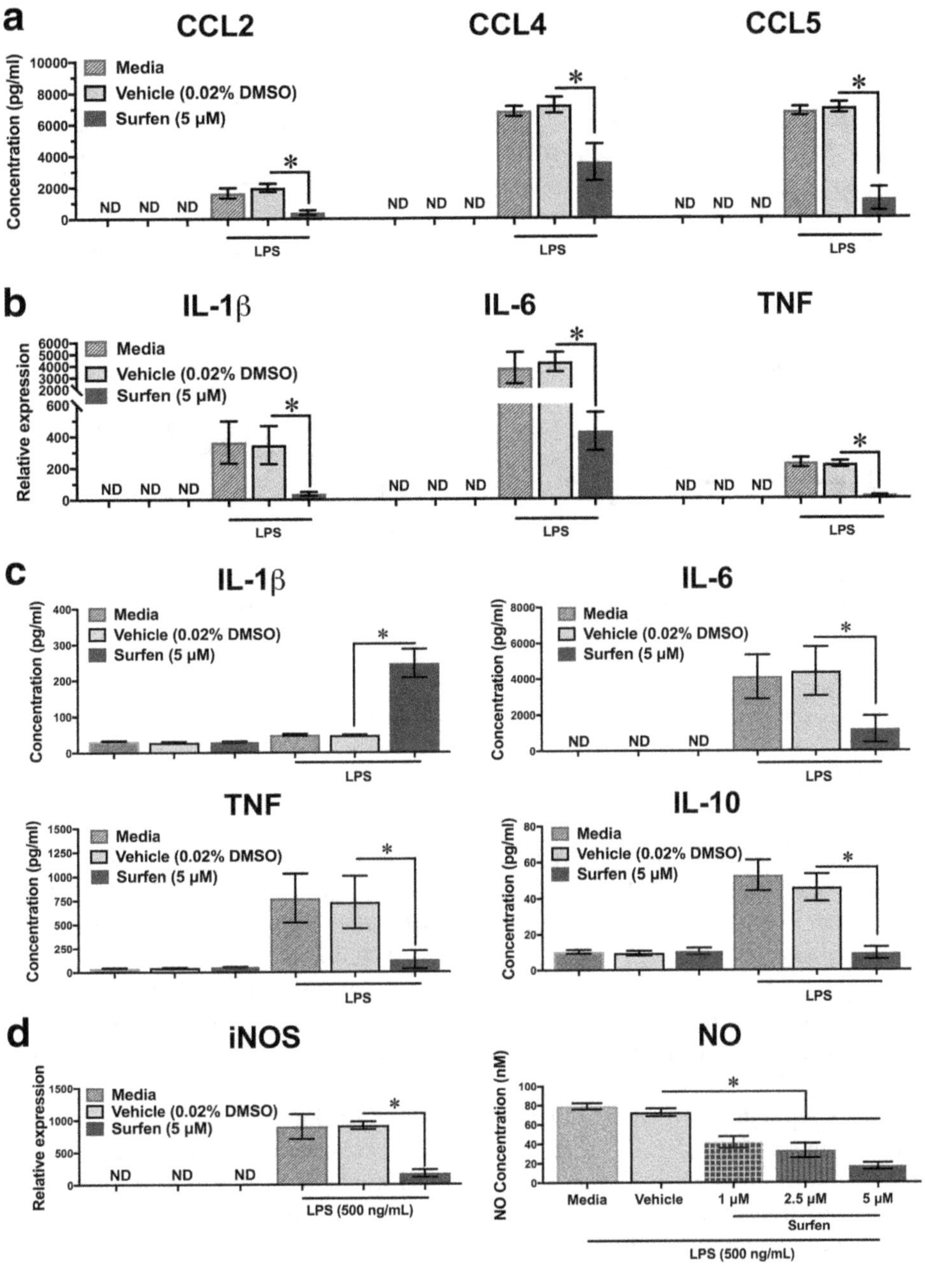

Fig. 1 Effects of surfen on factor expression by cultured bone marrow derived macrophages. **a** mRNA expression for selected chemokines. **b** mRNA expression and **c** protein concentration for selected cytokines. **d** mRNA expression for inducible NO synthase (iNOS) and NO production. Data compares cells exposed to media, vehicle or surfen. Bar indicates cells treated with LPS. Significance compares groups linked by cross bars (* = $P < 0.05$). ND = not detectable

with EAE (Additional file 3: Figure S2). These data show that surfen reduces infiltration of immune cells into the CNS during EAE.

During EAE, surfen treatment reduces the expression of the chemokines CCL3 and CCL5, with variable effects on CCL2 and CCL4

One mechanism by which surfen could reduce cellular infiltration into the CNS is to modify local chemokine expression. To explore this possibility, spinal cord extracts were analyzed for levels of the chemokines CCL2, CCL3, CCL4 and CCL5. Relative messenger (m)RNA expression was low in control groups (mice given CFA + PTX and vehicle or CFA + PTX and surfen). Pooled data from these controls showed mean expression for all chemokines of 0.038 ± 0.01 (mean ± sem, $n = 40$). During vehicle treated EAE, mRNA expression for CCL3 and CCL5 was significantly increased

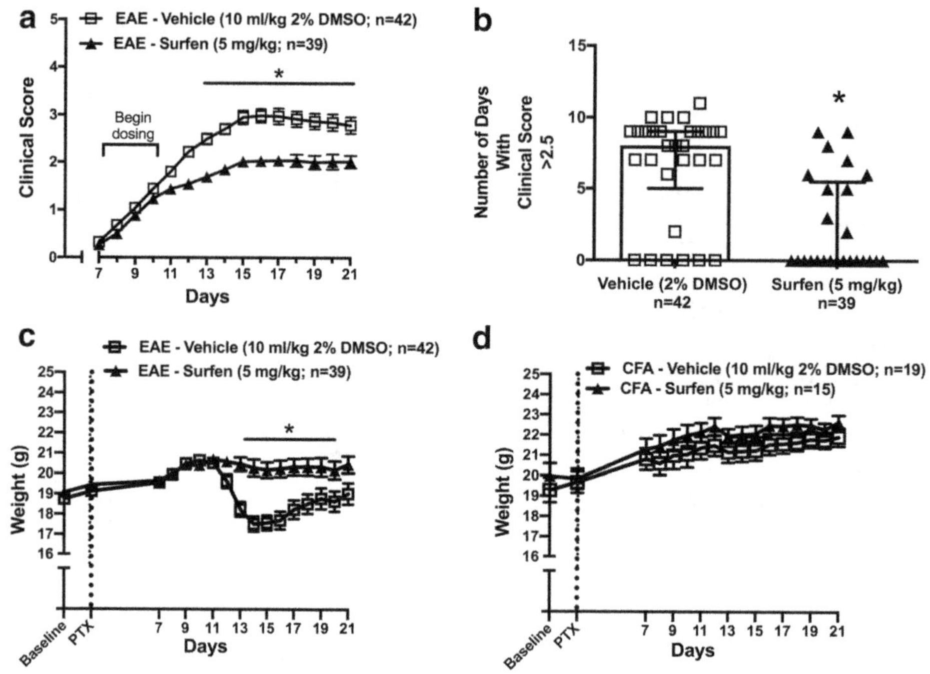

Fig. 2 Surfen ameliorates EAE. **a** Clinical scores in mice with EAE, either vehicle treated or surfen treated (dosage and numbers indicated). **b** Number of days spent with clinical scores above 2.5 in each group. **c** Changes in body weight in each group. **d** Changes in body weight in CFA + PTX controls treated with vehicle (CFA - Vehicle) or surfen (CFA - Surfen). Data are shown as mean ± SEM; significant data is marked for surfen versus vehicle, comparing time points (**a**,**c**) or grouped data (**b**); * = $P < 0.05$

(Fig. 4a). Mean expression varied between 1.44 (CCL2) and 2.14 (CCL3). Surfen treatment during EAE resulted in a significant reduction in mRNA expression for CCL3 and CCL5. Mean expression for CCL2 and CCL4 reduced to between 0.21 (CCL2) and 0.35 (CCL4), which was not significant (Fig. 4a). When protein concentrations were measured, significant increases occurred during vehicle treated EAE for CCL2, CCL3 and CCL5. Levels of these chemokines were significantly reduced by surfen treatment during EAE (Fig. 4b). Concentrations of CCL4 were unaltered. These reductions in chemokine expression provide a partial explanation for the reduced cellular infiltration induced by surfen treatment during EAE.

Surfen treatment modifies the expression of T cell regulators in EAE

As well as an impact on cellular infiltration, surfen may reduce disease by direct effects on T cell function within the CNS. To explore this possibility, proteins involved in different T cell responses were studied during EAE in surfen treated mice. mRNA expression of the T helper (Th) 1 transcription factor Tbet, Th2 transcription factor Gata3 and T regulatory (Treg) transcription factor FoxP3 were significantly increased during vehicle treated EAE and significantly reduced in surfen treated EAE (Fig. 5a). There were significant positive correlations between mRNA expression and clinical score for these transcription factors. For Tbet, the Spearman correlation coefficient (R) was 0.73 ($p = 0.01$), for GATA3 it was 0.68 ($p = 0.003$) and for FoxP3 it was 0.79 ($p = 0.003$). mRNA expression of the transcription factor RORγT which regulates Th17 responses was unaltered (data not shown). mRNA expression of the Th1 cytokine IL-12p40 and Th2/Treg cytokine IL-10 was also significantly increased during vehicle treated EAE, while the increase in mean expression of the Treg cytokine TGF-β was not significant. Expression for all three cytokines was significantly reduced in surfen treated EAE (Fig. 5a). In spite of reductions in mRNA for the Th2 factors Gata3 and IL-10, surfen treatment during EAE induced a significant increase in concentration of the Th2 cytokine IL-4 (Fig. 5b) but had no effect on the Th2 cytokines IL-5, IL-10 and IL-13 (data not shown). The reduction in mRNA expression for IL-12p40 was paralleled by significant reductions in protein concentration in surfen treated EAE (Fig. 5b). There was a non-significant trend for surfen to increase the concentration of IL12p70, with an increased mean in surfen treated CFA + PTX controls and surfen treated EAE. This is reflected in the significant reduction in the p40/p70 ratio during surfen treated EAE (Fig. 5b). During EAE, there was a significant increase in mRNA expression for Tumor Necrosis Factor (TNF), but not for Interleukin (IL)-1β or IL-6.

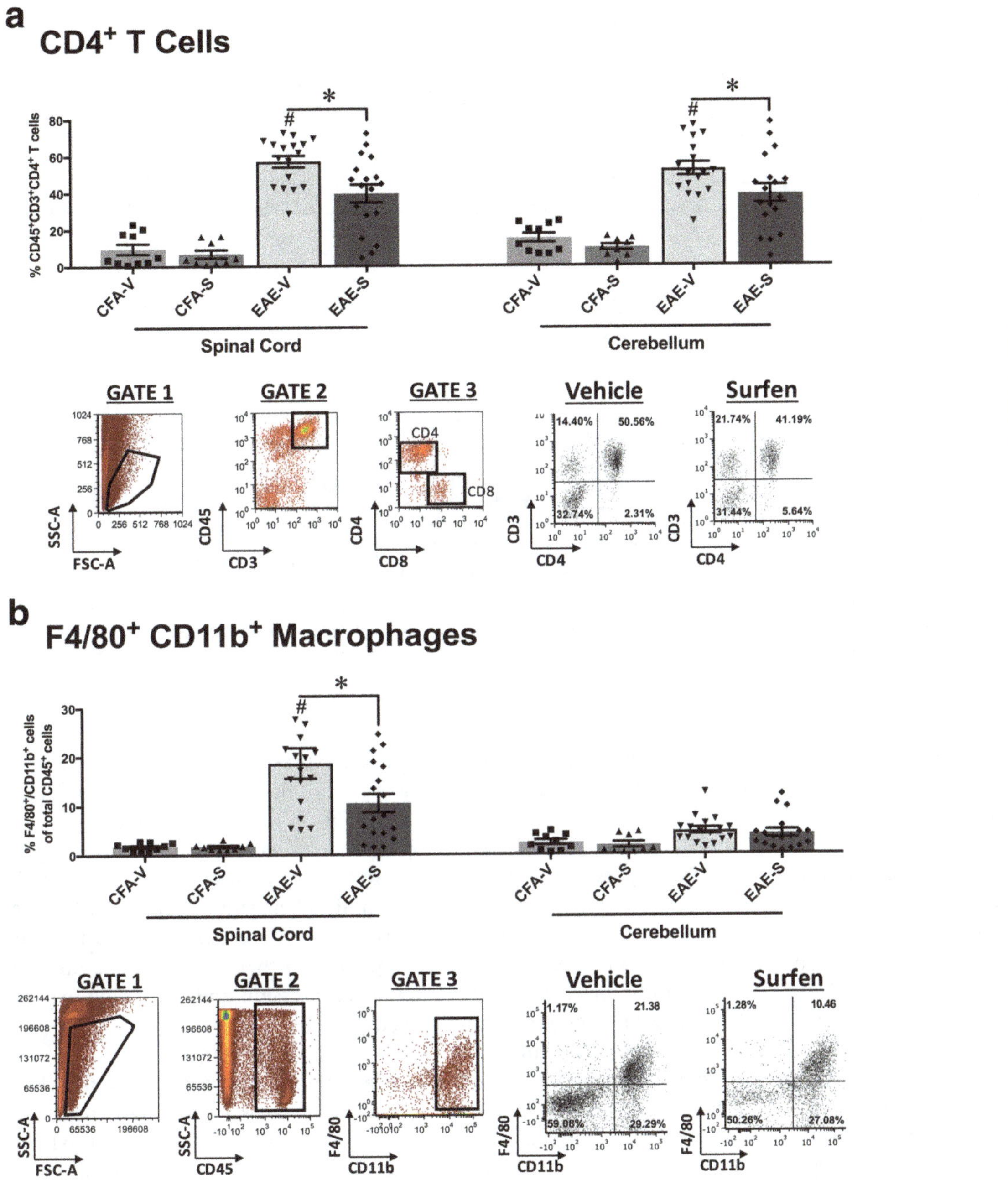

Fig. 3 During EAE, surfen reduces cellular infiltration into spinal cord and/or cerebellum. **a** CD4 positive T cells, **b** F4/80, CD11b positive macrophages. Upper panels show % changes in spinal cord and cerebellum for 4 groups. CFA + PTX controls treated with vehicle (CFA-V) or surfen (CFA-S) are compared to EAE treated with vehicle (EAE-V) or surfen (EAE-S). Lower panels illustrate the gating strategy used to calculate the data. Grouped data is shown as mean ± SEM; significant data is marked, comparing vehicle treated EAE with CFA-vehicle control (# = $P < 0.05$) or between groups as indicated by cross bars (* = $P < 0.05$)

The increase in TNF expression was suppressed by surfen treatment during EAE (Fig. 5c). Surfen did not alter protein levels for these cytokines (IL-1β: 156.5 ± 15.5 pg/ml (vehicle treated EAE, $n = 10$) v. 161.7 ± 14.94 pg/ml (surfen treated EAE, n = 10); IL-6: 91.17 ± 16.30 pg/ml (vehicle treated EAE, $n = 9$) v. 97.49 ± 9.93 pg/ml (surfen treated EAE, $n = 10$); TNF: 1046 ± 156.4 pg/ml (vehicle treated EAE, n = 10) v. 1302 ± 159.3 pg/ml (surfen treated EAE, n = 10). Surfen also had no effect on concentrations of IL-17A, IL-2 or Interferon (IFN)-γ (data not shown). mRNA expression for inducible nitric oxide synthase (iNOS) and arginase-1 were not significantly increased during EAE, and surfen had no effect on

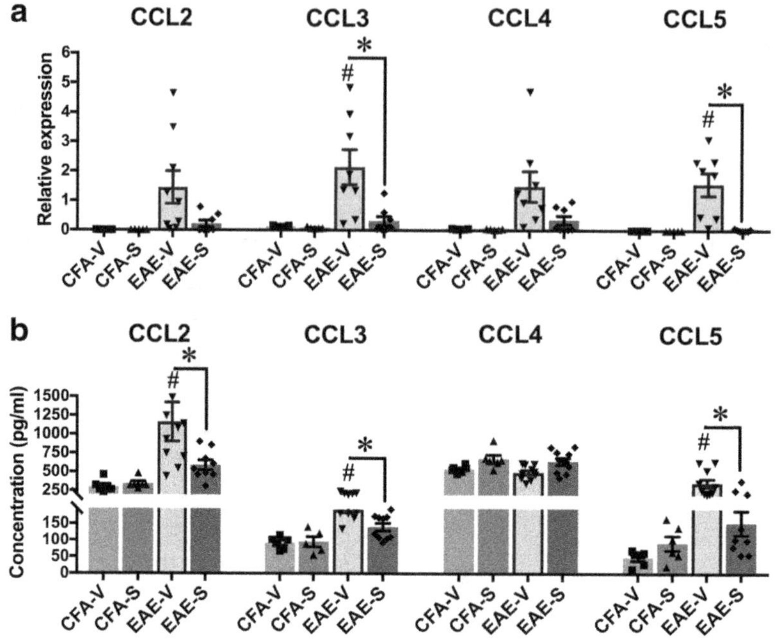

Fig. 4 Surfen selectively reduces chemokine expression during EAE. **a** mRNA expression, **b** protein concentration for selected chemokines. CFA + PTX controls treated with vehicle (CFA-V) or surfen (CFA-S) are compared to EAE treated with vehicle (EAE-V) or surfen (EAE-S). Significance is shown as mean ± SEM; significant data are marked, comparing vehicle treated EAE with CFA-vehicle (# = $P < 0.05$) or between groups as indicated by cross bars (* = $P < 0.05$)

their expression (Fig. 5c). These data suggest that surfen prolongs the Th2 response during EAE, which may contribute to disease suppression.

Surfen modulates proteoglycan (PG) expression during EAE

PG expression within the CNS is known to change within MS plaques and when modulated, it can impact disease severity during EAE [12, 27]. Therefore, surfen may influence EAE by modulating PG expression. The data show that surfen reduced mRNA expression of a number of PGs during EAE. Significant increases in mRNA expression occurred during vehicle treated EAE for 3 of the 6 heparan sulphate proteoglycans (HSPGs) studied: perlecan, serglycin and syndecan-1. The remaining 3 HSPGs were unaltered (syndecan-4, N-deacetylase/N-sulfotransferase-1 (NDST1) and agrin). However, compared to vehicle treated EAE, mice treated with surfen during EAE showed significant reductions in expression for all 6 HSPGs (Fig. 6a). The chondroitin sulphate proteoglycans (CSPGs) neurocan, aggrecan and versican were also studied. While there were no significant changes in expression during vehicle treated EAE, in surfen treated mice the level of aggrecan expression was significantly increased, matching levels in both CFA + PTX controls. By contrast, versican levels were significantly reduced, following the pattern noted for the HSPGs. Neurocan levels remained unchanged as a result of surfen treatment (Fig. 6b). The mRNA expression for each PG was also related to clinical scores both during vehicle treated EAE and surfen treated EAE (Fig. 7). In vehicle treated EAE, there were significant positive correlations between PG expression and clinical score for serglycin, syndecan-1 and syndecan-4. There was a significant negative correlation for aggrecan. Significant correlations were absent in surfen treated EAE, which may indicate that surfen ameliorates disease by lowering HSPG expression and increasing expression of the CSPG aggrecan.

Surfen inhibits remyelination in the LPC model

The later phases of MS have been modeled by injecting lysolecithin (lysophosphatidylcholine, LPC) into the corpus callosum to create a discrete region of demyelination, similar to a demyelinated MS plaque. LPC is generated by phospholipase A2, and can both act as a detergent, solubilizing lipid rich membranes such as myelin, and as a toxin to myelin forming oligodendrocytes [9]. It has been injected into various white matter tracts in rodents, including the dorsal columns of the spinal cord [14], the caudal cerebellar peduncle [29] and corpus callosum as here [16] to create a demyelinated focus that then undergoes progressive remyelination, which has been noted in certain MS plaques, and mimics the processes of repair. The LPC model was used to determine if surfen would promote or inhibit remyelination, and

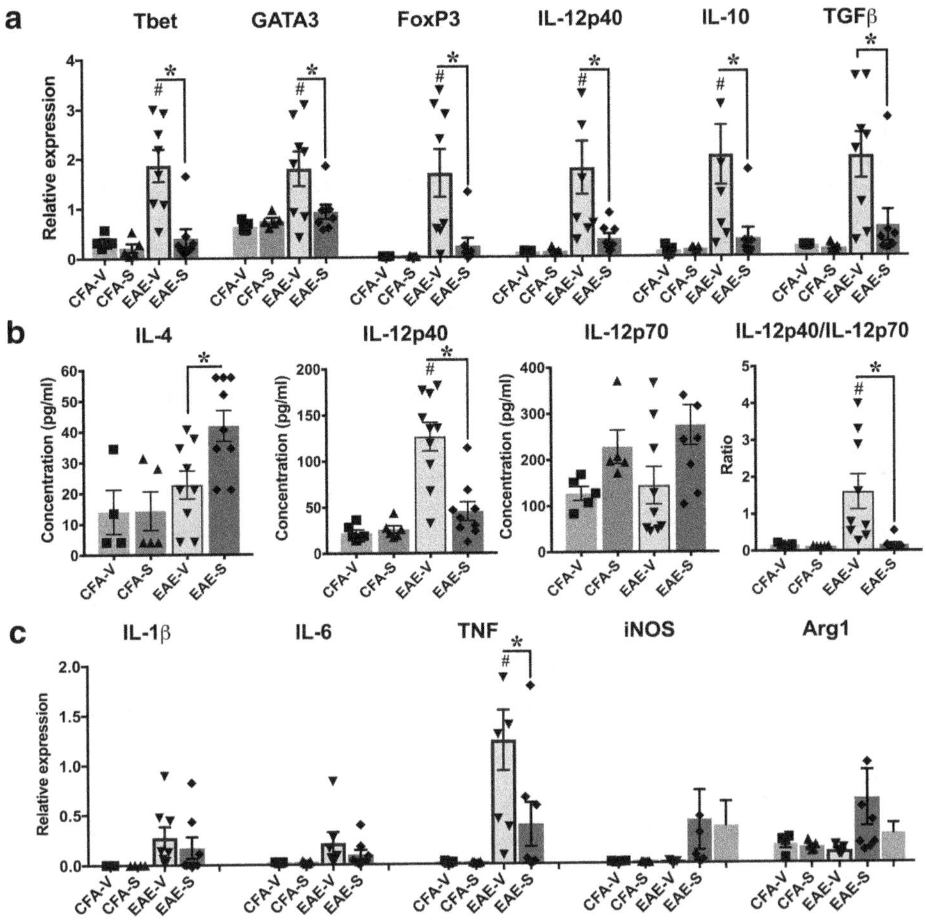

Fig. 5 Effect of surfen on T cell regulators during EAE. **a,c** mRNA expression for indicated regulators (see Results for details), **b** protein concentrations. Data compare CFA + PTX controls treated with vehicle (CFA-V) or surfen (CFA-S) to EAE treated with vehicle (EAE-V) or surfen (EAE-S). Significance is shown as mean ± SEM; significant data are marked, comparing vehicle treated EAE with CFA-vehicle (# = $P < 0.05$) or between groups as indicated by cross bars (* = $P < 0.05$)

potentially promote (or inhibit) repair during MS. When surfen was co-injected with LPC, lesion size was unaltered 7 days later (Additional file 4: Figure S3). This indicates that surfen does not interfere with the demyelinating action of LPC. Demyelination is maximal 2 days after LPC injection, when lesion size is at its peak. Subsequent remyelination proceeds rapidly between day 2 and 7; between day 7 and 21 there is little further reduction in lesion size (Fig. 8b, sham data). When surfen was injected into the lesion at day 2 it impeded remyelination, so that lesion size was virtually unchanged between day 2 and day 7. Remyelination did occur in the surfen injected group, but was considerably delayed. By day 14 in this group, lesion size was still significantly greater than the sham group, however the two groups converged at day 21 (Fig. 8b). When surfen was injected into the lesion at day 7, that is after most remyelination had occurred, then it had no significant effect on subsequent remyelination (Fig. 9). At day 14, there was a tendency for the lesion to increase in size after surfen injection at day 7, but the surfen data is too variable to show a significant increase (mean lesion size in the surfen group was 2.97 ± 0.90 mm^2 ($n = 10$) compared to 1.47 ± 0.14 mm^2 ($n = 6$) in the sham group). Therefore surfen impairs the recovery in lesion size when injected 2 days after LPC injection but not at 7 days. To confirm that the day 2 injection of surfen inhibits remyelination of axons rather than inducing axonal loss, ultrastructural examination of axons in the corpus callosum of day 7 lesions was performed. To assess remyelination, 5 mice were examined in each of 3 groups: healthy controls, mice injected with LPC (day 0) followed by vehicle on day 2, and mice injected with LPC (day 0) followed by surfen on day 2. G ratios were calculated from 30 to 40 axons in each mouse, where a G ratio of 1 indicates a denuded axon lacking a myelin sheath. The normal G ratio (in healthy controls) was 0.63 ± 0.01 (mean ± sem, $n = 193$), rising to 0.83 ± 0.01 ($n = 191$) in the LPC-vehicle group and 0.92 ± 0.01 (n = 191) in the LPC-surfen group. Both groups will have a higher G ratio than healthy controls, because remyelination produces thinner myelin

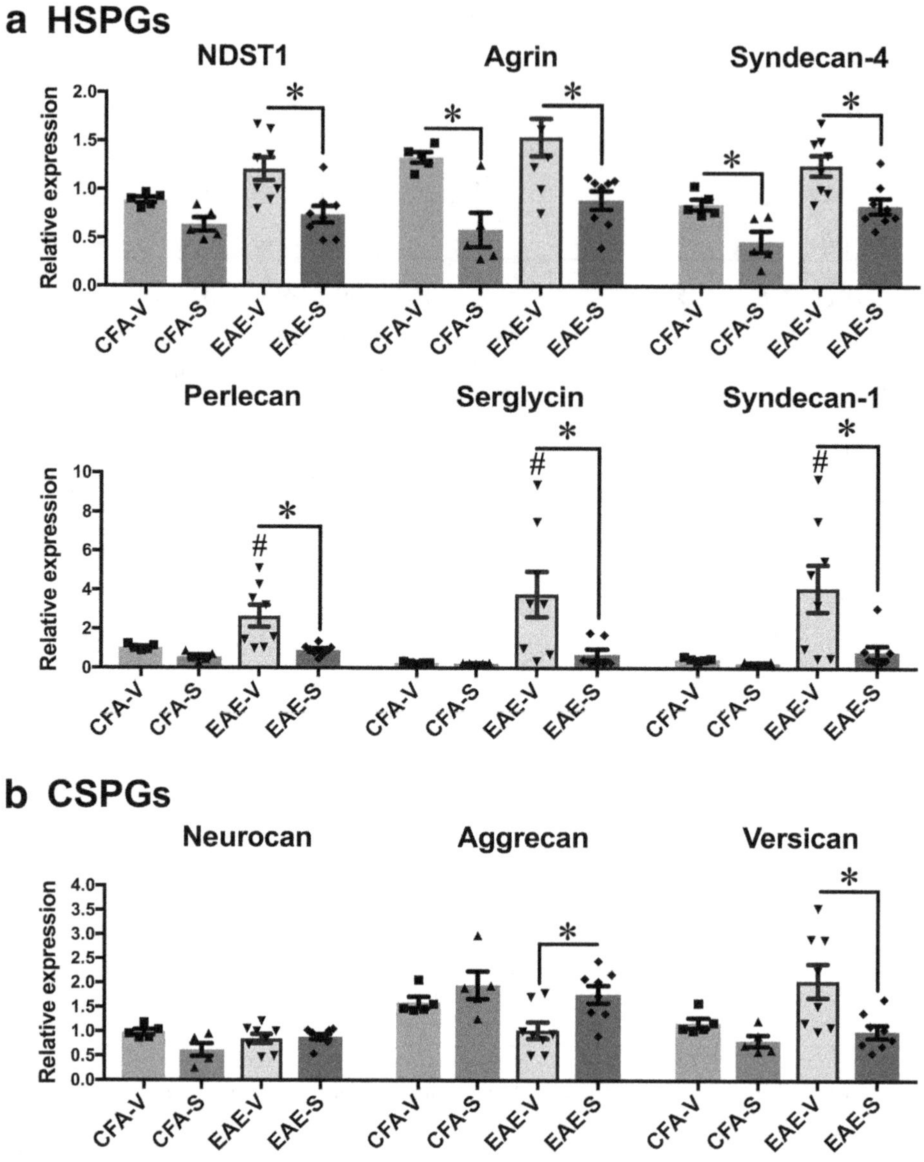

Fig. 6 Effect of surfen on proteoglycan mRNA expression during EAE. **a** Expression of HSPGs as indicated. **b** Expression of CSPGs as indicated. Data compare CFA + PTX controls treated with vehicle (CFA-V) or surfen (CFA-S) to EAE treated with vehicle (EAE-V) or surfen (EAE-S). Significance is shown as mean ± SEM; significant data are marked, comparing vehicle treated EAE with CFA-vehicle (# = $P < 0.05$) or between groups as indicated by cross bars (* = $P < 0.05$)

sheaths than normal. The percentage of denuded axons (with a G ratio of 1) in the vehicle group was 38.2%, nearly doubling to 73.3% in the surfen group. A significant increase in G ratio was found in both LPC treated groups compared to healthy controls as would be expected, but the G ratio in LPC injected mice co-injected with surfen was significantly higher than the vehicle controls. This indicates that surfen reduced remyelination at day 7, compared to controls injected with LPC alone (Fig. 10). Finally, the lesions were examined for expression of the macrophage-microglial marker Iba-1 and for CSPGs. As expected from the histological sections where macrophages filled the regions of demyelination (see Fig. 8a images), in day 7 mice Iba-1 expression (adjusted for area) was increased in both groups (LPC day 0/vehicle day 2, LPC day 0/surfen day 2), but it was significantly higher in the surfen treated mice compared to vehicle. To confirm this impression, we also counted cells based on DAPI-stained nuclei in the lesions, and found a significant increase in cell counts in the surfen treated group compared to vehicle. CSPG expression also increased in both groups, but was significantly higher in surfen treated mice compared to vehicle (Fig. 11). The ability of surfen to

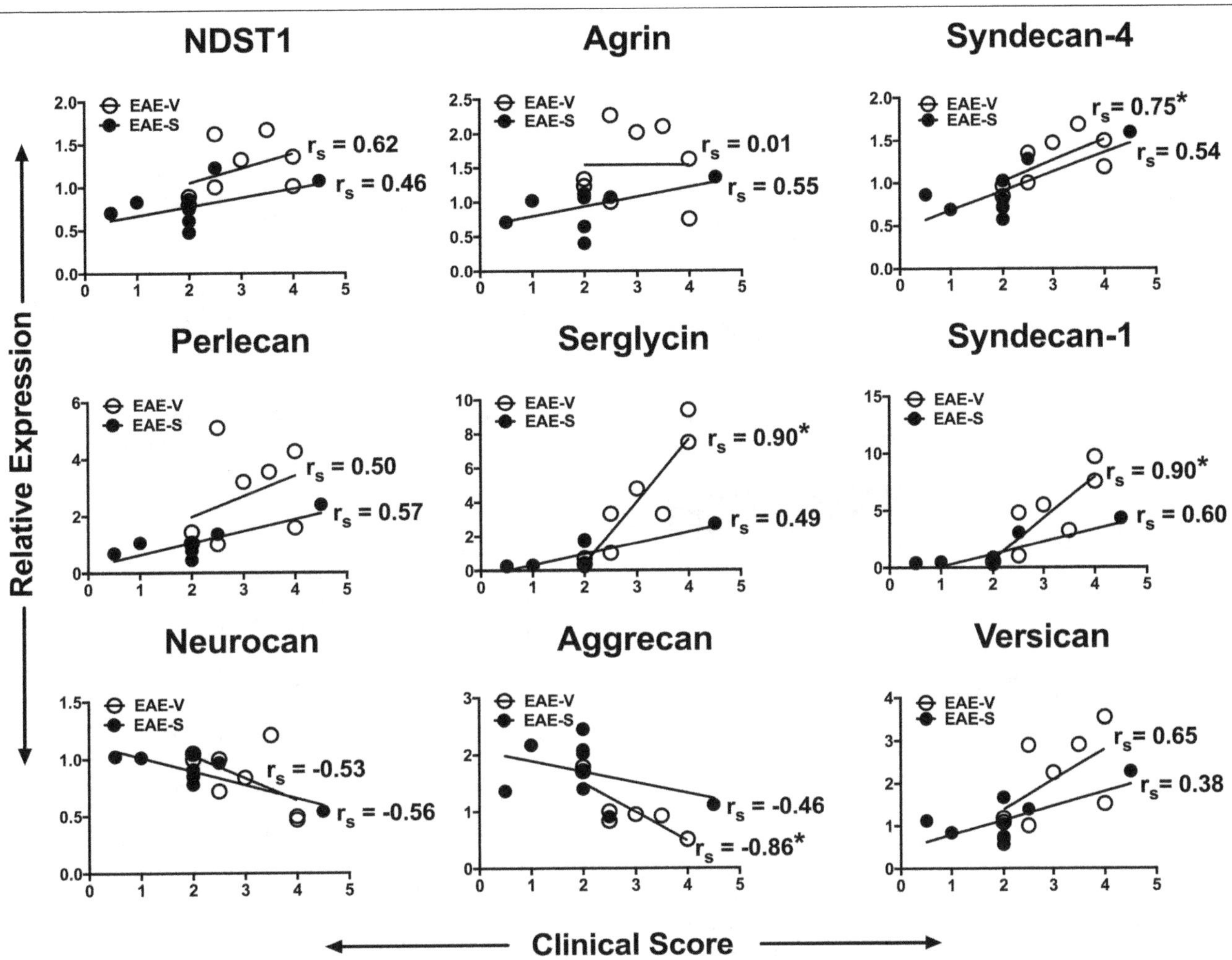

Fig. 7 Correlations between proteoglycan mRNA expression and clinical score during EAE. The data points relate mRNA expression to clinical score for individual mice with vehicle treated EAE (open circles) or surfen treated EAE (filled circles). Spearmann's correlation coefficient (r_s) for each group is shown. * indicates significance ($P < 0.05$)

inhibit remyelination may be related to this increase in macrophage-microglial cell density and/or CSPG expression.

Discussion

Proteoglycans (PGs) represent a potential therapeutic target in MS, because they regulate many aspects of the associated immune responses (which characterize relapsing disease) and remyelination (which by restoring the myelin sheath to axons may prevent or delay progressive disease). To date there are relatively few studies that examine how PG modifying agents like surfen impact disease models of MS. Two reports [12, 14] detail the impact of xyloside and fluorosamine, agents that inhibit the synthesis and secretion of CSPGs. The resulting reduction in tissue CSPGs enhanced remyelination following LPC injection into mouse spinal cord, and fluorosamine treatment also reduced clinical scores in EAE. Other work showed that a sulfated disaccharide derived from CSPGs reduces clinical scores in EAE and also inhibits cytokine secretion by isolated T cells [19, 31]. These studies appear to be contradictory, since they show that disease severity in EAE is reduced both when CSPG synthesis is inhibited, and when components of CSPGs are administered. Surfen has a potentially wider impact than these compounds, because it binds to a variety of GAG side chains on PGs. Its binding results in a fluorescence signal that was strongest for heparin followed by dermatan sulphate, heparan sulphate, and chondroitin sulphate. The binding strength correlates with the degree of sulfation on these GAGs, and binding to heparin was reduced when chemically modified heparins were used that have lower negative charge [20]. Therefore the binding of surfen depends on a charge based ionic interaction, in which positive charged quinoline rings on surfen are thought to bind to negatively charged sulphate and carboxyl groups on the GAG side chains of PGs. The binding of surfen to GAGs appears

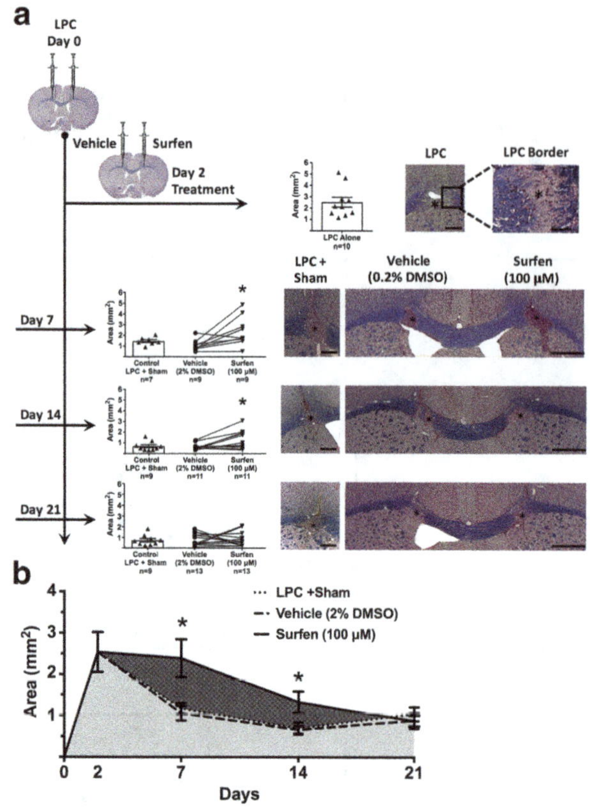

Fig. 8 Surfen injected 2 days after lysolecithin (lysophosphatidylcholine, LPC) delays remyelination of lesions in the corpus callosum. Surfen is administered 2 days after LPC injection. **a** Left sided linear graphic shows treatment schedule, while right sided panels show data for each time point, as well as representative images of lesions in the corpus callosum. **b** The area of the lesions is plotted against time from LPC injection for groups indicated. Data is shown as mean ± SEM; significant differences between matched surfen and vehicle injected groups are indicated (* = $P < 0.05$); Scale bars: LPC, LPC + Sham = 300 μm; LPC border = 100 μm, Vehicle/Surfen = 500 μm

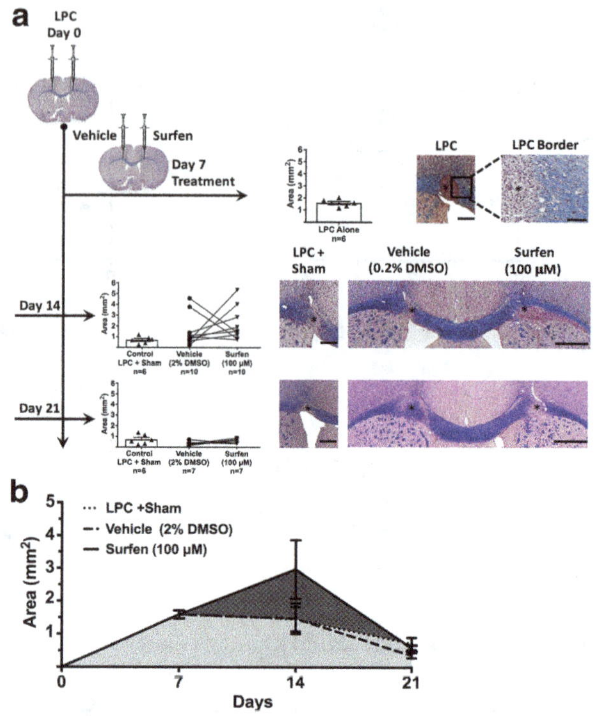

Fig. 9 Surfen has no significant effect on lesion size when administered 7 days after LPC injection. **a** Left sided linear graphic shows treatment schedule, while right sided panels show data for each time point, as well as representative images of lesions in the corpus callosum. **b** The area of the lesions is plotted against time from LPC injection for groups indicated. Data is shown as mean ± SEM; Scale bars: LPC, LPC + Sham = 300 μm; LPC border = 100 μm, Vehicle/Surfen = 500 μm

to cause its molecules to form stacked structures which exhibit an increase in fluorescence, thus providing a useful experimental readout for surfen binding.

What the present study shows is that surfen has a variety of effects on the inflammatory and remyelinating phases of MS, as modeled respectively in mice using EAE and the LPC injection models. Where then does surfen act in these models? In EAE surfen is administered peripherally, so it would have access to peripheral lymph nodes and other sources of circulating immune cells before they enter the CNS. However, surfen is a lipid soluble compound, with a Log P value of 2.48 (referring to the logarithm of P, the ratio of solute that dissolves in octanol compared to water). This gives it a high penetration across lipid bilayers, specifically through capillaries in the CNS which form a barrier to water soluble compounds (known as the blood-brain or blood-CNS barrier), but which allow free access to lipid soluble compounds, unless they are specifically extruded by efflux pumps [4]. Therefore it is reasonable to assume that surfen binds to a variety of targets in the CNS during EAE as well as the periphery. Clearly, the direct injection of surfen into the CNS during the LPC model bypasses the blood-brain barrier, and therefore the CNS is the main target in this model. The precise mechanism of action of surfen either on the periphery or in the CNS is unknown, but is likely to result from its direct binding to the GAG side chains of endogenous PGs on a variety of cells. When surfen binds to PGs associated with receptors on the surface of cells, it can prevent these receptors from interacting with a variety of chemokines, cytokines and growth factors. For instance, surfen reduces the ability of Vascular Endothelial Growth Factor to bind to its receptor, which reduces receptor phosphorylation and the resulting increase in dermal vascular permeability [30]. Therefore, surfen may act indirectly by inhibiting other factors from operating. However, surfen can also have direct effects on the functions of immune cells like T cells and macrophages. We have reported that surfen reduces murine T cell proliferation after T cells are stimulated with anti-CD3/

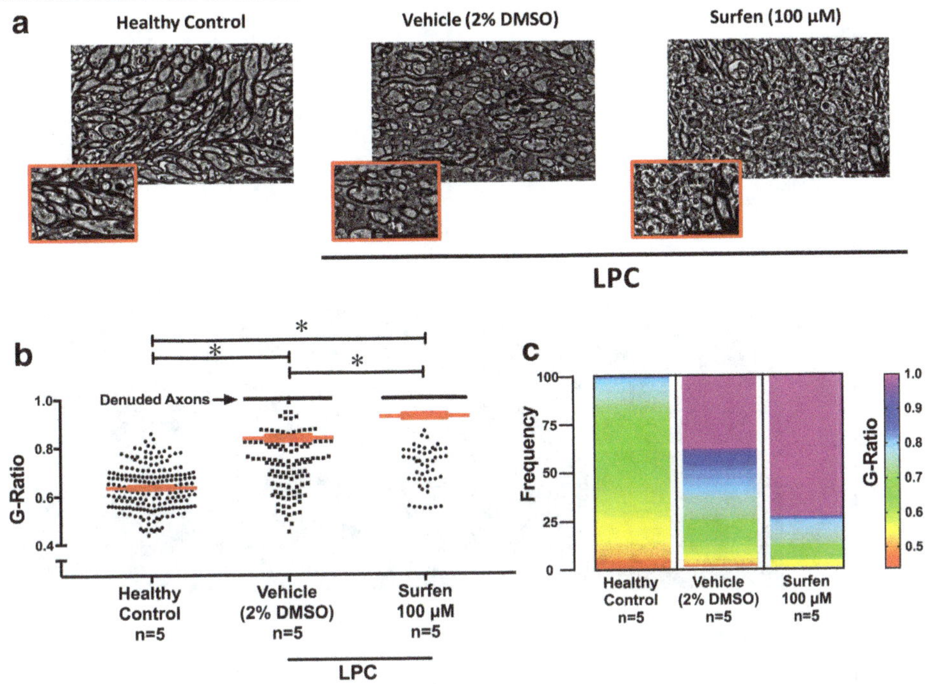

Fig. 10 Surfen injected 2 days after LPC prevents remyelination at day 7. **a** Representative electron micrographs for the normal corpus callosum and day 7 lesions in mice injected with vehicle or surfen 2 days after LPC. Scale bars = 50 µm. Higher magnification insets are also included with each micrograph. **b** Summary data for G-ratios. Left panel shows individual G ratios for axons in each group, with superimposed mean ± SEM. Significant differences between groups are indicated above linking cross bars (* = $P < 0.05$). **c** Frequency distribution plot using pseudocolor for each group. *N* indicates number of mice used to obtain the data

CD28 antibody-coated microbeads. When cell surface activation was bypassed, and T cells were activated with phorbyl myristate acetate or ionomycin, surfen had an opposite effect and it increased T cell proliferation, or, at lower doses had no effect [28]. This raises the possibility that the interaction between surfen and cell surface PGs has a direct agonist effect, triggering multiple signaling events in immune and other cell populations that directly alter their function. The first effect is probably steric, in that surfen simply prevents physical interactions from occurring between receptors and their chemokine and growth factor agonists. The second effect may depend on conformational changes in the PGs themselves, so that they act as primary receptors.

Given the wide variety of potential cellular targets for surfen, both in the CNS and in the periphery, its impact on cultured BMDM (Fig. 1) should reflect only part of its mechanisms of action in the animal models. In this regard, there were both similarities and differences when comparing the effect of surfen on LPS-stimulated (activated) BMDM and its actions during EAE. Surfen significantly reduced concentrations of the chemokines CCL2, CCL4 and CCL5 released by lipopolysaccharide (LPS)-stimulated BMDMs (Fig. 1a), while during EAE, reductions were seen for CCL2 and CCL5 but not CCL4 (Fig. 4b). In LPS-stimulated BMDMs, surfen significantly reduced mRNA expression for IL-1β, IL-6 and TNF (Fig. 1b). This differs somewhat from EAE, since surfen reduced mRNA expression for TNF but had no effect on IL-1β or IL-6 (Fig. 5c). Concentrations of IL-6, TNF and IL-10 produced by LPS-stimulated BMDMs were significantly reduced by surfen, while, by contrast, the concentration of IL-1β was significantly increased (Fig. 1c). These effects were not identified during EAE. In LPS-stimulated BMDMs, surfen significantly reduced the mRNA expression of inducible nitric oxide synthase (iNOS), and induced a dose dependent reduction in NO production (Fig. 1d). Changes in iNOS were not detected during EAE (Fig. 5c). It should be emphasized that brain intrinsic glial cells (such as microglia, astrocytes and oligodendrocyte precursor cells) play a vital role in the animal models that were used, including in the deposition by astrocytes of ECM molecules after injury, and work remains to be done in characterizing the impact of surfen on these cell types, both in vitro and in vivo.

During EAE, treatment with surfen resulted in a variety of downstream effects that contributed to a significant reduction in clinical scores (Fig. 2). Clinical scores were recorded for 21 days from induction, and then mice were killed in order to assess the impact of surfen on various parameters, so these results come from the

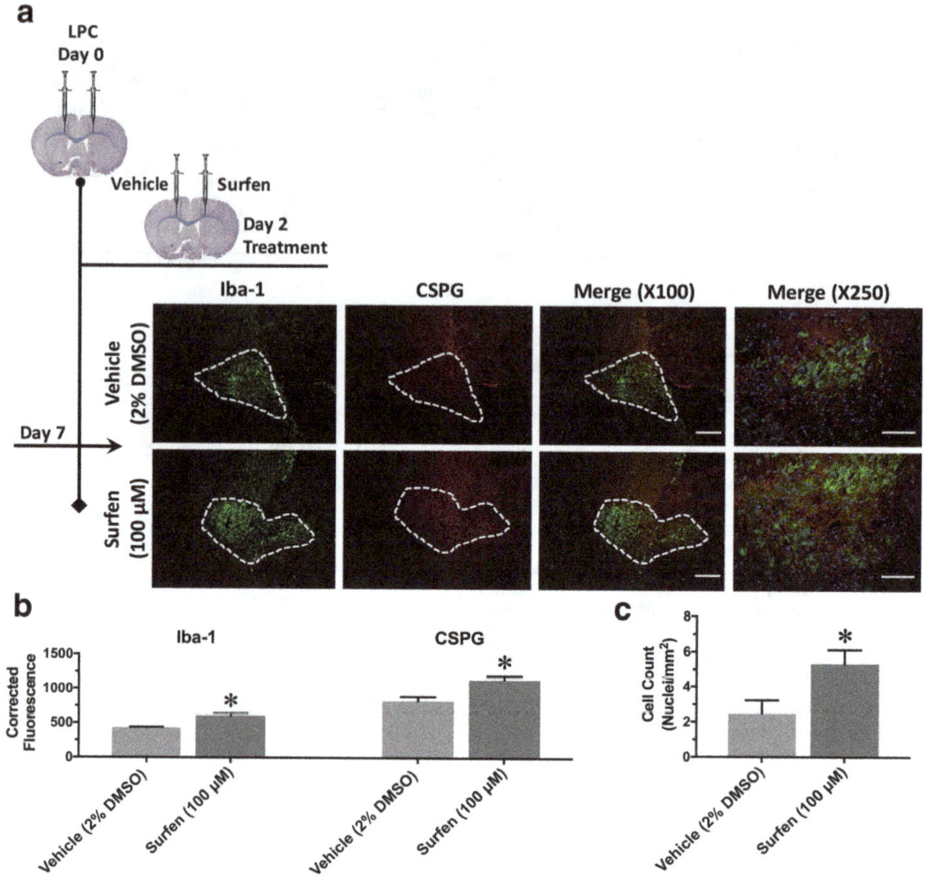

Fig. 11 Surfen injected 2 days after LPC increases local expression of CSPG and Iba-1 with increased cell counts at day 7. **a** Left sided linear graphic shows treatment schedule. Representative immunofluorescence images are shown for Iba-1,CSPGexpression in groups indicated. Merge image (×100 magnification)shows no overlap for Iba-1 and CSPG. Higher magnification merge image (×250) was used to visualize DAPI nuclear staining for cell counts. **b** Summary data for Iba-1 and CSPG expression. c. Summary data for cell counts. $N = 3$ mice per group significance compares surfen with vehicle ($* = P < 0.05$); Scale bars = 100 μm

chronic phase of EAE. In general, EAE consists of an early induction phase before clinical signs appear (days 0-7 from inoculation) followed by an acute phase in which scores increase (days 8-16) and a chronic phase where scores reach a plateau (days 17-21) [1]. In the spinal cord of mice with EAE, surfen reduced the number of infiltrating CD4 positive T cells and macrophages (Fig. 3). Surfen treatment also led to significant reductions in the messenger (m)RNA and/or protein expression of the chemokines CCL2, CCL3 and CCL5, with no significant effect on CCL4 (Fig. 4). There are multiple potential mechanism by which surfen could reduce the infiltration of CD4 positive T cells and macrophages into the CNS. Clues come from the reductions in chemokine expression induced by surfen (Fig. 4) and the intriguing albeit preliminary finding that surfen increased numbers and reduced proliferation of T cells in peripheral lymph nodes, although it had no effect on the proportion of CD4 positive T cells in splenic extracts (Additional file 3: Figure S2). This suggests that surfen is acting peripherally as well as centrally, to control T cell migration into the CNS, leading to 'trapping' of T cells in the peripheral lymph nodes, as well as reduced chemokine gradients for cellular migration of immune cells from circulating blood into the CNS.

T helper (Th) subsets were also evaluated in the context of EAE (Fig. 5). Broadly speaking, EAE is driven by Th1 and Th17 responses, while Th2 and T-regulatory (Treg) responses are associated with disease resolution. Surfen induced significant reductions in mRNA expression for Th1, Th2 and Treg transcription factors and associated downstream cytokines (Th1 cytokine IL12p40, Th2/Treg cytokine IL-10 and Treg cytokine TGFβ). At the protein level, the Th1 cytokine IL12p40 was also significantly reduced in surfen treated mice, which would tend to reduce EAE disease activity. By contrast, at the protein level, Th2 cytokines were either not changed (IL-5, IL-10, IL-13) or in the case of IL-4 significantly increased. In a previous study, it was shown that IL-4 levels peak during the acute phase of EAE but return to undetectable control levels during the chronic phase [11]. We therefore propose that, in addition to its effects on net cellular migration of T cells and macrophages into the CNS, surfen reduces disease activity through a combination of reduced Th1 responses and enhanced Th2 responses mediated by IL-4, whose levels remain elevated during the chronic phase of surfen treated EAE. If surfen acts in a similar manner to heparanase, an enzyme that inactivates PGs by cleaving heparan sulfate side chains, then our data is consistent with a report in which IL-4 and other Th2 cytokines were induced in ex vivo splenocytes taken from mice treated with heparanase [2]. The persistent elevation in IL-4 may also account for the tendency of surfen to reduce both IL12p40 and the ratio of IL12p40 to IL12p70 (with surfen tending to increase IL12p70 levels). A previous study showed that IL-4 stimulates production of IL-12p70 by dendritic cells and macrophages, while inhibiting IL12-p40 production [10]. The effects of surfen on cytokine expression were more muted in these mice. mRNA expression for Tumor Necrosis Factor (TNF) alone was significantly reduced by surfen, but protein expression was not changed. This likely reflects timing, as many of these cytokines would be past peak expression in the chronic phase of EAE.

Surfen treatment also changed the local expression of mRNA for a variety of PGs (Fig. 6). This data begins to unravel some of the complex effects of different classes of proteoglycan in EAE. mRNA for some of the HSPGs increased significantly during EAE (perlecan, serglycin and syndecan-1) while others were unchanged (syndecan-4, N-deacetylase/N-sulfotransferase-1 and agrin). However, surfen reduced mRNA expression for all six HSPGs, when the EAE groups (vehicle treated and surfen treated) were compared. When clinical scores were plotted as a function of mRNA levels, there were significant positive correlations for the HSPGs serglycin, syndecan-1 and syndecan-4 (Fig. 7). While it is known that HSPGs increase in the brains of patients with MS [27], this data provides evidence linking this expression to deleterious clinical effects. The role that HSPGs play as inhibitors of remyelination is also not well understood, but CSPG expression has been better studied [12, 14, 17]. The implication of these studies is that all CSPGs worsen disease. However, when we examined three CSPGs (neurocan, aggrecan and versican) we found no increases in mRNA expression during EAE, but when EAE groups (vehicle treated and surfen treated) were compared, surfen induced a significant increase in mRNA expression for aggrecan, a decrease for versican, and had no effect on neurocan. Versican expression was previously shown to increase in EAE, and to decrease when EAE was treated with fluorosamine [12], which parallels the effect of surfen. However, alone among the PGs examined, mRNA expression of the CSPG aggrecan had a negative correlation to clinical scores (Fig. 7). Aggrecan is a key component of perineuronal nets involved in synaptic transmission [8], so increased levels of aggrecan induced by surfen may contribute to axonal protection. This lends further nuance to the role of PGs in demyelinating disease of the CNS. While reductions in CSPGs have improved remyelination after administration of LPC [12, 14] our data suggests that in EAE the CSPG aggrecan is protective.

The impact of surfen on remyelination was assessed in the LPC model, and direct injection of surfen into the region of demyelination produced a prolonged delay in remyelination (Figs. 8-10). This inhibitory action was associated with increased local expression of CSPGs in the corpus callosum (Fig. 11), which is similar to the effect of surfen on aggrecan expression during EAE (Fig. 6). We speculate that surfen triggers the synthesis of CSPGs by local cells, either by binding directly to PGs on the cell surface, or by blocking the interaction of regulating factors (cytokines, chemokines, growth factors) with their receptors on these cells. Both astrocytes and macrophages in the CNS have been shown to be sources of CSPGs following LPC injection into the spinal cord [14] and are likely targets for surfen in this model. The increase in Iba-1 labeling as well as cell counts in the surfen group (Fig. 11) suggests that macrophages infiltrate these lesions in larger numbers, and are likely sources for the increase in CSPGs.Other work has shown that LPC injection into the spinal cord increases local expression of versican in the region of demyelination, but aggrecan levels were not changed in nearby grey matter [12]. Since aggrecan is largely confined to perineuronal nets in grey matter, it is unlikely to be found in a white matter tract such as the corpus callosum, and surfen probably increased levels of other CSPGs, with versican a likely candidate. However, in the context of MS plaques, both aggrecan and neurocan were expressed in CNS white matter [27], and both CSPGs inhibited the ability of oligodendrocytes to myelinate axons in tissue culture [17]. Although the two animal models reported here differ in many respects, perhaps the increase in CSPGs induced by surfen has a double effect. Some CSPGs (such as versican) are well known to inhibit remyelination, but others (such as aggrecan) may also be essential as protective factors during inflammation. This raises a dilemma with respect to manipulating PGs in MS using therapeutic agents like surfen, especially if the result is a generalized increase in CSPG expression. This may be therapeutically desirable when CSPGs like aggrecan increase to ameliorate the earlier inflammatory stages of MS, but therapeutically problematic when other CSPGs such as versican increase, that inhibit remyelination and repair in later phases of the disease.

Additional files

Additional file 1: Table S1. List of qRT-PCR primers used to determine mRNA expression (TIFF 1810 kb)

Additional file 2: Figure. S1. a,b. Surfen affects viability of cultured bone marrow derived macrophages (BMDMs) at higher doses (a as assessed by 7-ADD staining, b as assessed by MTT assay, doses indicated). c. Surfen (5 μM) binding to BMDMs is reduced by co-application of heparitinase-III and chondroitinase ABC, alone or in combination. Data is shown as mean ± SEM from 4 independent experiments. Significance compares surfen with vehicle unless otherwise indicated by cross bars (* = $P < 0.05$) (TIFF 1367 kb)

Additional file 3: Figure S2. During EAE, surfen increases lymph node cell count, but reduces proliferation in extracted CD4 positive T cells. Superficial cervical, axillary, brachial and inguinal lymph nodes were pooled from individual mice (n shown). Total cells were counted (a) and then isolated T cells were stimulated in vivo with anti-CD3, anti CD-28 T cell expander beads for 24 h, and proliferation assessed by Oregon Green staining (b). Spleens were also homogenized (n indicates number of mice, with one spleen per mouse) and cells stained with antibodies directed against surface markers and then analyzed by flow cytometry. The percentage of CD4 positive T cells among the extracts is shown (c) along with the gating strategy (d). Data compare EAE treated with vehicle (EAE-V) or surfen (EAE-S), and is shown as mean ± SEM. Significance compares surfen with vehicle (* = $P < 0.05$) (TIFF 1933 kb)

Additional file 4: Figure S3. Surfen injected at the same time as LPC has no effect on lesion size 7 days later. Left sided linear graphic shows treatment schedule, while right hand panel shows data for each group as well as representative images of lesions in the corpus callosum. Data is shown as mean ± SEM. Scale bars = 200 μm (TIFF 6018 kb)

Acknowledgements
This study was funded by the Canadian Institutes of Health Research (operating grant to SG), Natural Sciences and Engineering Research Council (discovery grant to DH) and Dalhousie Medical Research Foundation (research grant to AE).

Authors' contributions
JRW conducted the experiments, analyzed the data, prepared the figures and edited the manuscript. A-CL performed many of the experiments in Figs. 8, 9 and 11 and analyzed the data. DRC, AM, BEK and YK assisted with the experiments in Fig. 3. SAG contributed to the study design and provided funding. DWH and ASE conceived of the study and provided funding, while ASE wrote and edited the manuscript. All authors read and approved the final manuscript.

Competing interests
The authors declare that they have no competing interests.

Author details
[1]Department of Pathology, Dalhousie University, Sir Charles Tupper Medical Building, 5850 College Street, PO Box 15000, Halifax, NS B3H 4R2, Canada. [2]Department of Microbiology and Immunology, Dalhousie University, Sir Charles Tupper Medical Building, 5850 College Street, PO Box 15000, Halifax, NS B3H 4R2, Canada.

References

1. Barthelmes J, Tafferner N, Kurz J, de Bruin N, Parnham MJ, Geisslinger G et al (2016) Induction of experimental autoimmune encephalomyelitis in mice and evaluation of the disease-dependent distribution of immune cells in various tissues. J Vis Exp Doi:https://doi.org/10.3791/53933
2. Bitan M, Weiss L, Reibstein I, Zeira M, Fellig Y, Slavin S et al (2010) Heparanase upregulates Th2 cytokines, ameliorating experimental autoimmune encephalitis. Mol Immunol 47:1890–1898
3. Bjartmar C, Trapp B (2001) Axonal and neuronal degeneration in multiple sclerosis: mechanisms and functional consequences. Curr Opin Neurol 14: 271–278
4. Bodor N, Buchwald P (1999) Recent advances in the brain targeting of neuropharmaceuticals by chemical delivery systems. Adv Drug Deliv Rev 36: 229–254
5. Dyck SM, Karimi-Abdolrezaee S (2015) Chondroitin sulfate proteoglycans: key modulators in the developing and pathologic central nervous system. Exp Neurol 269:169–187
6. Fiander MDJ, Stifani N, Nichols M, Akay T, Robertson GS (2017) Kinematic gait parameters are highly sensitive measures of motor deficits and spinal cord injury in mice subjected to experimental autoimmune encephalomyelitis. Behav Brain Res 317:95–108
7. Foote AK, Blakemore WF (2005) Inflammation stimulates remyelination in areas of chronic demyelination. Brain 128:528–539
8. Giamanco KA, Morawski M, Matthews RT (2010) Perineuronal net formation and structure in aggrecan knockout mice. Neuroscience 170:1314–1327
9. Jeffrey ND, Blakemore WF (1995) Remyelination of mouse spinal cord axons demyelinated by local injection of lysolecithin. J Neurocytol 24:775–781
10. Kaliński P, Smits HH, Schuitemaker JH, Vieira PL, van Eijk M, de Jong EC et al (2000) IL-4 is a mediator of IL-12p70 induction by human Th2 cells: reversal of polarized Th2 phenotype by dendritic cells. J Immunol 165:1877–1881
11. Kennedy MK, Torrance DS, Picha KS, Mohler KM (1992) Analysis of cytokine mRNA expression in the central nervous system of mice with experimental autoimmune encephalomyelitis reveals that IL-10 mRNA expression correlates with recovery. J Immunol 149:2496–2505
12. Keough MB, Rogers JA, Zhang P, Jensen SK, Stephenson EL, Chen T et al (2016) An inhibitor of chondroitin sulfate proteoglycan synthesis promotes central nervous system remyelination. Nat Commun 7:11312
13. Kotter MR, Zhao C, van Rooijen N, Franklin RJM (2005) Macrophage-depletion induced impairment of experimental CNS remyelination is associated with a reduced oligodendrocyte precursor cell response and altered growth factor expression. Neurobiol Dis 18:166–175
14. Lau LW, Keough MB, Haylock-Jacobs S, Cua R, Doring A, Sloka S et al (2012) Chondroitin sulphate proteoglycans in demyelinated lesions impair remyelination. Ann Neurol 72:419–432
15. Livak KJ, Schmittgen TD (2001) Analysis of relative gene expression data using real-time quantitative PCR and the 2(–Delta Delta C(T)) method. Methods 25:402–408
16. Miron VE, Boyd A, Zhao J-W, Yuen TJ, Ruckh JM, Shadrach JL et al (2013) M2 microglia and macrophages drive oligodendrocyte differentiation during CNS remyelination. Nat Neurosci 16:1211–1218
17. Pendleton JC, Shamblott MJ, Gary DS, Belegu V, Hurtado A, Malone ML, McDonald JW (2013) Chondroitin sulfate proteoglycans inhibit oligodendrocyte myelination through PTPσ. Exp Neurol 247:113–121
18. Raine CS, Wu E (1993) Multiple sclerosis: remyelination in acute lesions. J Neuropath Exp Neurol 52:199–204
19. Rolls A, Cahalon L, Bakalash S, Avidan H, Lider O, Schwartz M (2006) A sulfated disaccharide derived from chondroitin sulfate proteoglycan protects against inflammation-associated neurodegeneration. FASEB J 20:547–549
20. Schuksz M, Fuster MM, Brown JR, Crawford BE, Ditto DP, Lawrence R et al (2008) Surfen, a small molecule antagonist of heparan sulfate. PNAS 105: 13075–13080
21. Setzu A, Lathia JD, Zhao C, Wells K, Rao MS, Ffrench-Constant C et al (2006) Inflammation stimulates myelination by transplanted oligodendrocyte precursor cells. Glia 54:297–303
22. Shute J (2012) Glycosaminoglycan and chemokine/growth factor interactions. Handbook Exper Pharmacol 207:307–324
23. Sobel RA, Ahmed AB (2001) White matter extracellular matrix chondroitin sulphate/dermatan sulphate proteoglycans in multiple sclerosis. J Neuropath Exp Neurol 60:1198–1207
24. Stromnes IM, Goverman JM (2006) Active induction of experimental allergic encephalomyelitis. Nat Protoc 1:1810–1819
25. Stys PK, Zamponi GW, van Minnen J, Geurts JG (2012) Will the real multiple sclerosis please stand up? Nat Rev Neurosci 13:507–514

26. Taylor S, Wakem M, Dijkman G, Alsarraj M, Nguyen M (2010) A practical approach to RT-qPCR-publishing data that conform to the MIQE guidelines. Methods 50:S1–S5
27. van Horssen J, Bö L, Dijkstra CD, de Vries HE (2006) Extensive extracellular matrix depositions in active multiple sclerosis lesions. Neurobiol Dis 24:484–491
28. Warford J, Doucette CD, Hoskin DW, Easton AS (2014) Murine T cell activation is regulated by surfen (*bis*-2-methyl-4-amino-quinolyl-6-carbamide). Biochem Biophys Res Commun 443:524–530
29. Woodruff RH, Franklin RJM (1999) Demyelination and remyelination of the caudal cerebellar peduncle of adult rats following stereotactic injections of lysolecithin, ethidium bromide and complement/anti-galactocerebroside: a comparative study. Glia 25:216–228
30. Xu D, Fuster MM, Lawrence R (2011) Esko JD (2011) Heparan sulfate regulates VEGF165- and VEGF121-mediated vascular hyperpermeability. J Biol Chem 286:737–745
31. Zhou J, Nagarkatti P, Zhong Y, Nagarkatti M (2010) Immune modulation by chondroitin sulfate and its degraded disaccharide product in the development of an experimental model of multiple sclerosis. J Neuroimmunol 223:55–64
32. Zimmerman DR, Dours-Zimmermann MT (2008) Extracellular matrix of the central nervous system: from neglect to challenge. Histochem Cell Biol 130:635–653

2

Astrocyte remodeling without gliosis precedes optic nerve axonopathy

Melissa L. Cooper, John W. Collyer and David J. Calkins*

Abstract

Astroyctes serve myriad functions but are especially critical in white matter tracts, where energy-demanding axons propagate action potentials great distances between neurons. Axonal dependence on astrocytes for even normal function accentuates the critical role astrocytes serve during disease. In glaucoma, the most common optic neuropathy, sensitivity to intraocular pressure (IOP) challenges RGC axons early, including degradation of anterograde transport to the superior colliculus (SC). Astrocyte remodeling presages overt axon degeneration in glaucoma and thus may present a therapeutic opportunity. Here we developed a novel metric to quantify organization of astrocyte processes in the optic nerve relative to axon degeneration in the DBA/2 J hereditary mouse model of glaucoma. In early progression, as axons expand prior to loss, astrocyte processes become more parallel with migration to the nerve's edge without a change in overall coverage of the nerve. As axons degenerate, astrocyte parallelism diminishes with increased glial coverage and reinvasion of the nerve. In longitudinal sections through aged DBA/2 J nerve, increased astrocyte parallelism reflected elevated levels of the astrocyte gap-junction protein connexin 43 (Cx43). In the distal nerve, increased Cx43 also indicated with a higher level of intact anterograde transport from retina to SC. Our results suggest that progression of axonopathy in the optic nerve involves astrocyte remodeling in two phases. In an early phase, astrocyte processes organize in parallel, likely through gap-junction coupling, while a later phase involves deterioration of organization as glial coverage increases and axons are lost.

Keywords: Neurodegeneration, Glaucoma, Glia, Astrocytes, Retinal ganglion cell, Connexin 43, Axonopathy

Introduction

Astrocytes serve myriad functions in the mammalian central nervous system; aside from providing structural support, they additionally maintain the extracellular environment, optimize neuronal signaling, and release neurotransmitters themselves [39, 57]. Astrocytes are especially critical in white matter tracts, where axons propagate energy demanding action potentials great distances from their nuclei [29, 45]. Due to this relationship, astrocyte-axon interactions are increasingly recognized as important both in neural homeostasis and in pathology. Astrocytes exhibit multiple phases of remodeling due to neurodegenerative stress, demonstrating nuanced responsiveness and providing depth to a previously binary 'reactive or quiescent' classification system [33, 45, 46, 51]. Intriguingly, early astrocyte responses to neurodegeneration are often highly beneficial to injured neurons [16, 27, 32, 50]. In the optic nerve, astrocytes provide biochemical support and maintain extracellular ion balance for retinal ganglion cell (RGC) axons, which transmit retinal signals to visual structures in the brain [1, 53]. Glaucomatous optic neuropathy (or simply glaucoma), a neurodegenerative disease projected to affect some 11 million people by 2020 [37], selectively targets RGCs and their axons. Although age is the greatest risk factor, intraocular pressure (IOP) remains the only modifiable risk factor [19, 54]. However, many patients continue to lose RGC axons despite IOP-lowering treatments [26]. RGC axons and the glia that support them are particularly sensitive to age-related stressors, such as deficits in metabolism and loss of anterograde axonal transport, both of which are common aspects of age-related neurodegenerative disease [2, 5, 7–9, 40]. Recent work has focused on early phases of axonal

* Correspondence: david.j.calkins@vanderbilt.edu
Department of Ophthalmology and Visual Sciences, The Vanderbilt Eye Institute, Vanderbilt University Medical Center, 1105 Medical Research Building IV, Nashville, TN 37232-0654, USA

pathology in order to abate axon susceptibility prior to overt loss [12, 35].

In neurodegenerative disease, a glial scar generally fills volume previously occupied by axons [45]. Such reactive gliosis contributes to remodeling within the optic nerve during glaucomatous progression, as in the DBA/2 J mouse model of hereditary glaucoma [3, 4, 22, 30, 43, 48]. However, earlier components of astrocyte remodeling presage overt axonal degeneration [11]. Early RGC axonopathy in animal models of glaucoma is characterized by enlargement of the optic nerve concurrent with expansion of individual axons, accumulation of hyperphosphorylated neurofilaments, and loss of anterograde transport from the retina to central brain targets [11, 13, 36]. In the DBA/2 J mouse, astrocyte processes retract from local axon bundles and redistribute from the center of the nerve to the edge before reclaiming additional coverage later in progression [11]. Early morphological remodeling may be reversible without leading to discernible axonal damage [33, 51]. Thus, understanding how astrocyte remodeling progresses early and its relationship to axonopathy may present novel therapeutic opportunities.

Here we measured defining features of astrocyte morphological remodeling that presage overt axonal degeneration in the optic nerve. We developed a novel method to quantify organization of astrocyte processes relative to their orientation during axonal degenerative progression [11, 30]. We find that astrocyte processes lose parallel orientation as axons are lost, coincident with changes in overall glial area and the distribution of astrocytes in the nerve. Diminished organization is closely related to axonal properties, rather than to changes in age or IOP. Parallelism closely relates both to astrocyte connectivity through gap junctions and maintenance of axonal anterograde transport.

Materials and methods

Animals and tissue preparation

The Vanderbilt University Medical Center Institutional Animal Care and Use Committee approved all animal work and experimental procedures. We obtained DBA/2 J and DBA/2 J-*Gpnmb⁺/SjJ* ('D2 control') mice from Jackson Laboratories (Bar Harbor, ME). A subset of DBA/2 J mice were bred in a pathogen-free facility and regularly backcrossed with fresh founders obtained from Jackson Laboratories to minimize genetic drift, as previously described [6, 21]. As described [11], 48 DBA/2 J optic nerves were used in the cross-sectional analyses within this study (Table 1). An additional 10 DBA/2 J mice and 8 D2 control mice were utilized in the immunolabeling portion of this study, all of which were harvested at 10 months. All mice were maintained on a 12 h light-dark cycle with standard rodent chow available ad libitum. We measured IOP monthly in a subset of these DBA/2 J mice representing 20 eyes using TonoPen XL rebound tonometry as previously described [11, 21]. Briefly, prior to measurement, the mice were anesthetized (Avertin, 1.3% tribromoethanol, 0.8% tert-amyl alcohol) and proparacaine ophthalmic solution (0.5% proparacaine hydrochloride, Bausch&Lomb, Tampa, FL) was applied topically to the eye. Monthly IOP for each eye was taken as the average of 25–30 Tono-Pen measurements recorded during a session.

Table 1 Nerves used for cross-sectional analysis

Age (mo.)	Cohort size
1.5	5
3	6
4	2
5	8
6	6
8	7
9	4
10	2
11	2
13	6

All mice were transcardially perfused with PBS followed by 4% paraformaldehyde in PBS. A 1–3 mm section of optic nerve proximal to the globe was isolated and post-fixed for 1 h in 4% paraformaldehyde. Nerves were prepared for embedding in Epon resin and semi-thin (1–2 μm) cross-sectioning as described previously [11, 14, 21, 25, 41, 42]. Cross-sections were imaged using an Olympus Provis AX70 microscope equipped with a motorized X-Y-Z stage, a digital video camera, and 100× oil-immersion, differential interference contrast optics. Photomicrographs were obtained *en montage* to represent the entire cross-section.

A subset of eyes and optic nerves from DBA/2 J and D2 control mice were enucleated and dissected from the optic chiasm for longitudinal sectioning and immunohistochemical staining. Tissue was cryoprotected in a sequence of 10, 20, and 30% sucrose/PBS overnight and subsequently embedded and frozen in Tissue-Plus O.C.T. Compound (Fisher Healthcare, Houston, TX). We labeled 10 μm cryosections with the following antibodies: anti-glial fibrillary acidic protein (GFAP; EMD Millipore, Billerica, MA, 1:500), and anti-Connexin-43 (Cx43; Alomone Labs, Jerusalem, Israel, 1:250). Immunolabeling was visualized using appropriate DyLight-conjugated secondary antibodies (Jackson Immunoresearch, West Grove, PA 1:200). Fluorescent montages were captured using an Olympus Provis AX70 microscope as described above. Confocal images were captured using an Olympus FV-1000 inverted microscope. Settings were kept constant for all sections so that comparisons in label intensity could be made.

Nerve and axon quantification

We measured cross-sectional nerve area in a total of 110 DBA/2 J optic nerves and axon density (axons/mm^2) in a subset of 46 DBA/2 J optic nerves as described previously [3, 6, 21]. Briefly, we randomly selected 25–30 non-overlapping frames representing a known area of nerve. Previously developed routines were used to identify and count each axon for which a single, intact myelin sheath could be identified. Nerves with pathology so severe that intact myelin sheaths were difficult for the program to detect were excluded. The mean axon density relationship for all frames was taken as the representative axon density for the nerve. In these same 46 nerves, we additionally determined the cross-sectional area for each identified axon within a myelin sheath. A range of 6000–40,000 measurements were used to calculate mean axon area (in um^2). We calculated correlation coefficients from best-fitting regression via Pearson's coefficient.

Quantification of glial area and process organization

Optic nerve sections were filtered using a suite of MATLAB routines (MathWorks, Natick, MA) to generate a binary image that highlighted glial processes (described in [11]). Glial area and center of mass (CoM) were calculated as described previously. Briefly, the sum of all identified processes was used to determine the percentage of the nerve occupied by glia; the CoM was obtained by dividing the binary image into 20 concentric rings from the edge to the center of the nerve, measuring the percent glial area within each, and determining which division delineated 50% of total glial area on either side. Thus, a nerve with an even distribution of glial area between edge and center has a CoM of 10; nerves with glial area biased towards the edge have a lower CoM, while nerves with glial area biased towards the center have a higher CoM.

Binary images were additionally used to quantify glial organization by measuring the overall parallelism of the cells' processes. The outer 20% of each nerve's area was first eroded in order to remove the disorganized glia along the nerve edge. This erosion maximized the signal-to-noise ratio and thus the robustness of the final organization parameter. Next, the eroded image was skeletonized and pruned, reducing each binary object to a one-pixel wide collection of segments. The length of each segment was determined as the maximum with constant orientation between corners, with each corner defining a branch point to a different orientation. The branch points between segments were then removed in order to calculate a vector for each segment. The magnitude (M) and the directional angle ($\boldsymbol{\theta}$) of each organizational vector were computed using Eqs. 1–2. These values were then used to calculate the horizontal (x) and vertical (y) components of each vector (Eqs. 3–4). This process was repeated as the eroded image was rotated one degree at a time until the sum of all vertical components reached an absolute minimum, indicating the orientation of maximal horizontal orientation of glial processes in the nerve. After finding this optimal rotational angle, the final organizational parameter was derived using Eq. 5. A parallelism percentage of 100% corresponds to a theoretical nerve that is perfectly organized, while 0% describes a nerve that is perfectly disorganized. Parallelism percentages above 50% were rarely observed because glial cell bodies typically have a rounded shape, and thus the vectors derived from their skeletons are not oriented parallel to one another.

$$M = \sqrt{(y_2 - y_1)^2 + (x_2 - x_1)^2} \tag{1}$$

$$\theta = \left| \arctan\left(\frac{y_2 - y_1}{x_2 - x_1}\right) \right|, \quad \text{for branch endpoints } (x_1, y_1), (x_2, y_2) \tag{2}$$

$$x\_comp = M \cos\theta \tag{3}$$

$$y\_comp = M \sin\theta, \quad \text{where } \theta \in [0, 90] \tag{4}$$

$$Parallelism = \left(1 - \frac{\min \sum_{i=1}^{n} y\_comp_i}{\max \sum_{i=1}^{n} x\_comp_i}\right) \times 100 \tag{5}$$

Tracing of anterograde axonal transport

Forty-eight hours prior to perfusion, a subset of animals were anesthetized with 2.5% isoflurane and bilaterally injected intravitreally with 2 µl of 0.5 mg cholera toxin subunit B (CTB) conjugated to Alexa Fluor 488 (Invitrogen) as previously described [13, 14]. Two days post-injection, animals were transcardially perfused with PBS followed by 4% paraformaldehyde in PBS. Brains were cryoprotected in 30% sucrose/PBS overnight, and 50 µm coronal midbrain sections were cut on a freezing sliding microtome. Serial superior colliculus sections were imaged using a Nikon Eclipse TI microscope (Nikon Instruments) and the intensity of the fluorescent CTB signal was quantified using ImagePro custom routines (Media Cybernetics) as previously described [13, 56]. CTB signal was normalized to background and alternating sections were analyzed for intensity. Intensity from each section was calculated to reconstruct a retinotopic map of intact anterograde transport across the superior colliculus. Intact transport for each map was defined as any region with an intensity ≥ 70% of the maximum CTB signal for that tissue.

Statistical analysis

Data for IOP and glial area analysis are presented as mean ± standard error of the mean (SEM) for each treatment. Statistical analysis and p-values for comparing means were obtained using Kruskal-Wallis one-way ANOVA or two-sided t-tests, and all data met criteria for normalcy as confirmed using the Shapiro-Wilk normality test; all datasets compared passed with $p \geq 0.22$. Correlations were calculated using the two-tailed Pearson product moment test and verified by linear regression analysis. Statistical tests were considered significant if $p < 0.05$. All statistical tests were performed with SigmaPlot 12.5 (Systat Software Inc., San Jose, CA). Numbers of samples and measurements along with actual p values of significance are indicated where appropriate in the text or figure legends.

Results

Optic nerve remodeling involves diminished astrocyte organization

Astrocyte processes retract from axon bundles prior to frank loss of axons in the myelinated segment of the DBA/2 J optic nerve [11]. Using the same cohort of nerves, here we report another interesting characteristic of astrocyte organization and orientation. Fig. 1a (left) shows a healthy nerve with high axon density (6.2×10^5 axons/mm^2) and a low fraction of its area covered by glia (11.4%). For this nerve, astrocyte processes appear to follow a parallel pattern of distribution (Fig. 1b). This pattern is consistent with astrocyte distribution in cross-section of healthy white matter tracts [28, 31]. However, a glaucomatous nerve with substantial loss of axons (2.4×10^5 axons/mm^2) and increased glial coverage (45.19%) demonstrates clear disorganization of astrocyte processes (Fig. 1a, right), with less apparent parallel orientation (Fig. 1c).

To quantify loss of parallelism in our cross-sections of proximal DBA/2 J optic nerve, we devised an algorithm that decomposes glial processes into horizontal and vertical vector components. Using a binary representation of each nerve in which glial processes are highlighted (Fig. 2a; see Fig. 7 of [11]), each nerve was rotated to maximize the orientation of glial processes along the horizontal axis (Fig. 2b). This normalizes images for nerve orientation. Following rotation (Fig. 2c), each process was skeletonized to simplify decomposition into vectors (Fig. 2d). Skeletons were decomposed by removing branch points, resulting in a population of vectors representing the orientation of each segment of astrocyte processes (Fig. 2e).

By collecting all such segments across the nerve, we generated a single representative value of astrocyte parallelism. For the collection of vectors (Fig. 3a), we

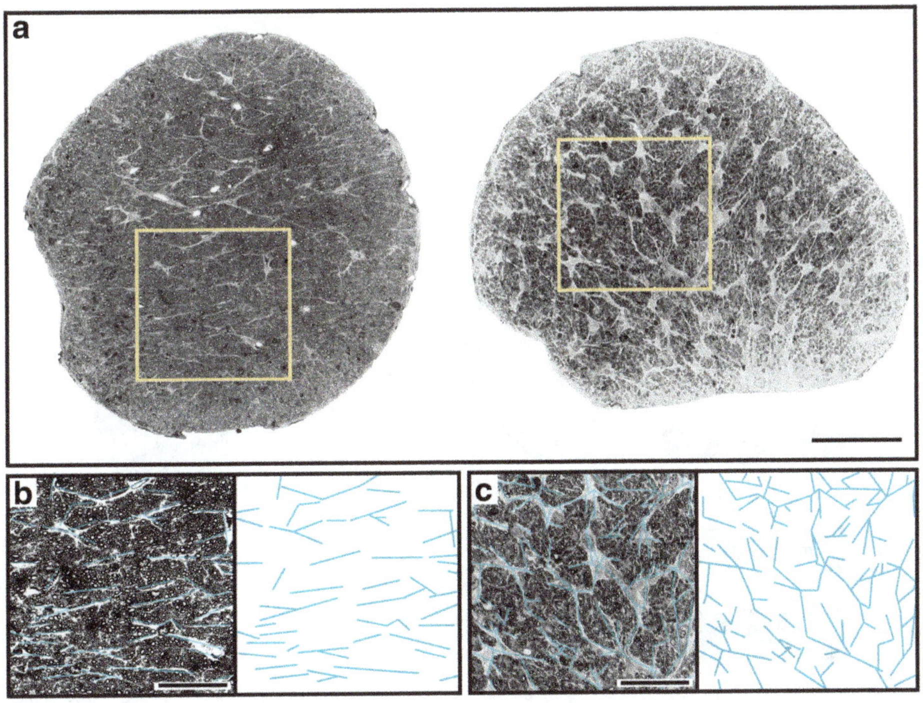

Fig. 1 Pathology alters glial orientation in the optic nerve. **a** Left: cross-section through DBA/2 J optic nerve prior to progression. Nerve has high axon packing density (6.2×10^5 axons/mm^2) and low glial coverage area (11.4% of total nerve area). Right: during progression axons are lost (2.4×10^5 axons/mm^2) and glial coverage increases (45.19%). **b** Higher magnification of inset from healthy nerve in **a** with highlighted glial processes demonstrating parallel orientation. **c** Inset from glaucomatous nerve in **a** with glial processes similarly highlighted. In this nerve, processes appear disordered, or oriented without a discernable pattern. Scale = 100 μm (**a**), 10 μm (**b**, **c**)

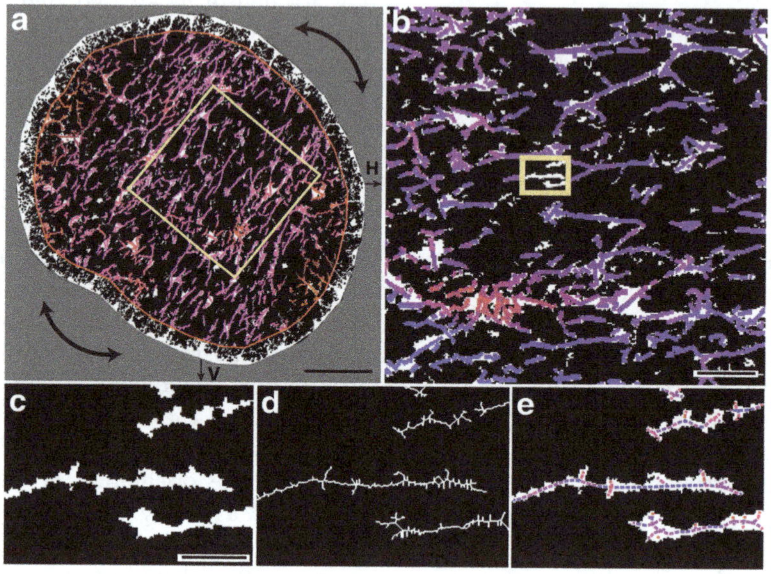

Fig. 2 Deconstruction of astrocyte processes into representative vectors. **a** Binary representation of an 8-month DBA/2 J nerve with glial processes highlighted to indicate coverage (white; 19.35% of nerve area). Colored overlay demonstrates result of algorithm to calculate vectors, with degree of orientation along the vertical axis (V) indicated by red tint and degree of orientation along the horizontal axis (H) indicated with blue tint. Our algorithm excludes the outer 20% of nerve area to minimize edge effects and rotates the image to maximize orientation along the horizontal axis, shown by the inset magnified in panel **b**. c Inset from **b** in higher magnification shows glial processes in binary image. **d** Same glial processes skeletonized for assigning vectors to segments of constant orientation. **e** Representative resultant vectors for each segment calculated from skeletonized image overlaid on original binary representation of glial processes. The length of each vector represents the pixel distance of each segment between branch points in the skeletonized image. Side branches less than threshold length or width were excluded (see Materials and methods). Scale = 100 μm (**a**), 10 μm (**b**), 2 μm (**c**, **d**, **e**)

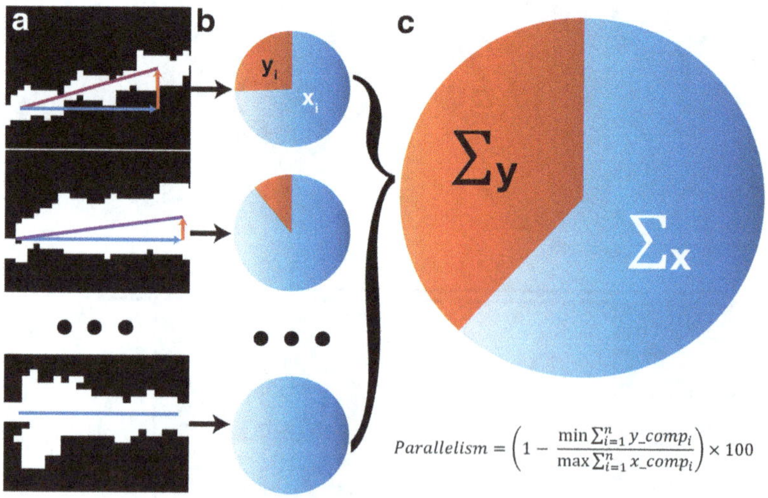

$$Parallelism = \left(1 - \frac{\min \sum_{i=1}^{n} y\_comp_i}{\max \sum_{i=1}^{n} x\_comp_i}\right) \times 100$$

Fig. 3 Method to quantify the overall parallelism of glial processes. **a** Binary high-magnification images of glial processes with increasing horizontal vector components (blue) compared to vertical (red). Resultant vector is the sum of these components (purple). **b** Individual pie charts depict the ratio of the length of the horizontal (blue, x_i) and vertical (red, y_i) components for each resultant vector. **c** The sum of the horizontal (x) and vertical (y) components for each nerve represents the degree of parallelism. The percent parallelism for each nerve is calculated from the ratio of the summed components following rotation to minimize vertical and maximize horizontal orientation. 100% corresponds to perfect parallelism and 0% corresponds to random orientation

summed the pixel length of all horizontal and vertical components (Fig. 3b). This summation defined a resultant vector representing the orientation and length of all vectors across the cross section (Fig. 3c). We defined the percent parallelism in each nerve using the ratio of summed horizontal and vertical components such that that a value of 100 indicates perfectly parallel orientation (i.e., no vertical component), while a value of 0 indicates random orientation due to equivalent vertical and horizontal components. This single value represents the organization across an entire nerve, providing a mechanism to analyze process organization in relation to other outcome measures.

Astrocyte processes in the DBA/2 J optic nerve redistribute spatially during progression, showing a tendency to retreat towards the edge prior to frank axon degeneration [11]. With progression, astrocyte processes once again fill in across the nerve. In Cooper et al. [11], we quantified this trend by defining a center of mass (CoM) based on division of the nerve into concentric rings, with values near 10 indicating an even distribution and values < 10 indicating bias towards the edge of the nerve (Fig. 4a). As glial area increases, the pattern of process distribution alters (Fig. 4b, c, d). We found that nerves with lower glial area tended to have an edge-distributed CoM (about 7), while nerves with higher glial area have a relatively even glial distribution (about 10; Fig. 4e). As CoM increased and glial coverage expanded, parallelism diminished as well (Fig. 4f,g).

Parallelism reflects early axonal changes

Next we examined how redistribution of astrocyte processes in the nerve is influenced by other predictors and indices of glaucomatous progression in the DBA/2 J nerves. Across our sample of optic nerves, we found that parallelism diminished only modestly with age (Fig. 5a); the relationship with IOP was even weaker (Fig. 5b). Cross-sectional nerve area (measured in mm^2) increases with age in the DBA/2 J mouse; this is linked eventually to axon loss and significant enlargement of cross-sectional area of surviving axons [11]. Here, we found that as the nerve enlarges, parallelism decreases significantly (Fig. 5c). Accordingly, since nerve expansion predicts both axon loss and axonal enlargement [11], increased axon size (Fig. 5d), diminished axon density (Fig. 5e), and loss of total number of axons all correlated with decreased parallelism (Fig. 5f). There is, however, a caveat to this conclusion.

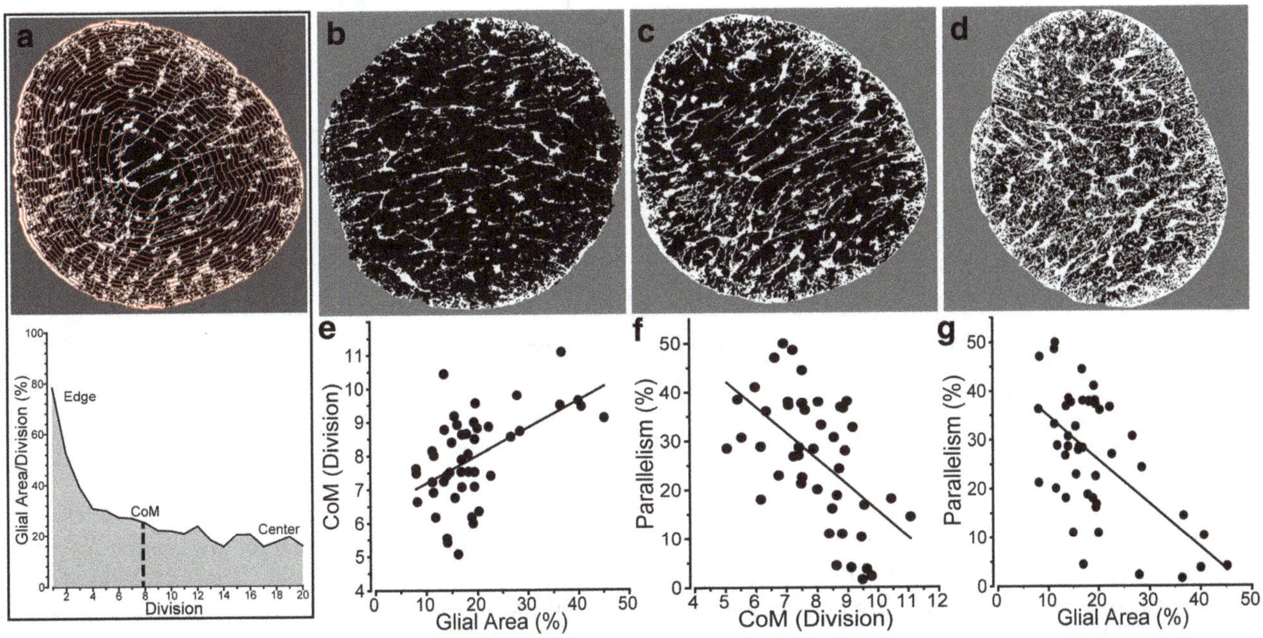

Fig. 4 Measuring the spatial distribution of astrocyte processes. **a** Modified from Cooper et al. [11]. Center of Mass (CoM) was calculated using a series of concentric circles (red) each delineating 5% of nerve area. From the first division at the edge of the nerve to the twentieth division at the center (graph below), the CoM represents the division at which half of the glial area resides on each side. **b** Cross-section through a young (1.5 month) DBA/2 J optic nerve shows slight bias of astrocyte center of mass (CoM) towards edge (CoM = 7.22), low coverage (11.2%), and high parallelism (48.6%). **c** A 3 month DBA/2 J nerve with higher CoM (8.55) and coverage (26.7%) shows less parallelism (30.6%). **d** A 5 month nerve with expansive glial coverage (40.6%) shows even astrocyte distribution (CoM = 9.44) and loss of parallelism (10.3%). **e** CoM increases significantly with glial area (modified from [11]; $r = 0.529$, $p < 0.001$). **f, g** Parallelism decreases with both increasing CoM ($r = -0.55$, $p < 0.001$) and expanding glial area ($r = -0.60$, $p < 0.001$). Scale = 100 μm (A-C)

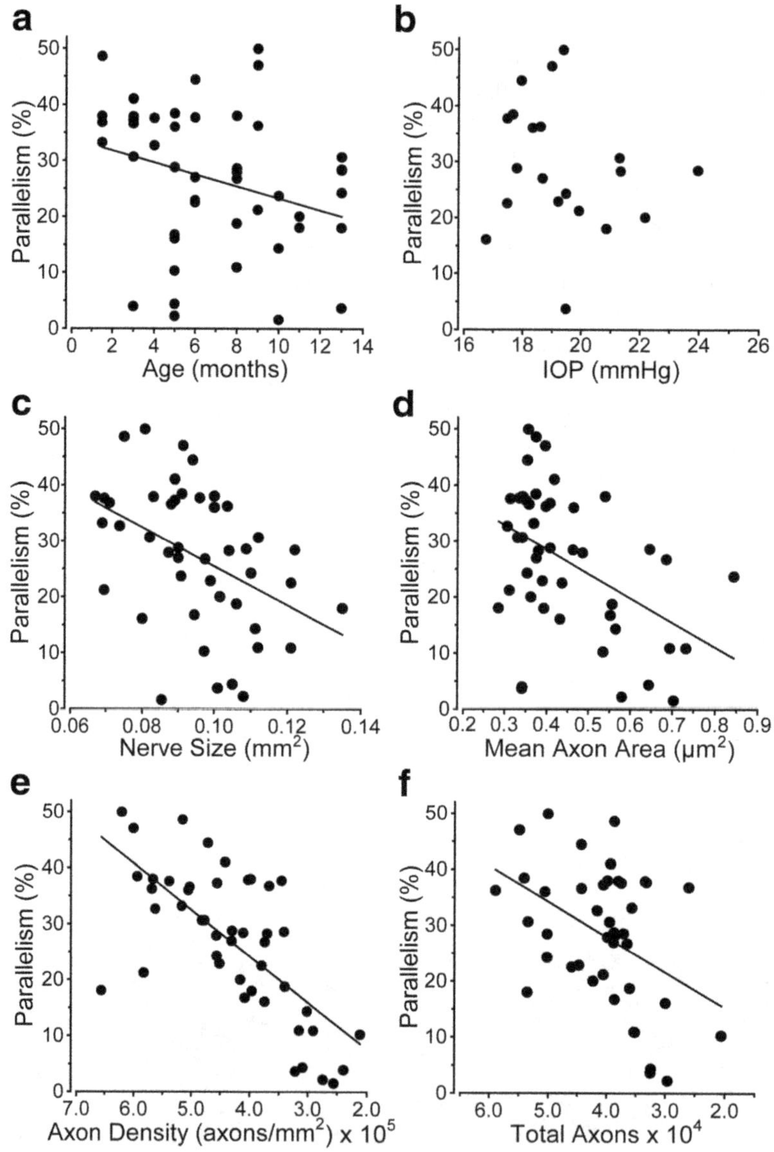

Fig. 5 Parallelism diminishes with markers of axon degeneration. **a** Parallelism decreases moderately as DBA/2 J mice age ($r = -0.293$, $p = 0.046$); there is no correlation with the mean lifetime IOP (**b**; $r = -0.193$, $p = 0.415$). **c** Parallelism rapidly diminishes with enlargement of the nerve ($r = -0.435$, $p = 0.003$). **d** Increased mean axon area is also correlated with decreased parallelism ($r = -0.457$, $p = 0.001$). **e** Parallelism demonstrates a tight correlation with diminished axon density ($r = -0.628$, $p < 0.001$). **f** As the total number of axons decreases, parallelism decreases ($r = -0.427$, $p = 0.005$)

While axons expand in area continuously from early to late progression in the DBA/2 J optic nerve, expansion is not associated with axon loss up to a critical threshold of about 0.50 μm^2 [11]. This early axon expansion is coincident with retraction of astrocyte processes towards the nerve edge and a temporary decrease in CoM (Fig. 6a, modified from [11]). For these same pre-degenerative nerves, we then examined parallelism. As axons expanded and astrocyte processes retracted towards the edge, parallelism increased (Fig. 6b). Intriguingly, these nerves at early stages of pathology exhibit glial distributions opposite that of the sample of nerves across all stages of degeneration (Fig. 6d). Moreover, the dependence of parallelism on CoM was slightly weaker for these pre-degenerative nerves than for the entire sample ($p = 0.071$; Fig. 6c, compare to Fig. 5e). For this subset of nerves, glial coverage did not change with axon size (Fig. 6d) or with parallelism (data not shown; $r = 0.0942$; $p = 0.0729$). These data indicate that while parallelism diminishes as axons degenerate later (Fig. 5e), early changes in the nerve prior to overt axon loss are associated with increased parallelism without a change in overall glial coverage.

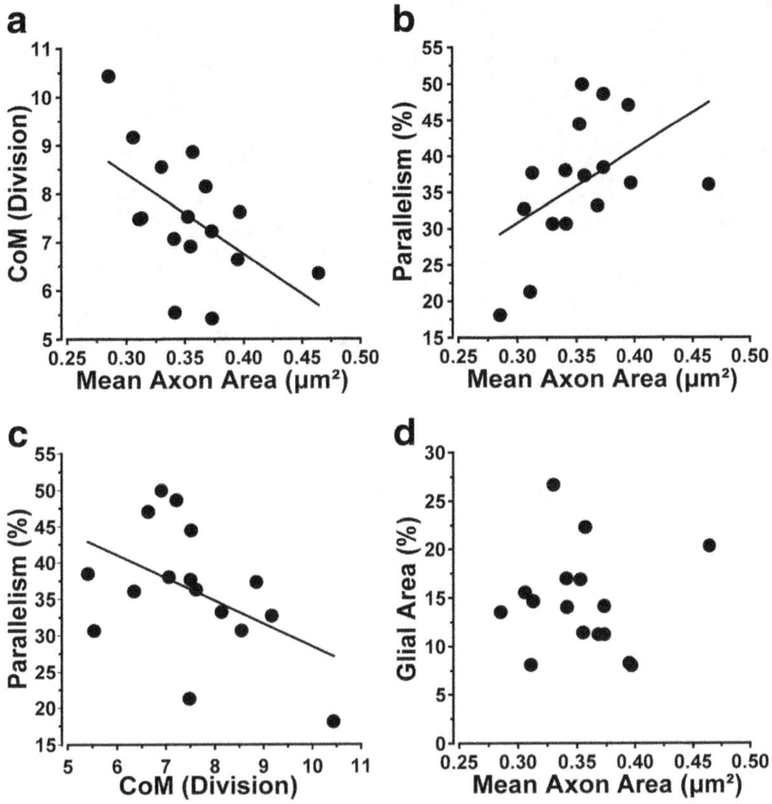

Fig. 6 Astrocytes become more parallel as axons expand early prior to loss. **a** Modified from Cooper et al. [11]. CoM decreases significantly as axons expand early in the DBA/2 J nerve prior to overt loss of axons ($r = 0.55$, $p < 0.001$). **b** As axons expand prior to outright loss, parallelism increases ($r = 0.50$, $p = 0.05$). **c** Parallelism tends to increase with decreasing CoM for the same set of nerves ($r = 0.47$; $p = 0.071$). **d** Glial coverage of the nerve does not change as axons expand prior to loss ($r = 0.006$, $p = 0.98$). All data collected from subset of nerves with highest axon sampling density below the threshold of axon size for which loss occurs (4.8–6.5 × 10^5 axons/mm^2; see [11])

Astrocyte cytoskeletal reorganization depends on location in the nerve

To determine how astrocyte reorganization reflects cytoskeletal changes, we measured the distribution of GFAP in discrete intervals along longitudinal sections through the aged (10 month) DBA/2 J optic nerve, spanning proximal to the nerve head (< 1 mm) and to more distal (> 4 mm; Fig. 7a insets 1 and 2). We then compared this distribution to CoM and parallelism redefined for immuno-labeling in longitudinal sections (see Materials and methods). On average, DBA/2 J nerves exhibited increased total nerve GFAP compared to the age-matched D2 control strain ($p < 0.001$; Fig. 7b). While at discrete points along the nerve GFAP in DBA/2 J was systematically higher, this trend did not translate to a significant difference within any one interval (Fig. 7c). The CoM for GFAP was significantly elevated in DBA/2 J compared to D2 nerves, indicating a more central distribution of astrocytes ($p < 0.001$; Fig. 7d). Moreover, unlike GFAP levels, CoM did significantly depend on location in the nerve (Fig. 7e), with GFAP-labeled processes distributing more towards the nerve center at distal locations compared to D2 nerves. This is a later hallmark of progression [11]. Additionally, we found that GFAP parallelism is elevated in the distal nerve of both DBA/2 J ($p = 0.015$) and D2 control compared to proximal nerve ($p = 0.003$; Fig. 7f). Finally, the CoM for distal segments of DBA/2 J nerve indicated edge-distributed astrocytes with increased parallelism ($p = 0.005$), while CoM in D2 nerves showed the opposite trend (Fig. 7g), though not significant ($p = 0.07$).

Parallelism reflects both astrocyte connectivity and RGC axonal function

Loss of anterograde axonal transport of cholera toxin B (CTB) from retina to superior colliculus (SC) is an early hallmark of axonopathy in the DBA/2 J and other models [13, 18, 25, 34, 51, 56]. Consistent with this pattern, while SC from D2 animals demonstrated mostly intact transport (75% intact), DBA/2 J SC exhibited severe deficits (Fig. 8a), with intact transport averaging only about 20% (22.784 ± 5.493), a highly significant difference ($p = 0.0015$, Fig. 8b). Astrocytes couple to one another through gap junctions to form a dense network

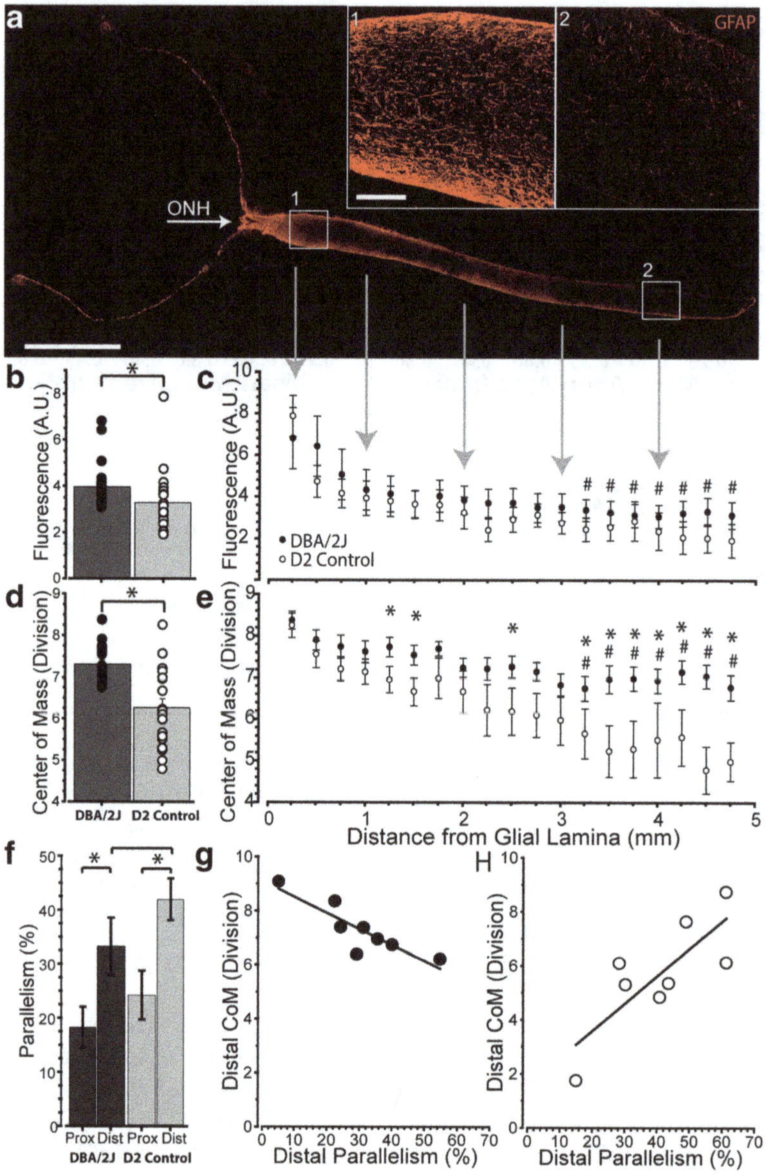

Fig. 7 Astrocyte GFAP redistributes throughout the optic nerve. **a**. Longitudinal section through 10-month DBA/2 J retina and optic nerve shows astrocytes labeled for GFAP (red). GFAP expression is highest at the optic nerve head (ONH), proximal optic nerve (1), and at the edges of the distal nerve (2). **b**. GFAP is significantly elevated in DBA/2 J nerves compared to D2 control nerves ($p < 0.001$). **c**. When analyzed in 0.25 mm segments, no one segment of DBA/2 J nerve contains significantly elevated GFAP compared to the same D2 control segment; however, the most proximal segment (0.25 mm) in both DBA/2 J and D2 control nerves contains significantly more GFAP than distal segments (#; $p < 0.001$). **d**. The CoM of GFAP within DBA/2 J nerves is significantly greater than D2 control nerves ($p < 0.001$). **e**. DBA/2 J nerves contain significantly altered GFAP CoM from D2 control nerves, and these differences occur most often within distal nerve segments (*; $p < 0.029$). **f**. GFAP parallelism is significantly greater in the distal compared to the proximal nerve in both the DBA/2 J ($p = 0.015$) and D2 control ($p = 0.003$). Additionally, GFAP within distal DBA/2 J nerves trends toward less parallelism than the equivalent segment of D2 control nerves ($p = 0.09$). **g**. DBA/2 J distal nerves tend to have a more edge-distributed center of mass when parallelism is greater ($p = 0.005$), indicating parallelism and center of mass are related. **h**. This relationship is trending toward the reverse in distal D2 control nerves ($p = 0.07$). Scale: 1 mm (A), 100 μm (A insets)

that is tightly modulated by axonal function and neuronal activity [38]. In these same animals, we examined levels of connexin 43 (Cx43), a marker for gap junctions between astrocytes [24]. Consistent with this role, both proximal and distal segments of DBA/2 J and D2 optic nerve show strong Cx43 colocalization with GFAP (Fig. 8c). Additionally, there are significantly more Cx43 puncta in proximal vs. distal segments in the DBA/2 J nerve ($p = 0.043$; Fig. 8d), similar to the distribution of GFAP (Fig. 7c). Additionally, Cx43 puncta are increased in DBA/2 J nerve compared to D2, though this is only significant for proximal segments ($p = 0.032$; Fig. 8d).

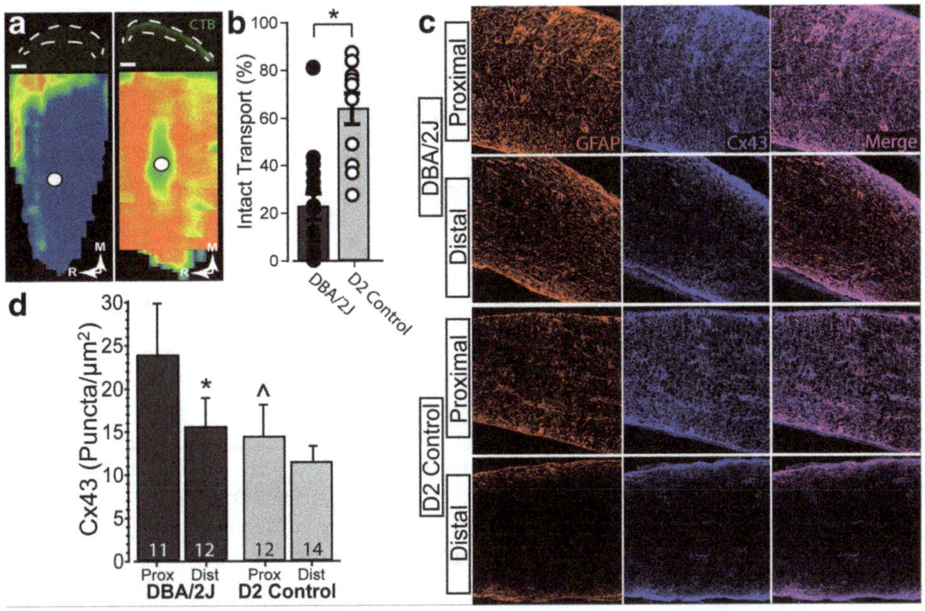

Fig. 8 Diminished anterograde transport in a sample of DBA/2 J nerves. **a** Top Left: Coronal section through superior colliculus of DBA/2 J mouse (between dashed white lines) following intravitreal injection of CTB (green). Bottom Left: Corresponding retinotopic map shows nearly depleted anterograde transport of CTB. Top Right: Coronal section through superior colliculus of D2 control mouse prepared as on left. Bottom Right: Corresponding retinotopic map shows a full complement of anterogradely transported CTB. **b** Transport of CTB from DBA/2 J eyes was near 20% (22.8 ± 5.5), significantly reduced from D2 control which is near 75% (74.896 ± 4.328) ($p = 0.0015$). **c** Confocal micrographs of proximal (left) and distal (right) DBA/2 J (top) and D2 control (bottom) optic nerves. Connexin 43 (Cx43, blue) and GFAP (red) colocalize, and both are elevated in proximal optic nerve. **d**. Density of Cx43 (puncta/μm^2) in proximal segment of DBA/2 J nerves is significantly elevated compared to both distal DBA/2 J (*; $p = 0.043$) and proximal D2 nerves (#; $p = 0.032$)

Higher Cx43 in the proximal segment predicted a greater degree of parallelism for GFAP-labeled astrocyte processes ($p = 0.04$; Fig. 9a, left). This was not so for the distal segment ($p = 0.77$; Fig. 9a, right), though overall parallelism was higher in this location (Fig. 7f). These differences may have functional significance for axons. Earlier we demonstrated that anterograde transport from retina to the SC in the DBA/2 J degrades in a distal (brain) to proximal (retina) pattern [13]. Here, while Cx43 in the proximal segment did not correlate with levels of intact axonal anterograde transport (Fig. 9b, left), increased Cx43 in the distal segment strongly correlated with this measure of axonal function ($p < 0.001$; Fig. 9b, right).

Discussion

Our results demonstrate several key features of astrocyte organization and its alterations through pathology. In cross-sections of healthy DBA/2 J optic nerve (Fig. 1), astrocyte processes organize in a similar direction, i.e., exhibit a high degree of parallelism as indicated by our metric (Figs. 2 and 3). As axon pathology increases with a commensurate increase in glial coverage of the nerve, parallelism diminishes and astrocytes distribute more evenly across the nerve (Fig. 4). Accordingly, axon density, total number of axons, and axon expansion all predict changes in astrocyte parallelism more accurately than independent measures of glaucoma progression in the DBA/2 J (i.e., IOP and age; Fig. 5). Earlier we reported that axons expand in mean cross-sectional area up to a threshold of about 0.5 mm^2 before their number begins to decline [11]. Concomitantly, astrocyte processes retreat towards the edge of the nerve, meaning center-of-mass (or CoM) diminishes. In these pre-degenerative nerves, as mean axon area increases towards the threshold for loss, astrocyte parallelism increases without a change in overall glial coverage of the nerve (Fig. 6). Once axon loss begins and density diminishes, parallelism decreases in kind (Fig. 5e), presumably as astrocyte processes re-invade axon bundles [51]. In total, these results from the DBA/2 J nerve indicate that astrocytes remodel biphasically. During early axon expansion prior to axonal loss, astrocyte processes increase in parallelism as CoM diminishes *independent from gliosis* (Fig. 6). Once axons are lost, gliosis involves diminished parallelism and uniform astrocyte distribution across the nerve (Fig. 4).

In longitudinal sections of nerve, we found that both GFAP and Cx43 - which marks astrocyte gap junctions [24] – are higher in proximal vs. distal segments (Figs. 7c, 8d). This is consistent with a more even distribution of astrocytes, as indicated by the higher CoM in the proximal vs. the distal segment (Fig. 7e). In earlier

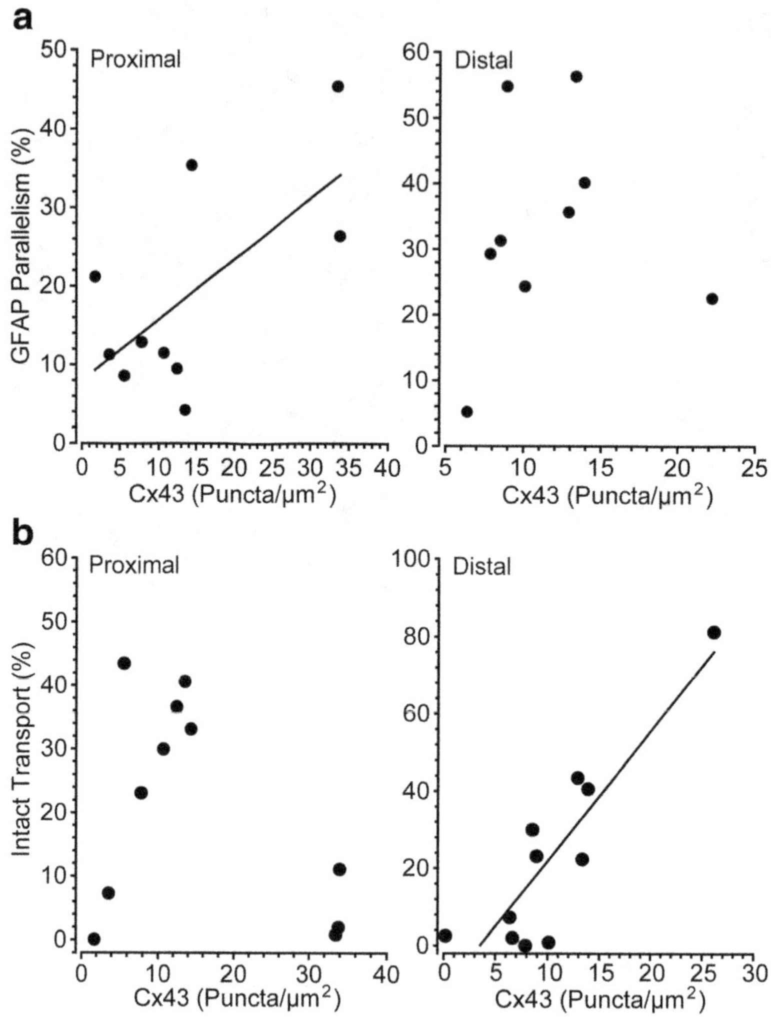

Fig. 9 RGC axon functional deficits are associated with astrocyte connectivity in DBA/2 J optic nerve. **a**. Higher levels of Cx43 are associated with a greater degree of parallelism of GFAP-labeled astrocyte processes in proximal segments of DBA/2 J nerve (left, $R = 0.66$; $p = 0.04$) but not distal (right, $R = 0.11$; $p = 0.77$). **b** Intact anterograde transport to the superior colliculus is well-predicted by levels of Cx43 in the distal optic nerve (right, $R = 0.88$; $p < 0.001$), but not proximal (left, $R = 0.39$; $p = 0.23$). Scale: 100 μm (**a**)

work, we demonstrated that anterograde axonal transport from retina to brain is an early harbinger of axon pathology in the DBA/2 J and degrades in distal-to-proximal fashion [13]. We found here that parallelism of GFAP-labeled astrocyte processes was higher in distal segments of our 10-month old DBA/2 J nerves (Fig. 7f). As parallelism increased in the distal segment, astrocytes redistributed towards the nerve edge, as indicated by a lower CoM (Fig. 7g). This pattern of remodeling reflects that seen in early stages of axonal pathology, indicating that astrocytes in the distal nerve may be reacting to pathology prior to those in the proximal nerve.

In the distal segment, nerves containing elevated Cx43 also demonstrated higher levels of intact transport, but did not show a relationship with parallelism (Fig. 9b). In contrast, levels of Cx43 in the proximal segment predicted parallelism with no clear relationship to transport (Fig. 9a). Thus, these results indicate that in the distal segment, where axonopathy has already begun [13], Cx43 in astrocytes better reflects axon function than astrocyte organization. This is consistent with findings showing that gap-junction coupling of the astrocyte network is tightly modulated by axonal function and neuronal activity [38]. Similarly, increased parallelism in the distal vs. proximal segment is reminiscent of our results from cross-sections of proximal nerve, where increased parallelism correlated with early expansion of axons prior to overt loss (Fig. 6b). Through gap-junction coupling, astrocytes may be able to more evenly distribute resources to those axons undergoing the highest degree of stress [17, 20, 36, 47].

Our results suggest that early progression in the optic nerve involves remodeling of astrocyte processes, first to a higher state of organization with increased parallelism (Fig. 6) and gap-junction coupling (Fig. 9) and then to gradual deterioration of organization as coverage increases and axons are lost (Figs. 4 and 5). Perhaps well-organized astrocyte processes lend structural stability to the nerve. In the optic nerve head, astrocytes form a continuously remodeling network that adapts to IOP exposure [44], with astrocyte actin and tubulin filaments gradually re-orienting as IOP increases [52]. With short exposures to elevated IOP, astrocyte processes retract towards the cell body [51]; astrocyte processes also may also fortify the edge of the nerve, as coverage in the center diminishes (Fig. 3 of Sun et al., 2013). As astrocyte processes re-invade the nerve center with longer IOP exposure, their organization diminishes [51]. With acute injury (nerve crush), astrocyte processes appear to detach from the edge [49], but this likely reflects the more severe nature of the injury. Similar to our results in the myelinated nerve, astrocyte remodeling following induced short-term elevations in pressure is most extensive distal from the sclera [55]. Portions of the optic nerve beyond the sclera itself are unlikely to be impacted directly by elevated IOP, and secondary changes could involve different structural mechanisms. This may be why we did not note a simple linear relationship between IOP and loss of parallelism (Fig. 5b), but did find strong correlations between measures of axonal degeneration and loss of parallelism (Figs. 5 and 6).

Perhaps the most important question is whether early astrocyte remodeling is protective or pathogenic. Cx43 is elevated in the optic nerve head and the retina in human glaucomatous tissue [23], and here we find that astrocyte remodeling is associated with increased Cx43 (Fig. 9). Intriguingly, we additionally find that elevated Cx43 is also associated with intact axonal anterograde transport (Fig. 9d). This suggests that the early phases of astrocyte remodeling involving increased connectivity may be a component of an endogenously protective mechanism, wherein these alterations within astrocytes positively influence the health of axons within the optic nerve. In late stages of neurodegeneration Cx43-mediated coupling helps disperse inflammatory cytokines through gap junctions [10, 15]. The data presented herein leads us to believe that Cx43 exhibits a multitude of functions, like astrocytes themselves. In these early stages of pathology, gap junctions allow astrocytes to couple with neighboring cells and share signals that may contribute to the redistribution of resources to those regions most at risk.

Conclusions

Early optic nerve pathology involves astrocyte process remodeling, first to a higher state of organization and gap-junction coupling and then to gradual deterioration of organization as coverage increases and axons are lost. Morphologically, therefore, astrocytes exhibit multiple phases of remodeling due to neurodegenerative stress. We find that these early astrocyte responses to neurodegeneration are associated with beneficial functional outcomes for neurons. This responsiveness includes elevation in the gap-junction protein Cx43. Together, these data provide evidence for an endogenously protective mechanism wherein astrocytes increase connectivity to positively influence optic nerve axonal health during neurodegenerative stress.

Acknowledgments

Supported by National Institutes of Health grants R01 EY17427, R01 EY024997, T32 EY021453, T32 EY007135, and P30 EY008126, Departmental Unrestricted and Senior Investigator Awards from Research to Prevent Blindness, Inc., the Melza M. and Frank Theodore Barr Foundation through the Glaucoma Research Foundation, and the Stanley Cohen Innovation Fund through Vanderbilt University Medical Center. Imaging supported through the Vanderbilt University Medical Center Cell Imaging Shared Resource core facility (Clinical and Translational Science Award Grant UL1 RR024975 from National Center for Research Resources). The authors would like to thank Victoria Vest for her programming expertise along with Wendi Lambert for her assistance with animal husbandry, tissue processing, and for editing the manuscript.

Authors' contributions

MC carried out each experiment, performed statistical analysis, and drafted the manuscript. JC participated in coding and experimental design. DC participated in the design of the study and reviewed the manuscript. All authors read and approved the final manuscript.

Competing interests

The authors declare that they have no competing interests.

References

1. Almeida A, Almeida J, Bolanos JP, Moncada S (2001) Different responses of astrocytes and neurons to nitric oxide: the role of glycolytically generated ATP in astrocyte protection. Proc Natl Acad Sci U S A 98:15294–15299. https://doi.org/10.1073/pnas.261560998
2. Baltan S, Inman DM, Danilov CA, Morrison RS, Calkins DJ, Horner PJ (2010) Metabolic vulnerability disposes retinal ganglion cell axons to dysfunction in a model of glaucomatous degeneration. J Neurosci 30:5644–5652. https://doi.org/10.1523/JNEUROSCI.5956-09.2010
3. Bosco A, Breen KT, Anderson SR, Steele MR, Calkins DJ, Vetter ML (2016) Glial coverage in the optic nerve expands in proportion to optic axon loss in chronic mouse glaucoma. Exp Eye Res 150:34–43. https://doi.org/10.1016/j.exer.2016.01.014
4. Bosco A, Inman DM, Steele MR, Wu G, Soto I, Marsh-Armstrong N, Hubbard WC, Calkins DJ, Horner PJ, Vetter ML (2008) Reduced retina microglial activation and improved optic nerve integrity with minocycline treatment in the DBA/2J mouse model of glaucoma. Invest Ophthalmol Vis Sci 49:1437–1446. https://doi.org/10.1167/iovs.07-1337
5. Boumezbeur F, Mason GF, de Graaf RA, Behar KL, Cline GW, Shulman GI, Rothman DL, Petersen KF (2010) Altered brain mitochondrial metabolism in healthy aging as assessed by in vivo magnetic resonance spectroscopy. J Cereb Blood Flow Metab 30:211–221. https://doi.org/10.1038/jcbfm.2009.197
6. Buckingham BP, Inman DM, Lambert W, Oglesby E, Calkins DJ, Steele MR, Vetter ML, Marsh-Armstrong N, Horner PJ (2008) Progressive ganglion cell degeneration precedes neuronal loss in a mouse model of glaucoma. J Neurosci 28:2735–2744. https://doi.org/10.1523/JNEUROSCI.4443-07.2008

7. Burgoyne CF (2011) A biomechanical paradigm for axonal insult within the optic nerve head in aging and glaucoma. Exp Eye Res 93:120–132. https://doi.org/10.1016/j.exer.2010.09.005
8. Calkins DJ (2013) Age-related changes in the visual pathways: blame it on the axon. Invest Ophthalmol Vis Sci 54: ORSF37–41 Doi https://doi.org/10.1167/iovs.13-12784
9. Cavallotti C, Pacella E, Pescosolido N, Tranquilli-Leali FM, Feher J (2002) Age-related changes in the human optic nerve. Can J Ophthalmol 37: 389–394
10. Chen YS, Green CR, Danesh-Meyer HV, Rupenthal ID (2015) Neuroprotection in the treatment of glaucoma–a focus on connexin43 gap junction channel blockers. Eur J Pharm Biopharm 95:182–193. https://doi.org/10.1016/j.ejpb.2015.01.031
11. Cooper ML, Crish SD, Inman DM, Horner PJ, Calkins DJ (2016) Early astrocyte redistribution in the optic nerve precedes axonopathy in the DBA/2J mouse model of glaucoma. Exp Eye Res 150:22–33. https://doi.org/10.1016/j.exer.2015.11.016
12. Crish SD, Dapper JD, Macnamee SE, Balaram P, Sidorova TN, Lambert WS, Calkins DJ (2013) Failure of axonal transport induces a spatially coincident increase in astrocyte Bdnf prior to synapse loss in a central target. Neuroscience 229:55–70. https://doi.org/10.1016/j.neuroscience.2012.10.069
13. Crish SD, Sappington RM, Inman DM, Horner PJ, Calkins DJ (2010) Distal axonopathy with structural persistence in glaucomatous neurodegeneration. P Natl Acad Sci USA 107:5196–5201. https://doi.org/10.1073/pnas.0913141107
14. Dapper JD, Crish SD, Pang IH, Calkins DJ (2013) Proximal inhibition of p38 MAPK stress signaling prevents distal axonopathy. Neurobiol Dis 59:26–37. https://doi.org/10.1016/j.nbd.2013.07.001
15. Decrock E, De Vuyst E, Vinken M, Van Moorhem M, Vranckx K, Wang N, Van Laeken L, De Bock M, D'Herde K, Lai CPet al (2009) Connexin 43 hemichannels contribute to the propagation of apoptotic cell death in a rat C6 glioma cell model. Cell Death Differ 16: 151–163 Doi https://doi.org/10.1038/cdd.2008.138
16. Falkowska A, Gutowska I, Goschorska M, Nowacki P, Chlubek D, Baranowska-Bosiacka I (2015) Energy metabolism of the brain, including the cooperation between astrocytes and neurons, especially in the context of glycogen metabolism. Int J Mol Sci 16:25959–25981. https://doi.org/10.3390/ijms161125939
17. Fazio MA, Grytz R, Bruno L, Girard MJ, Gardiner S, Girkin CA, Downs JC (2012) Regional variations in mechanical strain in the posterior human sclera. Invest Ophthalmol Vis Sci 53:5326–5333. https://doi.org/10.1167/iovs.12-9668
18. Formichella CR, Abella SK, Sims SM, Cathcart HM, Sappington RM (2014) Astrocyte reactivity: a biomarker for retinal ganglion cell health in retinal neurodegeneration. J Clin Cell Immunol 5. https://doi.org/10.4172/2155-9899.1000188
19. Gordon MO, Beiser JA, Brandt JD, Heuer DK, Higginbotham EJ, Johnson CA, Keltner JL, Miller JP, Parrish RK, Wilson MR et al (2002) The ocular hypertension treatment study - baseline factors that predict the onset of primary open-angle glaucoma. Arch Ophthalmol-Chic 120:714–720
20. Grytz R, Sigal IA, Ruberti JW, Meschke G, Downs JC (2012) Lamina Cribrosa thickening in early Glaucoma predicted by a microstructure motivated growth and remodeling approach. Mech Mater 44:99–109. https://doi.org/10.1016/j.mechmat.2011.07.004
21. Inman DM, Sappington RM, Horner PJ, Calkins DJ (2006) Quantitative correlation of optic nerve pathology with ocular pressure and corneal thickness in the DBA/2 mouse model of glaucoma. Invest Ophthalmol Vis Sci 47:986–996. https://doi.org/10.1167/iovs.05-0925
22. Jakobs TC, Libby RT, Ben Y, John SW, Masland RH (2005) Retinal ganglion cell degeneration is topological but not cell type specific in DBA/2J mice. J Cell Biol 171:313–325. https://doi.org/10.1083/jcb.200506099
23. Kerr NM, Johnson CS, Green CR, Danesh-Meyer HV (2011) Gap junction protein connexin43 (GJA1) in the human glaucomatous optic nerve head and retina. J Clin Neurosci 18:102–108. https://doi.org/10.1016/j.jocn.2010.06.002
24. Koulakoff A, Ezan P, Giaume C (2008) Neurons control the expression of connexin 30 and connexin 43 in mouse cortical astrocytes. Glia 56:1299–1311. https://doi.org/10.1002/glia.20698
25. Lambert WS, Ruiz L, Crish SD, Wheeler LA, Calkins DJ (2011) Brimonidine prevents axonal and somatic degeneration of retinal ganglion cell neurons. Mol Neurodegener 6:4. https://doi.org/10.1186/1750-1326-6-4
26. Leske MC, Heijl A, Hussein M, Bengtsson B, Hyman L, Komaroff E, Grp EMGT (2003) Factors for glaucoma progression and the effect of treatment - the early manifest Glaucoma trial. Arch Ophthalmol-Chic 121:48–56
27. Li L, Lundkvist A, Andersson D, Wilhelmsson U, Nagai N, Pardo AC, Nodin C, Stahlberg A, Aprico K, Larsson Ket al (2008) Protective role of reactive astrocytes in brain ischemia. J Cereb Blood Flow Metab 28: 468–481 https://doi.org/10.1038/sj.jcbfm.9600546
28. Liuzzi FJ, Miller RH (1987) Radially oriented astrocytes in the normal adult-rat spinal-cord. Brain res 403: 385-388 Doi. https://doi.org/10.1016/0006-8993(87)90081-3
29. Lundgaard I, Osorio MJ, Kress BT, Sanggaard S, Nedergaard M (2014) White matter astrocytes in health and disease. Neuroscience 276:161–173. https://doi.org/10.1016/j.neuroscience.2013.10.050
30. Lye-Barthel M, Sun D, Jakobs TC (2013) Morphology of astrocytes in a glaucomatous optic nerve. Invest Ophthalmol Vis Sci 54:909–917. https://doi.org/10.1167/iovs.12-10109
31. Miller JP, Liuzzi FJ (1986) Regional specialization of the radial glial cells of the adult frog spinal cord. J Neurocytol 15:187–196. https://doi.org/10.1007/bf01611655
32. Myer DJ, Gurkoff GG, Lee SM, Hovda DA, Sofroniew MV (2006) Essential protective roles of reactive astrocytes in traumatic brain injury. Brain 129:2761–2772. https://doi.org/10.1093/brain/awl165
33. Okada S, Nakamura M, Katoh H, Miyao T, Shimazaki T, Ishii K, Yamane J, Yoshimura A, Iwamoto Y, Toyama Yet al (2006) Conditional ablation of Stat3 or Socs3 discloses a dual role for reactive astrocytes after spinal cord injury. Nat Med 12: 829–834 https://doi.org/10.1038/nm1425
34. Park KK, Liu K, Hu Y, Smith PD, Wang C, Cai B, Xu B, Connolly L, Kramvis I, Sahin Met al (2008) Promoting axon regeneration in the adult CNS by modulation of the PTEN/mTOR pathway. Science 322: 963–966 https://doi.org/10.1126/science.1161566
35. Payne SC, Bartlett CA, Harvey AR, Dunlop SA, Fitzgerald M (2012) Myelin sheath Decompaction, axon swelling, and functional loss during chronic secondary degeneration in rat optic nerve. Invest Ophth Vis Sci 53:6093–6101. https://doi.org/10.1167/iovs.12-10080
36. Pazos M, Yang H, Gardiner SK, Cepurna WO, Johnson EC, Morrison JC, Burgoyne CF (2016) Expansions of the neurovascular scleral canal and contained optic nerve occur early in the hypertonic saline rat experimental glaucoma model. Exp Eye Res 145:173–186. https://doi.org/10.1016/j.exer.2015.10.014
37. Quigley HA, Broman AT (2006) The number of people with glaucoma worldwide in 2010 and 2020. Br J Ophthalmol 90:262–267. https://doi.org/10.1136/bjo.2005.081224
38. Rouach N, Glowinski J, Giaume C (2000) Activity-dependent neuronal control of gap-junctional communication in astrocytes. J Cell Biol 149:1513–1526
39. Rouach N, Koulakoff A, Abudara V, Willecke K, Giaume C (2008) Astroglial metabolic networks sustain hippocampal synaptic transmission. Science 322:1551–1555. https://doi.org/10.1126/science.1164022
40. Sandell JH, Peters A (2002) Effects of age on the glial cells in the rhesus monkey optic nerve. J Comp Neurol 445:13–28
41. Sappington RM, Carlson BJ, Crish SD, Calkins DJ (2010) The microbead occlusion model: a paradigm for induced ocular hypertension in rats and mice. Invest Ophthalmol Vis Sci 51:207–216. https://doi.org/10.1167/iovs.09-3947
42. Sappington RM, Pearce DA, Calkins DJ (2003) Optic nerve degeneration in a murine model of juvenile ceroid lipofuscinosis. Invest Ophthalmol Vis Sci 44:3725–3731
43. Schuettauf F, Rejdak R, Walski M, Frontczak-Baniewicz M, Voelker M, Blatsios G, Shinoda K, Zagorski Z, Zrenner E, Grieb P (2004) Retinal neurodegeneration in the DBA/2J mouse-a model for ocular hypertension. Acta Neuropathol 107:352–358. https://doi.org/10.1007/s00401-003-0816-9
44. Sigal IA, Yang H, Roberts MD, Grimm JL, Burgoyne CF, Demirel S, Downs JC (2011) IOP-induced lamina cribrosa deformation and scleral canal expansion: independent or related? Invest Ophthalmol Vis Sci 52:9023–9032. https://doi.org/10.1167/iovs.11-8183
45. Sofroniew MV (2009) Molecular dissection of reactive astrogliosis and glial scar formation. Trends Neurosci 32:638–647. https://doi.org/10.1016/j.tins.2009.08.002
46. Sofroniew MV (2005) Reactive astrocytes in neural repair and protection. Neuroscientist 11:400–407. https://doi.org/10.1177/1073858405278321
47. Strouthidis NG, Yang H, Downs JC, Burgoyne CF (2009) Comparison of clinical and three-dimensional histomorphometric optic disc margin anatomy. Invest Ophthalmol Vis Sci 50:2165–2174. https://doi.org/10.1167/iovs.08-2786

48. Sun D, Jakobs TC (2012) Structural remodeling of astrocytes in the injured CNS. Neuroscientist 18:567–588. https://doi.org/10.1177/1073858411423441
49. Sun D, Lye-Barthel M, Masland RH, Jakobs TC (2010) Structural remodeling of fibrous astrocytes after axonal injury. J Neurosci 30:14008–14019. https://doi.org/10.1523/JNEUROSCI.3605-10.2010
50. Sun D, Moore S, Jakobs TC (2017) Optic nerve astrocyte reactivity protects function in experimental glaucoma and other nerve injuries. J Exp Med 214:1411–1430. https://doi.org/10.1084/jem.20160412
51. Sun D, Qu J, Jakobs TC (2013) Reversible reactivity by optic nerve astrocytes. Glia 61:1218–1235. https://doi.org/10.1002/glia.22507
52. Tehrani S, Johnson EC, Cepurna WO, Morrison JC (2014) Astrocyte processes label for filamentous actin and reorient early within the optic nerve head in a rat glaucoma model. Invest Ophthalmol Vis Sci 55:6945–6952. https://doi.org/10.1167/iovs.14-14969
53. Tekkok SB, Brown AM, Westenbroek R, Pellerin L, Ransom BR (2005) Transfer of glycogen-derived lactate from astrocytes to axons via specific monocarboxylate transporters supports mouse optic nerve activity. J Neurosci Res 81:644–652. https://doi.org/10.1002/jnr.20573
54. Tuck MW, Crick RP (1998) The age distribution of primary open angle glaucoma. Ophthalmic Epidemiol 5:173–183
55. Wang R, Seifert P, Jakobs TC (2017) Astrocytes in the optic nerve head of glaucomatous mice display a characteristic reactive phenotype. Invest Ophthalmol Vis Sci 58:924–932. https://doi.org/10.1167/iovs.16-20571
56. Ward NJ, Ho KW, Lambert WS, Weitlauf C, Calkins DJ (2014) Absence of transient receptor potential vanilloid-1 accelerates stress-induced axonopathy in the optic projection. J Neurosci 34:3161–3170. https://doi.org/10.1523/JNEUROSCI.4089-13.2014
57. Zonta M, Angulo MC, Gobbo S, Rosengarten B, Hossmann KA, Pozzan T, Carmignoto G (2003) Neuron-to-astrocyte signaling is central to the dynamic control of brain microcirculation. Nat Neurosci 6:43–50. https://doi.org/10.1038/nn980

3

Dipeptide repeat proteins activate a heat shock response found in *C9ORF72*-ALS/FTLD patients

Daniel A. Mordes[1,2,3,4], Mercedes Prudencio[5†], Lindsey D. Goodman[6†], Joseph R. Klim[1,2,3], Rob Moccia[1,2,3,7], Francesco Limone[1,2,3], Olli Pietilainen[1,2,3], Kaitavjeet Chowdhary[1,2], Dennis W. Dickson[5], Rosa Rademakers[5], Nancy M. Bonini[6], Leonard Petrucelli[5] and Kevin Eggan[1,2,3*]

Abstract

A hexanucleotide (*GGGGCC*) repeat expansion in *C9ORF72* is the most common genetic contributor to amyotrophic lateral sclerosis (ALS) and frontotemporal lobar degeneration (FTLD). Reduced expression of the *C9ORF72* gene product has been proposed as a potential contributor to disease pathogenesis. Additionally, repetitive RNAs and dipeptide repeat proteins (DPRs), such as poly-GR, can be produced by this hexanucleotide expansion that disrupt a number of cellular processes, potentially contributing to neural degeneration. To better discern which of these mechanisms leads to disease-associated changes in patient brains, we analyzed gene expression data generated from the cortex and cerebellum. We found that transcripts encoding heat shock proteins (HSPs) regulated by the HSF1 transcription factor were significantly induced in *C9ORF72*-ALS/FTLD patients relative to both sporadic ALS/FTLD cases and controls. Treatment of human neurons with chemically synthesized DPRs was sufficient to activate a similar transcriptional response. Expression of *GGGGCC* repeats and also poly-GR in the brains of *Drosophila* lead to the upregulation of HSF1 and the same highly-conserved HSPs. Additionally, HSF1 was a modifier of poly-GR toxicity in *Drosophila*. Our results suggest that the expression of DPRs are associated with upregulation of HSF1 and activation of a heat shock response in *C9ORF72*-ALS/FTLD.

Keywords: Amyotrophic lateral sclerosis, *C9ORF72* repeat expansion, Dipeptide repeat proteins, Drosophila, Frontotemporal dementia, Frontotemporal lobar degeneration, HSF1, Heat shock response

Introduction

Amyotrophic lateral sclerosis (ALS) is an adult onset neurodegenerative disease characterized by the loss of upper and lower motor neurons and muscle atrophy. Patients become progressively paralyzed and develop difficulty speaking, swallowing, and eventually breathing. Survival is typically limited to 2–5 years from the time of onset, and current treatment options remain limited. About 90% of cases are seemingly "sporadic" without a family history of disease and about 10% are familial. Hundreds of distinct variants in more than a dozen genes, many of which act with high penetrance, can increase a person's risk of developing ALS [46, 51].

The most common genetic contributor to ALS is a hexanucleotide (*GGGGCC*) repeat expansion within the first intron of *C9ORF72* [14, 45]. Carriers of the *C9ORF72* expansion can also present with frontotemporal dementia (FTD), which is characterized by frontotemporal lobar degeneration (FTLD) of the brain. In many cases, these initially diverse diagnoses can progress towards the inclusion of neurological features from each condition leading many to believe they are spectrums of the same disorder [52]. In addition, both diseases can be characterized by the presence of TDP-43 positive inclusions [37].

Three distinct mechanisms have been proposed for how the *C9ORF72* expansion contributes to the development of ALS and FTLD. First, *C9ORF72*-ALS brains display

* Correspondence: eggan@mcb.harvard.edu
†Mercedes Prudencio and Lindsey D. Goodman contributed equally to this work.
[1]Department of Stem Cell and Regenerative Biology, Harvard University, Cambridge, MA 02138, USA
[2]Harvard Stem Cell Institute, Harvard University, Cambridge, MA 02138, USA
Full list of author information is available at the end of the article

reduced abundance of *C9ORF72* transcripts, suggesting that a loss-of-function mechanism may contribute to disease [14]. Although complete loss of C9ORF72 in mice leads to fatal autoimmunity and changes in microglia, no obvious signs of neurodegeneration or neural dysfunction have yet been reported in these animals [8, 23, 39]. Second, mutant transcripts containing the *GGGGCC* repeats form intranuclear RNA foci that may sequester RNA binding proteins and lead to nucleolar stress [14, 20]. Finally, dipeptide repeat proteins (DPRs) were unexpectedly found to be translated from both sense and antisense transcripts containing these repeats [34]. Several DPRs are toxic when overexpressed in model systems [11, 26, 33, 55], and have been shown to affect diverse cellular pathways, including RNA processing and nucleocytoplasmic transport [51, 52, 56].

The transcriptional response that occurs in various brain regions in ALS and FTLD patients has the potential to provide useful insights into whether genetic subgroups of patients display common or divergent mechanisms, and for validating proposed mechanisms through which mutations act. Here, we explored RNA-sequencing data from *C9ORF72* and sporadic patients, and identified distinct transcriptional responses in these two patient classes. We validate a *C9ORF72*-specific transcriptional signature in a large patient cohort. Additionally, we find that similar transcriptional changes occur in human neurons treated with DPRs and in gain-of-function *Drosophila* models.

Methods

Bioinformatics

The processed gene expression count matrix of the brain-derived RNA-seq datasets from Prudencio et al. were obtained via GEO (GSE67196). The data was analyzed using the R library "edgeR" as described by Prudencio et al., with modifications as follows [41, 47]. Statistical inference was performed with two methods which we refer to as "double cut-off" and "FDR". For the "double cut-off" method, as described by Prudencio et al., differentially expressed genes called by this approach had to pass two filters: one cut-off of absolute log2fold change > 2 and a second cut-off of unadjusted p-value < 0.05. For the "FDR" method, the false discovery rate was controlled using the Benjamini-Hochberg method [44] and all genes below a threshold FDR of 0.05 were considered to be significantly differentially expressed. Additionally, a generalized linear model (glmFit() in edgeR) was used to model the effect of gender rather than the exactTest() function, which resulted in slight differences in the number of differentially expressed genes found using the double cut-off method when compared to the original published analysis. Hypergeometric tests were used to compare sets of genes. Note that a pseudocount of 0.01 was used for plotting log2(CPM).

Protein-protein interaction networks were generated using GeNets hosted at the Broad Institute (apps.broadinstitute.org/genets) based on the InWeb network [28]. Associated gene ontology (GO) terms for biological process based on the GO Consortium were obtained with multiple testing correction for p-values using g:Profiler [43]. GO term clustering was performed with Revigo (reduce and visualize gene ontology, http://revigo.irb.hr/) [50] to support the identification of representative biological processes terms.

Brain samples

Protocols were approved by the Mayo Clinic IRB and Ethics Committee on Human Experimentation. Informed consent for post-mortem tissue was obtained from all individuals or the appropriate next-of-kin. The diagnosis of ALS and/or FTLD was based on neurological and pathological examination and *C9ORF72* repeat expansion status was determined using repeat-primed PCR and the cohort was described in Prudencio et al., including TDP-43 pathology [42]. See Additional file 1: Table S1 for patient characteristics. For transcript measurements by quantitative RT-PCR on human brains, total RNA was extracted and 500 ng of RNA with RNA integrity values (RIN) higher than 7, measured by an Agilent Bioanalyzer, and was used for reverse transcription to synthesize cDNA as previously described [41]. Using a SYBR green assay (Life Technologies) samples were run in triplicate on an ABI Prism 7900HT Real-Time PCR System (Applied Biosystems). Relative mRNA expression of examined genes was normalized to GAPDH and RPLP0 values, the endogenous transcript controls. Primer sequences are provided in Additional file 2: Table S2. Statistical differences were calculated by one-way ANOVA followed by Dunn's multiple comparison tests using GraphPad Prism. Associations between HSF1 and heat shock related transcripts were evaluated using a Spearman's test of correlation.

Neuron production and cell culture experiments

Neurons were generated from HuES-3-Hb9:GFP based on the following neuron differentiation protocol [6]. Human embryonic stem cells were cultured in mTeSR (Stemcell technologies) on matrigel (Corning)-coated plates. For motor neuron differentiation, the media was changed to 1:1 Neurobasal:DMEM/F12 (Life Technologies) supplemented with N2 (StemCell Technologies), B27 (Life technologies), Glutamax (Life Technologies), non-essential amino acids (Life technologies). For the first week, this neural media was supplemented with retinoic acid (Sigma Aldrich, 1 μM), smoothened agonist (SAG, DNSK, 1 μM), BMP inhibitor (LDN-193189,

DNSK, 100 nM) and TGF-beta inhibitor (SB431542, DNSK, 10 μM). Then, for the second week, this neural media was supplemented with retinoic acid, smoothened agonist, GSK3-beta inhibitor (SU-5402, DNSK, 4 μM), and gamma-secretase inhibitor (DAPT, DNSK, 5uM). Upon completion of the differentiation protocol, cells were dissociated with accutase (Innovative Cell Technologies) to single cells and sorted via flow-cytometry for GFP-positive cells to yield GFP-positive neurons, which were plated on poly-D-lysine(Sigma Aldrich)/laminin(Life Technologies)-coated plates. Neurons were maintained in Neurobasal medium supplemented with N2, B27, Glutamax, non-essential amino acids, and neurotrophic factors (BDNF, GDNF, CNTF), and allowed to mature for two weeks before experiments with dipeptide repeat proteins (DPRs). Recombinant biotin-tagged DPRs, (each 20 amino acids in length (poly-GA, poly-GP, or poly-GR with 10 repeats or scrambled control poly-GAPR with 5 repeats) were synthesize by Anaspec with > 95% purity and dissolved in DMSO (Sigma). Following DPR treatment, RNA was extracted after 24 h via an RNeasy Minikit (Qiagen), and cDNA prepared with iScript (Bio-Rad). qRT-PCR reactions were performed with iTaq SYBR green (Bio-Rad) on a C1000 touch thermal cycler with CFX real-time system (Bio-rad). Relative expression was normalized to GAPDH. Primers were designed from the MGH PrimerBank and synthesized by IDT. Primer sequences are provided in Additional file 2: Table S2. Viability was measured with CellTiter-Glo (Promega) on a Cytation3 reader (Biotek). All cell lines tested negative for mycoplasma using the MycoAlert detection kit (Lonza LT07–518).

Drosophila lines

Animals were raised and maintained at 18 °C on standard cornmeal-molasses food. The UAS-(G4C2)n transgenic models [9, 25], UAS-(GR)36 model [33], and the HSF overexpression (OE) mutant, HSF[+t8] [22], are previously defined. UAS-(GR)36, control, and mutant HSF[+t8] were obtained from Bloomington Drosophila Stock Center.

qPCR in the adult fly nervous system

UAS-(G4C2)n or UAS-(GR)36 transgenes were driven by elavGS, a drug-inducible Gal4 driver that expresses only in neurons. Crosses were setup and maintained at 24 °C. Female progeny with the desired genotype were collected and matured to 1-3d before being transferred to vials containing 40μg/ml of RU486. Animals were aged on RU486-infused food 16d while being flipped onto fresh drug-infused food every 2-days. Total RNA was collected from heads of frozen animals using Trizol, converted to cDNA using random primers, and analyzed by qPCR using SYBR Green. All primers were previously developed with the exception of dHSF1, dHSP70, dBAG3, dStip1, dFkbp4 (Fkbp59), and dChordc1 [5, 12]. Data was normalized to the housekeeping gene, RP49 [17]. Primer sequences are provided in Additional file 2: Table S2. Full genotypes for (G4C2)n are as follows: w1118/yw;; UAS-(G4C2)n, elavGS/+. (GR)36 animals, w1118/yw; UAS-(GR)36/+; elavGS/+, were compared to controls, w1118/yw;;. For analysis of HSF mutant expression, briefly, male HSF OE mutant flies were crossed to w1118 virgin females and maintained at 24 °C. Male progeny were collected and aged to 5d before analysis. Full genotype: w1118;; HSF[+t8]/+. Control w1118 males were maintained and aged in parallel.

External eye analysis

Scoring of the external eye phenotype for (G4C2)49 was done using a 0–8 scale previously defined where 0 = WT eye and 8 = lethality (extreme toxicity) [25]. (G4C2)49 expression causes an average degenerative score of 4–5 across multiple studies. Scoring of the external eye phenotype for (GR)36 was done using a 0–11 scale where 0 = WT eye and 11 = lethality (extreme toxicity) (Additional file 3: Figure S5). (GR)36 expression causes an average degenerative score of 5–6 across multiple studies.

For optimal eye phenotypes, crosses for (G4C2)n were setup and maintained at 24 °C and (GR)36 at 21 °C. Male progeny with the desired genotype were collected daily and matured to 1-2d before imaging on a Leica Apo16 microscope. Severity of the external eye phenotype was determined post-imaging while looking for changes in red pigmentation, ommatidial organization, and eye size. Full genotypes for (G4C2)n are as follows: "Control" = w1118;; UAS-(G4C2)n, Gmr-Gal4/+ and "HSF OE" = w1118;; UAS-(G4C2)n, Gmr-Gal4/HSF[+t8]. Full genotypes for (GR)36 are as follows: "Control" = w1118; UAS-(GR)36/+; Gmr-Gal4/+ and "HSF OE" = w1118; UAS-(GR)36/+; Gmr-Gal4/HSF[+t8].

Drosophila beta-galactosidase western blots

Western blots are as previously described [25].

Results

Identification of a *C9ORF72*-associated transcriptional signature in patient brain samples

There remains much to be learned concerning the mechanisms by which the repeat expansion in *C9ORF72* contributes to ALS and FTLD. Recently, RNA-sequencing datasets were generated from the frontal cortex as well as the cerebellum of sporadic ALS cases, *C9ORF72*-ALS cases and controls [41]. In Prudencio et al., a "double-cutoff method" was used for identifying genes whose expression was significantly changed in each class of ALS patient relative to controls (methods). Although such methods are useful for identifying changes in gene expression, they tend to be more sensitive to large fold-changes in less abundant transcripts, while modest fold-changes in abundant transcripts may go undetected (Additional file 4: Figure S1) [3, 29]. We reasoned that further analyses of these data might provide new insights into the disease mechanisms acting in *C9ORF72* and sporadic patients, respectively. Utilizing a false discovery rate (FDR) threshold of 5%, we sought to identify changes in abundantly-expressed transcripts and found 56 transcripts that were differentially expressed between *C9ORF72*-ALS cortex and controls at this confidence interval (Additional file 4: Figure S1, methods). Comparison of sporadic ALS patient and control cortex with these same metrics identified 65 differentially expressed transcripts, most (61) of which were downregulated. Consistent with the previous report that sporadic and *C9ORF72* ALS patients display distinct transcriptional signatures relative to controls, we found no overlap in the identity of transcripts that we identified as differentially expressed in the cortex of sporadic ALS and *C9ORF72* ALS patient classes (Fig. 1b) [41]. However, the majority of the genes we had found as likely to be differentially expressed in sporadic and *C9ORF72*-ALS patients had not been previously identified [41], validating the importance of reanalyzing these sequencing data using the methods we employed (Additional file 5: Table S3, Additional file 4: Figure S1, see Methods).

In *C9ORF72*-ALS, the cortex is characterized by distinct p62-positive DPR neuronal inclusions and the cerebellum contains abundant DPR inclusions [1, 30, 34, 41]. Hence, we reasoned that identifying transcripts with expression changes shared in both the frontal cortex and the cerebellum might lead us to genes and pathways that were reproducibly induced by the *C9ORF72* repeat expansion. Strikingly, 27 of the 56 transcripts differentially expressed in the *C9ORF72*-ALS cortex were also significantly changed in the *C9ORF72*-ALS cerebellum ($p = 2.93*10^{-40}$; Fig. 1c). Comparison of the fold expression changes in these 27 transcripts between these two regions in *C9ORF72*-ALS brains revealed a strong positive correlation ($R^2 = 0.88$). Notably, we identified increased abundance for 26 of these 27 transcripts in both brain regions relative to controls (Fig. 1d). The one exception was the *C9ORF72* transcript itself which showed reduced abundance (57% cortex, FDR = 0.0169; 42% cerebellum, FDR = $2.75*10^{-5}$), in agreement with previous studies of patient brains [14, 52, 53]. In contrast to a

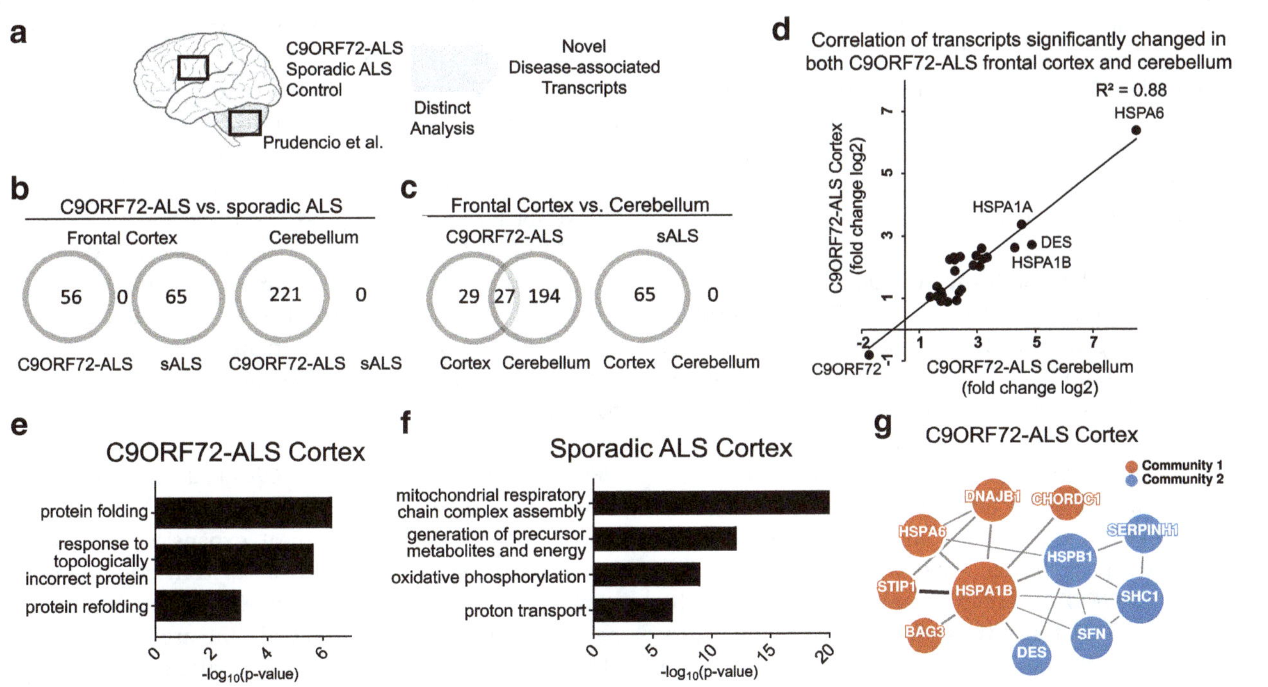

Fig. 1 Identification of specific cellular pathways perturbed in sporadic ALS and C9ORF72-ALS **a** Diagram of RNA-seq datasets obtained from the frontal cortex and cerebellum by Prudencio et al. **b** Comparison of the significant (FDR < 0.05) differentially expressed transcripts in C9ORF72-ALS (C9-ALS) and sporadic ALS (sALS). Note, there were no common transcripts between C9ORF72-ALS and sporadic ALS in either brain region. **c** Comparison of the differentially expressed transcripts by brain region. **d** Correlation of the fold change (log2) of changed transcripts in C9ORF72-ALS that were common to both brain regions (Spearman's R^2) **e**, **f** Gene ontology (GO) analysis revealed cellular processes affected in C9ORF72-ALS and sALS. **g** Protein-protein interaction analysis of proteins encoded by the transcripts changed in C9ORF72-ALS revealed a protein chaperone network

prior analysis, we detected no significant transcriptional changes between the cerebellum of sporadic ALS cases and controls (Fig. 1b), consistent with this region being histologically unremarkable in sporadic cases [2].

To determine if the transcripts significantly changed in *C9ORF72* and sporadic ALS cortex pointed to particular pathways that might be responding to disease processes, we carried out gene ontology (GO) analysis. Transcripts identified in *C9ORF72*-ALS were significantly associated with response to topologically incorrect proteins ($p = 2.13*10^{-6}$) and protein folding ($p = 4.57*10^{-7}$) (Fig. 1e). In contrast, differentially expressed transcripts detected in sporadic ALS were associated with functions in the mitochondrial respiratory chain complex assembly ($p = 8.53*10^{-21}$) and related terms (Fig. 1f), and included 9 members of the NADH dehydrogenase (complex I) enzyme and 6 components of cytochrome oxidase C (complex IV) (Additional file 6: Figure S2A). These findings suggest that the transcriptional responses in the *C9ORF72* and sporadic ALS cortex might be reflective of changes in protein and mitochondrial homeostasis, respectively. We also asked whether any of the *C9ORF72*-associated transcripts encoded proteins that interact in particular complexes. Using the InWeb protein-protein interaction network [28], analysis of the 56 differentially expressed transcripts from *C9ORF72* cortex identified an interaction network involving heat shock proteins (HSPs) and protein chaperones, with HSPA1B (HSP70) and HSPB1 (HSP27) at its hubs (Fig. 1g). Examination of protein interactions from the 221 transcripts differentially expressed in the *C9ORF72* cerebellum revealed a similar and expanded network of more than 80 interactors that was centered on the same core HSPs (Additional file 6: Figure S2B).

Activation of the HSF1 pathway in *C9ORF72*-ALS/FTLD

A well-established regulator of HSP and protein chaperone expression is the transcription factor heat shock factor 1 (HSF1) [57]. Hence, we wondered if the transcriptional response we observed in the *C9ORF72* brain might be at least in part mediated by activation of HSF1. To explore this possibility, we turned our attention to established HSF1 target genes previously identified by ChIP-seq and genome-wide methods [31, 32, 49]. Consistent with the notion that a portion of the response in *C9ORF72* patient brain was mediated by HSF1, 13 of the 27 transcripts identified as significantly changed in both the cerebellum and frontal cortex were among 812 genes bound by HSF1 after heat shock treatment across three human cell lines ($p = 1.22*10^{-12}$) [32], including several HSPs shown to be upregulated in the initial small *C9ORF72*-ALS cohort [41].

As a next step towards investigating whether activation of the HSF1 might be responsible for the induction of these genes in *C9ORF72* patients, we used quantitative RT-PCR to measure the transcript abundance of *HSF1* and 11 of these conserved HSP-associated transcripts in a much larger patient cohort that also included patients diagnosed with FTLD and both ALS and FTLD ($n = 56$ *C9ORF72*-ALS/FTLD, $n = 46$ sporadic ALS/FTLD, $n = 8$ controls). In the frontal cortex, expression of each of these 11 HSF1 target genes was significantly increased in the *C9ORF72*-ALS/FTLD cohort relative to controls ($p < 0.05$ or lower for each gene) and to sporadic cases ($p < 0.01$ or lower) (Fig. 2a, Additional file 7: Table S4). Next, we extended our expression analyses of these 11 HSF1 targets to the cerebellum, and again found that the abundance of each transcript gene was significantly elevated in *C9ORF72*-ALS/FTLD relative to both controls and sporadic ALS cases (Additional file 8: Figure S3A, Additional file 7: Table S4). For example, we found a significant, two orders of magnitude induction of the HSP70 transcript *HSPA1B* in *C9ORF72*-ALS/FTLD cases relative to controls. To investigate if the larger number of genes initially detected only in the *C9ORF72* cerebellum might also be reflective of a heat shock response, we examined another HSF1 target gene *CRYAB* and found it was significantly upregulated in both *C9ORF72* brain regions in this larger patient cohort (Fig. 2a, Additional file 8: Figure S3A).

Evaluation of *HSF1* expression in these same samples demonstrated that it was significantly more abundant in both the cortex and cerebellum relative to sporadic ALS cases ($P < 0.05$) (Fig. 2b). We found a strong and consistent correlation between the levels of *HSF1* and each of these *C9ORF72*-chaperome transcripts in both brain regions ($p < 0.0001$ for each gene, Additional file 8: Figure S3B). For instance, the relationship between the transcript levels of *HSF1* and *HSPB1* yielded an R^2 value of 0.73 (95% CI 0.63–0.81) in the cortex and 0.65 (95% CI 0.52–0.75) in the cerebellum. Taken together, these findings indicate that HSF1 is activated in *C9ORF72*-ALS and FTLD patient brains and suggests that it is regulating the expression of the HSPs we found to be induced there.

DPRs are sufficient to induce a *C9ORF72*-associated transcriptional changes

The *C9ORF72 GGGGCC* repeat expansion is translated from both sense and anti-sense transcripts through non-ATG translation to generate 5 distinct dipeptide repeat proteins (DPRs), e.g. poly-glycine-arginine (poly-GR) [18, 34, 52]. We wondered if DPRs alone were sufficient to induce the upregulation of C9ORF72 signature transcripts. Therefore, we tested the effects of synthetic DPRs in human stem cell-derived neurons [26]. GP_{10}, GA_{10} and a scrambled $GAPR_5$ control were not acutely toxic to the parental human stem cell line or stem-cell derived neurons. In contrast poly-GR_{10} resulted in a dose-dependent decrease in the viability of stem cell-derived neurons, but

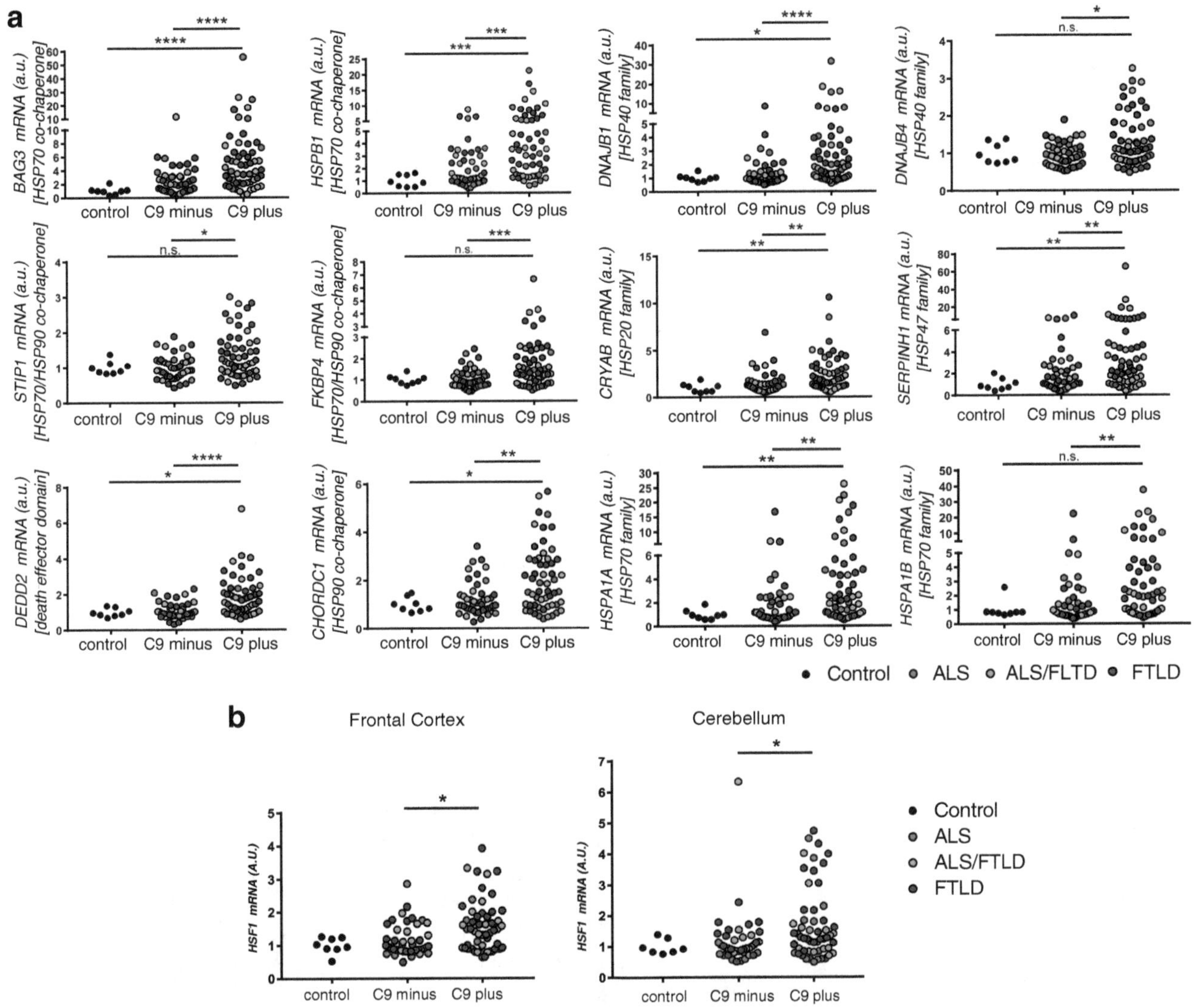

Fig. 2 Activation of HSF1 in C9ORF72-ALS, FTLD, and combined ALS/FTLD patients. **a** Quantitative real-time PCR (qRT-PCR) for HSF1 target genes in the frontal cortex of sporadic and C9ORF72-associated disease ($n = 56$ C9ORF72-ALS/FTLD, $n = 46$ sporadic ALS/FTLD, $n = 9$ controls) (one-way ANOVA with Bonferonni post-hoc test for multiple comparisons, *$p < 0.05$, **$p < 0.01$, ***$p < 0.001$). No significant changes were detected between the sporadic cases and controls (mean values for each gene are provided in Additional file: 3 Table S3). **b** qRT-PCR for HSF1 in the frontal cortex and cerebellum of these same cases

not the stem cell from which they were produced (Fig. 3b). In human neurons, we found that both poly-GA and poly-GR led to the significant upregulation of *HSPA1B* ($p < 0.01$), as well as additional C9ORF72 signature transcripts (Fig. 3c). Given that poly-GA is not associated with decreased viability in these conditions, this suggests that the observed transcriptional changes are not simply a consequence of general neuronal toxicity. There was a strong correlation ($R^2 = 0.58$) between the degree of induction of these transcripts in human neurons by poly-GR and the changes present specifically in *C9ORF72* brains. Upon measuring *HSF1*, there was a trend for increased levels with poly-GA and poly-GP, and the greatest increase was again observed with poly-GR (Fig. 3d). These findings support the notion that gain-of-function effects from DPRs are sufficient to induce HSF1 target genes that are upregulated in *C9ORF72*-associated disease.

Detection of *C9ORF72*-associated transcriptional changes in gain-of-function *Drosophila* models

To test for correlations in DPR production and altered HSF1 target gene expression in vivo, we evaluated a *Drosophila* gain-of-function transgenic model engineered to express 49 pure *GGGGCC* repeats driven by a drug-inducible neuronal-specific *ElavGS-GAL4* driver [25, 33]. Fly models expressing toxic GGGGCC repeats produce DPRs and RNA foci [16, 33, 54]. We found

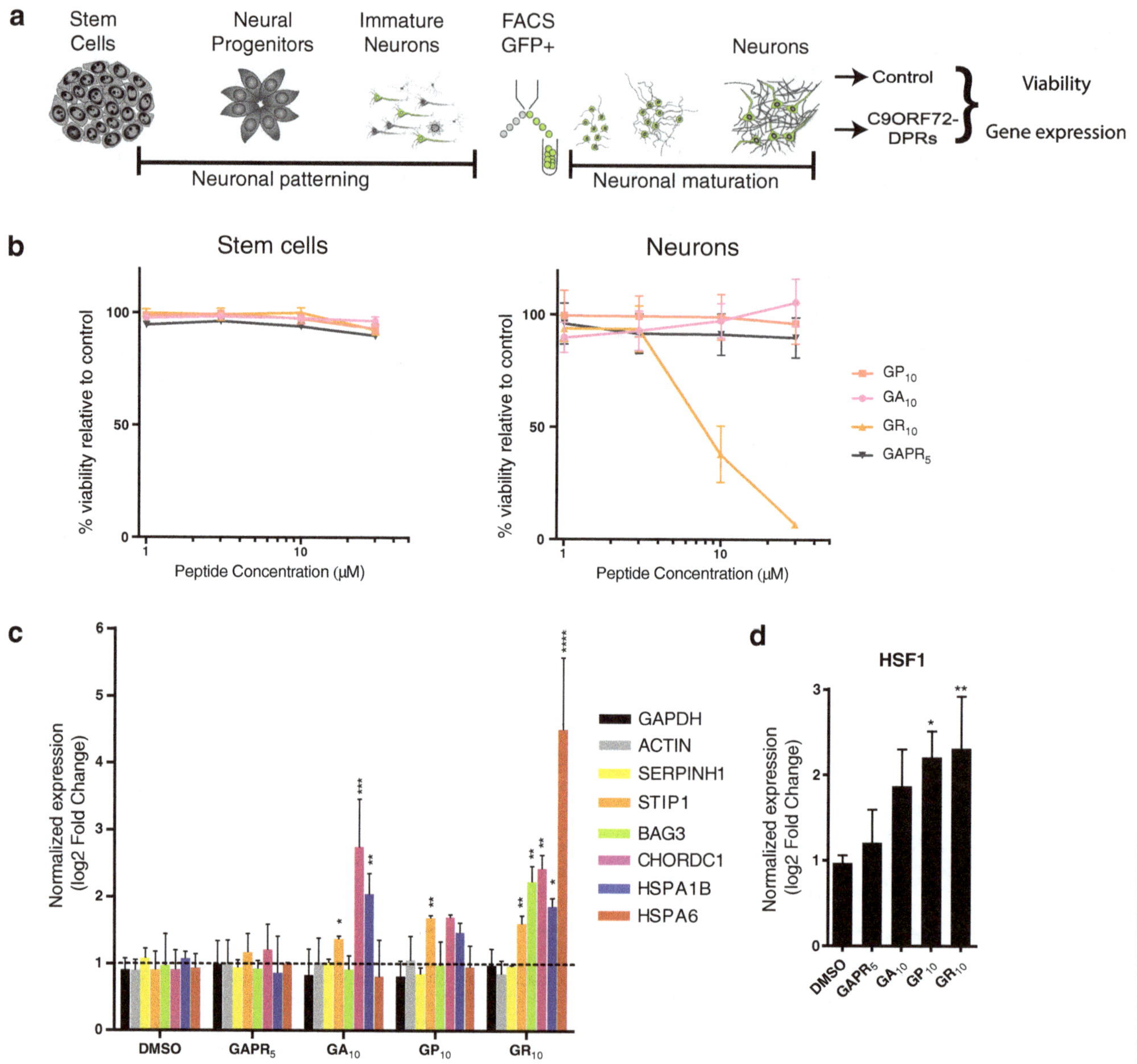

Fig. 3 DPRs induce expression of C9ORF72 signature transcripts in human neurons. **a** Diagram of generation of human neurons from stem cells. **b** Viability dose response curve of human stem cells and stem-cell derived neurons exposed to various DPRs ($n = 6$). **c, d** qRT-PCR of C9ORF72-chaperome transcripts (**c**) and HSF1 (**d**) in human stem cell-derived motor neurons following treatment with DPRs (poly-GA, poly-GP, poly-GR) or a scrambled poly-GAPR (5 uM for 24 h) normalized to control (DMSO-treated) neurons (mean ± SD, $n = 3$, one-way ANOVA with Dunnett's post-hoc test for upregulated genes in DPR-treated neurons compared to control, * $p < 0.05$, ** $p < 0.01$, *** $p < 0.001$, **** $p < 0.0001$)

significant increased expression of the *Drosophila* orthologs of conserved *C9ORF72*-associated HSPs and protein chaperones in flies expressing 49 repeats in neurons compared to controls (Fig. 4a). Upregulation of HSF1-associated genes was observed in the absence of significant animal death, arguing that the effect is specific to expression of $(GGGGCC)_{49}$. Note that these expression changes are likely to be an underestimation of the actual changes caused by the repeats in vivo since $(GGGGCC)_{49}$ was only expressed in neurons while gene expression changes were assayed using whole heads, including non-neuronal tissue. Additionally, we detected an increase in HSF1 expression similar to that observed in *C9ORF72* patient brains (Fig. 4a). This demonstrates that at least part of the transcriptional response to the *C9ORF72* repeat expansion is conserved in *Drosophila*, and is consistent with gain-of-function effects of the *C9ORF72* repeat expansion driving the expression of HSF1 target genes.

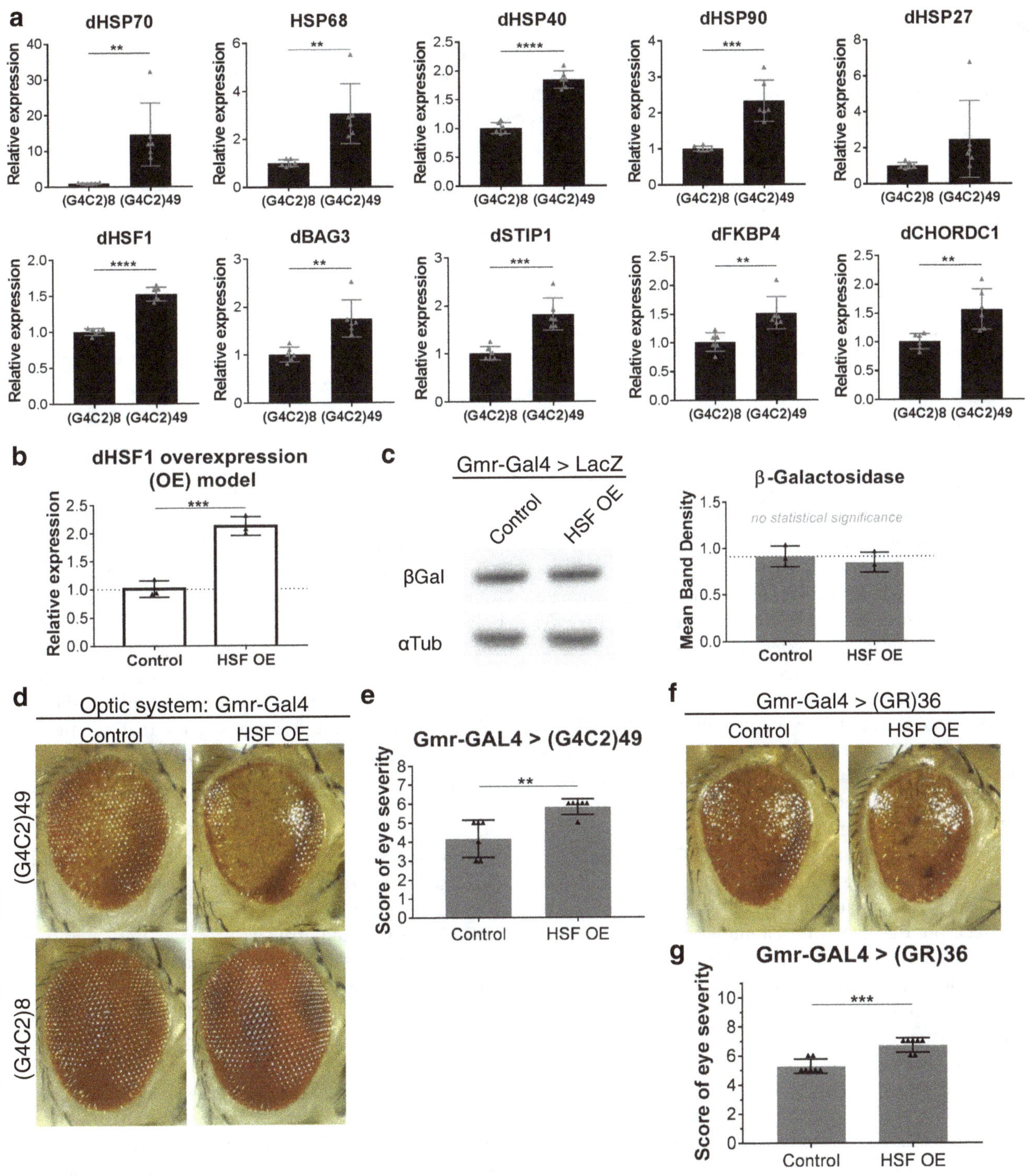

Fig. 4 (See legend on next page.)

(See figure on previous page.)

Fig. 4 a Control UAS-(G4C2)8 and expanded UAS-(G4C2)49 transgenes were expressed in the adult fly nervous system using the drug-inducible Gal4 driver, elavGS, for 16d. Quantitative PCR (qPCR) analysis of endogenous dHSF1 and HSF1-regulated genes revealed significant upregulation with (G4C2)49 expression compared to (G4C2)8 controls. Differences in expression are likely underestimated as the analyses include neuronal and non-neuronal tissue while (G4C2)n was expressed only in neurons. **b** qPCR analysis of a dHSF1 overexpression mutant fly line shows endogenous HSF is upregulated approximately 2-fold in mutant flies compared to control. **c** Western immunoblot analysis of expression of a control UAS-LacZ transgene confirmed that the HSF OE mutant did not affect the Gal4/UAS expression system. **d** (G4C2)49 was expressed in the optic system of control animals or HSF OE animals using Gmr-Gal4. (G4C2)49 causes toxicity seen by pigment loss, reduced eye size, and disruptions in the normal ommatidial organization. In HSF OE animals, toxicity of (G4C2)49 is enhanced – animals have increased pigment loss, increased disruption of ommatidial organization, and further reduced eye size. Expression of control (G4C2)8 in the fly optic system (Gmr-Gal4) of control and HSF OE animals does not affect the external eye. **e** Quantification of the external eye degenerative phenotype caused by (G4C2)49 expression shows enhancement in HSF OE animals versus control animals to be consistent and statistically significant ($n = 6$). Animals received a score between 0 (WT eye) and 8 (lethality caused by extreme degeneration in the optic system). (G4C2)49 expression causes an average score of 4 in controls. **f** Gmr-GAL4 driven expression of (GR)36 shows toxicity in control scenarios like (G4C2)49. HSF OE in these animals also causes enhanced toxicity (increased pigment loss, increased disruption of ommatidial organization, and reduced eye size) **g** Quantification of the external eye degenerative phenotype caused by (GR)36 expression shows enhancement in HSF OE animals versus control animals to be consistent and statistically significant ($n = 7$). Animals received a score between 0 (WT eye) and 11 (lethality caused by extreme degeneration in the optic system) while (GR)36 causes an average score of 5 in controls. (All plots: mean +/− SD, unpaired, student's t-test, *$p < 0.05$, **$p < 0.01$, ***$p < 0.001$, ****$p < 0.0001$)

Activation of the HSF1 pathway has been proposed to be protective in several neurodegenerative diseases associated with protein aggregation as a means to combat the cellular effects of toxic proteins [35]. Given that we observed an HSF1 heat shock response in *C9ORF72* patients and model systems, we wondered whether HSF1 may be a potential modifier of *C9ORF72* gain-of-function toxicity. To investigate this idea, we selected a fly line harboring an additional allele of the *Drosophila HSF1* ortholog (*dHSF*1) [22]. We confirmed increased *dHSF1* expression in this line and noted that it was comparable to the relative increase in *dHSF1* expression observed in response to the *GGGGCC* repeat expansion (Fig. 4b). The presence of additional *dHSF1* did not affect the expression of a control *LacZ* transgene (Fig. 4c). We next asked if this increase in *dHSF1* would have an effect on *GGGGCC*-mediated toxicity and used the *Gmr-Gal4* driver to specifically express the repeats in the fly optic system to assess the effect on the eye. Consistent with prior observations, $GGGGCC_{49}$ expression in the eye during development led to generation of animals with eye degeneration and disruption of the highly regular ommatidial structure, reduced eye size, and loss of pigment (Fig. 4d) [25, 33]. *dHSF1* upregulation by itself did not affect eye structure in the presence of a control $GGGGCC_8$ (Fig. 4d). Surprisingly, we found that $GGGGCC_{49}$-induced toxicity in the external eye was enhanced in the presence of *dHSF1* overexpression (Fig. 4d, e).

Among the repeat expansion encoded DPRs, arginine-rich DPRs are particularly toxic in model systems, including *Drosophila* [33]. Given that the expression of $GGGGCC_{49}$ is associated with the production of both DPRs and potentially toxic RNA, we assayed the transcriptional effects of poly-GR in vivo. There was significant upregulation of *dHSF1* and many HSF1-regulated transcripts in *Drosophila* expressing a poly-GR_{100} transgene in neurons compared to non-transgenic controls (Additional file 9: Figure S4). We additionally tested the effects of modulating *dHSF1* levels in the optic system of poly-GR *Drosophila* again using *Gmr-GAL4* to drive transgene expression. We observed exacerbation of poly-GR_{36} external eye toxicity in the presence of *dHSF1* upregulation (Fig. 4h, j). These results argue that the changes in toxicity caused by added *dHSF1* in the $GGGGCC_{49}$ model is in part due to the effects of GR-dipeptide. Taken together, these findings suggest that augmentation of HSF1 activity may enhance DPR-mediated toxicity in *Drosophila*.

Discussion

In this study, we have identified novel differentially expressed transcripts in *C9ORF72*-ALS based on analysis of two brain regions compared to controls. Every *C9ORF72*-associated transcript was not significantly altered in sporadic ALS, suggesting that the observed changes in this set of transcripts are not just an indicator of neuronal loss but rather reflective of *C9ORF72*-specific pathogenesis. Furthermore, we validated our *C9ORF72* transcriptional signature in a large ALS/FTLD patient cohort and gain-of-function models.

Our findings specifically link activation of the HSF1 pathway to *C9ORF72*-ALS/FTLD. The HSF1 pathway is highly conserved from budding yeast to mammals and is an important mediator of the compensatory response to disruptions in proteostasis, such as heat shock [49]. Impairment of HSF1 activity and loss of protein chaperone function have been reported to occur with ageing and in the setting of age-related neurodegeneration [7, 21, 35]. For instance, in models of poly-glutamine repeat-associated Huntington disease decreased expression of HSF1 target genes is observed and may contribute to protein aggregation [10]. Likewise, decreased expression of a particular set of protein chaperones, including HSP90, occurs in Alzheimer disease and Parkinson disease [7]. In *C9ORF72*-ALS/FTLD, we found robust increased expression of a family of protein chaperones and co-chaperones, consistent with activation of a heat shock response in this particular disease. Our study may provide the first evidence of increased, rather than impaired, activity of HSF1 based on human brain samples for a specific neurodegenerative disease. In addition, HSF1 is generally not thought to be regulated at the transcriptional level in the context of neurodegeneration. We found upregulation of HSF1 itself in *C9ORF72*-ALS/FTLD and a strong correlation between levels of HSF1 and its target genes. It will be important to examine transcriptional changes in HSF1 in post-mortem brain samples of additional neurodegenerative diseases.

Prior studies in model systems have suggested that HSF1 is a protective factor that helps neurons cope with cellular stress associated with misfolded proteins and protein aggregates [19]. Unexpectedly, we observed that having additional HSF1 in the developing eye in two *Drosophila* models of *C9ORF72*-ALS/FTLD was not beneficial. Additional studies in these *Drosophila* models that characterize the functional consequences of the loss of individual HSF1-associated protein chaperones and HSPs may be useful to further dissect the relationship between this pathway and *C9ORF72*-related pathology. Pharmacological activation of HSF1 has been proposed as a therapeutic strategy to enhance protein chaperone function and neuronal survival in neurodegenerative disease [36]. For instance, arimoclomol, which may act to enhance HSF1-pathway activation, has been shown to delay disease progression in an SOD1 overexpression mouse model [24]. A phase II clinical trial for arimoclomol was recently conducted for a subtype of familial ALS associated with mutations in SOD1 and was found to be well-tolerated [4]. Our findings suggest that additional pre-clinical studies may be warranted if this strategy is applied to other forms of ALS, especially the most common type of ALS, *C9ORF72*-ALS, and associated dementias. Additionally, the transcriptional differences present among distinct cohorts of ALS/FTLD patients re-emphasizes the potential importance of patient stratification by genotype for future clinical trials.

Several studies have aimed to identify the specific transcriptional changes and pathways affected by the *C9ORF72* repeat expansion in patient-based cellular models, including iPSC-derived neurons, with little concordance among them [13, 15, 27, 48]. Gene expression changes have also been explored in a few animal models for this disease. In a loss-of-function mouse model lacking both copies of *C9ORF72*, transcriptional analysis of the spinal cord from *C9ORF72–/–* animals revealed significant changes in several pathways related to inflammation [39]. On the other hand, gain-of-function bacterial artificial chromosome (BAC) transgenic mouse models harboring the human *C9ORF72* repeat expansion have been generated with varying phenotypes and transcriptional changes. In one model containing exons 1–6 of human *C9ORF72* with approximately 500 hexanucleotide repeats, no significant changes in the transcriptome of the frontal cortex at 6 months of age were reported [40]. In another BAC mouse model with 100–1000 repeats, immunomodulatory and extracellular matrix pathways were identified as being altered in the frontal cortex also at 6 months of age [38]. Although both of these BAC mouse models exhibit DPR inclusions in the nervous system that increase with age, evidence of neurodegeneration was not observed. One possibility is that DPRs did not reach sufficient levels in these models at the examined time points to induce neurodegeneration or the transcriptional changes described herein. Indeed, robust expression of DPRs using an adeno-associated viral vector with 66 repeats was sufficient to induce DPR aggregates, TDP-43-positive inclusions, neuronal loss, and behavioral deficits in mice [11]. However, gene expression studies have not yet been performed in this viral mouse model.

Using two gain-of-function *Drosophila* models, we found upregulation of many *Drosophila* orthologs of the same genes that were upregulated in *C9ORF72* patient brains. This is consistent with the notion that more potent expression of DPRs in models is essential to recapitulate *C9ORF72* transcriptional changes and disease phenotypes. Our approach and findings starting with unbiased transcriptional analysis of patient samples may be useful for the characterization and assessment of existing and new models employed to study *C9ORF72* disease.

Based on our findings, we propose the following model. The presence of the *C9ORF72* repeat expansions results in the production of various toxic DPRs. In early life, neurons can degrade DPRs or perhaps sequester them into protective p62-positive inclusions. With aging, there is a decreased capacity of neurons to maintain proteostasis, and environmental insults may be associated with additional proteotoxic stress. This leads to the gradual accumulation of DPRs and the activation of a heat shock response to increase protein chaperones, perhaps in an attempt to refold inherently unstructured DPRs. However, increased HSF1 activity may actually contribute to DPR-dependent toxicity. One possibility is that the resulting increased levels of protein chaperones may promote the solubility or the stability of toxic DPRs. This model could partially explain the variable disease penetrance and expressivity by which the C9ORF72 repeat expansion acts to cause ALS and/or FTLD. It could be that natural human variation in the HSF1 response influences when and where the repeat expansion results in neurodegeneration.

Conclusions

In summary, we have identified specific gene expression changes in *C9ORF72* disease that are consistent with the activation of a HSF1-associated transcriptional response. We found that the expression levels of HSF1 and protein chaperones are increased in *C9ORF72*-ALS/FTLD patients and in gain-of-function model systems. Our results suggest that DPRs encoded by the *C9ORF72* hexanucleotide repeat expansion are sufficient to lead to the upregulation of HSF1 and its target genes. The effects of the HSF1 pathway on *C9ORF72* pathogenesis in models of disease that express DPRs warrants further investigation.

Additional files

Additional file 1: Table S1. Characteristics of patient cohort for brain samples used in qPCR analysis. (PDF 154 kb)

Additional file 2: Table S2. Primer sequences for PCR. (PDF 167 kb)

Additional file 3: Figure S5. External eye quantification scale for (GR)36 animals. For quantification of the enhancement effects of increased expression of HSF in the eye, (GR)36 animals received a score between 0 (normal eye) and 11 (extreme toxicity causing lethality). Across multiple studies control Gmr-GAL4 > (GR)36 animals receive a score between 5 and 6. (PDF 1969 kb)

Additional file 4: Figure S1. Bioinformatic method comparison for gene expression analysis of C9ORF72-associated ALS and sporadic ALS (sALS) in the frontal cortex and cerebellum. (a-d) Gene density plots comparing the expression levels of differentially expressed transcripts as determined by the prior double cut-off method ($|\log2 \text{ fold change}| \geq 2$ and *p*-value < 0.05) and the FDR method (FDR < 0.05), which was used in Fig. 1 and subsequent analysis. Note, no significant changes were detected in the sALS cerebellum using with FDR method. (e) Venn diagrams demonstrating considerable differences in the designated disease-associated transcripts between these bioinformatics methods in both brain regions. (f) Table of the number of differentially expressed transcripts as determined by Prudencio et al., the double cut-off method and the FDR method used here. (PDF 216 kb)

Additional file 5: Table S3. Genes significantly changes in RNA-seq analysis from ALS patients. (XLSX 52 kb)

Additional file 6: Figure S2. Gene networks in C9ORF72-ALS and sporadic ALS. (a) Protein-protein interaction network derived from differentially expressed transcripts in C9ORF72-ALS cerebellum. Those transcripts that are differentially expressed in both the frontal cortex and the cerebellum in C9ORF72-ALS are highlighted by dashed yellow circles, and predominantly consist of heat shock proteins and protein chaperones. (b) Protein-protein interaction network derived from differentially expressed transcripts in the sporadic ALS cortex. (PDF 164 kb)

Additional file 7: Table S4. Values from qPCR analysis in brain samples. (PDF 178 kb)

Additional file 8: Figure S3. Activation of HSF1 in C9ORF72-ALS, FTLD, and combined ALS/FTLD patients. (a) Quantitative real-time PCR (qRT-PCR) for HSF1 target genes in the cerebellum of sporadic and C9ORF72-associated disease ($n = 56$ *C9ORF72*-ALS/FTLD, $n = 42$ sporadic ALS/FTLD, $n = 7$ controls) (one-way ANOVA with Bonferonni *post-hoc* test for multiple comparisons * $p < 0.05$, ** $p < 0.01$, *** $p < 0.001$. Note, no significant changes were detected between the sporadic cases and controls. (b) Correlation of HSF1 levels and HSF1 target gene levels in the frontal cortex and cerebellum in C9ORF72-ALS/FTLD. Spearman's R^2 values are plotted for each target gene, error bars denote 95% confidence interval, *p*-value < 0.0001 in all cases. (PDF 209 kb)

Additional file 9: Figure S4. poly-GR expression results in the upregulation of heat shock response genes and dHSF1 in the adult fly nervous system. UAS-(GR)36 was expressed in the adult fly nervous system using the drug-inducible Gal4 driver, elavGS, for 16d. qPCR analysis of endogenous HSF1-regulated genes and dHSF1 revealed significant upregulation of the *Drosophila* orthologs of many of the genes identified in patient studies, suggesting that poly-GR is contributing to the altered transcriptome in C9ORF72-ALS/FTLD patients. Control animals did not express a transgene. Differences in expression are likely underestimated as the analyses include neuronal and non-neuronal tissue while (GR)36 was expressed only in neurons. ($n = 6$, mean +/− SD, unpaired, student's t-tests, *p-value* * < 0.05, ** < 0.01). (PDF 389 kb)

Acknowledgments

We are grateful to all patients who donated tissues. We thank members of the Eggan laboratory and Camille Sindu for helpful discussion and Kasper Lage's group for supporting GeNets. We thank Kiki Lilliehook for comments on the manuscript.

This work was supported by the NINDS R01NS089742 (K.E.), R35-NS097275 (N.B.), R21NS084528 (L.P.), R01NS088689 (L.P.), R01NS063964 (L.P.); R01NS077402 (L.P.); P01NS084974 (L.P.); R35NS097273 (L.P.), NCI 5T32CA009216-34 (D.A.M), NIA P50AG016574 (L.P.), NIEHS R01ES20395 (L.P.), Project ALS (K.E.), Mayo Clinic Foundation (L.P.) and Robert Packard Center for ALS Research at Johns Hopkins (L.P.), Target ALS (L.P. and K.E.), a pilot project from 5P50AG005134 (D.A.M.), and grants from the ALS Association to D.A.M., M.P., L.P., and K.E.

Authors' contributions

KE and DAM: study design; DAM, RM, OP: bioinformatics analysis; MP and LP: brain PCR; RR and DWD: procurement and characterization of brain tissue samples; LDG and NMB: Drosophila studies; JRK, FL, DAM, KC: cell line studies; KE: supervision of study. DAM and KE: drafting of manuscript. All authors read and approved the final manuscript.

Competing interests

The authors declare that they have no competing interests.

Author details

[1]Department of Stem Cell and Regenerative Biology, Harvard University, Cambridge, MA 02138, USA. [2]Harvard Stem Cell Institute, Harvard University, Cambridge, MA 02138, USA. [3]Stanley Center for Psychiatric Research, Broad Institute of MIT and Harvard, Cambridge, MA 02142, USA. [4]Department of Pathology, Massachusetts General Hospital, Boston, MA 02114, USA. [5]Department of Neuroscience, Mayo Clinic, Jacksonville, FL 32224, USA. [6]Department of Biology, University of Pennsylvania, Philadelphia, PA 19104, USA. [7]Present address: Pfizer, Cambridge, MA 02139, USA.

References

1. Agosta F, Ferraro PM, Riva N, Spinelli EG, Domi T, Carrera P, Copetti M, Falzone Y, Ferrari M, Lunetta C, Comi G, Falini A, Quattrini A, Filippi M (2017) Structural and functional brain signatures of C9orf72 in motor neuron disease. Neurobiol Aging. https://doi.org/10.1016/j.neurobiolaging.2017.05.024
2. Al-Sarraj S, King A, Troakes C, Smith B, Maekawa S, Bodi I, Rogelj B, Al-Chalabi A, Hortobagyi T, Shaw CE (2011) p62 positive, TDP-43 negative, neuronal cytoplasmic and intranuclear inclusions in the cerebellum and hippocampus define the pathology of C9orf72-linked FTLD and MND/ALS. Acta Neuropathol 122:691–702. https://doi.org/10.1007/s00401-011-0911-2
3. Anders S, Huber W (2010) Differential expression analysis for sequence count data. Genome Biol 11:R106. https://doi.org/10.1186/gb-2010-11-10-r106
4. Benatar M, Wuu J, Andersen PM, Atassi N, David W, Cudkowicz M, Schoenfeld D (2018) Randomized, double-blind, placebo-controlled trial of arimoclomol in rapidly progressive SOD1 ALS. Neurology 90:e565–e574. https://doi.org/10.1212/WNL.0000000000004960

5. Berson A, Sartoris A, Nativio R, Van Deerlin V, Toledo JB, Porta S, Liu S, Chung CY, Garcia BA, Lee VM, Trojanowski JQ, Johnson FB, Berger SL, Bonini NM (2017) TDP-43 promotes neurodegeneration by impairing chromatin remodeling. Curr Biol 27:3579–3590 e3576. doi:https://doi.org/10.1016/j.cub.2017.10.024
6. Boulting GL, Kiskinis E, Croft GF, Amoroso MW, Oakley DH, Wainger BJ, Williams DJ, Kahler DJ, Yamaki M, Davidow L, Rodolfa CT, Dimos JT, Mikkilineni S, MacDermott AB, Woolf CJ, Henderson CE, Wichterle H, Eggan K (2011) A functionally characterized test set of human induced pluripotent stem cells. Nat Biotechnol 29:279–286. https://doi.org/10.1038/nbt.1783
7. Brehme M, Voisine C, Rolland T, Wachi S, Soper JH, Zhu Y, Orton K, Villella A, Garza D, Vidal M, Ge H, Morimoto RI (2014) A chaperome subnetwork safeguards proteostasis in aging and neurodegenerative disease. Cell Rep 9: 1135–1150. https://doi.org/10.1016/j.celrep.2014.09.042
8. Burberry A, Suzuki N, Wang JY, Moccia R, Mordes DA, Stewart MH, Suzuki-Uematsu S, Ghosh S, Singh A, Merkle FT, Koszka K, Li QZ, Zon L, Rossi DJ, Trowbridge JJ, Notarangelo LD, Eggan K (2016) Loss-of-function mutations in the C9ORF72 mouse ortholog cause fatal autoimmune disease. Sci Transl Med 8:347ra393. https://doi.org/10.1126/scitranslmed.aaf6038
9. Burguete AS, Almeida S, Gao FB, Kalb R, Akins MR, Bonini NM (2015) GGGG CC microsatellite RNA is neuritically localized, induces branching defects, and perturbs transport granule function. Elife 4:e08881. https://doi.org/10.7554/eLife.08881
10. Chafekar SM, Duennwald ML (2012) Impaired heat shock response in cells expressing full-length polyglutamine-expanded huntingtin. PLoS One 7: e37929. https://doi.org/10.1371/journal.pone.0037929
11. Chew J, Gendron TF, Prudencio M, Sasaguri H, Zhang YJ, Castanedes-Casey M, Lee CW, Jansen-West K, Kurti A, Murray ME, Bieniek KF, Bauer PO, Whitelaw EC, Rousseau L, Stankowski JN, Stetler C, Daughrity LM, Perkerson EA, Desaro P, Johnston A, Overstreet K, Edbauer D, Rademakers R, Boylan KB, Dickson DW, Fryer JD, Petrucelli L (2015) Neurodegeneration. C9ORF72 repeat expansions in mice cause TDP-43 pathology, neuronal loss, and behavioral deficits. Science 348:1151–1154. https://doi.org/10.1126/science.aaa9344
12. Colinet H, Lee SF, Hoffmann A (2010) Temporal expression of heat shock genes during cold stress and recovery from chill coma in adult Drosophila melanogaster. FEBS J 277:174–185. https://doi.org/10.1111/j.1742-4658.2009.07470.x
13. Cooper-Knock J, Bury JJ, Heath PR, Wyles M, Higginbottom A, Gelsthorpe C, Highley JR, Hautbergue G, Rattray M, Kirby J, Shaw PJ (2015) C9ORF72 GGGGCC expanded repeats produce splicing dysregulation which correlates with disease severity in amyotrophic lateral sclerosis. PLoS One 10:e0127376. https://doi.org/10.1371/journal.pone.0127376
14. DeJesus-Hernandez M, Mackenzie IR, Boeve BF, Boxer AL, Baker M, Rutherford NJ, Nicholson AM, Finch NA, Flynn H, Adamson J, Kouri N, Wojtas A, Sengdy P, Hsiung GY, Karydas A, Seeley WW, Josephs KA, Coppola G, Geschwind DH, Wszolek ZK, Feldman H, Knopman DS, Petersen RC, Miller BL, Dickson DW, Boylan KB, Graff-Radford NR, Rademakers R (2011) Expanded GGGGCC hexanucleotide repeat in noncoding region of C9ORF72 causes chromosome 9p-linked FTD and ALS. Neuron 72:245–256. https://doi.org/10.1016/j.neuron.2011.09.011
15. Donnelly CJ, Zhang PW, Pham JT, Haeusler AR, Mistry NA, Vidensky S, Daley EL, Poth EM, Hoover B, Fines DM, Maragakis N, Tienari PJ, Petrucelli L, Traynor BJ, Wang J, Rigo F, Bennett CF, Blackshaw S, Sattler R, Rothstein JD (2013) RNA toxicity from the ALS/FTD C9ORF72 expansion is mitigated by antisense intervention. Neuron 80:415–428. https://doi.org/10.1016/j.neuron.2013.10.015
16. Freibaum BD, Lu Y, Lopez-Gonzalez R, Kim NC, Almeida S, Lee KH, Badders N, Valentine M, Miller BL, Wong PC, Petrucelli L, Kim HJ, Gao FB, Taylor JP (2015) GGGGCC repeat expansion in C9orf72 compromises nucleocytoplasmic transport. Nature 525:129–133. https://doi.org/10.1038/nature14974
17. Gabler M, Volkmar M, Weinlich S, Herbst A, Dobberthien P, Sklarss S, Fanti L, Pimpinelli S, Kress H, Reuter G, Dorn R (2005) Trans-splicing of the mod(mdg4) complex locus is conserved between the distantly related species Drosophila melanogaster and D. Virilis. Genetics 169:723–736. https://doi.org/10.1534/genetics.103.020842
18. Gendron TF, Bieniek KF, Zhang YJ, Jansen-West K, Ash PE, Caulfield T, Daughrity L, Dunmore JH, Castanedes-Casey M, Chew J, Cosio DM, van Blitterswijk M, Lee WC, Rademakers R, Boylan KB, Dickson DW, Petrucelli L (2013) Antisense transcripts of the expanded C9ORF72 hexanucleotide repeat form nuclear RNA foci and undergo repeat-associated non-ATG translation in c9FTD/ALS. Acta Neuropathol 126:829–844. https://doi.org/10.1007/s00401-013-1192-8
19. Gomez-Pastor R, Burchfiel ET, Thiele DJ (2018) Regulation of heat shock transcription factors and their roles in physiology and disease. Nat Rev Mol Cell Biol 19:4–19. https://doi.org/10.1038/nrm.2017.73
20. Haeusler AR, Donnelly CJ, Rothstein JD (2016) The expanding biology of the C9orf72 nucleotide repeat expansion in neurodegenerative disease. Nat Rev Neurosci 17:383–395. https://doi.org/10.1038/nrn.2016.38
21. Hartl FU, Bracher A, Hayer-Hartl M (2011) Molecular chaperones in protein folding and proteostasis. Nature 475:324–332. https://doi.org/10.1038/nature10317
22. Jedlicka P, Mortin MA, Wu C (1997) Multiple functions of Drosophila heat shock transcription factor in vivo. EMBO J 16:2452–2462. https://doi.org/10.1093/emboj/16.9.2452
23. Jiang J, Zhu Q, Gendron TF, Saberi S, McAlonis-Downes M, Seelman A, Stauffer JE, Jafar-Nejad P, Drenner K, Schulte D, Chun S, Sun S, Ling SC, Myers B, Engelhardt J, Katz M, Baughn M, Platoshyn O, Marsala M, Watt A, Heyser CJ, Ard MC, De Muynck L, Daughrity LM, Swing DA, Tessarollo L, Jung CJ, Delpoux A, Utzschneider DT, Hedrick SM, de Jong PJ, Edbauer D, Van Damme P, Petrucelli L, Shaw CE, Bennett CF, Da Cruz S, Ravits J, Rigo F, Cleveland DW, Lagier-Tourenne C (2016) Gain of toxicity from ALS/FTD-linked repeat expansions in C9ORF72 is alleviated by antisense oligonucleotides targeting GGGGCC-containing RNAs. Neuron 90:535–550. https://doi.org/10.1016/j.neuron.2016.04.006
24. Kieran D, Kalmar B, Dick JR, Riddoch-Contreras J, Burnstock G, Greensmith L (2004) Treatment with arimoclomol, a coinducer of heat shock proteins, delays disease progression in ALS mice. Nat Med 10:402–405. https://doi.org/10.1038/nm1021
25. Kramer NJ, Carlomagno Y, Zhang YJ, Almeida S, Cook CN, Gendron TF, Prudencio M, Van Blitterswijk M, Belzil V, Couthouis J, Paul JW 3rd, Goodman LD, Daughrity L, Chew J, Garrett A, Pregent L, Jansen-West K, Tabassian LJ, Rademakers R, Boylan K, Graff-Radford NR, Josephs KA, Parisi JE, Knopman DS, Petersen RC, Boeve BF, Deng N, Feng Y, Cheng TH, Dickson DW, Cohen SN, Bonini NM, Link CD, Gao FB, Petrucelli L, Gitler AD (2016) Spt4 selectively regulates the expression of C9orf72 sense and antisense mutant transcripts. Science 353:708–712. https://doi.org/10.1126/science.aaf7791
26. Kwon I, Xiang S, Kato M, Wu L, Theodoropoulos P, Wang T, Kim J, Yun J, Xie Y, McKnight SL (2014) Poly-dipeptides encoded by the C9orf72 repeats bind nucleoli, impede RNA biogenesis, and kill cells. Science 345:1139–1145. https://doi.org/10.1126/science.1254917
27. Lagier-Tourenne C, Baughn M, Rigo F, Sun S, Liu P, Li HR, Jiang J, Watt AT, Chun S, Katz M, Qiu J, Sun Y, Ling SC, Zhu Q, Polymenidou M, Drenner K, Artates JW, McAlonis-Downes M, Markmiller S, Hutt KR, Pizzo DP, Cady J, Harms MB, Baloh RH, Vandenberg SR, Yeo GW, Fu XD, Bennett CF, Cleveland DW, Ravits J (2013) Targeted degradation of sense and antisense C9orf72 RNA foci as therapy for ALS and frontotemporal degeneration. Proc Natl Acad Sci U S A 110:E4530–E4539. https://doi.org/10.1073/pnas.1318835110
28. Li T, Wernersson R, Hansen RB, Horn H, Mercer J, Slodkowicz G, Workman CT, Rigina O, Rapacki K, Staerfeldt HH, Brunak S, Jensen TS, Lage K (2017) A scored human protein-protein interaction network to catalyze genomic interpretation. Nat Methods 14:61–64. https://doi.org/10.1038/nmeth.4083
29. Love MI, Huber W, Anders S (2014) Moderated estimation of fold change and dispersion for RNA-seq data with DESeq2. Genome Biol 15:550. https://doi.org/10.1186/s13059-014-0550-8
30. Mackenzie IR, Frick P, Grasser FA, Gendron TF, Petrucelli L, Cashman NR, Edbauer D, Kremmer E, Prudlo J, Troost D, Neumann M (2015) Quantitative analysis and clinico-pathological correlations of different dipeptide repeat protein pathologies in C9ORF72 mutation carriers. Acta Neuropathol 130: 845–861. https://doi.org/10.1007/s00401-015-1476-2
31. Mahat DB, Salamanca HH, Duarte FM, Danko CG, Lis JT (2016) Mammalian heat shock response and mechanisms underlying its genome-wide transcriptional regulation. Mol Cell 62:63–78. https://doi.org/10.1016/j.molcel.2016.02.025
32. Mendillo ML, Santagata S, Koeva M, Bell GW, Hu R, Tamimi RM, Fraenkel E, Ince TA, Whitesell L, Lindquist S (2012) HSF1 drives a transcriptional

program distinct from heat shock to support highly malignant human cancers. Cell 150:549–562. https://doi.org/10.1016/j.cell.2012.06.031

33. Mizielinska S, Gronke S, Niccoli T, Ridler CE, Clayton EL, Devoy A, Moens T, Norona FE, Woollacott IO, Pietrzyk J, Cleverley K, Nicoll AJ, Pickering-Brown S, Dols J, Cabecinha M, Hendrich O, Fratta P, Fisher EM, Partridge L, Isaacs AM (2014) C9orf72 repeat expansions cause neurodegeneration in Drosophila through arginine-rich proteins. Science 345:1192–1194. https://doi.org/10.1126/science.1256800
34. Mori K, Weng SM, Arzberger T, May S, Rentzsch K, Kremmer E, Schmid B, Kretzschmar HA, Cruts M, Van Broeckhoven C, Haass C, Edbauer D (2013) The C9orf72 GGGGCC repeat is translated into aggregating dipeptide-repeat proteins in FTLD/ALS. Science 339:1335–1338. https://doi.org/10.1126/science.1232927
35. Morimoto RI (2011) The heat shock response: systems biology of proteotoxic stress in aging and disease. Cold Spring Harb Symp Quant Biol 76:91–99. https://doi.org/10.1101/sqb.2012.76.010637
36. Neef DW, Jaeger AM, Thiele DJ (2011) Heat shock transcription factor 1 as a therapeutic target in neurodegenerative diseases. Nat Rev Drug Discov 10:930–944. https://doi.org/10.1038/nrd3453
37. Neumann M, Sampathu DM, Kwong LK, Truax AC, Micsenyi MC, Chou TT, Bruce J, Schuck T, Grossman M, Clark CM, McCluskey LF, Miller BL, Masliah E, Mackenzie IR, Feldman H, Feiden W, Kretzschmar HA, Trojanowski JQ, Lee VM (2006) Ubiquitinated TDP-43 in frontotemporal lobar degeneration and amyotrophic lateral sclerosis. Science 314:130–133. https://doi.org/10.1126/science.1134108
38. O'Rourke JG, Bogdanik L, Muhammad AK, Gendron TF, Kim KJ, Austin A, Cady J, Liu EY, Zarrow J, Grant S, Ho R, Bell S, Carmona S, Simpkinson M, Lall D, Wu K, Daughrity L, Dickson DW, Harms MB, Petrucelli L, Lee EB, Lutz CM, Baloh RH (2015) C9orf72 BAC transgenic mice display typical pathologic features of ALS/FTD. Neuron 88:892–901. https://doi.org/10.1016/j.neuron.2015.10.027
39. O'Rourke JG, Bogdanik L, Yanez A, Lall D, Wolf AJ, Muhammad AK, Ho R, Carmona S, Vit JP, Zarrow J, Kim KJ, Bell S, Harms MB, Miller TM, Dangler CA, Underhill DM, Goodridge HS, Lutz CM, Baloh RH (2016) C9orf72 is required for proper macrophage and microglial function in mice. Science 351:1324–1329. https://doi.org/10.1126/science.aaf1064
40. Peters OM, Cabrera GT, Tran H, Gendron TF, McKeon JE, Metterville J, Weiss A, Wightman N, Salameh J, Kim J, Sun H, Boylan KB, Dickson D, Kennedy Z, Lin Z, Zhang YJ, Daughrity L, Jung C, Gao FB, Sapp PC, Horvitz HR, Bosco DA, Brown SP, de Jong P, Petrucelli L, Mueller C, Brown RH Jr (2015) Human C9ORF72 Hexanucleotide expansion reproduces RNA foci and dipeptide repeat proteins but not neurodegeneration in BAC transgenic mice. Neuron 88:902–909. https://doi.org/10.1016/j.neuron.2015.11.018
41. Prudencio M, Belzil VV, Batra R, Ross CA, Gendron TF, Pregent LJ, Murray ME, Overstreet KK, Piazza-Johnston AE, Desaro P, Bieniek KF, DeTure M, Lee WC, Biendarra SM, Davis MD, Baker MC, Perkerson RB, van Blitterswijk M, Stetler CT, Rademakers R, Link CD, Dickson DW, Boylan KB, Li H, Petrucelli L (2015) Distinct brain transcriptome profiles in C9orf72-associated and sporadic ALS. Nat Neurosci 18:1175–1182. https://doi.org/10.1038/nn.4065
42. Prudencio M, Gonzales PK, Cook CN, Gendron TF, Daughrity LM, Song Y, Ebbert MTW, van Blitterswijk M, Zhang YJ, Jansen-West K, Baker MC, DeTure M, Rademakers R, Boylan KB, Dickson DW, Petrucelli L, Link CD (2017) Repetitive element transcripts are elevated in the brain of C9orf72 ALS/FTLD patients. Hum Mol Genet 26:3421–3431. https://doi.org/10.1093/hmg/ddx233
43. Reimand J, Arak T, Adler P, Kolberg L, Reisberg S, Peterson H, Vilo J (2016) G: profiler-a web server for functional interpretation of gene lists (2016 update). Nucleic Acids Res 44:W83–W89. https://doi.org/10.1093/nar/gkw199
44. Reiner A, Yekutieli D, Benjamini Y (2003) Identifying differentially expressed genes using false discovery rate controlling procedures. Bioinformatics 19:368–375
45. Renton AE, Majounie E, Waite A, Simon-Sanchez J, Rollinson S, Gibbs JR, Schymick JC, Laaksovirta H, van Swieten JC, Myllykangas L, Kalimo H, Paetau A, Abramzon Y, Remes AM, Kaganovich A, Scholz SW, Duckworth J, Ding J, Harmer DW, Hernandez DG, Johnson JO, Mok K, Ryten M, Trabzuni D, Guerreiro RJ, Orrell RW, Neal J, Murray A, Pearson J, Jansen IE, Sondervan D, Seelaar H, Blake D, Young K, Halliwell N, Callister JB, Toulson G, Richardson A, Gerhard A, Snowden J, Mann D, Neary D, Nalls MA, Peuralinna T, Jansson L, Isoviita VM, Kaivorinne AL, Holtta-Vuori M, Ikonen E, Sulkava R, Benatar M, Wuu J, Chio A, Restagno G, Borghero G, Sabatelli M, Consortium I, Heckerman D, Rogaeva E, Zinman L, Rothstein JD, Sendtner M, Drepper C, Eichler EE, Alkan C, Abdullaev Z, Pack SD, Dutra A, Pak E, Hardy J, Singleton A, Williams NM, Heutink P, Pickering-Brown S, Morris HR, Tienari PJ, Traynor BJ (2011) A hexanucleotide repeat expansion in C9ORF72 is the cause of chromosome 9p21-linked ALS-FTD. Neuron 72:257–268. https://doi.org/10.1016/j.neuron.2011.09.010
46. Robberecht W, Philips T (2013) The changing scene of amyotrophic lateral sclerosis. Nat Rev Neurosci 14:248–264. https://doi.org/10.1038/nrn3430
47. Robinson MD, McCarthy DJ, Smyth GK (2010) edgeR: a Bioconductor package for differential expression analysis of digital gene expression data. Bioinformatics 26:139–140. https://doi.org/10.1093/bioinformatics/btp616
48. Sareen D, O'Rourke JG, Meera P, Muhammad AK, Grant S, Simpkinson M, Bell S, Carmona S, Ornelas L, Sahabian A, Gendron T, Petrucelli L, Baughn M, Ravits J, Harms MB, Rigo F, Bennett CF, Otis TS, Svendsen CN, Baloh RH (2013) Targeting RNA foci in iPSC-derived motor neurons from ALS patients with a C9ORF72 repeat expansion. Sci Transl Med 5:208ra149. https://doi.org/10.1126/scitranslmed.3007529
49. Solis EJ, Pandey JP, Zheng X, Jin DX, Gupta PB, Airoldi EM, Pincus D, Denic V (2016) Defining the essential function of yeast Hsf1 reveals a compact transcriptional program for maintaining eukaryotic Proteostasis. Mol Cell 63:60–71. https://doi.org/10.1016/j.molcel.2016.05.014
50. Supek F, Bosnjak M, Skunca N, Smuc T (2011) REVIGO summarizes and visualizes long lists of gene ontology terms. PLoS One 6:e21800. https://doi.org/10.1371/journal.pone.0021800
51. Taylor JP, Brown RH Jr, Cleveland DW (2016) Decoding ALS: from genes to mechanism. Nature 539:197–206. https://doi.org/10.1038/nature20413
52. Todd TW, Petrucelli L (2016) Insights into the pathogenic mechanisms of chromosome 9 open reading frame 72 (C9orf72) repeat expansions. J Neurochem 138(Suppl 1):145 162. https://doi.org/10.1111/jnc.13623
53. Waite AJ, Baumer D, East S, Neal J, Morris HR, Ansorge O, Blake DJ (2014) Reduced C9orf72 protein levels in frontal cortex of amyotrophic lateral sclerosis and frontotemporal degeneration brain with the C9ORF72 hexanucleotide repeat expansion. Neurobiol Aging 35:1779 e1775–1779 e1713. https://doi.org/10.1016/j.neurobiolaging.2014.01.016
54. Zhang K, Donnelly CJ, Haeusler AR, Grima JC, Machamer JB, Steinwald P, Daley EL, Miller SJ, Cunningham KM, Vidensky S, Gupta S, Thomas MA, Hong I, Chiu SL, Huganir RL, Ostrow LW, Matunis MJ, Wang J, Sattler R, Lloyd TE, Rothstein JD (2015) The C9orf72 repeat expansion disrupts nucleocytoplasmic transport. Nature 525:56–61. https://doi.org/10.1038/nature14973
55. Zhang YJ, Gendron TF, Grima JC, Sasaguri H, Jansen-West K, Xu YF, Katzman RB, Gass J, Murray ME, Shinohara M, Lin WL, Garrett A, Stankowski JN, Daughrity L, Tong J, Perkerson EA, Yue M, Chew J, Castanedes-Casey M, Kurti A, Wang ZS, Liesinger AM, Baker JD, Jiang J, Lagier-Tourenne C, Edbauer D, Cleveland DW, Rademakers R, Boylan KB, Bu G, Link CD, Dickey CA, Rothstein JD, Dickson DW, Fryer JD, Petrucelli L (2016) C9ORF72 poly(GA) aggregates sequester and impair HR23 and nucleocytoplasmic transport proteins. Nat Neurosci 19:668–677. https://doi.org/10.1038/nn.4272
56. Zhang YJ, Jansen-West K, Xu YF, Gendron TF, Bieniek KF, Lin WL, Sasaguri H, Caulfield T, Hubbard J, Daughrity L, Chew J, Belzil VV, Prudencio M, Stankowski JN, Castanedes-Casey M, Whitelaw E, Ash PE, DeTure M, Rademakers R, Boylan KB, Dickson DW, Petrucelli L (2014) Aggregation-prone c9FTD/ALS poly(GA) RAN-translated proteins cause neurotoxicity by inducing ER stress. Acta Neuropathol 128:505–524. https://doi.org/10.1007/s00401-014-1336-5
57. Zou J, Guo Y, Guettouche T, Smith DF, Voellmy R (1998) Repression of heat shock transcription factor HSF1 activation by HSP90 (HSP90 complex) that forms a stress-sensitive complex with HSF1. Cell 94:471–480

4

Activity of translation regulator eukaryotic elongation factor-2 kinase is increased in Parkinson disease brain and its inhibition reduces alpha synuclein toxicity

Asad Jan[1*], Brandon Jansonius[3†], Alberto Delaidelli[2†], Forum Bhanshali[4], Yi Andy An[4], Nelson Ferreira[5], Lisa M. Smits[6], Gian Luca Negri[2], Jens C. Schwamborn[6], Poul H. Jensen[5], Ian R. Mackenzie[2], Stefan Taubert[4] and Poul H. Sorensen[2,3*]

Abstract

Parkinson disease (PD) is the second most common neurodegenerative disorder and the leading neurodegenerative cause of motor disability. Pathologic accumulation of aggregated alpha synuclein (AS) protein in brain, and imbalance in the nigrostriatal system due to the loss of dopaminergic neurons in the substantia nigra-pars compacta, are hallmark features in PD. AS aggregation and propagation are considered to trigger neurotoxic mechanisms in PD, including mitochondrial deficits and oxidative stress. The eukaryotic elongation factor-2 kinase (eEF2K) mediates critical regulation of dendritic mRNA translation and is a crucial molecule in diverse forms of synaptic plasticity. Here we show that eEF2K activity, assessed by immuonohistochemical detection of eEF2 phosphorylation on serine residue 56, is increased in postmortem PD midbrain and hippocampus. Induction of aggressive, AS-related motor phenotypes in a transgenic PD M83 mouse model also increased brain eEF2K expression and activity. In cultures of dopaminergic N2A cells, overexpression of wild-type human AS or the A53T mutant increased eEF2K activity. eEF2K inhibition prevented the cytotoxicity associated with AS overexpression in N2A cells by improving mitochondrial function and reduced oxidative stress. Furthermore, genetic deletion of the eEF2K ortholog *efk-1* in *C. elegans* attenuated human A53T AS induced defects in behavioural assays reliant on dopaminergic neuron function. These data suggest a role for eEF2K activity in AS toxicity, and support eEF2K inhibition as a potential target in reducing AS-induced oxidative stress in PD.

Keywords: eEF2K, Parkinson disease, Alpha synuclein, Oxidative stress, Neurotoxicity

Introduction

Parkinson disease (PD) is the most common neurodegenerative cause of motor disability and is estimated to affect around 10 million people worldwide [33, 53]. Clinically, it presents as a movement disorder characterized by resting tremor, rigidity, and bradykinesia, and in a substantial number of patients the motor disability is compounded by non-motor symptoms such as cognitive impairment and autonomic dysfunction [33, 53]. Neuropathologically, loss of dopamine producing neurons in the midbrain *substantia nigra* (SN)-*pars compacta*, and intraneuronal inclusions of aggregated α-synuclein (AS) protein in multiple brain regions are hallmark features in PD [33, 53]. AS is a 14 kDa cytosolic protein (encoded by the *SNCA* gene) with putative roles in synaptic vesicle recycling, mitochondrial functions, and chaperone activity [39, 71]. Deposition of AS in the form of inclusions in neurons and/or nerve terminals, also known as Lewy body pathology, is also seen in other neurodegenerative diseases such as Alzheimer disease (AD), Lewy body dementia (LBD), and in

* Correspondence: ajan@aias.au.dk; psor@mail.ubc.ca
†Brandon Jansonius and Alberto Delaidelli contributed equally to this work.
1 Aarhus Institute of Advanced Studies, Department of Biomedicine, Aarhus University, Høegh-Guldbergs Gade 6B, DK-8000 Aarhus, Denmark
2 Department of Pathology and Laboratory Medicine, University of British Columbia, Vancouver, Canada
Full list of author information is available at the end of the article

oligodendrocytes in Multiple system atrophy (MSA) [67]. Idiopathic (non-inheritable) PD accounts for a vast majority of cases, while 5–10% of clinically diagnosed PD is attributable to genetic factors [53]. Missense mutations in *SNCA* resulting in N-terminal amino acid substitutions in the AS protein, or multiplications in *SNCA* gene locus leading to increased AS expression are the earliest known causes of autosomal-dominant inherited forms of PD [53, 54, 62]. There are additional genes associated with familial PD including autosomal-dominant and recessive inheritance (reviewed by [33, 53]), underlining the complex etiologic nature of PD.

Driven by the neuropathology and genetics, the neurotoxicity of AS has been a major area of research in PD towards the elucidation of disease-associated mechanisms and discovery of novel therapies. Based on studies in animal models and cell cultures, including neuronal cultures, substantial evidence implicates AS aggregation in triggering different alterations including synaptic dysfunction, calcium dyshomeostasis, mitochondrial impairment, endoplasmic reticulum (ER) stress, defective autophagy, neuroinflammation, and oxidative stress [27, 39, 59, 71]. In a broader perspective, a pathological role for dysregulation of some of these cellular mechanisms is also supported by the discovery of other genetic factors causing PD. For instance, autosomal-dominant mutations in leucine-rich repeat kinase 2 (*LRRK2*), which account for the most common cause of inherited PD [53], are associated with defective autophagy and mitochondrial dysfunction [68]. Similarly, mutations in *PARK2* (Parkin, an E3 ubiquitin ligase), *PINK1* (PTEN-induced putative kinase 1) and *PARK7* (DJ-1, a protein deglycase), which are associated with early onset (age less than 40 years) PD [33, 53], directly or indirectly affect mitochondrial function either by regulating mitophagy (Parkin and PINK1) or protecting mitochondria from oxidative stress (DJ-1) [5, 59]. Some studies have also reported that mitochondrial complex I protein expression and/or activity is reduced in PD substantia nigra [29, 60] and platelets [21]. Additionally, cultures of induced pluripotent stem cells (iPSCs) derived from PD patients show defects in oxygen consumption and mitochondrial function [3, 56]. Furthermore, exposure to several chemical toxins that inhibit complex I is well documented to induce dopaminergic neuron degeneration and a parkinsonian phenotype in humans (e.g., 1-methyl-4-phenyl-1,2,3,6-tetrahydropyridine, MPTP) and in animals (e.g., MPTP, rotenone, paraquat etc.) [33, 59].

The eukaryotic elongation factor-2 kinase (eEF2K), also known as calcium/calmodulin dependent kinase III, is an important regulatory molecule in cellular protein synthesis and also in diverse forms of synaptic plasticity [23]. Upon activation, eEF2K phosphorylates its major known substrate, the eukaryotic elongation factor-2 (eEF2), on threonine-56 (Thr56), thus leading to the dissociation of eEF2 from ribosomes and stalling of mRNA translation during the elongation phase [34, 57]. eEF2K activity is increased under condition of nutrient stress via the energy sensor AMP-activated kinase (AMPK), which positively regulates eEF2K activity by phosphorylation on serine residue 398 [34, 42]. We and others have observed increased eEF2K expression and/or activity in AD post-mortem brains [28, 43, 46], and in the brains of transgenic AD mice [28, 46]. We have also shown that eEF2K inhibition prevents the toxicity of amyloid-β (Aβ) oligomers in neuronal cultures by activating the NRF2 antioxidant response, and attenuates human Aβ-induced deficits in neuronal function in *C. elegans* [28].

Mitochondrial defects (directly or indirectly associated with the aggregation of AS protein) and oxidative stress are implicated in PD pathogenesis [5, 59], and eEF2K inhibition reduces reactive oxygen species (ROS) levels in cells [10, 28]. Therefore, we hypothesized that eEF2K inhibition may mitigate AS induced neurotoxicity by reducing oxidative stress. To test this hypothesis, we first examined markers of eEF2K activity,[1] i.e., phosphoryalation of eEF2 on serine residue 56, in postmortem PD brains in order to establish its relevance to human pathology, and subsequent to the induction of AS pathology in transgenic mouse M83 line expressing PD-associated mutant *Ala53Thr* (A53T) AS [20, 58]. Then, we probed the effects of eEF2K inhibition on cytotoxicity, mitochondrial function and oxidative stress in AS overexpressing dopaminergic N2A cells, and on dopaminergic neuronal function in *C. elegans* expressing mutant A53T AS. By using multiple experimental approaches, we elucidate the relevance of eEF2K in AS toxicity, and discuss the potential utility of eEF2K inhibition in PD and related synucleinopathies.

Materials and methods

Reagents and biochemical assays

Plasmids for overexpression of AS in mammalian cells were obtained under MTA from Addgene, and included human wild type AS (pHM6-alphasynuclein-WT, Addgene #40824) and human mutant A53T AS (pHM6-alphasynuclein-A53T, Addgene #40825). Additional reagents and biochemical assays employed during these studies include: pool of small interference RNAs (SiRNAs) targeting mouse eEF2K (Santa Cruz, #sc-39,012), Cell Titer Glo ATP measurement kit (Promega, #G7570), Lactate dehydrogenase (LDH) fluorometric assay (Novus Biologicals, #NBP2–54851), Seahorse Mito stress test kit (Agilent, #103015–100), 2′,7′-dichlorodihydrofluorescein diacetate (DCFDA) fluorescent ROS reagent (ThermoFisher, #D399), and MitoTracker Green fluorescent reagent for mitochondrial mass (ThermoFisher, #M7514). Biochemical assays (LDH and ATP), Seahorse assays and flow cytometry assays were performed according to manufacturer's recommendations and are also outlined in details below.

Immunohistochemistry (IHC) and immunofluorescence studies on postmortem human brain sections

Five-micrometer formalin-fixed paraffin embedded separate post-mortem sections from midbrain and hippocampus of control or PD patients were provided by the laboratory of IM (co-author), as approved by the University of British Columbia Ethics Committee. Anonymized brain sections from 3 control individuals and 6 clinically and pathologically confirmed PD patients were obtained at autopsy and used in these experiments (Additional file 1: Table S1).

IHC on brain sections from human tissue was performed after deparaffinization and antigen retrieval. The following antibodies were employed to stain serial tissue sections, as indicated: antibody against phospho-eEF2 (Thr56) (Novus Biologicals, #NB100–92518) [28, 42], and antibody against phospho-alpha synuclein (pSer129; EMD Millipore, #MABN826), using the alkaline phosphatise conjugated streptavidin-biotin ABC kit (Vector Labs, # AK-5000). For destaining/bleaching neuromelanin in substantia nigra in the midbrain sections, the IHC protocol was modified slightly, as described [52] . Briefly, sections mounted on slides were incubated in a 60 °C degrees oven for 30 min and then were transferred into ambient distilled water. Then, the slides were placed in 0.25% potassium permanganate solution for 5 min. Subsequently, the slides were rinsed with distilled water. This was followed by incubation in 5% oxalic acid until section became clear. A final rinse in distilled water was performed before proceeding with the normal IHC staining as described above. Sections were counterstained with hematoxylin (Vector Labs, #H-3401). High resolution panoramic images of tissue sections for p-eEF2 and p-ASyn IHC analysis were acquired using a Leica Aperio digital slide scanner. IHC staining for p-eEF2 was quantified by manual counting of the DAB (3,3′-diaminobenzidine; Vector Labs, #SK-4100) positive cells.

For the detection of p-eEF2 (T56) and p-ASyn (S129) in the same tissue section, i.e., colocalization studies, immunofluorescence labelling was performed. For this purpose, after incubation of the tissue sections with primary antibodies as in the staining protocol described above, Alexa Fluor conjugated secondary fluorescent antibodies (Alexa Fluor 488 Goat anti-Mouse IgG, Thermo Fisher # A32723 and Alexa Fluor 594 Goat anti-Rabbit IgG, Thermo Fisher # R37119) were used for the detection. Image acquisition was performed using a Nikon Eclipse TE2000 confocal microscope.

Animal studies

Husbandry

Transgenic M83$^{+/+}$ PD mice [B6; C3-Tg (Prnp-SNCA*A53T) 83Vle/J] were kindly provided by the laboratory of Benoit Gaisson at the Centre for Translation Research in Neurodegenerative Diseases, University of Florida, USA to the laboratory of PHJ (co-author). These mice express the mutant human A53T AS under the direction of the mouse prion protein promoter [20]. The mice were housed at the Aarhus University Bartholin animal facility under conditions of 12 h light/dark cycles and received ad libitum standard laboratory chow diet. All procedures were performed in accordance with National rules and the European Communities Council Directive for the care and handling of laboratory animals. Both male and female mice were used for biochemical analyses. All genotypes were determined by PCR.

Intramuscular injections of alpha synuclein fibrils

Fibrillar mouse AS was prepared essentially according to an established protocol [58]. Tg M83$^{+/+}$ were bilaterally injected with recombinant mouse AS preformed fibrils (PFF) as described [58]. Briefly, 2–3 month-old mice were anesthetized with isoflurane (1–5%) inhalation and injected intramuscularly into the hindlimb biceps femoris bilaterally. The inoculum (5 μL of 2 mg/mL PFF or PBS) was injected using a 10-μL Hamilton syringe with a 25-gauge needle. Separate syringes were used for each type of inoculums (PBS or PFF) to avoid any cross-contamination. After the injection, mice were allowed to recover under close observation before being returned to their original cage.

Hindlimb clasping

Assessment of hindlimb clasping behaviour was performed with a modified tail suspension test [22]. Freely moving, non-anesthesized, Tg M83$^{+/+}$ were held by the tail and lifted in air for 10 s. Severity of clasping was assessed as follows: 1) No clasping (score 0), hindlimbs were consistently spread outward and away from the abdomen; 2) Mild clasping (score 1), one hindlimb was retracted toward the abdomen for more than 50% of the time; 3) Moderate clasping (score 2), both hindlimbs were partially retracted toward the abdomen for more than 50% of the time suspended; and 4) Severe clasping (score 3), hindlimbs were entirely retracted and touching the abdomen for more than 50% of the time suspended.

Quantitative RT-PCR

Total RNA from the whole brain homogenates was extracted using a commercial kit (Qiagen, #74134), and cDNA was synthesized using high capacity reverse transcriptase kit (Applied Biosystems, #4368814). The following gene specific primer pairs were used in qRT-PCR: Mouse *eef2k* (forward, 5'-CGCTTTGTACCGGGGATTCT-3′; reverse, 5′- AAGG

ATGGTCCTCCCACAGT-3′) and Mouse *Gapdh* (forward, 5′- CCCTTAAGAGGGATGCTGCC-3′; reverse, 5'-TACG GCCAAATCCGTTCACA-3′). The data were analyzed by relative ΔΔCT quantification method using *Gapdh* CT values as internal reference in each sample.

Cell culture

Midbrain organoid cultures

Midbrain organoids were generated with a modified protocol as reported previously [49], from human iPSCs essentially as described [3]. After 35 days of differentiation, RNA from snap frozen wild type or A53T mutation carrying organoids was isolated using a commercial kit (Qiagen, # 74104), and cDNA was synthesized using Applied Biosystems high capacity reverse transcriptase kit (Thermo Fisher, # 4368814). Following gene specific primer pairs were used in qRT-PCR: Human *EEF2K*, forward 5′- CCCAAGCAGGTGGACATCAT-3′ and reverse 5'-TTGCCCTCGATGTAGTGCTC-3′ and human glyceraldehyde 3-phosphate dehydrogenase (*GAPDH*), forward 5′- GACAGTCAGCCGCATCTTCT -3′ and reverse 5′- ACCAAATCCGTTGACTCCGA -3′.

N2A cultures

N2A neuroblastoma cells were obtained from ATCC (#CCL-131), and maintained in DMEM (4.5 g/L glucose; Gibco, #11965–084) supplemented with 1% antibiotic-antimycotic solution (Gibco, #15240062) and 10% Fetal Bovine Serum (FBS), Cells were cultured in 6-well (500, 000 cells/well) 12-well (250,000 cells/well) or 96-well (50,000 cells/well) plates. DNA plasmid transfections were performed using Lipofectamine 2000 (Invitrogen, #11668019), and Lipofectamine RNAiMAX (Invitroge, #13778150) for siRNAs, according to the recommended procedures. After 24 h, cells were briefly washed with phosphate-buffer saline (PBS) and allowed to differentiate into neurons in a modified culture medium [59] containing DMEM (Gibco, #21969035) supplemented with 500 μM L-glutamine, 1% antibiotic-antimycotic, 2% FBS and 500 μM Dibutyryladenosine 3′,5′-cyclic monophosphate (db cAMP; Sigma, #D0627) [28, 63]. Unless indicated otherwise, differentiated N2A cells which were mock transfected, or transfected with AS plasmids (ASyn-WT or ASyn-A53T; Addgene plasmid #40824 and #40825 respectively) +/− eEF2K kd, were used in the various assays described below after 72–76 h post-transfection.

Cytotoxicity assays

For the lactate dehydrogenase (LDH) release, 50 μl of culture medium was collected from each well into sterile tubes and cell debris was removed by centrifugation (1100 rpm, 10 min; 4 °C) in a tabletop centrifuge. Then, 5 μl of the supernatant were carefully transferred into a 96-well black microplate cooled and kept on ice. Then, the assay reagents, as recommended by the manufacturer were added to the wells. Fluorescence (Ex/Em = λ535/λ587 nm) was measured in a Tecan microplate reader equipped with necessary filters at room temperature. Measurements were acquired in a kinetics mode every minute, after 5 s of gentle shaking, over 20 min. Stabilized fluorescence signal from each sample was collected and analyzed. For the propidium iodide (PI) cell death detection assay, the cells were gently trypsinized (0.05% Trypsin-EDTA; Gibco, #25300054), centrifuged (1100 rpm, 5 min, 4 °C) and resuspended in 500 μl of sterile ice-cold PBS containing 20% FBS and 0.001% PI (ThermoFisher, #P3566). After transferring into FACS tubes, on ice, the cells were analyzed on a FACSCalibur-Tangerine flow cytometry instrument, as described [28]. Cellular ATP levels were measured using a bioluminescence firefly luciferase assay (Cell Titer Glo, Promega) with minor modifications to the manufacturer's instructions. Briefly, the cells were resuspended in the assay mix by thorough pipetting and transferred into a 96-well white assay plate, previously cooled on ice. Then luminescence signal was measured in a Tecan microplate reader at room temperature. Measurements were acquired in a kinetics mode every 3 min, after 5 s of gentle shaking, over 30 min. Stabilized luminescence signal from each sample was collected and analyzed.

Mitochondrial respiration and cellular mitochondrial content

Cellular oxygen consumption rate (OCR) was measured using the Seahorse Mito stress kit according to the supplier's instructions. Apart from the basal OCR, a combination of pharamcological agents (components of the Seahorse Mito Stress test) enables the assessment of different aspects of cellular respiration. These include non-mitochondrial (NM) respiration, maximal respiration (MR) and spare respiratory capacity (SRC). Optimal cell density and concentrations of drugs for the assay were established according to the kit instructions/parameters. Then, 30,000 cells/well were seeded in a 96-well microplate (included in the kit) and transfections were carried out (Mock, ASyn-WT or ASyn-A53, all ± eEF2K siRNA). OCR measurements were performed in a Seahorse XF analyzer according to the assay guidelines. Basal OCR was measured over 20 min (4 cycles, 5 min/cycle), followed by exposure to oligomycin, ATP synthase inhibitor (2 μM), carbonilcyanide p-triflouromethoxyphenylhydrazone-FCCP, oxidative phosphorylation uncoupler (0.5 μM) and rotenone/antimycin, complex I and III inhibitor respectively (0.5 μM). After injection with each drug, OCR was measured over 15 min (4 cycles, 5 min/cycle). After the assay completion, the cells were gently rinsed with PBS and homogenized by pipetting in ice cold 50 μl RIPA lysis buffer

(25 mM Tris-HCl pH 7.6, 150 mM NaCl, 1% NP-40, 1% sodium deoxycholate, 0.1% SDS, protease inhibitors and phosphatase inhibitors cocktail). Then, the cell lysate was transferred into microtubes, centrifuged (10,000 rpm, 10 min, 4 °C) and 25 μl of supernatant was transferred into a 96-well assay plate. Total protein in samples was determined by BCA protein assay (Pierce, #23225). OCR data was normalized to the protein content/well.

Mitochondrial content (mass) in differentiated N2A cells ± eEF2K kd was determined by labelling with Mitotracker fluorescent dye, and by quantification of mitochondrial DNA copy number. For the Mitotracker assay, cells were incubated with 50 nM Mitotracker Green FM reagent for 30 min in fresh medium. The cells were trypsinized, and centrifuged as described under the PI assay, and resuspended in 500 μl of sterile ice-cold PBS containing 20% FBS. Control cells without Mitotracker dye treatment were used as the background fluorescence signal. Separately, mitochondrial DNA (mtDNA) quantification was carried out by RT-PCR as described [47]. Briefly, nuclear DNA and mtDNA were isolated from differentiated N2A cells ± eEF2K using a Qiagen All Prep kit (#80204). Isolated samples were sonicated, then diluted to contain either 10 ng or 1 ng of DNA. This was used as an internal control to ensure that the ratio of mtDNA to nuclear DNA remained constant at different concentrations. qPCR was run on a Quant Studio 6 instrument using Fast SYBR Green Master Mix (ThermoFisher, #4309155). The primer sequences used for qPCR are as follows: mouse mitochondrial marker- *mMito* (forward, 5'-CTAGAAACCCCGAAACCAAA-3'; reverse, 5'-CCAGCTATCACCAAGCTCGT-3') and mouse beta-2-microglobulin- *mB2M* (forward, 5'-ATGGGAAGC CGAACATACTG-3'; reverse: 5'-CAGTCTCAGTGGGG GTGAAT-3'). In each sample, mtDNA was quantified as a ratio of mtDNA to nuclear DNA (mtDNA/N) and were expressed as mtDNA copy numbers.

ROS measurements

For ROS detection, cells were incubated with 5 μg/mL 2, 7-dichlorofluorescein diacetate- DCFDA for 30 min in fresh medium. The cells were gently trypsinized (0.05% Trypsin-EDTA), centrifuged (1100 rpm, 5 min, 4 °C) and resuspended in 500 μl of sterile ice-cold PBS containing 20% FBS and 0.001% PI. After transferring into FACS tubes, on ice, the cells were analyzed on a FACSCalibur-Tangerine flow cytometry instrument as described previously [28]. During the analysis, dead cells were excluded from analysis based on PI staining. Control cells without DCDFA treatment were used as the background fluorescence signal.

Western blotting

Whole brain tissue homogenates from euthanized M83$^{+/+}$ mice were prepared in RIPA buffer (25 mM Tris-HCl pH 7.6, 150 mM NaCl, 1% NP-40, 1% sodium deoxycholate, 0.1% SDS, protease inhibitors and phosphatase inhibitors cocktail). For cellular assays, the cells were washed (ice cold PBS, 2–3 times) and lysed in RIPA buffer. Then, the mouse brain homogenates or cell lysates were briefly sonicated on ice and centrifuged (12,000 rpm, 15 min, 4 °C). Supernatant was collected and protein quantitation was done using BCA protein assay (Pierce, #23225). Then 25–40 μg of total proteins per sample were electrophoresed on 8% or 10% Bis-Tris acrylamide gels. Proteins were transferred onto a nitrocellulose membrane, incubated in blocking buffer (Li-Cor, #927–50,100]), and probed with following primary antibodies: eEF2K (Abcam, #46787), p-eEF2 Thr56 (Cell Signalling, #2331), eEF2 (Cell Signalling, #2332), ASyn (Santa Cruz #sc-12,767), p-ASyn Ser129 (Abcam, #168381, MJF-R13), and GAPDH (Cell Signaling 2118). Detection was performed using goat anti-mouse (Li-Cor, #925–32,210) or goat anti-rabbit (Li-Cor, #925–68,071) secondary antibodies conjugated with fluorescent infrared dyes using an Odyssey scanner (Li-Cor). Densitometry analysis was performed using ImageJ (NIH) [28].

C. elegans studies

Nematode strains and culture methods

C. elegans strains N2 wild-type (referred to as WT-N2), RB2588 *efk-1(ok3609)*, [28] (referred to as efk-1$_{del}$), JVR107 *Pdat-1::a-synuclein[A53T]*, [12] ((referred to as ASyn (A53T)), and STE120 *efk-1(ok3609); Pdat-1::a-synuclein[A53T]* ((generated herein, referred to as ASyn (A53T)/efk-1$_{del}$)) were grown on Nematode Growth Medium (NGM) lite plates at 20 °C and with *E. coli* OP50 as food source, as described [28]. We used standard sodium hypochlorite bleaching and L1 stage starvation to generate synchronized populations, which were then allowed to grow for 72 h, i.e. until day two of adulthood; all assays were performed at that stage.

Dopamine-dependent behaviour assays

Ethanol avoidance assay

Ethanol avoidance assays were done as described [12], on an unseeded 15 mm × 60 mm plate divided into four quadrants with a circle of 1 cm in diameter in between. Then, 1cm^3 agarose chunks were soaked in ice-cold ethanol overnight, and placed 0.5 cm from the edge of the plate in the centre of two opposing quadrants, while the other two quadrants remained untreated. Ethanol was allowed to diffuse in media for 2 h. Actively growing day 2 old adult worms were washed five times with M9 buffer, and 150–200 worms were placed in the centre of the plate, and allowed to move for 1 h at 20 °C. Then, worms were counted manually and ethanol avoidance was calculated as [(number of worms in control quadrants) – (number of worms in ethanol quadrants))/(total number of worms)]. Three assay plates were used for each strain, and a minimum of three biological replicates was performed.

Pharyngeal pumping assay

The pharyngeal pumping rate was measured by manually counting the number of pumps made by each worm on seeded plate for 30 s using a Leica M205FA microscope. A total of 10–15 worms were used for each replicate. The assay was repeated at least three times on separate worms.

Area-restricted searching assay

Area-restricted searching assays were done as described [13]. Worms were washed very quickly to remove bacteria, and 10–15 worms were placed on an unseeded plate. To record the turning frequency, worms were videotaped at intervals of 5 and 30 min for one minute using a MoticamX camera mounted on a Leica M205FA microscope. Videotapes were analyzed manually to count the number of high-angled turns, i.e. those that exceeded 90°, including reversals and omega turns. The area-restricted searching ratio was calculated as [(number of turns/worm at 5 min)/(number of turns per worm at 30 min)]. A minimum of three replicates was performed for this assay.

Statistics

The data were analyzed in Graphpad Prism software (version 5) or Microsoft Excel 2010, and graphs were made in Microsoft Excel 2010. Statistical differences between two sets of data were calculated by Mann-Whitney nonparametric test or unpaired T-test, as indicated in the figure legends. Multiple column datasets were analyzed by One-way ANOVA followed by Bonferonni *posthoc* analysis. Longitudinal analysis was performed by Two-way ANOVA.

Results

eEF2K expression and activity are increased in PD brain

Using postmortem brain sections from midbrain and hippocampus of controls and PD patients (Additional file 1: Table S1), we performed immunohistochemistry (IHC) analysis of eEF2 phosphorylation on threonine residue 56 (p-eEF2, T56), which reflects eEF2K activity [42, 57]. In parallel, using serial sections, we also assessed the phosphorylation of AS on serine residue 129 (p-ASyn, S129) by IHC, as it is a robust marker for AS Lewy pathology (~ 90% S129 phosphorylated AS is found in inclusions) [2, 65]. To avoid ambiguity with neuromelanin pigment found in dopaminergic neurons in substantia nigra (SN) with DAB IHC staining, we employed a modified IHC protocol [52] in order to effectively destain/bleache neuromelanin in midbrain sections without adversely affecting p-eEF2 (T56) IHC staining (Additional file 1: Figure S1a-b). Our data show that p-eEF2 (T56) immunostaining is increased in SN and periaqueductal gray (PAG) matter (gray matter surrounding cerebral aqueduct) in PD midbrain sections compared to controls (Fig. 1a-b; additional controls shown in Additional file 1: Figure S2a; additional PD cases are shown in Additional file 1: Figure S3a; quantitation of p-eEF2 IHC staining is presented in Fig. 3a). We observed that p-eEF2 IHC staining was predominantly in neurons in SN and PAG in PD cases, and in some glial cells in SN (for instance in PD-2, Fig. 1b; PD-3 and PD-4, Additional file 1: Figure S3a). As expected, we observed Lewy body pathology (p-ASyn, S129) characteristic of PD in both of these midbrain regions in PD cases but not in controls (Fig. 1a-b; Additional file 1: Figure S2a, S3a). Accordingly, Lewy body inclusion pathology was seen in most PD cases both in SN and PAG, with some lewy neurites in SN (PD-2, Fig. 1b; PD-6, Additional file 1: Figure S3a) and PAG area (PD-2, Fig. 1b; PD-3 and PD-5, Additional file 1: Figure S3a). Then, by using immunofluorescence, we assessed whether p-eEF2 (T56) immunopositivity potentially colocalizes with p-ASyn (S129), or p-eEF2 (T56) is a possible component of lewy body pathology. While we observed some neurons in PD SN which were clearly positive for both p-eEF2 (T56) and p-ASyn (S129), we also found substantial p-eEF2 (T56) immunopositivity in cells without p-ASyn (S129) and vice versa (Additional file 1: Figure S4b).

Previous reports, including our own published data, show that phosphorylation of eEF2 (p-eEF2, T56) is strongly increased in postmortem hippocampus and mesial temporal cortex in AD, the major neurodegenerative disease with dementia [28, 43, 46]. Among the PD cases examined here, PD-1 and PD-5 were also clinically diagnosed with PD with dementia (PDD), which is usually seen in longstanding PD [1, 2]. Therefore, we assessed p-eEF2 (T56) in postmortem hippocampus sections from control and PD cases. We found increased p-eEF2 IHC staining in hippocampal CA1 and CA2 (CA, *cornu ammonis*) fields in PD cases compared to controls, predominantly in neurons (Fig. 2a-b; additional controls shown in Additional file 1: Figure S5a-b; additional PD cases shown in Additional file 1: Figure S6a, panoramic views; Additional file 1: Figure S7a-b, magnified field views; quantitation of p-eEF2 IHC staining in areas CA1-CA2 is presented in Fig. 3a). There was little or none p-eEF2 immunopositivity in CA3 and dentate gyrus (DG) in all PD cases, except PD-1 and PD-3 (CA3, Additional file 1: Figure S7a-b). We also assessed Lewy body pathology in hippocampal sections from these control and PD cases, since Lewy pathology in hippocampus is found at advanced neuropathological stages of PD (Braak PD staging, stages 4–6) [1, 36]. Our IHC analysis for p-ASyn (S129) showed varying degrees of Lewy body inclusions (PD-1 and PD-2, Fig. 2b; PD-3 and PD-6, Additional file 1: Figure S7b) and Lewy neurites pathology (PD-1 and PD-2, Fig. 2b; PD-6, Additional file 1: Figure S7b), with pronounced involvement of hippocampal

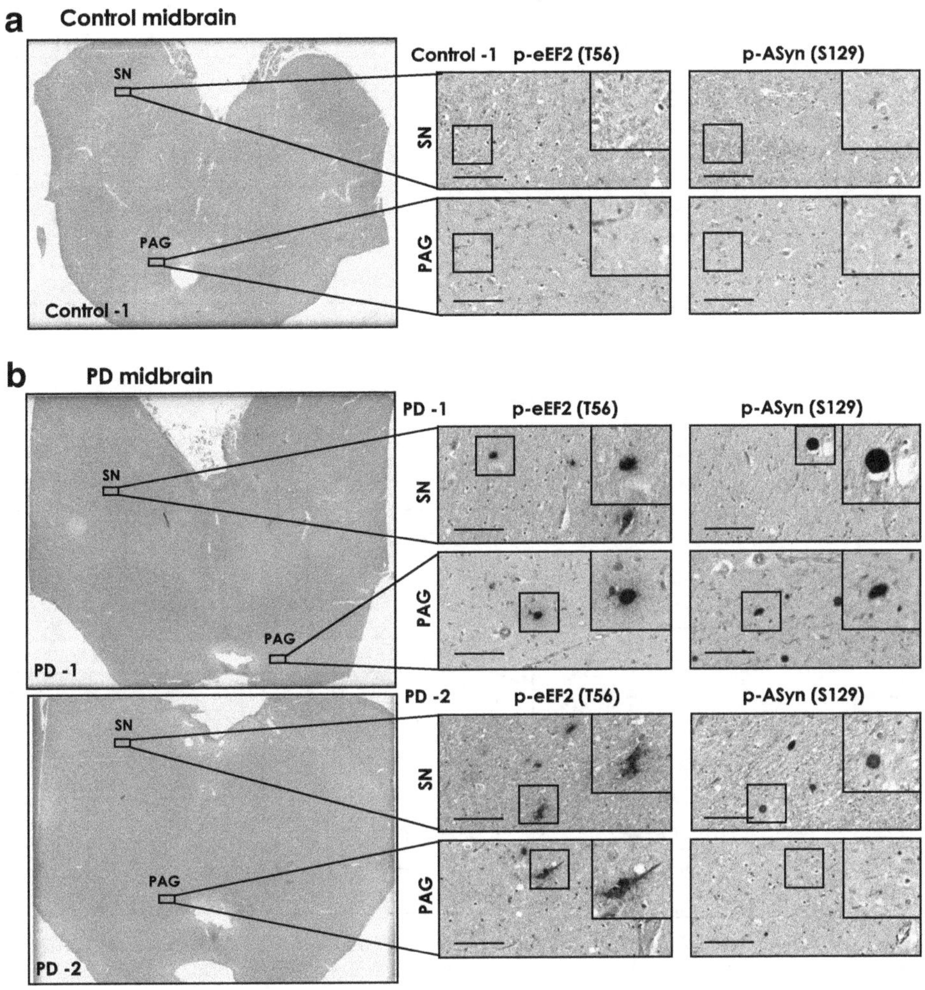

Fig. 1 Immunostaining for phospho-eEF2 (p-eEF2, Thr56) and phospho-AS (p-ASyn, Ser129) in postmortem control and PD midbrain serial sections. **a**-**b** p-eEF2 (T56) and p-ASyn (S129) IHC in postmortem midbrain serial sections from one control (**a**) and two PD cases (**b**). IHC staining for p-eEF2 is predominantly seen in neurons in both cases, and possibly glial cells in substantia nigra in PD-2. Substantia nigra in both cases shows involvement by lewy body-LB pathology (p-ASyn, S129); while in periaqueductal gray matter, LB inclusions are seen in PD-1 and some lewy neurites are seen in PD-2. Additional control and PD midbrain IHC data are presented in Additional file 1: Figure S2-S3, and case details are included in Additional file 1: Table S1. (SN- substantia nigra; PAG- periaqueductal gray matter; scale bar, 100 μm; insets show 40x magnified view in each image)

CA2 field in most PD cases (Fig. 2a-b and Additional file 1: Figure S7a-b).

We also queried multiple transcriptome datasets publicly available in the National Center for Biotechnology Information (NCBI) Gene Expression Omnibus (GEO) platform for eEF2K mRNA expression in PD brain. Significantly increased eEF2K mRNA expression was found in Striatum (Fig. 3b, GEO accession # GSE28894), medial substantia nigra (Fig. 3c, GEO accession # GSE8397), and dorsal nucleus of vagus (dmX) (Fig. 3d, GEO accession # GSE43490). Collectively, these data provide strong evidence for aberrant eEF2K expression and activity in PD brain. Finally, we also performed quantitative PCR in cultured midbrain organoids derived from human iPSCs [3, 49], and found significantly increased eEF2K mRNA expression in A53T mutant AS carrying organoids compared to wild type controls (Fig. 3e).

eEF2K expression and activity are increased in M83$^{+/+}$ transgenic PD mouse brains subsequent to induction of AS neuropathology

To further establish the relevance of eEF2K to AS-related pathology in PD, we analyzed brain eEF2K expression in transgenic PD M83$^{+/+}$ mice, subsequent to induction of AS pathology by intramuscular injection of pre-formed fibrillar PFF AS [20, 58]. Within 8–10 weeks post-injection, the PFF AS injected M83$^{+/+}$ mice show profound motor neuron loss, AS inclusions, progressive motor deficits and reduced survival at much earlier ages than native M83$^{+/+}$ mice [58]. For these analyses, PFF AS injected M83$^{+/+}$ mice (injected at 2–3 months of age) were used after 8–10 weeks

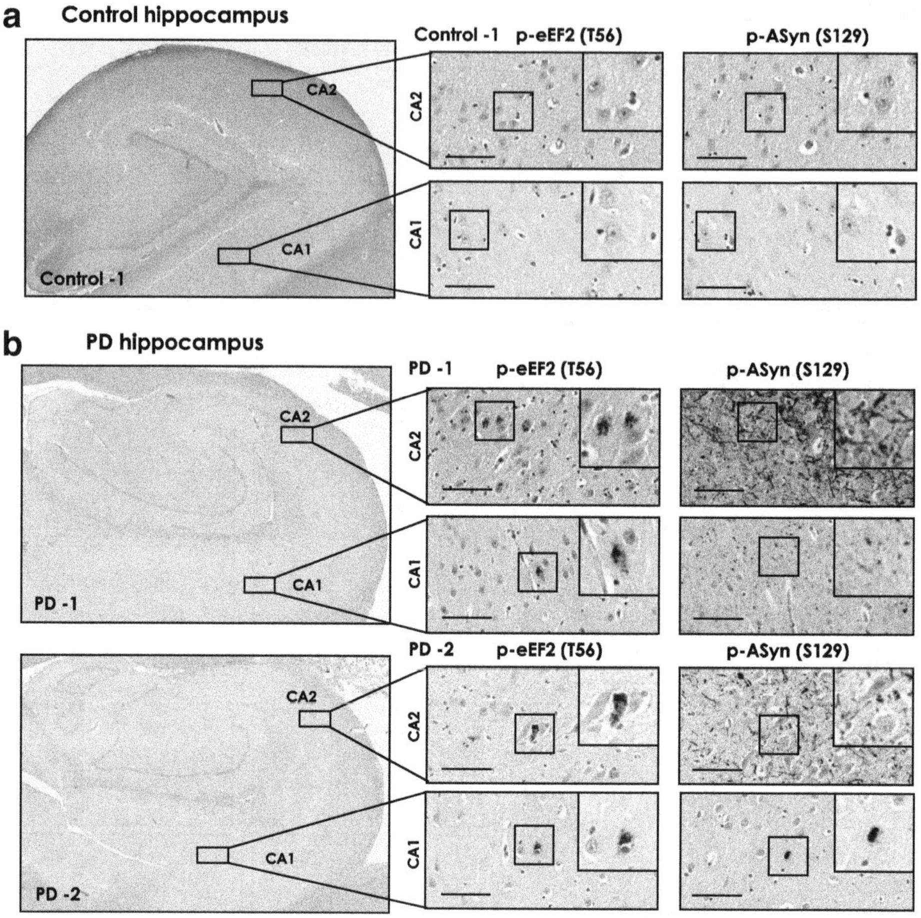

Fig. 2 Immunostaining for phospho-eEF2 (p-eEF2, Thr56) and phospho-AS (p-ASyn, Ser129) in postmortem control and PD hippocampus serial sections. **a-b** p-eEF2 (T56) and p-ASyn (S129) IHC in postmortem hippocampus serial sections from one control (**a**) and two PD cases (**b**). IHC staining for p-eEF2 in PD cases is seen predominantly in CA1 and CA2 neurons. Lewy body inclusions and neurites (p-ASyn, S129) are seen in both PD cases, with pronounced involvement of CA2. IHC data concerning CA3 and dentate gyrus from PD-1 and PD-2 are included in Additional file 1: Figure S7a. Additional control and PD hippocampus IHC data are presented in Additional file 1: Figure S5-S7, and case details are included in Additional file 1: Table S1 (CA1 and CA2- hippocampal cornu ammonis fields 1 and 2 respectively; scale bar, 100 μm; insets show 40× magnified view in each image)

post-injection when typical motor abnormalities such as hindlimb paralysis (Additional file 1: Figure S8a) and severe hindlimb clasping behaviour (Additional file 1: Figure S8b-c) were evident. Our data show that compared to PBS injected $M83^{+/+}$ mice, brain eEF2K mRNA expression is remarkably increased (~ 5–6 fold) in PFF AS injected $M83^{+/+}$ moribund (clasping score 3, see Materials and Methods) mice (Fig. 4a). Accordingly, we also found increased eEF2K activity (p-eEF2, T56) and induction of pathological AS phosphorylation (p-ASyn, S129) by western blotting in PFF AS injected $M83^{+/+}$ (Fig. 4b-c). These data further support our hypothesis regarding a role of eEF2K in AS neurotoxicity.

AS overexpression increases eEF2K activity, while eEF2K inhibition reduces AS cytotoxicity in dopaminergic N2A cells

As mentioned above, AS-induced neurotoxicity is considered to play an important role in neurodegeneration in PD [39, 71]. Indeed, overexpression of AS in cultured cells promotes AS aggregation, increases oxidative stress, and reduces cell survival [4, 8]. This has been observed for the wild-type and mutant forms of AS, including the A53T mutant AS, which accelerates AS aggregation and pathology [39, 41]. To study the effects of eEF2K inhibition on AS toxicity, we employed differentiated mouse neuroblastoma N2A cells overexpressing either wild-type AS (ASyn-WT) or the A53T mutant (ASyn-A53T) +/– siRNA mediated eEF2K knockdown (kd), and measured cytotoxicity in these cells. Differentiated N2A cells exhibit many features of mature dopaminergic neurons including functional neurotransmitter receptors [63], and are widely used to study the toxicity of amyloid proteins [14, 28].

Overexpression of ASyn-WT or ASyn-A53T increased p-eEF2 (T56) levels in N2A cells, which was reduced by eEF2K kd (Fig. 5a-b). We then assessed AS cytotoxicity by measuring the activity of lactate dehyrogenase (LDH) in

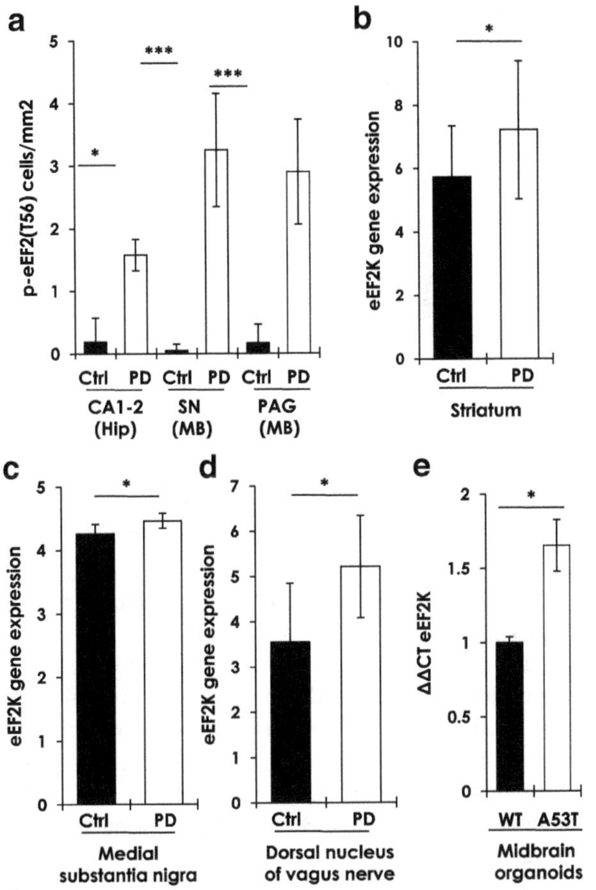

Fig. 3 eEF2K expression and activity in PD brain. **a** Quantitation of p-eEF2 (T56) IHC (3,3'-Diaminobenzidine-DAB staining) in postmortem hippocampus- Hip (CA1 and CA2 fields) and midbrain- MB (SN-substantia nigra, and PAG-peri-aqueductal gray matter) sections from 3 control and 6 PD cases (Additional file 1: Table S1; counts from at least 6 high power fields from each control or PD section; Mann–Whitney test, $*p < 0.05$, $***p < 0.005$; error bars indicate Mean ± S.D.). **b-d** eEF2K mRNA expression in control and PD striatum (**b**), medial substantia nigra (**b**) and dorsal nucleus of vagus nerve (**d**). The following publicly available transcriptomic profile datasets were analyzed on the National Center for Biotechnology Information (NCBI) Gene Expression Omnibus (GEO) platform: Striatum (**b**)- dataset GEO accession # GSE28894, Illumina human Ref-8 v2.0 expression beadchip platform, probe ID ILMN_1789171, controls $n = 15$ and PD $n = 15$; Medial substantia nigra (**c**)- dataset GEO accession # GSE8397, Affymetrix Human Genome U133B Array, probe ID 225546_at, controls $n = 8$ and PD $n = 15$; Dorsal nucleus of vagus (**d**)- dataset GEO accession # GSE43490, Agilent-014850 Whole Human Genome Microarray, probe ID A_24_P716162, controls $n = 6$ and PD $n = 7$. (Mann–Whitney test, $*p < 0.05$; error bars in 3b-d indicate Mean ± S.D.). **e** Relative eEF2K mRNA expression in human iPSCs derived cultured midbrain control (WT, $n = 3$) or A53T ($n = 2$) mutation carrying organoids (T-test, $*p < 0.05$; error bars indicate Mean ± S.D.)

the culture medium. LDH is a cytoplasmic enzyme released under conditions of cell membrane damage and during toxic stress in neuronal cultures [37]. As expected, overexpression of ASyn-WT or ASyn-A53T led to increased LDH release (72 h post-transfection), which was reduced significantly by eEF2K kd in both ASyn-WT or ASyn-A53T expressing cells (Fig. 5c). Next, we measured cytotoxicity in these cultures by labelling with propidium iodide (PI), another cell permeable marker of cell death. Overexpression of ASyn-WT or ASyn-A53T resulted in increased cell death (72 h post-transfection), as measured by flow cytometry analysis of PI staining, and eEF2K kd significantly improved viability in these cultures (Fig. 5d).

eEF2K inhibition mitigates AS induced mitochondrial dysfunction and oxidative stress in N2A cells

Next, we assessed whether the cytoprotective effects of eEF2K inhibition against AS toxicity are mediated by changes in mitochondrial function, since AS inhibits mitochondrial respiration and complex I activity [8, 55]. First, we characterized cellular respiration (oxygen consumption rate, OCR) in differentiated N2A cells following eEF2K kd without ASyn overexpression. This is important since eEF2K regulates highly energy consuming process of elongation during mRNA translation, and we wanted to assess if possible metabolic reprogramming in cells due to eEF2K inhibition does not impair mitochondrial function [15, 34]. Intriguingly, N2A cells with eEF2K kd exhibited significantly higher OCR under basal conditions, and maximal respiration subsequent to the treatment with FCCP (uncoupler of oxidative phosphorylation) than control cells (Additional file 1: Figure S9a). To investigate if the increased respiration in eEF2K kd cells under basal conditions is linked to an increase in the mitochondrial mass, we quantified mitochondrial content in control and eEF2K kd cells. However, there were no significant differences in mitochondrial mass by flow cytometry analysis using the fluorescent Mitotracker reagent (Additional file 1: Figure S9b), or by mitochondrial mtDNA quantification (Additional file 1: Figure S9c). These data demonstrate healthy mitochondrial function in eEF2K kd cells, and suggest that, compared to control cells, cellular respiration in eEF2K kd cells is increased predominantly due to enhanced mitochondrial respiration (Additional file 1: Figure S9a; compare changes in basal respiration and maximal respiration in control vs. eEF2K kd cells) without significant changes in mitochondrial content (Additional file 1: Figure S9b-c).

Having established that eEF2K kd per se does not negatively affect mitochondrial function in N2A cells, we proceeded to assess the effects of eEF2K kd on AS induced mitochondrial dysfunction [8, 27]. We investigated this activity in differentiated N2A cells with overexpression of ASyn-WT or ASyn-A53T +/− eEF2K kd (72 h post-transfection). There was a noticeable reduction in basal OCR in cells overexpressing ASyn-WT, or ASyn-A53T compared to mock transfected cells

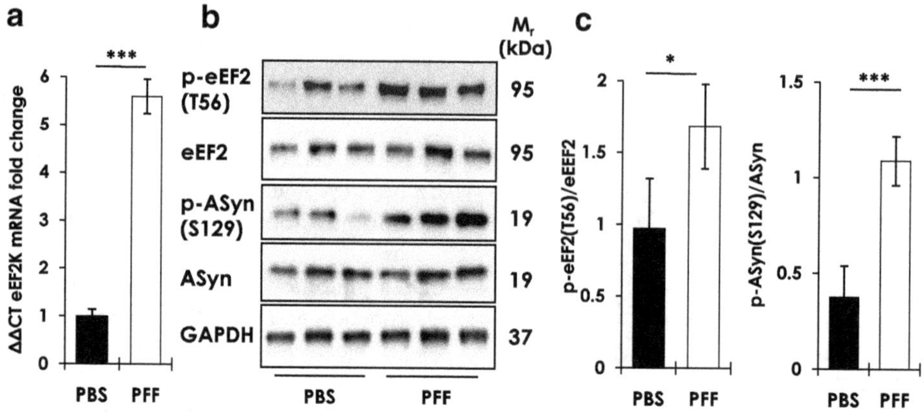

Fig. 4 Brain eEF2K expression and activity in transgenic M83$^{+/+}$ PD mice. **a** eEF2K mRNA levels in whole brain homogenates from transgenic M83$^{+/+}$ PD mice intramuscularly (IM) injected bilaterally with phosphate buffered saline (PBS, $n = 10$) or pre-formed fibrillar (PFF, $n = 13$) mouse wild type AS. (Mann–Whitney test, ***$p < 0.005$; error bars indicate Mean ± S.D.). **b-c** Western blot analysis of p-eEF2 (T56) and p-ASyn (S129) in whole brain homogenates from transgenic M83$^{+/+}$ PD mice intramuscularly (IM) injected bilaterally with phosphate buffered saline (PBS) or pre-formed fibrillar (PFF) mouse wild type AS (**b**), and corresponding densitometry analysis (**c**) ($n = 7$/group; Mann–Whitney test, *$p < 0.05$, ***$p < 0.005$; error bars indicate Mean ± S.D.)

(Fig. 6a). eEF2K kd led to significant improvement of the OCR under all conditions (compare Mock control vs. Mock+sieEF2K, ASyn-WT vs. ASyn-WT + sieEF2K and ASyn-A53T vs. ASyn-A53T + sieEF2K; Fig. 6a). Then, we measured cellular ATP levels under identical conditions, and found that overexpression of ASyn-WT or ASyn-A53T significantly reduced cellular ATP content reflecting AS toxicity (Fig. 6b). While eEF2K kd had negligible effect on ATP content in mock transfected cells, it attenuated the loss of ATP in ASyn overexpressing cells (compare ASyn-WT vs. ASyn-WT + sieEF2K and ASyn-A53T vs. ASyn-A53T + sieEF2K; Fig. 6b). Together, these data suggest that transient AS (WT or A53T) overexpression is associated with mitochondrial dysfunction in these dopaminergic cultures, which is rescued by eEF2K kd.

Mitochondrial dysfunction, including complex I inhibition, is associated with increased production of reactive oxygen species (ROS) and oxidative stress in cells [44]. As mentioned earlier, these processes, i.e., impaired mitochondrial function and increased ROS, are also implicated in AS toxicity [4]. Indeed, previous studies have shown that ROS levels are increased in AS overxpressing cells [27, 32]. Accordingly, we found that overexpression of ASyn-WT or ASyn-A53T increased ROS levels compared with mock transfected cells, as measured by flow cytometry analysis of the ROS detection reagent, DCFDA (Fig. 6c). Moreover, we found that eEF2K kd significantly reduced ROS in these cultures, in line with previously reported effects of eEF2K inhibition on cellular ROS levels [10, 28]. Collectively, these data suggest a role of eEF2K in AS toxicity (Fig. 5a-b), and demonstrate that eEF2K inhibition reduces AS toxicity by improving mitochondrial function and reducing ROS (Fig. 6a-c).

Deletion of efk-1 *improves dopaminergic neuronal function in a C. elegans model of AS neurotoxicity*

To assess the in vivo impact of eEF2K inhibition as a means of improving AS-mediated neurotoxicity, we used a *C. elegans* model of PD. *C. elegans* possess four bilaterally symmetric pairs of dopaminergic neurons that are critical for adaptations to mechanosensory stimuli, and for the regulation of complex behaviours such as foraging, movement, and egg-laying [50, 69]. Accordingly, this worm model is widely used in PD research to investigate the significance of specific mutations and variations, and to screen for candidate disease-modifying small molecules [70]. We studied a previously generated *C. elegans* strain that transgenically expresses human AS A53T mutant, which results in age-related degeneration of dopaminergic neurons and in defects in dopaminergic function in these worms [12]. Using this strain, we assessed dopaminergic neuron function with or without concomitant deletion of *efk-1*, the eEF2K ortholog in worms [(ASyn (A53T) and ASyn (A53T)/efk-1_{del} strains; see Materials and Methods)]. We assessed the effects of *efk-1* deletion in A53T AS expressing worms in three behavioural responses that are considered to be mediated predominantly by dopaminergic neurons in worms: ethanol avoidance, pharyngeal pumping, and area restricted searching (see Materials and Methods). We hypothesized that, in view of the cytoprotective effects of eEF2K inhibition against AS toxicity in cultured dopaminergic N2A cells (Figs. 5-6), *efk-1* deletion would improve AS-A53T-induced dopaminergic neuron dysfunction in worms.

In ethanol avoidance assays, worms exhibit an aversive response to acute ethanol exposure and this response is dependent on adequate sensory motor co-ordination [40]. Notably, *efk-1* deletion alone had no significant effects on this response (Fig. 7a; compare WT (N2) worms with efk-1_{del}), while, as previously reported,

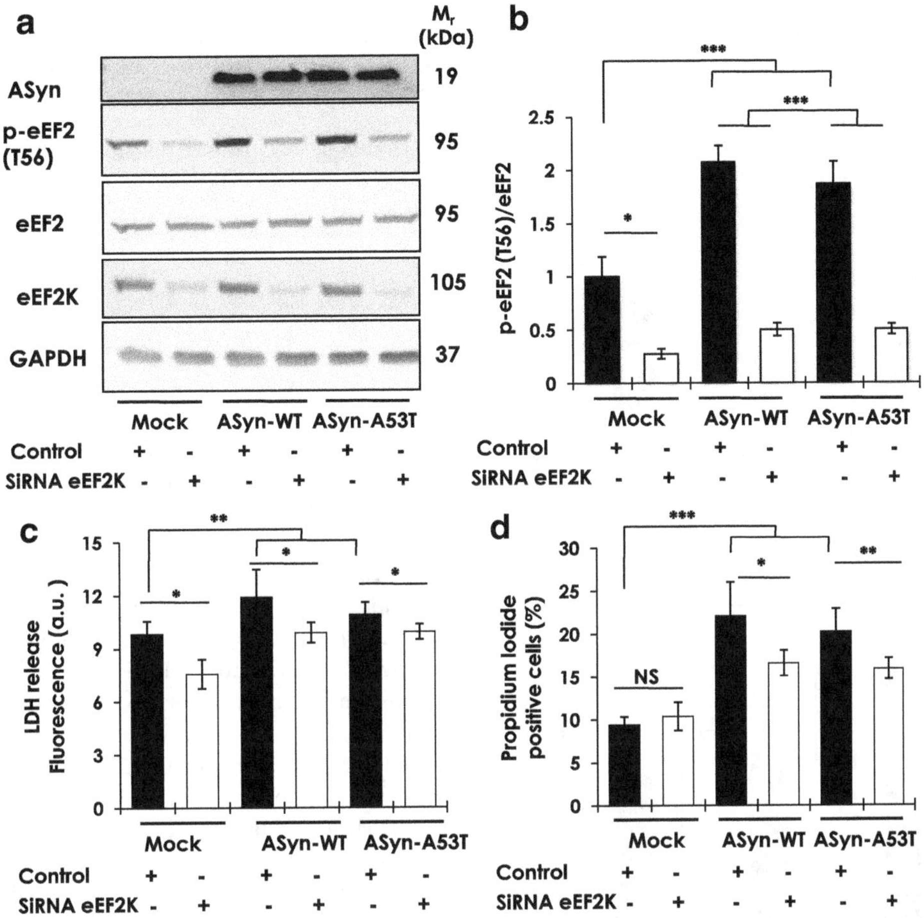

Fig. 5 Effects of eEF2K inhibition on human AS cytotoxicity in differentiated N2A cells. **a**-**b** Western blot analysis of p-eEF2 (T56) levels in N2A cells subsequent to transient overexpression of human wild type or mutant A53T AS, with or without siRNA mediated eEF2K knockdown (**a**), and corresponding densitometry analysis (**b**) ($n = 6$–9/group from three independent experiments; One-way ANOVA *post-hoc* Bonferroni test, $^*p < 0.05$, $^{***}p < 0.005$; error bars indicate Mean ± S.E.M). c Measurements of cytotoxicity by lactate dehydrogenase-LDH release in the culture medium (**c**) and FACS analysis of propidium iodide-PI staining (**d**) in N2A cells subsequent to transient overexpression of human wild type or mutant A53T AS, with or without siRNA mediated eEF2K knockdown ($n = 9$–12/group from three independent experiments; One-way ANOVA *post-hoc* Bonferroni test, $^*p < 0.05$, $^{**}p < 0.01$, $^{***}p < 0.005$, NS = not significant; error bars indicate Mean ± S.D.)

expression of ASyn-A53T led to a worsened response (Fig. 7a) [12]. Importantly, loss of *efk-1* completely rescued the reduced ethanol avoidance of ASyn-A53T expressing worms [(Fig. 7a; compare ASyn (A53T) with ASyn (A53T)/efk-1_{del})]. In pharyngeal pumping assays, rhythmic contractions (pumping) of the pharynx serve as marker of neuromuscular function and rely on a complex neural integration within the autonomic activity [64]. This response is essential for feeding and generation of consequent isthmus peristalsis. As expected, we observed no difference in the pharyngeal pumping activity between wild type worms and worms lacking *efk-1* [(Fig. 7b; compare WT (N2) with efk-1_{del})]. ASyn-A53T expressing worms showed a modest, but significant, reduction in pumping activity, which was restored significantly in ASyn-A53T worms with *efk-1* deletion [(Fig. 7b; compare ASyn (A53T) with ASyn (A53T)/efk-1_{del})]. Finally, the area-restricted search behaviour reflects foraging, such that the worms show an adaptive response by reducing turning frequency to the presence of food; this response is mediated by neural circuits involving dopaminergic and glutamatergic signalling [24]. As seen with the other two assays, *efk-1* deletion alone negligibly affected the performance of worms in the area restricted search assay [(Fig. 7c; compare WT (N2) worms with efk-1_{del})], whereas ASyn-A53T mutant expressing worms showed significant defects in this assay (Fig. 7c) as reported previously [12]. Critically, this defect was completely rescued in ASyn-A53T worms lacking *efk-1* [(Fig. 7c; compare ASyn (A53T) with ASyn (A53T)/efk-1_{del})]. Taken together, *efk-1* deletion improves three independent behaviours known to rely dominantly on normal dopaminergic neuron function. These data support our hypothesis and demonstrate that *efk-1* deletion mitigates the deleterious effects of ASyn (A53T) on the

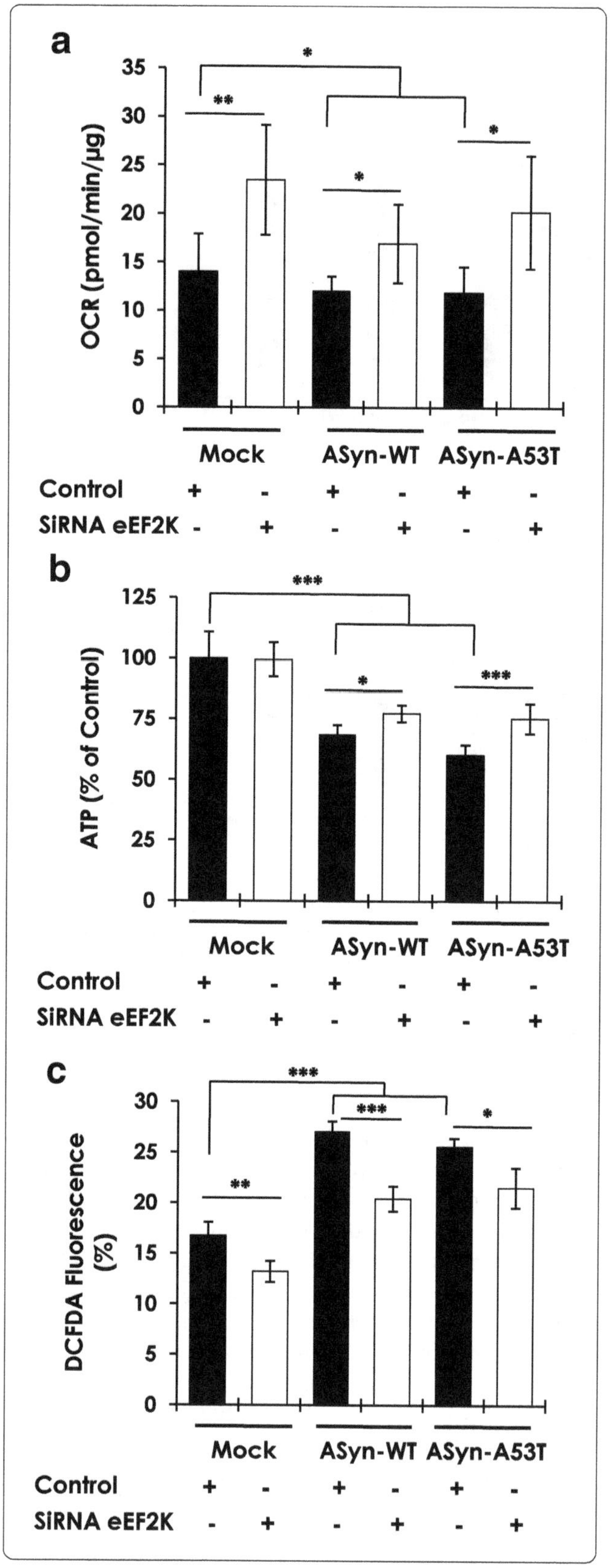

Fig. 6 Effects of eEF2K inhibition on mitochondrial dysfunction and oxidative stress induced by human AS in differentiated N2A cells. **a-b** Measurements of basal oxygen consumption rate-OCR (**b**) and ATP levels (**c**) in N2A cells subsequent to transient overexpression of human wild type or mutant A53T AS, with or without siRNA mediated eEF2K knockdown ($n = 9$–12/group from three independent experiments; Unpaired T-test, $*p < 0.05$, $**p < 0.01$, $***p < 0.005$; error bars indicate Mean ± S.D.). **c** Flow cytometry analysis of reactive oxygen species (ROS), measured by DCFDA staining, in N2A cells subsequent to transient overexpression of human wild type or mutant A53T AS, with or without siRNA mediated eEF2K knockdown ($n = 9$/group from three independent experiments; Unpaired T-test, $*p < 0.05$, $**p < 0.01$, $***p < 0.005$; error bars indicate Mean ± S.D.)

function of neural circuits involving dopaminergic neurons in *C. elegans*, and further point to an in vivo role for eEF2K signaling in AS-mediated neurotoxicity.

Discussion

Principally driven by the early genetic findings in inherited PD and PD neuropathology, a significant effort in the discovery of novel therapies in PD and other synucleinopathies has been to target AS production and/or aggregation [39, 71]. Although such studies have shown promising results in preclinical research, their translation into clinically implementable therapies has yet to be realized [71]. An additional area of research in potential therapies in PD has been to address AS neurotoxicity, and to target cellular mechanisms that potentially render neurons susceptible to AS neurotoxicity [38].

Our data suggest that eEF2K is one possible mechanism that is pathologically involved in AS-mediated toxicity, and that its inhibition represents a novel therapeutic strategy in PD. Our findings demonstrate that eEF2K activity is increased in postmortem PD midbrain (substantia nigra and periaqueductal gray matter) and in hippocampus (CA1 and CA2 regions), with the concomitant presence of Lewy pathology (phosphorylation of AS on Ser-129). Additionally, analysis of publicly available microarray datasets revealed increased eEF2K expression in striatum, medial substantia nigra and dorsal nucleus of vagus (dmX) in PD. Hence, dysregulated eEF2K expression and/or activity are observed in multiple brain regions that are affected in PD. We further show that induction of aggressive AS pathology in $M83^{+/+}$ transgenic PD mice, by intramuscular PFF AS injection, is associated with enhanced brain eEF2K expression and activity. In addition, transient overexpression of AS (WT or A53T mutant) is associated with cytotoxicity and oxidative stress in dopaminergic N2A cells, and leads to eEF2K activation in these cultures. Moreover, eEF2K inhibition mitigated the cytotoxic effects of AS overexpression in cells and prevented the deficits in dopaminergic function in *C. elegans* due to transgenic AS-A53T expression. These observations are supported by previous reports showing that eEF2K

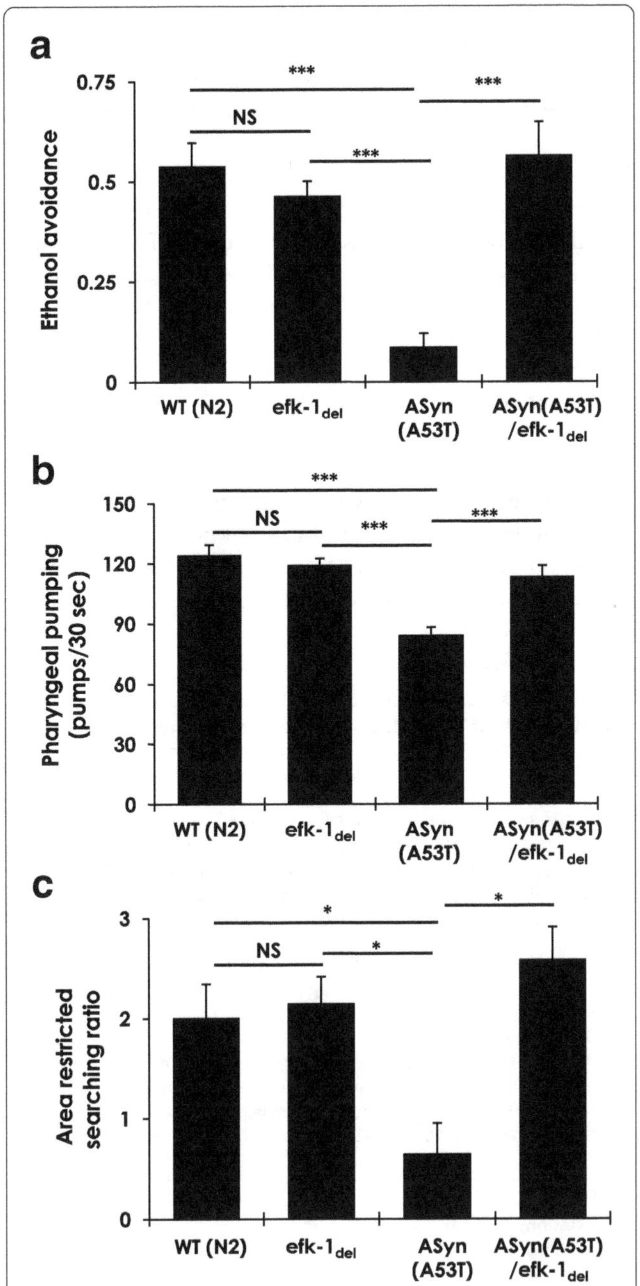

Fig. 7 Effects of efk-1 deletion on ethanol avoidance, pharyngeal pumping, and area restricted searching behavior in *C. elegans* expressing human AS-A53T. **a-c** Analysis of ethanol avoidance ($n = 100$–150 worms/measurement) (**a**), pharyngeal pumping ($n = 10$–15 worms/measurement) (**b**), and area restricted searching behavior ($n = 10$–15 worms/measurement) (**c**) in control (wild type N2) worms, in *efk-1(ok3609)* null mutant worms (efk-1_{del}), in worms expressing human mutant AS-A53T (*Pdat-1::a-synuclein[A53T]*), and in *efk-1(ok3609)* null mutant worms expressing AS-A53T (*efk-1(ok3609); Pdat-1::a-synuclein[A53T]*). Statistical analysis: one-way ANOVA with post-hoc Bonferroni test; $*p < 0.05$, $***p < 0.005$, NS = not significant; error bars indicate mean ± S.E.M. from at least three independent experiments

inhibition reduces oxidative and ER stress, processes associated with AS toxicity [6, 10, 28].

It is noteworthy that brain areas showing increased eEF2K activity in PD cases examined here are part of distinct neurotransmitter networks that are affected at different neuropathological stages in PD [7, 65]. Considering the neuronal populations found in these distinct anatomical brain areas and their connectivity, it has been postulated that the clinical spectrum of PD symptoms (i.e., motor, autonomic or cognitive) may arise depending on the extent of Lewy pathology and/or cell loss [7, 33]. From a neurological perspective, it is commonly thought that the lesions in the striatum or substantia nigra underlie the motor symptoms due to neurotransmitter imbalance in the nigrostriatal system causing defective motor control and muscle tone, and this assertion is supported by the studies in animal models [18]. Furthermore, the loss of cholinergic projections from dorsal nucleus of vagus (dmX) is implicated in the autonomic dysfunction in PD [65]. The periaqueductal gray (PAG) matter is also affected with AS inclusions in PD, Dementia with Lewy bodies (DLB), and Multiple system atrophy (MSA) [61]. This cell dense region harbours many distinct neuronal populations with projections linking forebrain and lower brain stem, and in mammals is involved in autonomic control, cardiovascular function, pain modulation, wakefulness, rapid eye movement (REM) sleep and vocalization [55]. Finally, Lewy body pathology is present in hippocampus at advanced neuropathological stages in PD, and thought to underlie cognitive symptoms [7, 33, 65].

The significance of enhanced eEF2K expression and/or activity in the aforementioned brain areas in PD remains unknown. Given the critical role of eEF2K in dendritic mRNA transaltion and synaptic integrity [34], it is plausible that aberrant eEF2K activity may underlie the dysfunction in these neuronal populations. Supporting this, some studies suggest a role for eEF2K in synaptic plasticity, in particular mGluR5-mediated long-term depression [66], a mechanism purported to underlie synaptic dysfunction in AD and other neuropsychiatric conditions [11]. Furthermore, eEF2K activity is also increased upon exposure to excitatory stimuli in neuronal cultures [23, 35, 66], and in response to nutrient deprivation (by energy sensor AMP-activated kinase). However, it remains to be established whether some of the aforementioned stimuli enhancing eEF2K activity also underlie increased eEF2K activity in PD. In this regard, activity of AMP-kinase, an important regulator of eEF2K in response to metabolic stimuli, is increased in cells and/or rodents after exposure to mitochondrial toxins (e.g., MPTP, rotenone) [9, 36]. In postmortem PD brain, activated AMPK has been detected near the rim of Lewy bodies in the cytoplasm as opposed to nuclear staining in controls [30]. However, the beneficial effects of AMPK inhibition in PD models have not been conclusively established [17], and in some studies

AMPK activation is protective [51]. A recent report showed aberrations in the expression of factors controlling protein synthesis (e.g., ribosomal proteins, translation initiation and elongation factors) in postrmortem PD brain, including reduced eEF2 levels in PD midbrain and cortex [19], supporting the notion of dysregulated mRNA translation in PD. Determining whether increased eEF2K activity plays a role in the synaptic defects of PD, or occurs due to aberrations within the translational machinery, represents a challenging task due to the complex nature of PD etiology and the possible involvement of multiple neurotransmitter systems as the disease progresses. For simplicity, it is plausible to suggest that increased eEF2K activity may be part of some stress-adaptive pathway, which plays a protective role in the short term under disturbed cellular homeostasis. However, chronic overactivation of this pathway in pathological states may be detrimental due to aberrations in mRNA translation and dendritic protein synthesis [28, 46].

From a therapeutic perspective, development of novel eEF2K inhibitors is actively being pursued towards novel experimental therapies in cancer due to its role in metabolic adaptations in cancer cells for survival under nutrient deprivation, including nervous system malignancies [16, 34, 42]. Here, we show that eEF2K inhibition augments mitochondrial respiration, reduces oxidative stress and prevents AS toxicity in dopaminergic N2A cells. The mechanism of increased mitochondrial function subsequent to eEF2K inhibition in dopaminergic N2A cells remains to be deciphered. We previously reported that eEF2K inhibition in dopaminergic N2A cells induces an NRF2 antioxidant response, and blocks the toxicity of Aβ oligomers in neuronal cultures [28]. NRF2 is a master regulator of cellular redox homeostasis under physiological and pathological conditions due to its ability in controlling the expression of antioxidant genes [31]. However, NRF2 is also known to regulate cellular metabolism (e.g., glutamine biogenesis), and affects mitochondrial structure and function such as ATP production, fatty acid oxidation and structural integrity [26, 48]. Accordingly, cells and mitochondria derived from NRF2 knockout mice show reduced respiration, lower ATP levels and impairments in mitochondrial fatty acid oxidation [25, 45]. Furthermore, several small molecules activators of NRF2 pathway have shown beneficial effects in restoring mitochondrial function under conditions of redox stress in cell cultures, and also in models of neurodegenerative diseases [26]. One such therapeutic molecule, dimethyl fumarate (DMF, Tecfidera), used to treat multiple sclerosis, exerts anti-inflammatory and antioxidant effects in cell culture and animal studies by activating NRF2 antioxidant response [1]. DMT administration prevents neurodegeneration in mice treated with MPTP [71], a mitochondrial toxin associated with chemically induced parkinsonism in humans and animals [1]. In this context, our findings raise the possibility that eEF2K can also be targeted in PD to mitigate AS-induced oxidative stress, and potentially neuronal dysfunction in this disease.

Conclusion

By employing multiple experimental models, our data support the relevance of eEF2K in PD, and of eEF2K inhibition in mitigating AS-induced oxidative stress and neuronal dysfunction. We anticipate that our findings will stimulate further mechanistic studies and a careful evaluation of eEF2K inhibition in PD, and potentially other neurodegenerative diseases.

Endnotes

[1]The term eEF2K activity in this manuscript denotes phosphorylation of eEF2, the major known substrate for eEF2K, on serine residue 56 assessed by immunohistochemistry, immunofluorescence or western blot.

Additional file

Additional file 1: Table S1. Control and PD cases; **Figure S1.** Melanin bleaching in postmortem midbrain sections and immunostaining for phospho-eEF2 (p-eEF2, Thr56); **Figure S2.** Immunostaining for phospho-eEF2 (p-eEF2, Thr56) and phospho-AS (p-ASyn, Ser129) in postmortem control midbrain sections; **Figure S3.** Immunostaining for phospho-eEF2 (p-eEF2, Thr56) and phospho-AS (p-ASyn, Ser129) in postmortem PD midbrain sections; **Figure S4.** Detection of phospho-eEF2 (p-eEF2, Thr56) and phospho-AS (p-ASyn, Ser129) in postmortem control and PD midbrain sections by immunofluorescence; **Figure S5.** Immunostaining for phospho-eEF2 (p-eEF2, Thr56) and phospho-AS (p-ASyn, Ser129) in postmortem control hippocampus sections; **Figure S6.** Immunostaining for phospho-eEF2 (p-eEF2, Thr56) in postmortem PD hippocampus sections-Panoramic views; **Figure S7.** Immunostaining for phospho-eEF2 (p-eEF2, Thr56) and phospho-AS (p-ASyn, Ser129) in postmortem PD hippocampus sections; **Figure S8.** Effects of intramuscularly injected pre-formed fibrillar (PFF) AS on motor phenotype and survival of transgenic M83+/+ PD mice and **Figure S9.** Mitochondrial respiration and mitochondrial mass in differentiated N2A cells subsequent to eEF2K knockdown. (PDF 2444 kb).

Abbreviations

AD: Alzheimer disease; AS: Alpha synuclein; eEF2: Eukaryotic elongation factor-2; eEF2K: Eukaryotic elongation factor-2 kinase; MPTP: 1-methyl-4-phenyl-1,2,3,6-tetrahydropyridine; PD: Parkinson disease; PFF: Pre-formed fibrils; ROS: Reactive oxygen species

Acknowledgements

The authors would like to thank following individuals their help and assistance during the study: (BCCRC) Amy Li, Jordan Cran, Bo Rafn, and Shawn Chafe, (PHJ lab) Rikke Hahn Kofoed.

Funding

This work was supported by funding to AJ in the form of AIAS-COFUND fellowship from European Union's Horizon 2020 Research and Innovation Programme under the Marie Skłodowska-Curie agreement (grant #754513) and the Lundbeckfonden, Denmark (grant #R250–2017-1131), Research grants to PHS from the Ride2Survive Brain Cancer Impact Grant of the Canadian Cancer Society and Brain Canada (grant #703205) and funds from the BC Cancer Foundation, Research support to ST by the Canadian Research Chair in Transcriptional Regulatory Networks and Canadian Institutes of Health Research Project Grant (grant #PJT-153199), NSERC USRA scholarship to YAN, and support to PHJ by Lundbeckfonden Grant (grant # DANDRITE-R248-2016-2518 and R171-2014-591).

Authors' contributions

AJ, AD, BJ, ST and PHS designed the research, AJ, AD, BJ, FB, YAN, LMS and NF performed research, GLN helped with experimental design and dataset analysis, IM provided human postmortem research material, JCS provided research material from iPSCs derived midbrain organoids, and AJ, ST and PHS wrote the manuscript. AD and BJ contributed equally to this work. All authors read and approved the final manuscript.

Authors' information

AJ was formerly a Postdoctoral Fellow in the research laboratory of PHS at the University of British Columbia (Canada), and since October 2017 is affiliated with Aarhus University (Denmark) as AIAS-COFUND Junior Research Fellow.

Competing interests

The authors declare that they have no competing interests.

Author details

[1]Aarhus Institute of Advanced Studies, Department of Biomedicine, Aarhus University, Høegh-Guldbergs Gade 6B, DK-8000 Aarhus, Denmark. [2]Department of Pathology and Laboratory Medicine, University of British Columbia, Vancouver, Canada. [3]British Columbia Cancer Research Centre, 675 West 10th Avenue, Vancouver, BC V5Z 1L3, Canada. [4]Centre for Molecular Medicine and Therapeutics, BC Children's Hospital Research Institute, Department of Medical Genetics, University of British Columbia, Vancouver, BC V5Z 4H4, Canada. [5]Danish Research Institute of Translational Neuroscience, Department of Biomedicine, Aarhus University, Ole Worms Allé 3, DK-8000 Aarhus, Denmark. [6]Developmental and Cellular Biology, Luxembourg Centre for Systems Biomedicine (LCSB), University of Luxembourg, 7, avenue des Hauts-Fourneaux, 4362 Esch-sur-Alzette, Luxembourg.

References

1. Ahuja M, Ammal Kaidery N, Yang L, Calingasan N, Smirnova N, Gaisin A, Gaisina IN, Gazaryan I, Hushpulian DM, Kaddour-Djebbar I et al (2016) Distinct Nrf2 Signaling Mechanisms of Fumaric Acid Esters and Their Role in Neuroprotection against 1-Methyl-4-Phenyl-1,2,3,6-Tetrahydropyridine-Induced Experimental Parkinson's-Like Disease. J Neurosci 36:6332–6351. https://doi.org/10.1523/JNEUROSCI.0426-16.2016
2. Anderson JP, Walker DE, Goldstein JM, de Laat R, Banducci K, Caccavello RJ, Barbour R, Huang J, Kling K, Lee M et al (2006) Phosphorylation of Ser-129 is the dominant pathological modification of alpha-synuclein in familial and sporadic Lewy body disease. J Biol Chem 281:29739–29752. https://doi.org/10.1074/jbc.M600933200
3. Arias-Fuenzalida J, Jarazo J, Qing X, Walter J, Gomez-Giro G, Nickels SL, Zaehres H, Scholer HR, Schwamborn JC (2017) FACS-assisted CRISPR-Cas9 genome editing facilitates Parkinson's disease modeling. Stem Cell Rep 9: 1423–1431. https://doi.org/10.1016/j.stemcr.2017.08.026
4. Behbehani MM (1995) Functional characteristics of the midbrain periaqueductal gray. Prog Neurobiol 46:575–605
5. Bose A, Beal MF (2016) Mitochondrial dysfunction in Parkinson's disease. J Neurochem 139(Suppl 1):216–231. https://doi.org/10.1111/jnc.13731
6. Boyce M, Py BF, Ryazanov AG, Minden JS, Long K, Ma D, Yuan J (2008) A pharmacoproteomic approach implicates eukaryotic elongation factor 2 kinase in ER stress-induced cell death. Cell Death Differ 15:589–599. https://doi.org/10.1038/sj.cdd.4402296
7. Braak H, Del Tredici K, Rub U, de Vos RA, Jansen Steur EN, Braak E (2003) Staging of brain pathology related to sporadic Parkinson's disease. Neurobiol Aging 24:197–211
8. Chinta SJ, Mallajosyula JK, Rane A, Andersen JK (2010) Mitochondrial alpha-synuclein accumulation impairs complex I function in dopaminergic neurons and results in increased mitophagy in vivo. Neurosci Lett 486:235–239. https://doi.org/10.1016/j.neulet.2010.09.061
9. Choi JS, Park C, Jeong JW (2010) AMP-activated protein kinase is activated in Parkinson's disease models mediated by 1-methyl-4-phenyl-1,2,3,6-tetrahydropyridine. Biochem Biophys Res Commun 391:147–151. https://doi.org/10.1016/j.bbrc.2009.11.022
10. Chu HP, Liao Y, Novak JS, Hu Z, Merkin JJ, Shymkiv Y, Braeckman BP, Dorovkov MV, Nguyen A, Clifford PM et al (2014) Germline quality control: eEF2K stands guard to eliminate defective oocytes. Dev Cell 28:561–572. https://doi.org/10.1016/j.devcel.2014.01.027
11. Collingridge GL, Peineau S, Howland JG, Wang YT (2010) Long-term depression in the CNS. Nat Rev Neurosci 11:459–473. https://doi.org/10.1038/nrn2867
12. Cooper JF, Dues DJ, Spielbauer KK, Machiela E, Senchuk MM, Van Raamsdonk JM (2015) Delaying aging is neuroprotective in Parkinson's disease: a genetic analysis in C. Elegans models. NPJ Parkinsons Dis 1:15022. https://doi.org/10.1038/npjparkd.2015.22
13. Cooper JF, Machiela E, Dues DJ, Spielbauer KK, Senchuk MM, Van Raamsdonk JM (2017) Activation of the mitochondrial unfolded protein response promotes longevity and dopamine neuron survival in Parkinson's disease models. Sci Rep 7: 16441. https://doi.org/10.1038/s41598-017-16637-2
14. Dahlgren KN, Manelli AM, Stine WB Jr, Baker LK, Krafft GA, LaDu MJ (2002) Oligomeric and fibrillar species of amyloid-beta peptides differentially affect neuronal viability. JBiolChem 277:32046–32053
15. De Gassart A, Martinon F (2017) Translating the anticancer properties of eEF2K. Cell Cycle 16:299–300. https://doi.org/10.1080/15384101.2016.1254974
16. Delaidelli A, Negri GL, Jan A, Jansonius B, El-Naggar A, Lim JKM, Khan D, Zarni Oo H, Carnie CJ, Remke M et al (2017) MYCN amplified neuroblastoma requires the mRNA translation regulator eEF2 kinase to adapt to nutrient deprivation. Cell Death Differ 24:1564–1576. https://doi.org/10.1038/cdd.2017.79
17. Domise M, Vingtdeux V (2016) AMPK in neurodegenerative diseases. EXS 107:153–177. https://doi.org/10.1007/978-3-319-43589-3_7
18. Duty S, Jenner P (2011) Animal models of Parkinson's disease: a source of novel treatments and clues to the cause of the disease. Br J Pharmacol 164: 1357–1391. https://doi.org/10.1111/j.1476-5381.2011.01426.x
19. Garcia-Esparcia P, Hernandez-Ortega K, Koneti A, Gil L, Delgado-Morales R, Castano E, Carmona M, Ferrer I (2015) Altered machinery of protein synthesis is region- and stage-dependent and is associated with alpha-synuclein oligomers in Parkinson's disease. Acta Neuropathol Commun 3:76. https://doi.org/10.1186/s40478-015-0257-4
20. Giasson BI, Duda JE, Quinn SM, Zhang B, Trojanowski JQ, Lee VM (2002) Neuronal alpha-synucleinopathy with severe movement disorder in mice expressing A53T human alpha-synuclein. Neuron 34:521–533
21. Haas RH, Nasirian F, Nakano K, Ward D, Pay M, Hill R, Shults CW (1995) Low platelet mitochondrial complex I and complex II/III activity in early untreated Parkinson's disease. Ann Neurol 37:714–722. https://doi.org/10.1002/ana.410370604
22. Hatzipetros T, Kidd JD, Moreno AJ, Thompson K, Gill A, Vieira FG (2015) A Quick Phenotypic Neurological Scoring System for Evaluating Disease Progression in the SOD1-G93A Mouse Model of ALS. J Vis Exp. https://doi.org/10.3791/53257
23. Heise C, Gardoni F, Culotta L, di Luca M, Verpelli C, Sala C (2014) Elongation factor-2 phosphorylation in dendrites and the regulation of dendritic mRNA translation in neurons. Front Cell Neurosci 8:35. https://doi.org/10.3389/fncel.2014.00035
24. Hills T, Brockie PJ, Maricq AV (2004) Dopamine and glutamate control area-restricted search behavior in Caenorhabditis elegans. J Neurosci 24:1217–1225. https://doi.org/10.1523/JNEUROSCI.1569-03.2004
25. Holmstrom KM, Baird L, Zhang Y, Hargreaves I, Chalasani A, Land JM, Stanyer L, Yamamoto M, Dinkova-Kostova AT, Abramov AY (2013) Nrf2 impacts cellular bioenergetics by controlling substrate availability for mitochondrial respiration. Biol Open 2:761–770. https://doi.org/10.1242/bio.20134853
26. Holmstrom KM, Kostov RV, Dinkova-Kostova AT (2016) The multifaceted role of Nrf2 in mitochondrial function. Curr Opin Toxicol 1:80–91. https://doi.org/10.1016/j.cotox.2016.10.002 S2468-2020(16)30025-0
27. Hsu LJ, Sagara Y, Arroyo A, Rockenstein E, Sisk A, Mallory M, Wong J, Takenouchi T, Hashimoto M, Masliah E (2000) Alpha-synuclein promotes mitochondrial deficit and oxidative stress. Am J Pathol 157:401–410
28. Jan A, Jansonius B, Delaidelli A, Somasekharan SP, Bhanshali F, Vandal M, Negri GL, Moerman D, MacKenzie I, Calon F et al (2017) eEF2K inhibition blocks Abeta42 neurotoxicity by promoting an NRF2 antioxidant response. Acta Neuropathol 133:101–119. https://doi.org/10.1007/s00401-016-1634-1
29. Janetzky B, Hauck S, Youdim MB, Riederer P, Jellinger K, Pantucek F, Zochling R, Boissl KW, Reichmann H (1994) Unaltered aconitase activity, but

decreased complex I activity in substantia nigra pars compacta of patients with Parkinson's disease. Neurosci Lett 169:126–128
30. Jiang P, Gan M, Ebrahim AS, Castanedes-Casey M, Dickson DW, Yen SH (2013) Adenosine monophosphate-activated protein kinase overactivation leads to accumulation of alpha-synuclein oligomers and decrease of neurites. Neurobiol Aging 34:1504–1515. https://doi.org/10.1016/j.neurobiolaging.2012.11.001
31. Johnson DA, Johnson JA (2015) Nrf2–a therapeutic target for the treatment of neurodegenerative diseases. Free Radic Biol Med 88:253–267. https://doi.org/10.1016/j.freeradbiomed.2015.07.147
32. Junn E, Mouradian MM (2002) Human alpha-synuclein over-expression increases intracellular reactive oxygen species levels and susceptibility to dopamine. Neurosci Lett 320:146–150
33. Kalia LV, Lang AE (2015) Parkinson's disease. Lancet 386:896–912. https://doi.org/10.1016/S0140-6736(14)61393-3
34. Kenney JW, Moore CE, Wang X, Proud CG (2014) Eukaryotic elongation factor 2 kinase, an unusual enzyme with multiple roles. Adv Biol Regul 55: 15–27. https://doi.org/10.1016/j.jbior.2014.04.003
35. Kenney JW, Sorokina O, Genheden M, Sorokin A, Armstrong JD, Proud CG (2015) Dynamics of elongation factor 2 kinase regulation in cortical neurons in response to synaptic activity. J Neurosci 35:3034–3047. https://doi.org/10.1523/JNEUROSCI.2866-14.2015
36. Kim TW, Cho HM, Choi SY, Suguira Y, Hayasaka T, Setou M, Koh HC, Hwang EM, Park JY, Kang SJ et al (2013) (ADP-ribose) polymerase 1 and AMP-activated protein kinase mediate progressive dopaminergic neuronal degeneration in a mouse model of Parkinson's disease. Cell Death Dis 4: e919. https://doi.org/10.1038/cddis.2013.447
37. Koh JY, Choi DW (1987) Quantitative determination of glutamate mediated cortical neuronal injury in cell culture by lactate dehydrogenase efflux assay. J Neurosci Methods 20:83–90
38. Kones R (2010) Mitochondrial therapy for Parkinson's disease: neuroprotective pharmaconutrition may be disease-modifying. Clin Pharmacol 2:185–198. https://doi.org/10.2147/CPAA.S12082 cpaa-2-185
39. Lashuel HA, Overk CR, Oueslati A, Masliah E (2013) The many faces of alpha-synuclein: from structure and toxicity to therapeutic target. Nat Rev Neurosci 14:38–48. https://doi.org/10.1038/nrn3406
40. Lee J, Jee C, McIntire SL (2009) Ethanol preference in C. Elegans. Genes Brain Behav 8:578–585. https://doi.org/10.1111/j.1601-183X.2009.00513.x
41. Lee MK, Stirling W, Xu Y, Xu X, Qui D, Mandir AS, Dawson TM, Copeland NG, Jenkins NA, Price DL (2002) Human alpha-synuclein-harboring familial Parkinson's disease-linked Ala-53 –> Thr mutation causes neurodegenerative disease with alpha-synuclein aggregation in transgenic mice. Proc Natl Acad Sci U S A 99:8968–8973. https://doi.org/10.1073/pnas.132197599
42. Leprivier G, Remke M, Rotblat B, Dubuc A, Mateo AR, Kool M, Agnihotri S, El-Naggar A, Yu B, Somasekharan SP et al (2013) The eEF2 kinase confers resistance to nutrient deprivation by blocking translation elongation. Cell 153:1064–1079. https://doi.org/10.1016/j.cell.2013.04.055
43. Li X, Alafuzoff I, Soininen H, Winblad B, Pei JJ (2005) Levels of mTOR and its downstream targets 4E-BP1, eEF2, and eEF2 kinase in relationships with tau in Alzheimer's disease brain. FEBS J 272:4211–4220. https://doi.org/10.1111/j.1742-4658.2005.04833.x
44. Lin MT, Beal MF (2006) Mitochondrial dysfunction and oxidative stress in neurodegenerative diseases. Nature 443:787–795. https://doi.org/10.1038/nature05292
45. Ludtmann MH, Angelova PR, Zhang Y, Abramov AY, Dinkova-Kostova AT (2014) Nrf2 affects the efficiency of mitochondrial fatty acid oxidation. Biochem J 457:415–424. https://doi.org/10.1042/BJ20130863
46. Ma T, Chen Y, Vingtdeux V, Zhao H, Viollet B, Marambaud P, Klann E (2014) Inhibition of AMP-activated protein kinase signaling alleviates impairments in hippocampal synaptic plasticity induced by amyloid beta. J Neurosci 34: 12230–12238. https://doi.org/10.1523/JNEUROSCI.1694-14.2014
47. Malik AN, Czajka A, Cunningham P (2016) Accurate quantification of mouse mitochondrial DNA without co-amplification of nuclear mitochondrial insertion sequences. Mitochondrion 29:59–64. https://doi.org/10.1016/j.mito.2016.05.003
48. Mitsuishi Y, Taguchi K, Kawatani Y, Shibata T, Nukiwa T, Aburatani H, Yamamoto M, Motohashi H (2012) Nrf2 redirects glucose and glutamine into anabolic pathways in metabolic reprogramming. Cancer Cell 22:66–79. https://doi.org/10.1016/j.ccr.2012.05.016
49. Monzel AS, Smits LM, Hemmer K, Hachi S, Moreno EL, van Wuellen T, Jarazo J, Walter J, Bruggemann I, Boussaad I et al (2017) Derivation of Human Midbrain-Specific Organoids from Neuroepithelial Stem Cells. Stem Cell Reports 8:1144–1154. https://doi.org/10.1016/j.stemcr.2017.03.010
50. Nass R, Blakely RD (2003) The Caenorhabditis elegans dopaminergic system: opportunities for insights into dopamine transport and neurodegeneration. Annu Rev Pharmacol Toxicol 43:521–544. https://doi.org/10.1146/annurev.pharmtox.43.100901.135934
51. Ng CH, Guan MS, Koh C, Ouyang X, Yu F, Tan EK, O'Neill SP, Zhang X, Chung J, Lim KL (2012) AMP kinase activation mitigates dopaminergic dysfunction and mitochondrial abnormalities in Drosophila models of Parkinson's disease. J Neurosci 32:14311–14317. https://doi.org/10.1523/JNEUROSCI.0499-12.2012
52. Orchard GE, Calonje E (1998) The effect of melanin bleaching on immunohistochemical staining in heavily pigmented melanocytic neoplasms. Am J Dermatopathol 20:357–361
53. Poewe W, Seppi K, Tanner CM, Halliday GM, Brundin P, Volkmann J, Schrag AE, Lang AE (2017) Parkinson disease. Nat Rev Dis Primers 3:17013. https://doi.org/10.1038/nrdp.2017.13
54. Polymeropoulos MH, Lavedan C, Leroy E, Ide SE, Dehejia A, Dutra A, Pike B, Root H, Rubenstein J, Boyer R et al (1997) Mutation in the alpha-synuclein gene identified in families with Parkinson's disease. Science 276:2045–2047
55. Reeve AK, Ludtmann MH, Angelova PR, Simcox EM, Horrocks MH, Klenerman D, Gandhi S, Turnbull DM, Abramov AY (2015) Aggregated alpha-synuclein and complex I deficiency: exploration of their relationship in differentiated neurons. Cell Death Dis 6:e1820. https://doi.org/10.1038/cddis.2015.166
56. Ryan SD, Dolatabadi N, Chan SF, Zhang X, Akhtar MW, Parker J, Soldner F, Sunico CR, Nagar S, Talantova M et al (2013) Isogenic human iPSC Parkinson's model shows nitrosative stress-induced dysfunction in MEF2-PGC1alpha transcription. Cell 155:1351–1364. https://doi.org/10.1016/j.cell.2013.11.009
57. Ryazanov AG (2002) Elongation factor-2 kinase and its newly discovered relatives. FEBS Lett 514:26–29
58. Sacino AN, Brooks M, Thomas MA, McKinney AB, Lee S, Regenhardt RW, McGarvey NH, Ayers JI, Notterpek L, Borchelt DR et al (2014) Intramuscular injection of alpha-synuclein induces CNS alpha-synuclein pathology and a rapid-onset motor phenotype in transgenic mice. Proc Natl Acad Sci U S A 111:10732–10737. https://doi.org/10.1073/pnas.1321785111
59. Schapira AH (2008) Mitochondria in the aetiology and pathogenesis of Parkinson's disease. Lancet Neurol 7:97–109. https://doi.org/10.1016/S1474-4422(07)70327-7
60. Schapira AH, Cooper JM, Dexter D, Jenner P, Clark JB, Marsden CD (1989) Mitochondrial complex I deficiency in Parkinson's disease. Lancet 1:1269
61. Seidel K, Mahlke J, Siswanto S, Kruger R, Heinsen H, Auburger G, Bouzrou M, Grinberg LT, Wicht H, Korf HW et al (2015) The brainstem pathologies of Parkinson's disease and dementia with Lewy bodies. Brain Pathol 25:121–135. https://doi.org/10.1111/bpa.12168
62. Spillantini MG, Schmidt ML, Lee VM, Trojanowski JQ, Jakes R, Goedert M (1997) Alpha-synuclein in Lewy bodies. Nature 388:839–840. https://doi.org/10.1038/42166
63. Tremblay RG, Sikorska M, Sandhu JK, Lanthier P, Ribecco-Lutkiewicz M, Bani-Yaghoub M (2010) Differentiation of mouse Neuro 2A cells into dopamine neurons. J Neurosci Methods 186:60–67. https://doi.org/10.1016/j.jneumeth.2009.11.004
64. Trojanowski NF, Raizen DM, Fang-Yen C (2016) Pharyngeal pumping in Caenorhabditis elegans depends on tonic and phasic signaling from the nervous system. Sci Rep 6:22940. https://doi.org/10.1038/srep22940
65. Uchihara T, Giasson BI (2016) Propagation of alpha-synuclein pathology: hypotheses, discoveries, and yet unresolved questions from experimental and human brain studies. Acta Neuropathol 131:49–73. https://doi.org/10.1007/s00401-015-1485-1
66. Um JW, Kaufman AC, Kostylev M, Heiss JK, Stagi M, Takahashi H, Kerrisk ME, Vortmeyer A, Wisniewski T, Koleske AJ et al (2013) Metabotropic glutamate receptor 5 is a coreceptor for Alzheimer abeta oligomer bound to cellular prion protein. Neuron 79:887–902. https://doi.org/10.1016/j.neuron.2013.06.036

67. Vekrellis K, Xilouri M, Emmanouilidou E, Rideout HJ, Stefanis L (2011) Pathological roles of alpha-synuclein in neurological disorders. Lancet Neurol 10:1015–1025. https://doi.org/10.1016/S1474-4422(11)70213-7
68. Wang X, Yan MH, Fujioka H, Liu J, Wilson-Delfosse A, Chen SG, Perry G, Casadesus G, Zhu X (2012) LRRK2 regulates mitochondrial dynamics and function through direct interaction with DLP1. Hum Mol Genet 21:1931–1944. https://doi.org/10.1093/hmg/dds003
69. White JG, Southgate E, Thomson JN, Brenner S (1986) The structure of the nervous system of the nematode Caenorhabditis elegans. Philos Trans R Soc Lond Ser B Biol Sci 314:1–340
70. Wolozin B, Gabel C, Ferree A, Guillily M, Ebata A (2011) Watching worms whither: modeling neurodegeneration in *C. elegans*. Prog Mol Biol Transl Sci 100:499–514. https://doi.org/10.1016/B978-0-12-384878-9.00015-7
71. Wong YC, Krainc D (2017) Alpha-synuclein toxicity in neurodegeneration: mechanism and therapeutic strategies. Nat Med 23:1–13. https://doi.org/10.1038/nm.4269

5

Ablation of tau causes an olfactory deficit in a murine model of Parkinson's disease

Leah C. Beauchamp[1,2], Jacky Chan[1], Lin W. Hung[1], Benjamin S. Padman[3], Laura J. Vella[1], Xiang M. Liu[1], Bradley Coleman[4], Ashley I. Bush[1], Michael Lazarou[3], Andrew F. Hill[4,5], Laura Jacobson[1,2] and Kevin J. Barnham[1,2*]

Abstract

Parkinson's disease is diagnosed upon the presentation of motor symptoms, resulting from substantial degeneration of dopaminergic neurons in the midbrain. Prior to diagnosis, there is a lengthy prodromal stage in which non-motor symptoms, including olfactory deficits (hyposmia), develop. There is limited information about non-motor impairments and there is a need for directed research into these early pathogenic cellular pathways that precede extensive dopaminergic death in the midbrain. The protein tau has been identified as a genetic risk factor in the development of sporadic PD. Tau knockout mice have been reported as an age-dependent model of PD, and this study has demonstrated that they develop motor deficits at 15-months-old. We have shown that at 7-month-old tau knockout mice present with an overt hyposmic phenotype. This olfactory deficit correlates with an accumulation of α-synuclein, as well as autophagic impairment, in the olfactory bulb. This pathological feature becomes apparent in the striatum and substantia nigra of 15-month-old tau knockout mice, suggesting the potential for a spread of disease. Initial primary cell culture experiments have demonstrated that ablation of tau results in the release of α-synuclein enriched exosomes, providing a potential mechanism for disease spread. These alterations in α-synuclein level as well as a marked autophagy impairment in the tau knockout primary cells recapitulate results seen in the animal model. These data implicate a pathological role for tau in early Parkinson's disease.

Keywords: Tau, Parkinson's disease, Olfaction, Autophagy, Neurodegeneration

Introduction

Parkinson's disease (PD) is a neurodegenerative disease primarily associated with neuronal degeneration of the Substantia Nigra pars compacta (SN). The disease results in severe motor deficits, as the degenerating neurons cannot provide sufficient dopamine, a neurotransmitter that helps control movement, to the axonal terminals located in the striatum. It is established that in addition to the overt motor deficits PD is associated with significant non-motor disturbances, including psychiatric symptoms, dementia, rapid eye movement (REM) sleep behaviour disorder, constipation and a reduced ability to smell odours (hyposmia) [27]. Hyposmia occurs in the prodromal phase of disease and is highly prevalent in both idiopathic and familial PD [34]. Although hyposmia is reported in as many as 90% of idiopathic PD cases [17], little is known about the underlying pathogenesis.

By virtue of its sporadic occurrence, the precise cause(s) of PD is unknown, however a range of genetic and environmental factors that increase the risk of PD developing have been identified. The dominant risk factor that relates to onset of PD is age [54]. The genetic risk factor with the highest population attributable risk (PAR) percent is the *SNCA* gene (12%) encoding the protein α-synuclein (α-syn) [60]. α-syn is the major constituent of Lewy bodies, an evident histopathological feature of PD, and as a result there is a large body of research dedicated to understanding its role in PD. Pathological staging by Braak et al. demonstrates that α-syn accumulation begins in the brainstem and the olfactory system (stage I), before following a topographical spread across the brain, reaching the nigrostriatal system in stage III [10].

The gene with the second highest PAR (8%) is *MAPT*, which encodes for the microtubule-associated protein, tau [60]. Tau has been implicated as a major contributor

* Correspondence: kbarnham@unimelb.edu.au
[1]The Florey Institute of Neuroscience and Mental Health, The University of Melbourne, Parkville, VIC 3010, Australia
[2]The Department of Pharmacology and Therapeutics, The University of Melbourne, Parkville, VIC 3010, Australia
Full list of author information is available at the end of the article

to disease pathogenesis in a number of neurodegenerative diseases including Alzheimer's disease where the presence of neurofibrillary tangles (NFTs) consisting of hyper-phosphorylated tau is a defining characteristic. NFTs are also a feature of PD brain, a finding first reported by Lewy himself (reviewed in [24]), and since reproduced a number of times [6, 32]. Despite the genetic and histopathological indications, the role tau plays in PD pathogenesis has not been well characterized.

One of the established biological functions of tau is promotion of the assembly of tubulin into microtubules, thereby stabilising the microtubule structure [18]. Tau has an intrinsically disordered structure that is subject to a number of post-translational modifications (PTMs) [30]. It has been demonstrated that the microtubule assembly role of tau is regulated by phosphorylation, and hyperphosphorylation leads to suppression of this function [3, 43]. It has been hypothesized that abnormal PTMs are a mechanism by which the function of tau is altered, resulting in loss of function, potentially via microtubule destabilisation [61].

The first line of tau$^{-/-}$ mice were generated by Harada et al. and although these animals were shown to have defective microtubule stability and organisation, they were viable and appeared macroscopically normal [25]. However, it has since been demonstrated that behavioural and motor impairments developed in these animals in an age-dependent manner. Lei et al. performed extensive behavioural and neurological investigations into tau$^{-/-}$ animals and showed that these mice display multiple features congruent with PD including an age-dependent motor and cognitive phenotype, iron accumulation and dopaminergic neurodegeneration of the SN [41, 42]. The findings in this study suggest dysfunction of tau is a key pathological event that eventuates in the hallmark pathological feature reported in the PD brain.

The appearance of motor symptoms associated with PD is reflective of advanced disease, as 50–70% of the dopaminergic neurons in the SN have perished by this stage [15, 38]. The advanced disease state currently aligned with diagnosis is a hindrance to the development of neuroprotective drugs and there is a need to develop methods to detect and diagnose patients much earlier in the prodromal phase of disease. As hyposmia is among the first symptoms to appear at the beginning of the prodromal phase, it follows that neuropathology in the olfactory system is an important feature of disease.

Studying olfactory deficits in animal models of PD is valuable in enhancing the understanding of the various mechanisms that may be contributing to PD-related hyposmia. Many animal models have been tested for a hyposmic phenotype [63, 65], and mice overexpressing human α-syn have demonstrated an age-dependent odour detection deficit [73]. Due to the age-dependent nature of the behavioural phenotype in the tau$^{-/-}$ mice, we sought to determine if hyposmia, an early process in the pathogenic pathway of PD, is associated with loss of tau function, using the tau$^{-/-}$ mice as a model.

Methods

Mice

Animals were housed according to standard animal care protocols. Rodent chow and water was available ad libitum. Mice were kept on a 12:12 h light dark cycle and all testing was performed during the light phase of the circadian cycle. Sv129B/6 tau$^{-/-}$ mice were bred in house. Wild type (WT) littermate controls (Sv129B/6 tau$^{+/+}$) were used in this study. All studies were conducted in a blinded fashion. All methods conformed to the Australian National Health and Medical Research Council published code of practice for animal research and all experimentation was approved by The Florey Animal Ethics Committee (AEC number: 12–094 and 15–092). Animal numbers (broken down by genotype and sex) are provided in Additional file 1: Table S1. Animals were genotyped as part of the breeding strategy and confirmation of tau ablation was performed on tissue via Western Blot (Additional file 1: Figure S2).

Odour detection test

The Odour Detection Test (ODT) was adapted from [53]. Mice were habituated to vehicle canisters in their home cage for 3 days prior to testing (day 1: single vehicle cannisters; day 2: two vehicle cannisters; day 3: two vehicle cannisters). The test (day 4) was comprised of four 5-min trials (1 h inter-trial interval (ITI)) performed in the home cage in which the mice were exposed to two canisters per trial; one vehicle (400 μL, MilliQ water + 0.1% Tween20) and one novel odour of either 0 (vehicle), 1:10^8, 1:10^6 or 1:10^4 dilutions (400 μL, MilliQ water + 0.1% Tween20 + orange essential oil (In Essence, Australia)). Animals were videoed, and videos manually scored (the scorer was blinded to the experimental conditions) and percentage investigation time was calculated based on the equation: (time spent with novel odour/combined time investigating either canister) X 100. An animal was deemed to be 'smelling' if their nose was within a 1–2 cm proximity to the either end of the cannister and appeared to be investigating the cannister (neck extended, whiskers forward). Normal mice will spend more time investigating a novel odour; as such this test determines the concentration at which can detect a novel odour by comparing time spent investigating the two canisters.

Rota rod

Mice were trained for three sessions on the Rota Rod (Panlab, Spain) 24 h prior to testing. Session 1 was set speed (4 rpm for 2 mins), session 2 was set speed (4 rpm for 2 mins) and session 3 was accelerating (4–40 rpm for 2 mins). During training if the mouse fell off the Rota

Rod it was placed back on until 2 min had lapsed. On the test day the Rota Rod was set to accelerating mode (4–40 rpm) over a 5 min trial. Mice were allowed three attempts and the average time of latency to fall was recorded.

Pole test

Mice were placed vertically (nose up) on a pole (45 cm) that was wrapped in self-adhesive bandage (NexCare, Australia) with a squash ball placed on top to prevent animals climbing and sitting on the top of the pole. Two lines were drawn on the pole to identify a segment of set length (22 cm). One day prior to testing animals were habituated to the pole and allowed five consecutive trials. On the day of testing animals were allowed a further five consecutive attempts which were recorded. Time to turn (animal to complete a 180° rotation) and time to complete were recorded. A successful pole test was defined by an animals ability to complete a full 360 degree rotation and descend the pole nose first using their limbs to 'walk' (animals failed if they slid or jumped down the pole).

Tissue preparation

Animals were euthanized with a lethal dose of sodium pentobarbitone (100 mg/kg, Lethobarb, Jurox, Rutherford, NSW, Australia), and transcardially perfused with cold 0.1 M phosphate-buffered saline (PBS) (Sigma-Aldrich, St. Louis, Missouri, MO, USA), pH 7.4.

The left-brain hemisphere was dissected for regions containing the striatum (caudate nucleus and putamen (CPU)), substantia nigra par compacta (SN) and olfactory bulbs (OB). These fractions were homogenized using a probe sonicator (10 s) in radioimmunoprecipitation assay (RIPA) lysis buffer (150 mM NaCl, 1% nonyl phenoxypolyethoxylethanol (NP-40), 0.5% sodium deoxycholate (DOC), 50 mM Tris (pH 8.0) + protease and phosphatase inhibitors (Complete Mini Protease Inhibitor Cocktail & PhosSTOP Phosphatase Inhibitor Cocktail, Roche Diagnostic)) and butylated hydroxytoluene (BHT) (1:5; tissue weight (mg): buffer volume (μL)). Homogenates were then centrifuged at 10,000 *g* for 20 min at 4°C. The clarified supernatant was collected (cell lysate) and total protein concentrations were determined using the bicinchoninic acid (BCA) assay (Pierce; Rockford, USA) according to the manufacturer's directions and made to 2 μg/μl aliquots and used for Western Blots.

Western blotting

Samples were mixed with 4X sample buffer (25 M Tris (pH 6.8), 20% SDS, Glycerol, 100 mg Bromo Blue) containing 100 mM dithiothreitol (DTT), boiled for 5 min and centrifuged at 10000 *g* for 5 mins. Protein was electrophoresed at 270 V for 25 min on 4–20% polyacrylamide gels (BioRad; USA) and transferred on to 0.45 μm (pore-size) nitrocellulose membranes (BioRad; USA). Membranes were blocked in tris-buffered saline with 0.05% Tween20 (TBS-T) containing 5% low-fat milk powder (Diploma, Australia) for 1 h at room temperature, incubated with primary antibodies overnight at 4 °C, and incubated with secondary antibodies for 2 h at room temp. All antibodies (BD Biosciences anti- α-syn, catalogue number: 610786, dilution 1:5000; Novus Biological anti-p62/SQSTM1, catalogue number: 3868, dilution 1:2000; Cell Signalling Technology anti-LC3B(D11)-XP, catalogue number: H00008878-MO1, dilution 1:2000) were diluted in TBS-T containing 5% low-fat milk powder. Membranes were washed in TBS-T for 21 min (3 X 7 min) before and after incubation with secondary antibodies. Proteins were detected using enhanced chemiluminescence (ECL) (BioRad) and visualised with the ChemiDoc (BioRad; USA) and analysed via densitometry (ImageLab 5.2.1, BioRad; USA). Cell lysates were normalised to automated total protein measurement via ChemiDoc stain-free detection software.

Primary cortical neuron preparation

Primary cortical neurons were isolated from embryonic brain cortices harvested from tau$^{-/-}$ and WT pregnant mice at 14 days of gestation. The neurons were plated in T75 flasks at a density of 150,000 cells/cm^2 in Neurobasal Medium (cat# 21103049; Life Technologies), and supplement with B-27 serum-free supplement (cat# 10889038; Life Technologies), Glutamax supplement (cat# 35050061; Life Technologies), gentamicin (cat# 15710072; Life Technologies) and incubated at (humidified, 37 °C, 5% CO_2) for 6 days.

Exosome isolation

Exosomes were isolated from cell culture media by differential ultracentrifugation. Culture supernatants were collected, and cellular debris was removed by centrifugation at 2000 *g* for 10 min. The supernatant was then centrifuged at 10,000 *g*, for 30 min at 4 °C. The supernatant was collected and centrifuged 100,000 *g* for 1 h at 4 °C to pellet exosomes. The supernatant was discarded and exosome containing pellets resuspended in filtered PBS and re-centrifuged at 100,000 *g* for 1 h at 4 °C to pellet exosomes. The pellet was resuspended in 50 μl PBS.

Electron microscopy

Exosomes were fixed with 2% glutaraldehyde/PBS, for 30 min at room temperature. 6 μl was applied to a glow-discharged 200 mesh copper grid coated with carbon-Formvar film (ProSciTech, QLD, Australia) and allowed to absorb for 5 min. Grids were washed 2 × with milliQ water and contrasted with 1.5% uranyl acetate. Transmission electron microscopy (TEM) was performed on a Tecnai G^2 F30 (FEI, Eindhoven, NL) transmission electron microscope operating at 300 kV (Bio21 Molecular Science and Biotechnology Institute, Parkville, VIC, Australia) across 15,000× – 36,000× magnification. Electron micrographs were captured with a Gatan UltraScan® 1000 2 k × 2 k CCD camera (Gatan, Inc., Pleasanton, CA, USA).

Immunofluorescence confocal microscopy

Cells were cultured on Laminin/Poly-D-Lysine coated glass coverslips for 9 days before experimental treatment. Samples were fixed with 4% (*w*/*v*) paraformaldehyde (PFA) in 0.1 M phosphate buffer (15 min), rinsed three times with PBS, permeabilized with 0.1% (*v*/*v*) Triton X-100 in PBS (10 min) then blocked with 3% (v/v) goat serum in 0.1% (v/v) Triton X-100/PBS (10 min). The samples were incubated with a rabbit monoclonal LC3B antibody (Cell Signaling Technologies) diluted in 3% (v/v) goat serum in 0.1% (v/v) Triton X-100/PBS for 2 h at room temperature, rinsed three times with PBS, then incubated at room temperature for 2 h with secondary antibodies conjugated to Alexa-Fluor-555 (ThermoFisher). The coverslips were then incubated 0.1% (v/v) Triton X-100/PBS containing 1 μM Hoechst 33,342 (ThermoFisher) and 1 μM DiO (Sigma Aldrich) for 15 min to visualise the cells independently of LC3B staining. The samples were three times with PBS, then mounted using a TRIS buffered DABCO-glycerol mounting medium. All samples were imaged in 3D by optical sectioning using an inverted Leica SP8 confocal laser scanning microscope equipped with an 63×/1.40NA objective (Oil immersion, HC PLAPO, CS2; Leica microsystems), using a z-stack range of 4.8 μm and a voxel size of 180 nm laterally (x,y) and 300 nm axially (z). All figure images were acquired at ambient room temperature using a Leica HyD Hybrid Detector (Leica Microsystems) and the Leica Application Suite X (LASX v2.0.1). All images are displayed as z-stack maximum projections.

Confocal image analysis

3D image data were processed and analysed using automated image segmentation in Imaris (V8.0; Bitplane). Autophagic vacuole volume was normalized to the cellular volume rather than number of nuclei, as the number of nuclei did not provide a robust measure of cells per image. For volumetric quantification of LC3B positive autophagic vacuoles, images were segmented using 1 μm diameter background subtraction, 150 nm surface smoothing, a manual intensity threshold of 12 (arbitrary), and seeded region growing segmentation (1 μm diameter seed). Cellular volume was quantified by segmentation of DiO staining, using 360 nm surface smoothing and a manual intensity threshold of 10 (arbitrary). Segmented structures smaller than 10 voxels were excluded to remove shot noise.

Statistical analysis

All data are presented as the means ± S.E.M., and statistical differences evaluated by Student's *t* test for two sample testing. Odour detection tests were evaluated using a Two-way ANOVA test with repeated measures (one factor repetition) with Fisher LSD post-hoc comparisons for multiple testing, details of ANOVAs and testing of parametric assumptions (Additional file 1: Table S2). For all analyses, $p < 0.05$ was considered to be statistically significant.

Results

7-month-old tau$^{-/-}$ mice have an olfactory deficit that is accompanied by autophagic impairment and accumulation of α-synuclein in the olfactory bulb

In order to test whether a loss of tau can impair olfactory capability, 7-month-old tau$^{-/-}$ mice and their WT littermates underwent an ODT (Fig. 1a). This test showed that 7-month-old tau$^{-/-}$ mice showed no preference for investigating the canister containing the novel odour, unlike their WT littermates who showed a significant preference for the novel odour (main effect of genotype $p = 0.003$). At the strongest odour concentration (1:10^4), a one sample t test with a hypothetical mean of 50% (chance) demonstrated that WT animals were performing significantly above chance, whereas tau$^{-/-}$ animals were not (WT $p = 0.0001$, tau$^{-/-}$$p = 0.32$) (Additional file 1: Table S3). The inability of tau$^{-/-}$ mice to differentiate between a novel odour and a vehicle canister is evidence of a hyposmic phenotype in these animals. In PD, hyposmia occurs prior to the onset of motor deficits. In order to ascertain whether the hyposmia observed in these mice similarly occurs prior to the onset of motor deficits that have previously been reported for these animals, the 7-month-old tau$^{-/-}$ mice underwent motor testing (Fig. 1b). At 7-months-old no difference in motor function was observed between tau$^{-/-}$ and WT mice on either the Rota Rod ($p = 0.15$) or Pole Test (time to turn $p = 0.76$; time to complete $p = 0.88$).

Accumulation and aggregation of protein is a characteristic feature of neurodegenerative diseases and may be the result of impaired clearance mechanisms in affected neurons. Macroautophagy, a major pathway for degradation and recycling of cellular material has been reported to be impaired in PD [45] and implicated in the accumulation of α-syn that is a characteristic feature of the disease [21, 22, 35, 40]. Microtubules, which are reported to be stabilised by tau, play a key role in the endo-lysosomal trafficking process required for autophagic degradation [13, 69]. Autophagosome lysosome fusion is mediated by a number of factors including SNARE Stx17, the HOPS complex and mammalian Atg8 family proteins [29, 31, 33, 49, 50]. Atg8 family members are conjugated to phosphatidylethanoamine on autophagosomal membrane during autophagosome biogenesis, and degraded

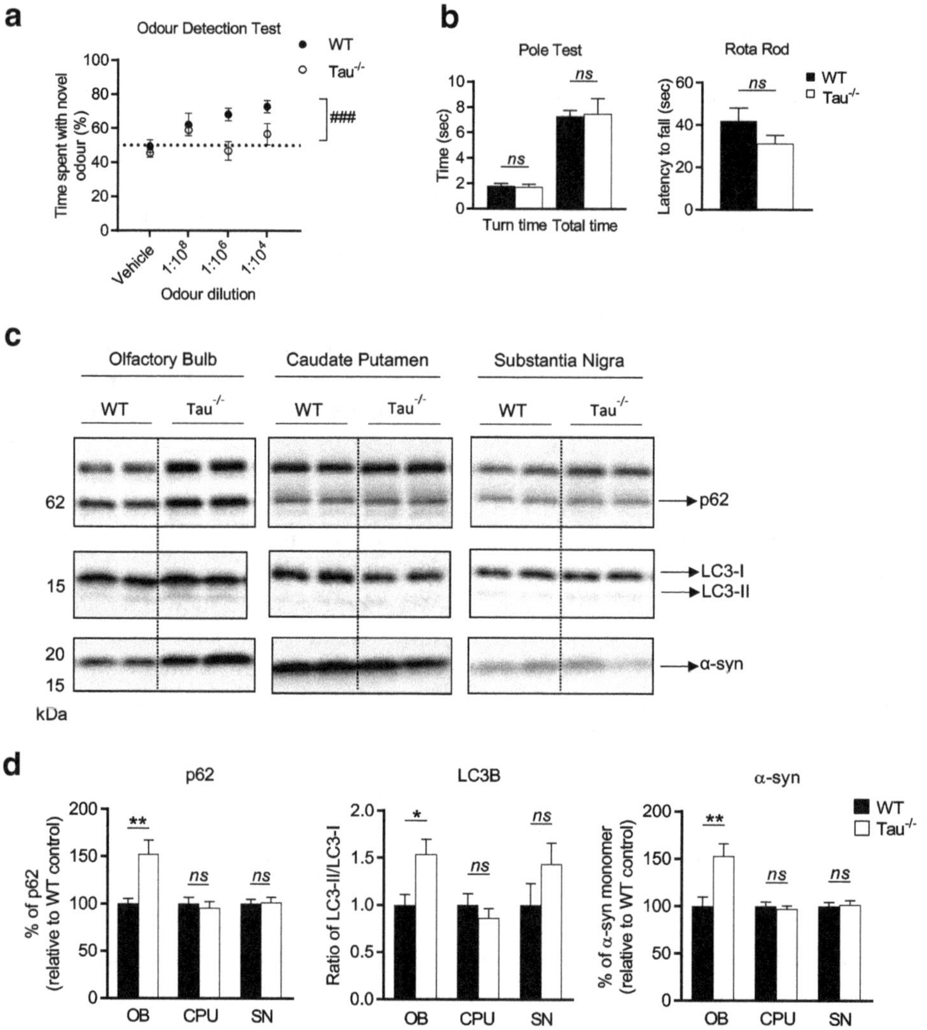

Fig. 1 Olfactory deficit, motor performance and pathological features in 7-month-old tau$^{-/-}$ mice. **a** Odour detection test performed on 7-month-old tau$^{-/-}$ (n = 10–11) and littermate WT controls (n = 10–12). **b** Motor evaluation of 7-month-old tau$^{-/-}$ (n = 10) and littermate WT control (n = 11), including Rota Rod and Pole Test performance. **c** Representative western blots of cell lysate from olfactory bulb, caudate putamen and substantia nigra from 7-month-old tau$^{-/-}$ (n = 6) and littermate WT controls (n = 6) immunoblotted for p62, LC3B and α-syn. **d** Quantification of western blot densitometry presented as % of p62 relative to WT control, ratio of LC3-II/I relative to WT control and % of α-syn relative to WT control. Cell lysate for western blots normalised to automated total protein measurement via ChemiDoc stain-free detection software. ODT analysed by two-way repeated measures ANOVA (one factor repetition) with Fisher LSD post-hoc comparisons. # represents significant main effect of genotype, ### $p < 0.001$. Motor tests analysed by unpaired two-sided t test. Western blot analysed by unpaired two-sided t test from 3 independent repeats, * $p < 0.05$, ** $p < 0.01$, *** $p < 0.001$, **** $p < 0.0001$, *ns*: not significant. Full western blot images presented in Additional file 1: Figure S3

upon lysosomal fusion with the autophagosome [62]. When analysed by SDS-PAGE, the lapidated form of the LC3B (LC3-II) migrates faster than the cleaved precursor form (LC3-I). As such, an increase in the ratio of LC3-II/LC3-I is often used as a marker of compromised autophagy-mediated degradation [36].

We therefore used LC3B levels to monitor autophagy in tau$^{-/-}$ OB tissue and determine if ablation of tau resulted in alterations to autophagy. A significant increase in LC3-II/I ratio (p = 0.01) was detected in the OB of 7-month old tau$^{-/-}$ mice compared to WT mice (Fig. 1d). This increase in the ratio of LC3-II/I was accompanied by a significant 50% increase in the level of p62 (an autophagy receptor that is basally turned over via autophagy) in tau$^{-/-}$ mice (p = 0.003) (Fig. 1d) further suggesting 7 mo tau$^{-/-}$ animals have an impairment in the autophagy pathway.

Hyposmia as seen in the human condition has been correlated with an accumulation of aggregated α-syn within Lewy bodies, as demonstrated in Braak staging [10]. Given the suggested autophagy impairment in the tau$^{-/-}$ mice it was of interest to probe the OB for protein accumulation.

Consistent with a PD-like phenotype there was an increase of α-syn in the OB at 7-months-old (p = 0.03) (Fig. 1d).

The midbrain (CPU and SN) of these animals was also analysed for LC3B, p62 and α-syn. In line with there being no overt motor deficit, there were no detectable differences in the aforementioned protein levels evident in these brain regions (Fig. 1d). CPU: p62 $p = 0.65$, LC3-II/I $p = 0.40$, α-syn $p = 0.60$; SN: p62 $p = 0.89$, LC3-II/I $p = 0.19$, α-syn $p = 0.83$.

15-month-old tau$^{-/-}$ mice have a motor deficit that is accompanied by autophagic impairment and accumulation of α-synuclein in the midbrain

At 15 months old tau$^{-/-}$ mice continued to display an odour detection deficiency, however WT mice were also displaying a hyposmic phenotype at this age, as demonstrated by a there being no main effect of genotype of $p = 0.54$ (Fig. 2a) when compared to tau$^{-/-}$ mice and no significant difference to a hypothetical mean of 50% at any of the odour concentrations (Additional file 1: Table S3). The onset of motor impairment in these mice is reported to occur at 12 months, and is accompanied by dopaminergic neuronal degeneration in the SN and iron accumulation in dopaminergic neurons [41]. Based on this data we examined 12-month-old tau$^{-/-}$ mice and found no significant difference in motor performance compared to WT controls, however there was still a robust olfactory deficit in tau$^{-/-}$ mice (Additional file 1: Figure S1). As such, mice were further aged to 15-months-old and at this point tau$^{-/-}$ performed significantly different on both the Rota Rod ($p < 0.0001$) and Pole Test (time to turn $p = 0.004$, total time $p = 0.03$) than WT controls (Fig. 2b).

Based on this behavioural deficit, we examined the autophagic markers and α-syn levels in the OB, CPU and SN of animals at 15-months-old. At this age the is no detectable difference in the OB between tau$^{-/-}$ and WT mice (p62 $p = 0.13$, LC3-II/I $p = 0.47$, α-syn $p = 0.73$) (Fig. 2d). Although there was no difference in the level of p62 in either the CPU ($p = 0.15$) or the SN ($p = 0.91$), tau$^{-/-}$ mice had a significant increase in the ratio of LC3-II/I in both brain regions (CPU $p = 0.04$, SN $p = 0.03$), indicative of impaired autophagy (Fig. 2d). In line with the early pathological features demonstrated in the OB of young animals, there was a congruent increase in α-syn in the CPU of older tau$^{-/-}$ mice ($p = 0.02$) (Fig. 2d).

Overall these data suggest that in this animal model there are changes in protein levels that align with a behavioural phenotype in the olfactory system that eventually present in the midbrain alongside a motor deficit.

Tau disruption and impaired autophagic clearance promotes the release of α-syn in association with exosomes

To further investigate whether a loss of tau can cause an impairment in autophagy, we harvested primary cortical neurons from tau$^{-/-}$ mice and their WT littermates and compared their autophagic flux. As we observed in the mouse tissue, there was a significant increase ($p = 0.04$) in the LC3-II/I ratio in the tau$^{-/-}$ neurons as compared with WT neurons (Fig. 3a). Immunocytochemistry was also used to assess autophagosome number in WT and tau$^{-/-}$ neurons (Fig. 3b). Quantitation of LC3B positive structures using semi-automated 3D image analysis revealed a significant increase in autophagosome number in tau$^{-/-}$ neurons under basal conditions ($p = 0.04$) (Fig. 3c). Treatment with the autophagosome biogenesis inhibitor wortmannin resulted in no significant difference in the number of LC3B structures between WT and tau$^{-/-}$, and an overall decrease of LC3B structures supporting that the structures represent autophagosomes. The data suggest that either there was a decrease in the lysosomal turnover of autophagosomes in tau$^{-/-}$, or an increase in the amount of autophagy under basal conditions.

Impairment of autophagosome maturation or fusion with a lysosome has been suggested to result in fusion of autophagosomes to MVBs [64]. Once formed, MVBs can fuse with the plasma membrane to release their intraluminal vesicles as exosomes into the extracellular space. Exosomes are small vesicles released by cells and are major regulators of cell-to-cell communication in both pathological and normal conditions [57, 59]. Exosomes have been implicated in prion disease progression by promoting the cell-to-cell spread of pathological forms of the prion protein [23, 67]. The temporal displacement in the onset of disease relevant symptoms in the tau$^{-/-}$ mice suggests a phenotype that is present at an earlier age in the OB spreads to the CPU/SN at an older age. Could this disease spread be facilitated through an exosome mediated mechanism? To test if loss of tau function could possibly contribute to exosome mediated disease spread we compared exosomes released into media from tau$^{-/-}$ and WT mouse primary cortical cell cultures. Tau deletion resulted in an increase in the number of exosomes released into the media ($p < 0.0001$) (Fig. 1d) and an increase in the enrichment of α-syn within these exosomes ($p = 0.049$) (Fig. 1e). Isolated extracellular vesicles were verified as exosomes using a number of positive and negative exosome markers (Additional file 1: Figure S5C).

Discussion

Variants of *MAPT* represent a risk factor in idiopathic PD and hyper-phosphorylation of tau is a consistent feature of many neurodegenerative diseases. Despite this evidence, the role tau plays in pathogenesis of PD has not been well characterised. Similarly, accumulation and aggregation of α-syn are histopathological hallmarks of PD brain and follow a defined pattern of spread with disease progression [10], however the mechanism(s) of protein aggregation and spread remain elusive. Our study demonstrates that a loss of the protein tau, via genetic knock out, resulted in a functional olfactory deficit coinciding with α-syn accumulation

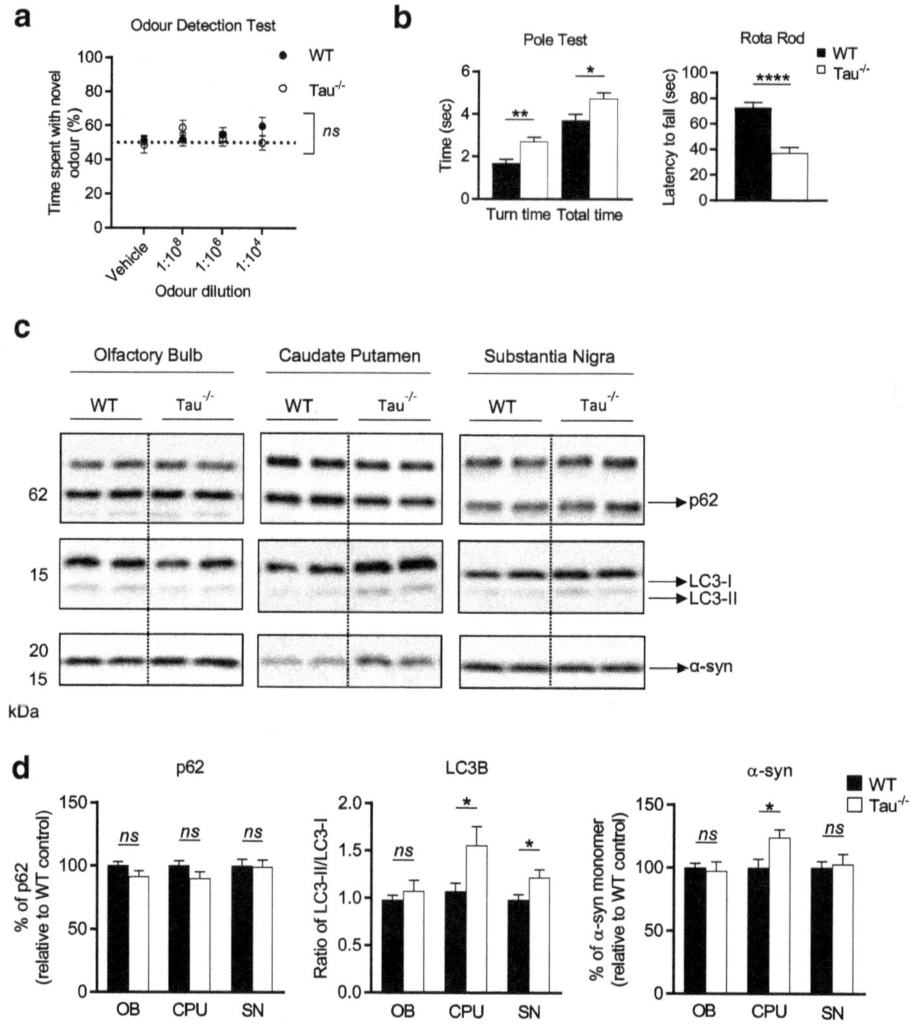

Fig. 2 Olfactory deficit, motor performance and pathological features in 15-month-old tau$^{-/-}$ mice. **a** Odour detection test performed on 15-month-old tau$^{-/-}$ ($n = 13$) and littermate WT controls ($n = 8$). **b** Motor evaluation of 15-month-old tau$^{-/-}$ ($n = 11$) and littermate WT control ($n = 8$), including Rota Rod and Pole Test performance. **c** Representative western blots of cell lysate from olfactory bulb, caudate putamen and substantia nigra from 15-month-old tau$^{-/-}$ ($n = 6$) and littermate WT controls ($n = 6$) immunoblotted for p62, LC3B and α-syn. **d** Quantification of western blot densitometry presented as % of p62 relative to WT control, ratio of LC3-II/I relative to WT control and % of α-syn relative to WT control. Cell lysate for western blots normalised to automated total protein measurement via ChemiDoc stain-free detection software. ODT analysed by two-way repeated measures ANOVA (one factor repetition) with Fisher LSD post-hoc comparisons. Motor tests analysed by unpaired two-sided t test. Western blot analysed by unpaired two-sided t test from 3 independent repeats, * $p < 0.05$, ** $p < 0.01$, *** $p < 0.001$, **** $p < 0.0001$, *ns*: not significant. Full western blot images presented in Additional file 1: Figure S4

and autophagic impairments that began in the olfactory bulb and appeared in the midbrain 8 months later. These finding suggest that dysfunction of tau is an early pathological event in the neurodegenerative cascade associated with PD.

In this study, odour detection tests revealed an inability of 7-month-old tau$^{-/-}$ mice to detect a novel odour. There have been numerous studies interrogating the tau$^{-/-}$ mouse as potential model of PD [1, 16, 28, 41, 42, 48, 68]. Although there have been no published investigations into the olfactory capacity of tau$^{-/-}$ mice to date, two tau-overexpressing models have reported olfactory dysfunction. Tα1-3RT tau transgenic mice that overexpress human tau and P301S tau mice that overexpress human mutant tau both demonstrate functional olfactory deficits [46, 72]. Although the exact cause of hyposmia has not been determined, there appeared to be a relationship between Lewy pathology and olfactory function [47, 51]. The delayed onset of motor impairment in this study (15-months-old) compared to published findings in this animal model (12-months-old) may be the result of genetic modifiers, as there have been

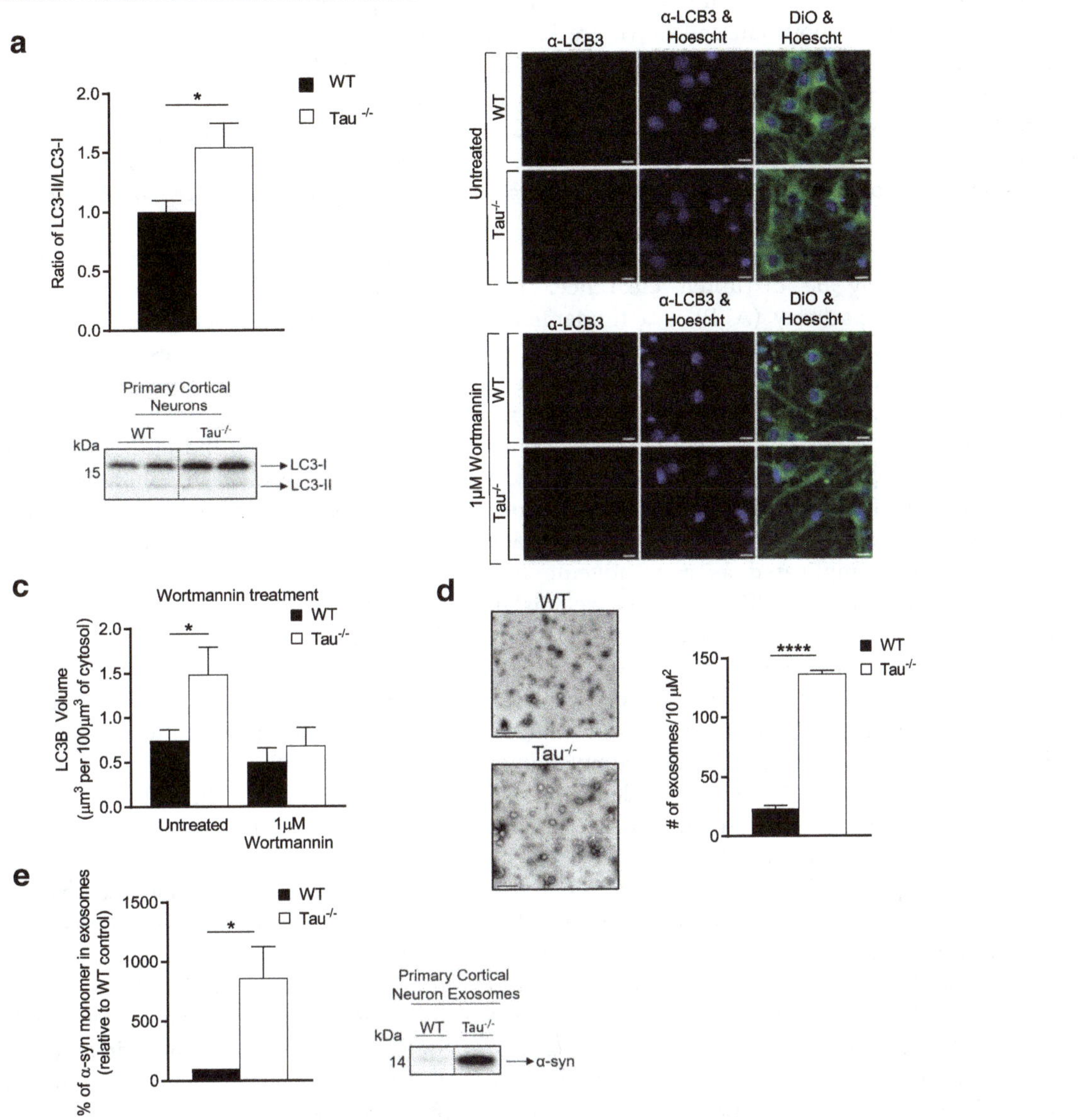

Fig. 3 Tau$^{-/-}$ primary cortical neurons display autophagic impairment and have an increase in the release of α-synuclein enriched exosomes. **a** Quantification of western blot densitometry presented as ratio of LC3-II/I of tau$^{-/-}$ primary cortical neurons ($n = 5$) and WT primary cortical neurons ($n = 5$). **b** Representative images of tau$^{-/-}$ and WT primary cortical neurons immunostained for LC3B and post-stained with DiO and Hoechst 33,342 after incubation with either culture medium (untreated) or 1 μM Wortmannin for 8 h, scale bars: 10 μm. **c** Quantification of the number of LCB3 positive autophagosomes per 100 μm^3 of DiO stained cytosol, in untreated and Wortmannin treated WT ($n = 5$) and tau$^{-/-}$ ($n = 5$) primary cortical neurons. **d** Representative electron micrograph images of tau$^{-/-}$ ($n = 3$) and WT ($n = 3$) exosome enriched cell culture media (scale bars: 200 μm) with quantitation of number of exosomes per 10 μM^2. **e** Quantification of western blot densitometry from exosomes isolated from tau$^{-/-}$ ($n = 2$) and WT ($n = 2$) primary cortical neurons, presented as % of α-syn relative to WT control and representative western blot. Cell lysate for western blots normalised to automated total protein measurement via ChemiDoc stain-free detection software. Immunocytochemistry data analysed by one-way ANOVA. Western blot analysed by unpaired two-sided t test from 3 independent repeats, * $p < 0.05$, ** $p < 0.01$, *** $p < 0.001$, **** $p < 0.0001$, *ns*: not significant. Full western blot images presented in Additional file 1: Figure S5

differing results between models on different background strains in tau$^{-/-}$ animals [42, 48]. The major motor and non-motor findings in the work by Lei et al. were reported in tau$^{-/-}$ mice on the Sv129B/6 background strain. Shortly after this study, a number of groups were able to recapitulate the motor deficit in a pure black 6 (B6) background strain, however when it came to the non-motor phenotype (cognition), the B6 animals appeared to have either a delayed onset or no apparent phenotype [42, 48]. Based on this, it was deemed appropriate to use the background strain with demonstrated non-motor features. This background effect is one factor that may also explain a lack of olfactory capacity in WT controls at 15-months-old and requires further investigation.

Protein aggregates appear across multiple levels of the olfactory system [5] and both tau and α-syn are known to accumulate in neurodegenerative disease [10, 66]. Braak staging references an initial increase of α-syn in the anterior olfactory nucleus in human tissue, and in this study, there was an accumulation of α-syn in the olfactory bulb of hyposmic $tau^{-/-}$ mice before midbrain pathological features appeared.

One explanation of the accumulation of α-syn in the $tau^{-/-}$ mice may be disrupted clearance. The autophagy-lysosome pathway (ALP) is a fundamental mechanism used to remove misfolded and aggregated proteins [12, 55]. Defects in the ALP have been linked to PD [11, 52] and other neurodegenerative disorders (for review see: [70]). Increasing evidence suggests that dysregulation of autophagy results in the accumulation of abnormal proteins and/or damaged organelles, and impairments in the autophagy pathway have been implicated as a pathogenic feature of PD, as observed in PD brains as well as in animal models of PD [2, 7, 8]. Data from this study suggests there was impairment in autophagy in the olfactory bulb of 7-month-old $tau^{-/-}$ mice, a deficit that appears in the midbrain in 15-month-old animals, correlating with motor deficits and α-syn accumulation in these brain regions. Although there is evidence of disrupted autophagic flux in 15-month-old animals, as demonstrated by an increase in the LC3II-I ratio, there was no notable change in p62 levels in the midbrain. While this was initially surprising, Sahani et al. have demonstrated in vivo that in distressed cells, there is an initial decrease in p62, but the cells were able to restore the level of p62 to basal levels [56]. Authors demonstrate that there are three major factors that control the expression level: autophagic degradation, transcriptional upregulation and availability of lysosomal-derived amino acids. Based on this, it is concluded that expression level of p62 does not always inversely correlate with autophagic activity and should only be taken in conjunction with other autophagic markers.

Many of the steps involved in autophagy require a functional cytoskeletal network. Disruption of dynein function leads to the accumulation of autophagosomes, suggesting that impairments to microtubule transport disrupt autophagosome-lysosome fusion [37, 71]. Tau is a microtubule-associated protein with a proposed role in microtubule stability; therefore, microtubule destabilisation following tau dysfunction is a potential mechanism of autophagy disruption. Data from this study demonstrates that ablation of tau in vivo lead to increases in the autophagy marker LC3B, suggestive of autophagy deficits that may lead to protein accumulation. It appears that although there is an increase in α-syn levels in the CPU at 15 months of age, the SN has no detectable difference between the WT and $tau^{-/-}$ animals. Shimozawa et al. have investigated the distribution and spread of α-syn and they demonstrated a retrograde spread of pathology from the CPU to the SN [58]. It is possible that in this study the tissue has been collected at a time point that is reflective of the beginning of pathological pathways in the midbrain, reflected by the accumulation of α-syn only in the CPU. Autophagy deficits were confirmed in primary cortical neurons of $tau^{-/-}$ neurons, supporting the principle that tau disruption results in altered autophagy.

α-syn aggregates are a histopathological hallmark of PD brain and follow a defined pattern of spread across the brain with disease progression. It was recently demonstrated that injection of exogenous α-syn into the brains of healthy animals could induce α-syn propagation in a "prion-like" manner and induce a PD phenotype [39, 44]. The specific mechanisms underlying the propagation of α-syn across the brain have however remained elusive.

Recent studies have shown that α-syn can be secreted via exosomes [4, 14, 20], although non-exosomal release of α-syn has also been described [14, 26]. Exosomes are the released form of intraluminal vesicles that are generated from invaginated membranes of multivesicular bodies (MVB) (reviewed in [9]). Exosome release is enhanced by impaired autophagosome-lysosome fusion, a key step in autophagy, as illustrated by genetic and pharmacological manipulations [19, 40]. The mechanism of this effect is not clear, although it has been proposed that autophagosomes may fuse with MVBs to subsequently effect fusion with the plasma membrane and release [14, 19, 22, 40]. Our study indicates that disruption of tau lead to autophagic impairment appearing initially in the olfactory bulb and later in the midbrain. Defective autophagy results in an accumulation of α-syn and in combination with autophagic impairments may drive the release of α-syn enriched exosomes, which may be an important mediator of α-syn spread.

Conclusion

This study has demonstrated a link between tau ablation and autophagic disruption that coincides with α-syn accumulation and related behavioural deficits beginning in the olfactory system and eventuating in the midbrain. This implicates dysfunction of tau as an early pathological event in PD and signifies the value of $tau^{-/-}$ mice as an age-dependent model of both prodromal and clinically overt Parkinson's disease.

Additional file

Additional file 1: Supplementary data **Table S1.** Animal numbers (genotype and sex). **Table S2.** ODT ANOVA factors. Normality test: Shapiro-Wilk. **Table S3.** ODT one sample t test, hypothetical mean = 50% (chance). **Figure S1.** ODT (A) and motor evaluation (B) of 12-month-old tau−/− (*n* = 12) and WT (*n* = 12). ODT analysed by two-way repeated measures ANOVA (one factor repetition) with Fisher LSD post-hoc comparisons. # represents significant main effect of genotype, ## $p < 0.01$. Motor tests analysed by unpaired two-sided t test. Ns = not significant. **Figure S2.** Western blot confirmation of tau ablation in 7- and 15-month old tissue. A) Tau antibody (Dako, catalogue number: A0024, dilution 1:10,000) confirmed tau ablation B) Protein loading in all wells confirmed by GAPDH (Cell Signaling Technology, catalogue number 2118, dilution 1:10,000). **Figure S3.** Full Western Blots of 7 mo WT (+) and Tau−/− (−) cell lysate. A, B, C: immunoblot of p62 from OB, CPU and SN respectively. D, E, F: immunoblot of LCB3 from OB, CPU and SN respectively. G, H, I: immunoblot of α-synuclein from OB, CPU and SN respectively. Red box indicates the section represented in Figures. **Figure S4.** Full Western Blots of 15 mo WT (+) and Tau−/− (−) cell lysate. A, B, C: immunoblot of p62 from OB, CPU and SN respectively. D, E, F: immunoblot of LCB3 from OB, CPU and SN respectively. G, H, I: immunoblot of α-synuclein from OB, CPU and SN respectively. Red box indicates the section represented in Figures. **Figure S5.** A) Full Western Blots of PCN for LC3B from WT (+) and Tau−/− (−) cell lysate. B) Full Western Blot of PCN-derived exosomes for α-synuclein from WT (+) and Tau−/− (−) cells. C) Exosome verification using exosome negative markers (GM130 & bcl-2), exosome positive marker (Tsg101) and microvesicle marker (Flotillin) in primary cortical neuron cell lysate and exosomes. (PDF 1104 kb)

Abbreviations
ALP: Autophagy-lysosome pathway; BCA: Bicinchonic acid; BHT: Butylated hydroxytoluene; CPU: Caudate putamen; DTT: Dithiothreitol; ECL: Enhanced chemiluminescence; ITI: Inter-trial interval; Knockout: −/−; MVB: Multivesicular bodies; NFT: Neurofibrillary tangle; OB: Olfactory bulb; ODT: Odour detection test; PAR: Population attributable risk; PBS: Phosphate-buffered saline; PD: Parkinson's disease; PFA: Paraformaldehyde; PTM: Post-translational modification; REM: Rapid eye movement; RIPA: Radioimmunoprecipitation assay; S.E.M: Standard error of the mean; SN: Substantia nigra; TBS: Tris-buffered saline; TEM: Transmission electron microscopy; WT: Wildtype; α-syn: Alpha synuclein

Funding
NHMRC grants APP10331193; APP1002373; 628946.

Authors' contributions
LB performed animal behaviour and brain tissue western blots, had substantial input in the design of the experiment as well as a major contributor in writing the manuscript. JC made substantial contributions to acquisition and interpretation of animal behaviour and brain tissue data. LWH and BC performed primary cell culture and exosome isolation and counts. BSP and XML performed the primary cell culture, Wortmannin treatment and IF analysis. AB, ML, LJV, LJ and AFH made substantial contributions to the conception and design of the study, interpretation of data and critically revising the manuscript for important intellectual content. KJB made substantial contributions to the conception and design of the study, interpretation of data, and was a major contributor in writing and critically revising the manuscript for important intellectual content. All authors have read and approved the final manuscript.

Competing interests
The authors declare that they have no competing interests.

Author details
[1]The Florey Institute of Neuroscience and Mental Health, The University of Melbourne, Parkville, VIC 3010, Australia. [2]The Department of Pharmacology and Therapeutics, The University of Melbourne, Parkville, VIC 3010, Australia. [3]Monash Biomedicine Discovery Institute, Monash University, Clayton, VIC 3800, Australia. [4]The Department of Biochemistry and Molecular Biology, Bio21 Institute, The University of Melbourne, Parkville, VIC 3010, Australia. [5]The Department of Biochemistry and Genetics, La Trobe Institute for Molecular Science, La Trobe University, Bundoora, VIC 3083, Australia.

References

1. Ahmed T, Van der Jeugd A, Blum D, Galas MC, D'Hooge R, Buee L, Balschun D (2014) Cognition and hippocampal synaptic plasticity in mice with a homozygous tau deletion. Neurobiol Aging 35:2474–2478. https://doi.org/10.1016/j.neurobiolaging.2014.05.005
2. Alegre-Abarrategui J, Wade-Martins R (2009) Parkinson disease, LRRK2 and the endocytic-autophagic pathway. Autophagy 5:1208–1210
3. Alonso AC, Zaidi T, Grundke-Iqbal I, Iqbal K (1994) Role of abnormally phosphorylated tau in the breakdown of microtubules in Alzheimer disease. Proc Natl Acad Sci U S A 91:5562–5566
4. Alvarez-Erviti L, Seow Y, Schapira AH, Gardiner C, Sargent IL, Wood MJ, Cooper JM (2011) Lysosomal dysfunction increases exosome-mediated alpha-synuclein release and transmission. Neurobiol Dis 42:360–367. https://doi.org/10.1016/j.nbd.2011.01.029
5. Attems J, Jellinger KA (2006) Olfactory tau pathology in Alzheimer disease and mild cognitive impairment. Clin Neuropathol 25:265–271
6. Bancher C, Braak H, Fischer P, Jellinger KA (1993) Neuropathological staging of Alzheimer lesions and intellectual status in Alzheimer's and Parkinson's disease patients. Neurosci Lett 162:179–182
7. Bandyopadhyay U, Cuervo AM (2007) Chaperone-mediated autophagy in aging and neurodegeneration: lessons from alpha-synuclein. Exp Gerontol 42:120–128. https://doi.org/10.1016/j.exger.2006.05.019
8. Banerjee R, Beal MF, Thomas B (2010) Autophagy in neurodegenerative disorders: pathogenic roles and therapeutic implications. Trends Neurosci 33:541–549. https://doi.org/10.1016/j.tins.2010.09.001
9. Bellingham SA, Guo BB, Coleman BM, Hill AF (2012) Exosomes: vehicles for the transfer of toxic proteins associated with neurodegenerative diseases? Front Physiol 3:124. https://doi.org/10.3389/fphys.2012.00124
10. Braak H, Del Tredici K, Rub U, de Vos RA, Jansen Steur EN, Braak E (2003) Staging of brain pathology related to sporadic Parkinson's disease. Neurobiol Aging 24:197–211
11. Cheung ZH, Ip NY (2009) The emerging role of autophagy in Parkinson's disease. Molecular brain 2:29. https://doi.org/10.1186/1756-6606-2-29
12. Ciechanover A (2005) Proteolysis: from the lysosome to ubiquitin and the proteasome. Nat Rev Mol Cell Biol 6:79–87. https://doi.org/10.1038/nrm1552
13. Cleveland DW, Hwo SY, Kirschner MW (1977) Purification of tau, a microtubule-associated protein that induces assembly of microtubules from purified tubulin. J Mol Biol 116:207–225
14. Danzer KM, Kranich LR, Ruf WP, Cagsal-Getkin O, Winslow AR, Zhu L, Vanderburg CR, McLean PJ (2012) Exosomal cell-to-cell transmission of alpha synuclein oligomers. Mol Neurodegener 7:42. https://doi.org/10.1186/1750-1326-7-42
15. Dauer W, Przedborski S (2003) Parkinson's disease: mechanisms and models. Neuron 39:889–909
16. Dawson HN, Ferreira A, Eyster MV, Ghoshal N, Binder LI, Vitek MP (2001) Inhibition of neuronal maturation in primary hippocampal neurons from tau deficient mice. J Cell Sci 114:1179–1187
17. Doty RL, Deems DA, Stellar S (1988) Olfactory dysfunction in parkinsonism: a general deficit unrelated to neurologic signs, disease stage, or disease duration. Neurology 38:1237–1244
18. Drubin DG, Kirschner MW (1986) Tau protein function in living cells. J Cell Biol 103:2739–2746
19. Ejlerskov P, Rasmussen I, Nielsen TT, Bergstrom AL, Tohyama Y, Jensen PH, Vilhardt F (2013) Tubulin polymerization-promoting protein (TPPP/p25alpha) promotes unconventional secretion of alpha-synuclein through exophagy by impairing autophagosome-lysosome fusion. J Biol Chem 288:17313–17335. https://doi.org/10.1074/jbc.M112.401174
20. Emmanouilidou E, Melachroinou K, Roumeliotis T, Garbis SD, Ntzouni M, Margaritis LH, Stefanis L, Vekrellis K (2010) Cell-produced alpha-synuclein is secreted in a calcium-dependent manner by exosomes and impacts neuronal survival. J Neurosci 30:6838–6851. https://doi.org/10.1523/JNEUROSCI.5699-09.2010
21. Fader CM, Colombo MI (2009) Autophagy and multivesicular bodies: two closely related partners. Cell Death Differ 16:70–78. https://doi.org/10.1038/cdd.2008.168
22. Fader CM, Sanchez D, Furlan M, Colombo MI (2008) Induction of autophagy promotes fusion of multivesicular bodies with autophagic vacuoles in k562 cells. Traffic 9:230–250. https://doi.org/10.1111/j.1600-0854.2007.00677.x
23. Fevrier B, Vilette D, Archer F, Loew D, Faigle W, Vidal M, Laude H, Raposo G (2004) Cells release prions in association with exosomes. Proc Natl Acad Sci U S A 101:9683–9688. https://doi.org/10.1073/pnas.0308413101

24. Goedert M, Spillantini MG, Del Tredici K, Braak H (2013) 100 years of Lewy pathology. Nat Rev Neurol 9:13–24. https://doi.org/10.1038/nrneurol.2012.242
25. Harada A, Oguchi K, Okabe S, Kuno J, Terada S, Ohshima T, Sato-Yoshitake R, Takei Y, Noda T, Hirokawa N (1994) Altered microtubule organization in small-calibre axons of mice lacking tau protein. Nature 369:488–491. https://doi.org/10.1038/369488a0
26. Hasegawa T, Konno M, Baba T, Sugeno N, Kikuchi A, Kobayashi M, Miura E, Tanaka N, Tamai K, Furukawa K et al (2011) The AAA-ATPase VPS4 regulates extracellular secretion and lysosomal targeting of alpha-synuclein. PLoS One 6: e29460 Doi https://doi.org/10.1371/journal.pone.0029460
27. Hawkes CH, Del Tredici K, Braak H (2010) A timeline for Parkinson's disease. Parkinsonism Relat Disord 16:79–84. https://doi.org/10.1016/j.parkreldis.2009.08.007
28. Ikegami S, Harada A, Hirokawa N (2000) Muscle weakness, hyperactivity, and impairment in fear conditioning in tau-deficient mice. Neurosci Lett 279: 129–132
29. Itakura E, Kishi-Itakura C, Mizushima N (2012) The hairpin-type tail-anchored SNARE syntaxin 17 targets to autophagosomes for fusion with endosomes/lysosomes. Cell 151:1256–1269. https://doi.org/10.1016/j.cell.2012.11.001
30. Jeganathan S, von Bergen M, Mandelkow EM, Mandelkow E (2008) The natively unfolded character of tau and its aggregation to Alzheimer-like paired helical filaments. Biochemistry 47:10526–10539. https://doi.org/10.1021/bi800783d
31. Jiang P, Nishimura T, Sakamaki Y, Itakura E, Hatta T, Natsume T, Mizushima N (2014) The HOPS complex mediates autophagosome-lysosome fusion through interaction with syntaxin 17. Mol Biol Cell 25:1327–1337. https://doi.org/10.1091/mbc.E13-08-0447
32. Joachim CL, Morris JH, Kosik KS, Selkoe DJ (1987) Tau antisera recognize neurofibrillary tangles in a range of neurodegenerative disorders. Ann Neurol 22:514–520. https://doi.org/10.1002/ana.410220411
33. Kabeya Y, Mizushima N, Ueno T, Yamamoto A, Kirisako T, Noda T, Kominami E, Ohsumi Y, Yoshimori T (2000) LC3, a mammalian homologue of yeast Apg8p, is localized in autophagosome membranes after processing. EMBO J 19:5720–5728. https://doi.org/10.1093/emboj/19.21.5720
34. Kertelge L, Bruggemann N, Schmidt A, Tadic V, Wisse C, Dankert S, Drude L, van der Vegt J, Siebner H, Pawlack H et al (2010) Impaired sense of smell and color discrimination in monogenic and idiopathic Parkinson's disease. Movement disorders : official journal of the Movement Disorder Society 25: 2665–2669. https://doi.org/10.1002/mds.23272
35. Klionsky DJ, Ohsumi Y (1999) Vacuolar import of proteins and organelles from the cytoplasm. Annu Rev Cell Dev Biol 15:1–32. https://doi.org/10.1146/annurev.cellbio.15.1.1
36. Kliosnky D (2016) Guidelines for the use and interpretation of assays for monitoring autophagy (3rd edition) (vol 12, pg 1, 2015) Autophagy 12: 443–443 Doi https://doi.org/10.1080/15548627.2016.1147886
37. Kochl R, Hu XW, Chan EY, Tooze SA (2006) Microtubules facilitate autophagosome formation and fusion of autophagosomes with endosomes. Traffic 7:129–145. https://doi.org/10.1111/j.1600-0854.2005.00368.x
38. Lang AE, Lozano AM (1998) Parkinson's disease. First of two parts. N Engl J Med 339:1044–1053. https://doi.org/10.1056/NEJM199810083391506
39. Lee HJ, Bae EJ, Lee SJ (2014) Extracellular alpha–synuclein-a novel and crucial factor in Lewy body diseases. Nat Rev Neurol 10:92–98. https://doi.org/10.1038/nrneurol.2013.275
40. Lee HJ, Cho ED, Lee KW, Kim JH, Cho SG, Lee SJ (2013) Autophagic failure promotes the exocytosis and intercellular transfer of alpha-synuclein. Exp Mol Med 45:e22. https://doi.org/10.1038/emm.2013.45
41. Lei P, Ayton S, Finkelstein DI, Spoerri L, Ciccotosto GD, Wright DK, Wong BX, Adlard PA, Cherny RA, Lam LQ et al (2012) Tau deficiency induces parkinsonism with dementia by impairing APP-mediated iron export. Nat Med 18:291–295. https://doi.org/10.1038/nm.2613
42. Lei P, Ayton S, Moon S, Zhang Q, Volitakis I, Finkelstein DI, Bush AI (2014) Motor and cognitive deficits in aged tau knockout mice in two background strains. Mol Neurodegener 9:29. https://doi.org/10.1186/1750-1326-9-29
43. Lindwall G, Cole RD (1984) Phosphorylation affects the ability of tau protein to promote microtubule assembly. J Biol Chem 259:5301–5305
44. Luk KC, Kehm V, Carroll J, Zhang B, O'Brien P, Trojanowski JQ, Lee VM (2012) Pathological alpha-synuclein transmission initiates Parkinson-like neurodegeneration in nontransgenic mice. Science 338:949–953. https://doi.org/10.1126/science.1227157
45. Lynch-Day MA, Mao K, Wang K, Zhao M, Klionsky DJ (2012) The role of autophagy in Parkinson's disease. Cold Spring Harbor perspectives in medicine 2:a009357. https://doi.org/10.1101/cshperspect.a009357
46. Macknin JB, Higuchi M, Lee VM, Trojanowski JQ, Doty RL (2004) Olfactory dysfunction occurs in transgenic mice overexpressing human tau protein. Brain Res 1000:174–178. https://doi.org/10.1016/j.brainres.2004.01.047
47. McShane RH, Nagy Z, Esiri MM, King E, Joachim C, Sullivan N, Smith AD (2001) Anosmia in dementia is associated with Lewy bodies rather than Alzheimer's pathology. J Neurol Neurosurg Psychiatry 70:739–743
48. Morris M, Hamto P, Adame A, Devidze N, Masliah E, Mucke L (2013) Age-appropriate cognition and subtle dopamine-independent motor deficits in aged tau knockout mice. Neurobiol Aging 34:1523–1529. https://doi.org/10.1016/j.neurobiolaging.2012.12.003
49. Nakatogawa H, Ichimura Y, Ohsumi Y (2007) Atg8, a ubiquitin-like protein required for autophagosome formation. mediates membrane tethering and hemifusion Cell 130:165–178. https://doi.org/10.1016/j.cell.2007.05.021
50. Nguyen TN, Padman BS, Usher J, Oorschot V, Ramm G, Lazarou M (2016) Atg8 family LC3/GABARAP proteins are crucial for autophagosome-lysosome fusion but not autophagosome formation during PINK1/Parkin mitophagy and starvation. J Cell Biol 215:857–874. https://doi.org/10.1083/jcb.201607039
51. Olichney JM, Murphy C, Hofstetter CR, Foster K, Hansen LA, Thal LJ, Katzman R (2005) Anosmia is very common in the Lewy body variant of Alzheimer's disease. J Neurol Neurosurg Psychiatry 76:1342–1347. https://doi.org/10.1136/Jnnp.2003.032003
52. Pan T, Kondo S, Le W, Jankovic J (2008) The role of autophagy lysosome pathway in neurodegeneration associated with Parkinson's disease. Brain : a journal of neurology 131:1969–1978. https://doi.org/10.1093/brain/awm318
53. Petit GH, Berkovich E, Hickery M, Kallunki P, Fog K, Fitzer-Attas C, Brundin P (2013) Rasagiline Ameliorates Olfactory Deficits in an Alpha-Synuclein Mouse Model of Parkinson's Disease. PloS one 8: Doi ARTN e60691 541371/Journalpone.0060691
54. Reeve A, Simcox E, Turnbull D (2014) Ageing and Parkinson's disease: why is advancing age the biggest risk factor? Ageing Res Rev 14:19–30. https://doi.org/10.1016/j.arr.2014.01.004
55. Rubinsztein DC (2006) The roles of intracellular protein-degradation pathways in neurodegeneration. Nature 443:780–786. https://doi.org/10.1038/nature05291
56. Sahani MH, Itakura E, Mizushima N (2014) Expression of the autophagy substrate SQSTM1/p62 is restored during prolonged starvation depending on transcriptional upregulation and autophagy-derived amino acids. Autophagy 10:431–441. https://doi.org/10.4161/auto.27344
57. Schneider A, Simons M (2013) Exosomes: vesicular carriers for intercellular communication in neurodegenerative disorders. Cell Tissue Res 352:33–47. https://doi.org/10.1007/s00441-012-1428-2
58. Shimozawa A, Ono M, Takahara D, Tarutani A, Imura S, Masuda-Suzukake M, Higuchi M, Yanai K, Hisanaga SI, Hasegawa M (2017) Propagation of pathological alpha-synuclein in marmoset brain. Acta neuropathologica communications 5:12. https://doi.org/10.1186/s40478-017-0413-0
59. Simons M, Raposo G (2009) Exosomes–vesicular carriers for intercellular communication. Curr Opin Cell Biol 21:575–581. https://doi.org/10.1016/j.ceb.2009.03.007
60. Simon-Sanchez J, Schulte C, Bras JM, Sharma M, Gibbs JR, Berg D, Paisan-Ruiz C, Lichtner P, Scholz SW, Hernandez DG et al (2009) Genome-wide association study reveals genetic risk underlying Parkinson's disease. Nat Genet 41:1308–U1368. https://doi.org/10.1038/ng.487
61. Spillantini MG, Goedert M (2001) Tau and Parkinson disease. Jama 286: 2324–2326
62. Tanida I, Ueno T, Kominami E (2004) LC3 conjugation system in mammalian autophagy. Int J Biochem Cell Biol 36:2503–2518. https://doi.org/10.1016/j.biocel.2004.05.009

63. Taylor TN, Caudle WM, Shepherd KR, Noorian A, Jackson CR, Iuvone PM, Weinshenker D, Greene JG, Miller GW (2009) Nonmotor symptoms of Parkinson's disease revealed in an animal model with reduced monoamine storage capacity. J Neurosci 29:8103–8113. https://doi.org/10.1523/JNEUROSCI.1495-09.2009
64. Tian Y, Chang JC, Greengard P, Flajolet M (2014) The convergence of endosomal and autophagosomal pathways: implications for APP-CTF degradation. Autophagy 10:694–696. https://doi.org/10.4161/auto.27802
65. Tillerson JL, Caudle WM, Parent JM, Gong C, Schallert T, Miller GW (2006) Olfactory discrimination deficits in mice lacking the dopamine transporter or the D2 dopamine receptor. Behav Brain Res 172:97–105. https://doi.org/10.1016/j.bbr.2006.04.025
66. Tsuboi Y, Wszolek ZK, Graff-Radford NR, Cookson N, Dickson DW (2003) Tau pathology in the olfactory bulb correlates with Braak stage, Lewy body pathology and apolipoprotein epsilon4. Neuropathol Appl Neurobiol 29:503–510
67. Vella LJ, Sharples RA, Nisbet RM, Cappai R, Hill AF (2008) The role of exosomes in the processing of proteins associated with neurodegenerative diseases. European biophysics journal : EBJ 37:323–332. https://doi.org/10.1007/s00249-007-0246-z
68. Watt AD, Crespi GA, Down RA, Ascher DB, Gunn A, Perez KA, McLean CA, Villemagne VL, Parker MW, Barnham KJ et al (2014) Anti-Abeta antibody target engagement: A response to Siemers et al. Acta neuropathologica 128: 611–614 Doi https://doi.org/10.1007/s00401-014-1333-8
69. Weingarten MD, Lockwood AH, Hwo SY, Kirschner MW (1975) A protein factor essential for microtubule assembly. Proc Natl Acad Sci U S A 72:1858–1862
70. Wong E, Cuervo AM (2010) Autophagy gone awry in neurodegenerative diseases. Nat Neurosci 13:805–811. https://doi.org/10.1038/nn.2575
71. Yamamoto M, Suzuki SO, Himeno M (2010) The effects of dynein inhibition on the autophagic pathway in glioma cells. Neuropathology : official journal of the Japanese Society of Neuropathology 30:1–6. https://doi.org/10.1111/j.1440-1789.2009.01034.x
72. Yang S, Kuan WL, Spillantini MG (2016) Progressive tauopathy in P301S tau transgenic mice is associated with a functional deficit of the olfactory system. Eur J Neurosci 44:2396–2403. https://doi.org/10.1111/ejn.13333
73. Zhang S, Xiao Q, Le W (2015) Olfactory dysfunction and neurotransmitter disturbance in olfactory bulb of transgenic mice expressing human A53T mutant alpha-synuclein. PLoS One 10:e0119928. https://doi.org/10.1371/journal.pone.0119928

6

The presubiculum is preserved from neurodegenerative changes in Alzheimer's disease

Christina E. Murray[1,7], Priya Gami-Patel[1], Eleni Gkanatsiou[2], Gunnar Brinkmalm[2], Erik Portelius[2,3], Oliver Wirths[4], Wendy Heywood[5], Kaj Blennow[2,3], Jorge Ghiso[6], Janice L. Holton[1], Kevin Mills[5], Henrik Zetterberg[2,3,7], Tamas Revesz[1] and Tammaryn Lashley[1*]

Abstract

In the majority of affected brain regions the pathological hallmarks of Alzheimer's disease (AD) are β-amyloid (Aβ) deposits in the form of diffuse and neuritic plaques, tau pathology in the form of neurofibrillary tangles, neuropil threads and plaque-associated abnormal neurites in combination with an inflammatory response. However, the anatomical area of the presubiculum, is characterised by the presence of a single large evenly distributed 'lake-like' Aβ deposit with minimal tau deposition or accumulation of inflammatory markers. Post-mortem brain samples from sporadic AD (SAD) and familial AD (FAD) and two hereditary cerebral amyloid diseases, familial British dementia (FBD) and familial Danish dementia (FDD) were used to compare the morphology of the extracellular proteins deposited in the presubiculum compared to the entorhinal cortex. The level of tau pathology and the extent of microglial activation were quantitated in the two brain regions in SAD and FAD. Frozen tissue was used to investigate the Aβ species and proteomic differences between the two regions. Consistent with our previous investigations of FBD and FDD cases we were able to establish that the 'lake-like' pre-amyloid deposits of the presubiculum were not a unique feature of AD but they also found two non-Aβ amyloidosis. Comparing the presubiculum to the entorhinal cortex the number of neurofibrillary tangles and tau load were significantly reduced; there was a reduction in microglial activation; there were differences in the Aβ profiles and the investigation of the whole proteome showed significant changes in different protein pathways. In summary, understanding why the presubiculum has a different morphological appearance, biochemical and proteomic makeup compared to surrounding brain regions severely affected by neurodegeneration could lead us to understanding protective mechanisms in neurodegenerative diseases.

Keywords: Alzheimer's disease, Presubiculum, Amyloid, Tau, Neuroinflammation

Introduction

The hippocampus and surrounding parahippocampal region are important for memory function and are severely affected early in Alzheimer's disease (AD) [2, 84]. The pathology observed in the hippocampus consists of marked neuronal loss, severe β-amyloid (Aβ) plaque deposition, neurofibrillary tangle (NFT) formation and a neuroinflammatory reaction. However, one area within the parahippocampus, the presubiculum, appears to have a different pathological profile in comparison to other areas of the medial temporal region [2, 36, 37, 84]. In AD, diffuse 'lake-like' Aβ deposits appear in the presubiculum early in the disease process corresponding to Thal phases 2 and 3 with the morphology of the deposits not changing through to end stage disease, Thal stage 5 [74].

The hippocampus proper is formed from the dentate gyrus, the CA3/4, CA2, CA1 areas and the subiculum. The adjacent parahippocampal region is connected to the hippocampus via the perforant pathway [4, 10, 79]. The parahippocampus is made up of the pre- and parasubiculum, transsubiculum and entorhinal cortex [17]. It has been shown that the presubiculum has different pathological properties to the hippocampal formation in AD [2, 37, 84], in the form that the presubiculum

* Correspondence: T.Lashley@ucl.ac.uk
[1]The Queen Square Brain Bank for Neurological Disorders, Department of Molecular Neuroscience, UCL Institute of Neurology, London WC1N 3BG, UK
Full list of author information is available at the end of the article

contained a 'lake-like amyloid deposit' composed of Aβ that filled the anatomical area instead of forming defined Aβ plaques [37]. Thioflavin S and Congo-red staining, which highlight misfolded protein aggregates in an amyloid β-sheet conformational state, confirmed that the Aβ deposited in the presubiculum was diffuse or pre-amyloid in nature [2, 75, 84]. A further number of observational differences were seen between the presubiculum and neighbouring hippocampal areas in that, only sparse NFTs, no activated glial cells and no amyloid-associated proteins such as apolipoprotein E or apolipoprotein J (clusterin) were detected [2, 36, 37, 84]. Conversely, the neighbouring entorhinal cortex had severe neuronal loss, dense core amyloid plaques, frequent NFT's, activated microglia and activated astrocytes [2, 36, 37, 84]. These previous studies used silver impregnation techniques to identify the amyloid and NFTs together with semi-quantitative methods of analysis.

The amyloid plaques present in AD are composed of aggregated Aβ peptides. Aβ is formed from cleavage of the amyloid precursor protein (APP) and a number of different Aβ peptide species are released due to secretases cleaving at different sites [11, 64, 71]. Whereas in the two hereditary neurodegenerative diseases, familial British dementia (FBD) and familial Danish dementia (FDD), both are characterised by extra-cellular amyloid and pre-amyloid deposits. In FBD a point mutation, while in FDD a decamer duplication insertion, abolishes the stop codon of the *BRI2* gene [23, 30, 31, 77, 80, 81] resulting in elongated precursor proteins, from which the amyloid peptides amyloid-Bri (ABri) and amyloid-Dan (ADan) are released in FBD and FDD, respectively. Similar to AD, there are numerous ABri and ADan amyloid plaques as well as diffuse plaques and also severe tau pathology in medial temporal lobe structures in both diseases, allowing for comparison with AD.

In this study we investigated whether the unique morphological appearance of deposited Aβ in the presubiculum was protein-specific or due to different tissue factors found in the two different brain regions. To achieve these aims we investigated the morphological appearance of three amyloid forming extracellular peptides found in the presubiculum in SAD, FAD, FBD and FDD using immunohistochemical methods. To determine whether the presubiculum is protected against neurodegeneration and neuroinflammation, in SAD and FAD we quantitated the level of total tau pathology, the number of neurofibrillary tangles and levels of microglial activation compared to the neighbouring entorhinal cortex using immunohistochemical methods. We used laser capture microdissection paired with mass spectrometry to determine the Aβ peptide species that form the extracellular parenchymal deposits in the presubiculum compared to the amyloid plaques found in the entorhinal cortex in SAD and FAD. Laser capture microdissection teamed with label-free proteomics were used to identify altered protein expression or pathways that could be responsible for the differences between the presubiculum and entorhinal cortex.

Material and methods

Cases

All sporadic AD cases (SAD; $n = 19$) and familial AD cases (FAD; $n = 11$ (8 *PS1* and 3 *APP* mutations) were obtained through the brain donation program of the Queen Square Brain Bank for Neurological Disorders (QSBB), Department of Molecular Neuroscience, UCL Institute of Neurology. The FBD ($n = 4$) and FDD ($n = 4$) brains were donated to the QSBB, the Neuropathology Department, Århus Kommunehospital, Århus, Denmark or the Division of Neuropathology Department, UCL Institute of Neurology. The criteria for the neuropathological diagnosis of FBD and FDD have been previously described [30, 31] while for that of AD standard diagnostic criteria were used [9, 52, 74]. The demographic data for all cases are shown in Table 1. Ethical approval for the study was obtained from the Local Research Ethics Committee of the National Hospital for Neurology and Neurosurgery.

Immunohistochemistry

Eight-micron-thick formalin-fixed paraffin-embedded tissue sections from the hippocampal/parahippocampal region, taken from the level of the lateral geniculate body, were cut from the cases listed in Table 1. Sections were deparaffinised in xylene and rehydrated using graded alcohols. Immunohistochemistry for all antibodies required pre-treatment with a pressure cooker for 10 min in citrate buffer pH 6.0. Aβ, ABri and ADan immunohistochemistry also required formic acid pre-treatment prior to pressure cooking. Endogenous peroxidase activity was blocked in 0.3% H_2O_2 in methanol for 10 min and non-specific binding with 10% dried milk solution. Tissue sections were incubated with primary antibodies; Aβ (1:100; Dako), 1–57 N-terminal $A\beta_{pE3}$ (1:1000; Synaptic Systems), 2–48 N-terminal $A\beta_{pE3}$ (1:100; Synaptic Systems), pE-Aβ (1:200; Synaptic Systems), Aβ-pE11 (1:100; Synaptic Systems), Aβ4-x (1:200; [83]); Aβ1–5 (1:500; Synaptic systems 218,231), ABri (338; 1:1000), ADan (5282; 1:1000), AT8 (1:600; Thermo), Iba1 (1:1000; Wako), CD68 (1:100, DAKO), CR3–43 (1:150, DAKO), Annexin A1 (1:4000; Abcam), Annexin 2 (1:2000; Abcam), DOCK2 (1:100; Abcam) and INPPD5 (1:200; Proteintech) for 1 h at RT, followed by biotinylated anti-rabbit IgG (1:200; DAKO) or biotinylated anti-mouse IgG (1:200; DAKO) for 30 min at RT and Avidin-Biotin complex (30 min; Dako). Colour was developed with di-aminobenzidine/H_2O_2 [42]. All antibodies were commercially available apart from anti-ABri

Table 1 Demographics of cases used in the study

Cases	Disease group	Gene/ Mutations	Age at onset	Age at death	Disease duration	Sex	Post-mortem delay (hours)	Fixation time (weeks)	Braak and Braak stage	Thal phase	CERAD score
1	SAD	–	63	73	10	M	31	7.14	6	5	Frequent
2	SAD	–	51	63	12	F	16	4.00	6	5	Frequent
3*	SAD	–	51	62	11	F	63	2.71	6	5	Frequent
4	SAD	–	65	70	5	F	47	4.29	5	5	Moderate
5	SAD	–	64	77	13	M	90	3.14	6	5	Frequent
6	SAD	–	49	62	13	F	77	8.00	6	5	Frequent
7	SAD	–	72	88	16	M	86	3.29	6	5	Frequent
8	SAD	–	52	69	17	M	35	6.14	6	5	Frequent
9	SAD	–	65	72	7	M	39	3.00	5	5	Moderate
10	SAD	–	76	85	9	F	90	3.86	6	5	Frequent
11	SAD	–	55	64	9	M	77	3.43	6	5	Frequent
12	SAD	–	69	74	5	F	94	3.00	6	5	Frequent
13	SAD	–	80	85	5	M	129	n/a	5	5	Moderate
14	SAD	–	46	52	6	F	52	2.57	6	5	Frequent
15	SAD	–	49	54	6	F	48	4.29	6	5	Frequent
16	SAD	–	67	72	5	M	91	4.14	6	5	Frequent
17	SAD	–	65	79	14	F	23	3.43	6	5	Frequent
18	SAD	–	52	68	16	M	35	3.00	6	5	Frequent
19*	SAD	–	58	68	10	M	52	3.86	6	5	Frequent
SAD summary			*60.5 (10)*	*70.4 (9.8)*	*9.9 (4.1)*	*10 M:9F*	*61.8 (30)*	*4.1 (1.5)*	*5.8 (0.4)*	*5 (0)*	*Frequent*
20*	FAD	*PS1 Intron 4*	35	52	17	F	33	n/a	6	5	Frequent
21	FAD	*PS1 S132A*	61	70	9	M	n/a	4.29	5	5	Frequent
22	FAD	*PS1 Intron 4*	42	51	9	M	43	4.00	6	5	Frequent
23*	FAD	*APP V717 L*	48	59	11	F	90	n/a	6	5	Frequent
24	FAD	*APP V717I*	60	66	6	M	68	3.14	6	5	Frequent
25	FAD	*PS1 A434T/ T291A*	42	47	5	M	44	4.29	5	5	Frequent
26	FAD	*PS1 R278I*	46	66	20	F	32	4.86	6	5	Frequent
27	FAD	*PS1 I202F*	48	59	11	F	26	4.00	6	5	Frequent
28	FAD	*PS1 E120K*	33	37	4	F	24	6.00	6	5	Frequent
29	FAD	*APP V717I*	44	56	12	F	16	4.29	6	5	Frequent
30	FAD	*PS1 Intron 4*	39	47	8	F	n/a	n/a	6	5	Frequent
FAD summary			*45.3 (8.9)*	*55.5 (9.9)*	*10.2 (4.9)*	*4 M:7F*	*53.7 (43.7)*	*4.4 (0.8)*	*5.8 (0.4)*	*5*	*Frequent*
31	FBD	*BRI2*	57	68	11	F	6.5	3.00	5	n/a	n/a
32	FBD	*BRI2*	n/a	56	n/a	F	n/a	n/a	5	n/a	n/a
33	FBD	*BRI2*	n/a	65	n/a	F	n/a	n/a	5	n/a	n/a
34	FBD	*BRI2*	n/a	60	n/a	M	n/a	n/a	5	n/a	n/a
FBD summary			*57*	*62.3 (5.3)*	*11*	*1 M:3F*	*6.5*	*3.00*	*5*	*n/a*	*n/a*
36	FDD	*BRI2*	25	43	18	M	n/a	n/a	5	n/a	n/a
37	FDD	*BRI2*	34	60	26	F	n/a	n/a	5	n/a	n/a
38	FDD	*BRI2*	40	58	18	M	n/a	n/a	5	n/a	n/a
39	FDD	*BRI2*	21	53	32	M	n/a	n/a	5	n/a	n/a
FDD summary			*30 (8.6)*	*53.5 (7.6)*	*23.5 (6.8)*	*2 M:1F*	*n/a*	*n/a*	*5*	*n/a*	*n/a*

All cases were used for morphological analysis of the presubiculum. '*' cases used for proteomics

and anti-ADan which have been previously validated [30, 31]. Stained sections were digitised using a Leica slide scanner with a 40× objective.

Thioflavin S immunofluorescence

Sections from the hippocampal/parahippocampal region were cut from all cases and were incubated with 0.1% Thioflavin-S (Sigma) solution for 7 min. The sections were differentiated in 70% ethanol and washed in Tris-buffered-saline. The standard immunohistochemistry protocol was applied to the sections to stain for Aβ, ABri and ADan, replacing di-aminobenzidine with TSA plus TMR system (Perkin Elmer) to provide the fluorescent signal. Sections were viewed with a Leica TCS4D confocal microscope using a 3-channel scan head and argon/krypton laser.

Laser capture microscopy

To investigate differences in the Aβ species profile between the presubiculum and entorhinal cortex in the AD cases, ten-micron-thick frozen tissue sections were sampled from the hippocampal/parahippocampal region at the level of the lateral geniculate body from SAD cases (cases 3 and 19) and FAD cases (case 20 (*PS1* mutation) and case 23 (*APP* mutation)) (highlighted in Table 1). Sections were mounted onto PEN-membrane slides (Leica) coated with polyethylene naphthalate, fixed with 4% paraformaldehyde (PFA), and treated in formic acid for 5 min before the immunohistochemistry protocol for Aβ was performed. The Leica DM6000B laser capture microdissection (LCM) microscope was used to firstly dissect the Aβ-positive areas of the presubiculum from three sections per each case (average area per case 1.6 μm^2) and 300 amyloid plaques (average area per case 2.0 μm^2) from the neighbouring entorhinal cortex. Samples were collected from both regions for matrix-assisted laser desorption/ionization-time-of-flight (MALDI-TOF) mass spectrometric analysis to identify the Aβ peptides present in both brain regions. Samples were also collected from both brain regions via LCM to investigate the whole proteome.

Mass spectrometry

To identify the Aβ peptides in the laser-captured presubiculum lesions and amyloid plaques from entorhinal cortex samples were aspirated with 70% formic acid, centrifuged and aspirated again. Samples were vortexed and dried before being resuspended in 5 µl 0.1% FA/20% acetonitrile (ACN). To prepare the matrix, 0.5 µl of the seedlayer (20 g/L α-cyano-4-hydroxycinnamic acid (CHCA) in 90% acetone/10% methanol with 0.005% trifluoroacetic acid [TFA]) was added to the probe. An aliquot sample (2 µl) was mixed with 1 µl sample matrix [15 g/L CHCA] in ACN and 0.1% TFA [1:1]) before being placed on the probe. The different Aβ peptides in each sample were determined using MALDI-TOF-MS [56].

To investigate the proteome in the laser-captured presubiculum and entorhinal cortex, samples were homogenised in 50 mM Ambic buffer with 2% ASB-14 using the Precellys 24 homogenizer (Bertin Instruments). The total protein concentration was determined by BCA protein assay (Thermofisher). Due to the low amount of protein present in the laser captured material samples had to be pooled. A sample pool of each disease group was created with equal protein concentration from each case. Samples were fractionated to look at soluble and insoluble proteins. Samples were spun at maximum speed for ten minutes at 4 °C and the supernatant containing the soluble proteins was removed. The remaining pellet was resuspended in ice cold acetone, vortexed and left at − 20 °C for at least an hour. Samples were vortexed and spun at 14000 g for ten minutes at 4 °C, the supernatant was removed. The pellets containing the insoluble proteins were air-dried and re-suspended in 70% formic acid and vortexed and dried in a speed-vac. Ice-cold acetone was added to the original soluble protein supernatants and left at − 20 °C overnight. The supernatants were vortexed and spun at 14000 g for ten minutes at 4 °C. The supernatant was removed and the remaining pellet was dried. Dried supernatants and pellets were reconstituted in 100 mM Tris/8 M Urea/2% ASB-14, pH 7.79, vortexed and left shaking for one hour to resolubilise the proteins. Dithioerythritol (30 mg/ml, Sigma) was added, vortexed and left shaking for a further hour as a reducing agent. To prevent the formation of disulphide bonds iodoacetamide (36 mg/ml, Sigma) was added to alkylate the proteins, before the addition of H_2O. 1 µg Trypsin-LysC enzyme (Promega Trypsin/Lys-C Mix, Mass Spec Grade cat no. V5073) was added to digest the proteins and was left for three-four hours at 37 °C. The digested samples were diluted 1:1 in 0.2% TFA and 5 pmol of Waters MassPREP enolase digestion standard (part no. 186002325) was added to the digest. Peptides were cleaned in Agilent C18 Bond Elut 96 well plates (Part no. A496011C). The wells were primed with 50% ACN/0.1% TFA and then washed twice with 0.1% TFA. The diluted digest samples were added to the wells and allowed to drip through. The residual salts were washed away using 3% ACN/0.1% TFA and peptides eluted using 2 × 50% ACN/0.1% TFA.

The digested cleaned peptides were reconstituted in 3% ACN/0.1% TFA. MS^e Label-free mass spectrometry was performed as previously described [6] with a SYNAPT G2-Si High Definition machine with 2D fractionation. Four fractions were run for each sample and 0.5 µg of protein was injected per fraction per run. The order of samples were randomised to avoid technical bias. The raw data was processed using Progenesis QI for proteomics (Nonlinear Dynamics, UK). Peptides were identified with an MS^e

search against the UniProt reviewed human proteome with the following parameters: missed cleavages, max one; max protein mass, 800,000 kDa; modifications of carbamidomethyl C, oxidation M, demidation N and Q. The ion matching requirements were set as follows: three fragments/peptide, five fragments/protein, one peptide/protein. Proteins that had been identified with only one unique peptide were excluded from the analysis. Protein identification and normalised abundance was exported into excel for further bioinformatics.

Bioinformatics

Proteins that had > 1.5-fold change in expression between regions were put into publicly available databases to assess the biological processes, molecular functions and cell components that were enriched in each region. Webgestalt was used to assess the enriched gene ontology terms [87].

Morphological analysis

Sequential sections were immunohistochemically stained for Aβ, AT8, Iba1, CD68 and CR3–43. Sections stained with Aβ were used to identify the 'lake-like' deposit in the presubiculum and entorhinal cortex in each case. Bland-Altman plots were used to determine the intra- and inter-rater reliability for the number of randomized snapshot areas required for the quantitation of the different immunohistochemical preparations [5]. Using Image J software (https://imagej.net/) and setting the threshold to include only di-aminobenzidine staining, twenty randomised snapshots from an identified region of interest, each measuring 1500 μm × 1000 μm, were generated, using a python script, from the pre-marked presubiculum and the entorhinal cortex. Images were captured using Leica Image scope. The twenty snapshots were then used to determine the mean 'areal fraction' for each immunohistochemical preparation, defined by the ratio of the area occupied by positive immunohistochemical staining and the field of interest [25]. Iba1, CD68 and CR3–43 immunohistochemical preparations were used for the assessment of the microglial response while AT8 immunohistochemistry was employed to determine the phosphorylated tau load, comprising NFTs, neuropil threads (NTs) and plaque-associated abnormal neurites. In addition, the number of NFTs, identified as large filamentous tau-positive structures in the neuronal cytoplasm [57], were also determined in both the presubiculum and entorhinal cortex. NFTs were systematically counted with any partial NFTs being excluded.

Statistical analysis

Statistical analysis was performed using GraphPad Prism 5 software (GraphPad Software Inc. USA). Continuous variables were analysed using either a two-tailed *t*-test or a Mann-Whitney U test, as appropriate while continuous variables between several groups were compared using the Kruskal-Wallis test. The statistical significance level was established at $p < 0.05$.

Results

Comparison of the pathological characteristics in the presubiculum and entorhinal cortex in AD, FDB and FDD

The pathology observed in the presubiculum was morphologically different from that in the entorhinal cortex in all cases of SAD and FAD investigated (Fig. 1). In the presubiculum Aβ deposited as hazy, diffuse 'lake-like' lesions in the parenchyma (Fig. 1a and d arrows and 1b and 1e, higher magnification) whereas large numbers of 'mature' Aβ amyloid cored plaques with well-defined edges were present in the entorhinal cortex (Fig. 1c and f). A similar difference in the morphology of the parenchymal deposits between these two anatomical areas was observed in two other cerebral amyloid diseases, FBD and FDD. Accordingly diffuse, 'lake-like' ABri and ADan deposits were seen in the presubiculum (Fig. 1g and j, arrows, shown at higher magnification Fig. 1h and k) and well-defined amyloid plaques in the entorhinal cortex (Fig. 1i and l) of FBD and FDD, respectively.

Aβ, ABri or ADan immunohistochemistry combined with Thioflavin-S staining revealed that the extracellular proteins found in the lake-like peptide deposits of the presubiculum (Fig. 2b, arrow) were Thioflavin-S negative in all cases (Fig. 2c) indicating that such deposits were of pre-amyloid nature in both SAD and FAD. In contrast, the plaque-like lesions of the entorhinal cortex were positive for both Aβ (Fig. 2e) and Thioflavin S (Fig. 2f) indicative of amyloid conformation of the Aβ species.

Tau deposition and NFT frequency in FAD and SAD

The phosphorylated tau load comprising all tau-positive lesions was significantly greater in the entorhinal cortex compared to the presubiculum in both SAD (*p* < *0.0001*) and FAD (*p* = *0.001*) (Table 2; Figs. 2h, l and 3). Furthermore, there were significantly more NFTs in the entorhinal cortex compared to the presubiculum in both AD groups (SAD: $p < 0.0001$; FAD: $p = 0.001$) (Table 2; Figs. 2h, l and 3).

Microglial activation in FAD and SAD

Neuroinflammation is a prominent feature of neurodegenerative diseases. In this study we assessed the extent of neuroinflammatory response by determining the density of three microglia markers in the presubiculum and entorhinal cortex. The Iba1 marker, a calcium binding protein that detects total numbers of microglia, was used to assess any homeostatic microglia present [8, 69]. The CD68 and CR3–43 antibodies both detect activated microglia, phagocytic microglia and antigen presenting microglia, respectively [8, 39]. The density of the resident microglia, as detected

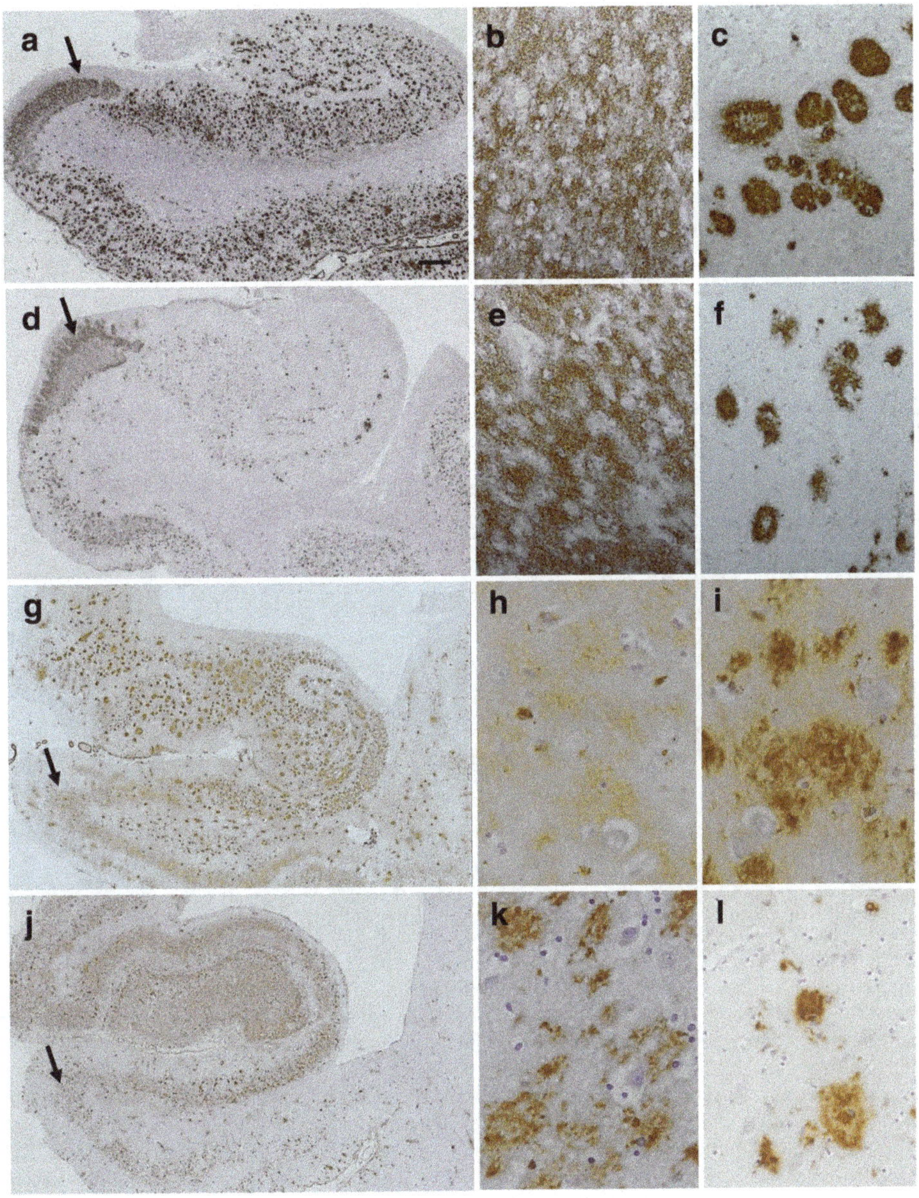

Fig. 1 Pathological analysis of the presubiculum in familial and sporadic Alzheimer's disease (AD; **a-f**), familial British dementia (FBD; **g-i**) and familial Danish dementia (FDD; **j-l**). Aβ immunohistochemistry demonstrates large diffuse, 'lake-like' deposits in the presubiculum in both familial AD (case 26; **a**, arrow; **b**, presubiculum at higher magnification) and sporadic AD (case 2; **d**, arrow; **e** presubiculum at higher magnification). In both disease types well-defined Aβ plaques were present in the entorhinal cortex as shown in sporadic AD (**c** and **f**). The ABri-positive (case 31; **g-i**) and ADan-positive (case 36; **j-l**) parenchymal deposits show similar morphological patterns in FBD and FDD, respetively. Bar in a represents 1000 μm in **a**,**d**,**g**, and **j**; 50 μm in all remaining images

by Iba1 immunohistochemistry, was similar in the presubiculum and the entorhinal cortex in FAD ($p = 0.92$) (Table 2). Whereas a similar analysis in SAD showed that more microglia were present in the presubiculum than in the entorhinal cortex ($p = 0.03$) (Table 2; Figs. 2i, m and 4). However, CD68 ($p < 0.0001$ and $p = 0.02$ in SAD and FAD respectively) and CR3–43 ($p = 0.0003$ and $p = 0.02$ in SAD and FAD respectively) preparations showed that the area density of the microglia was significantly reduced in the presubiculum compared with the entorhinal cortex in both the SAD and FAD groups (Table 2; Figs. 2j-o and 4).

Identification of Aβ species in FAD and SAD

LCM and MALDI-TOF-MS were utilised to examine whether the biochemical profile of the Aβ species found

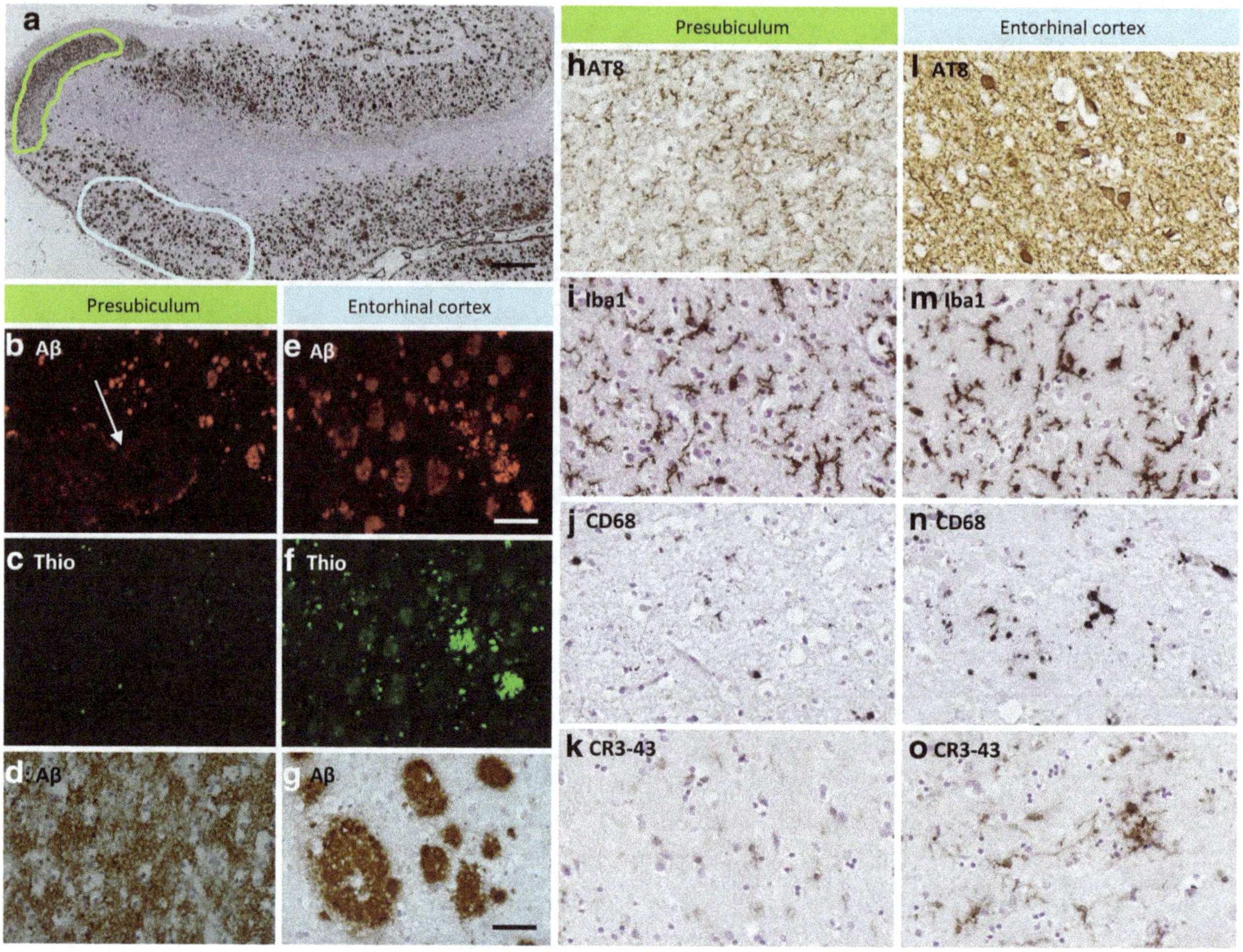

Fig. 2 Pathological comparisons of the presubiculum and entorhinal cortex in Alzheimer's disease. The image demonstrates the anatomy of the hippocampus and illustrates the difference in Aβ deposition between the presubiculum (green outline) and entorhinal cortex (blue outline). Fluorescent Aβ immunohistochemistry shows that the Aβ peptide is deposited in a diffuse manner in the presubiculum (**b**, white arrow) whereas defined Aβ plaques are shown in the entorhinal cortex (**e**). Thioflavin S staining highlights the Aβ plaques in the entorhinal cortex (**f**), whereas the presubiculum is negative for the Thioflavin S stain demonstrating the Aβ in the presubiculum contains pre-amyloid deposits (**c**). Tau immunohistochemistry shows a difference between the presubiculum (**h**) and entorhinal cortex (**l**) in the density of neuropil threads and neurofibrillary tangles. The microglial marker, Iba1, shows the total number of microglia being equal between the two regions (**l** and **m**), whereas CD68 and CR3-43 highlight the increase in the number of activated microglia in the entorhinal cortex (**n** and **o**) compared to the presubiculum (**j** and **k**). Bar in 'a' represents 1000 μm in **a**; 100 μm in **b**, **c**, **e**, and **f**; 50 μm in **d**, **g** and **h-o**

in the presubiculum were different from species present in amyloid plaques isolated from the entorhinal cortex. These studies showed no difference in the profile of the Aβ peptide species between the SAD and FAD cases (Fig. 5). Full length $A\beta_{1-42}$, numerous N-terminally truncated peptides and post-translationally modified peptide Aβ species with pyroglutamate at positions 3 or 11 were identified in the entorhinal cortex. This was in contrast to the Aβ peptides identified in the presubiculum where full length $A\beta_{1-42}$ and the N-terminally truncated $A\beta_{4-42}$ were identifed. No pyroglutamate post-translationally modified Aβ species were identified in the presubiculum in either SAD or FAD (Fig. 5). To validate the differences in Aβ species present in the entorhinal cortex compared to the presubiculum immunohistochemical methods utilising antibodies raised against N-terminally truncated and pyroglutamate modified Aβ species were employed. All antibodies (1–57 N-terminal $A\beta_{pE3}$, 2–48 N-terminal $A\beta_{pE3}$, pE-Aβ, Aβ-pE11, Aβ4-x, Aβ1-x) labelled the Aβ plaques in the entorhinal cortex and some degree of positve staining in the presubiculum was observed (Fig. 6a-f). Positive immunohistochemical staining for these Aβ species in the presubiculum indicates that the Aβ peptides are present in the presubiculum but the amount may differ between the two regions, making them undetectable by MALDI-TOF MS or that the

Table 2 Statistical analysis of the immunohistochemical quantification

		AT8		NFT's		Iba1		CD68		CR3-43	
		Presubiculum	Entorhinal cortex	Presubiculum	Entorhinal cortex	Presubiculum	Entorhinal cortex	Presubiculum	Entorhinal cortex	Presubiculum	Entorhinal cortex
SAD	Mean	11.30%	41.20%	15	41	4.10%	3.40%	1%	1.80%	2.50%	5.90%
	Range	0.9–35.6%	1.9–81%	8–27	12–73	0.3–8.9%	0.5–8.9%	0.1–2.6%	0.4–6.1%	0.2–18.6%	1–44.9%
	SD	9.50%	23.80%	6	16	2.70%	2.60%	0.90%	1.50%	4.10%	9.80%
FAD	Mean	13.30%	42.20%	16	34	5.60%	5.30%	1%	1.60%	2.20%	4.10%
	Range	1.3–26.3%	3.1–68.9%	3–32	2–68	0.9–17.9%	2–9.6%	0.6–2.2%	0.7–5%	0.1–8.6%	0.2–18.6%
	SD	9.10%	24.30%	10	23	5.10%	2.30%	0.50%	1.30%	2.60%	5.40%

Table shows the mean percentages, range and standard deviation of the immunhistochemical analysis using AT8, to quantitate the numbers of NFTs and total phosphorylated tau load; Iba1, CD68 and CR3-43 to quantitate the numbers of microglia in both the presubiculum and entorhinal cortex

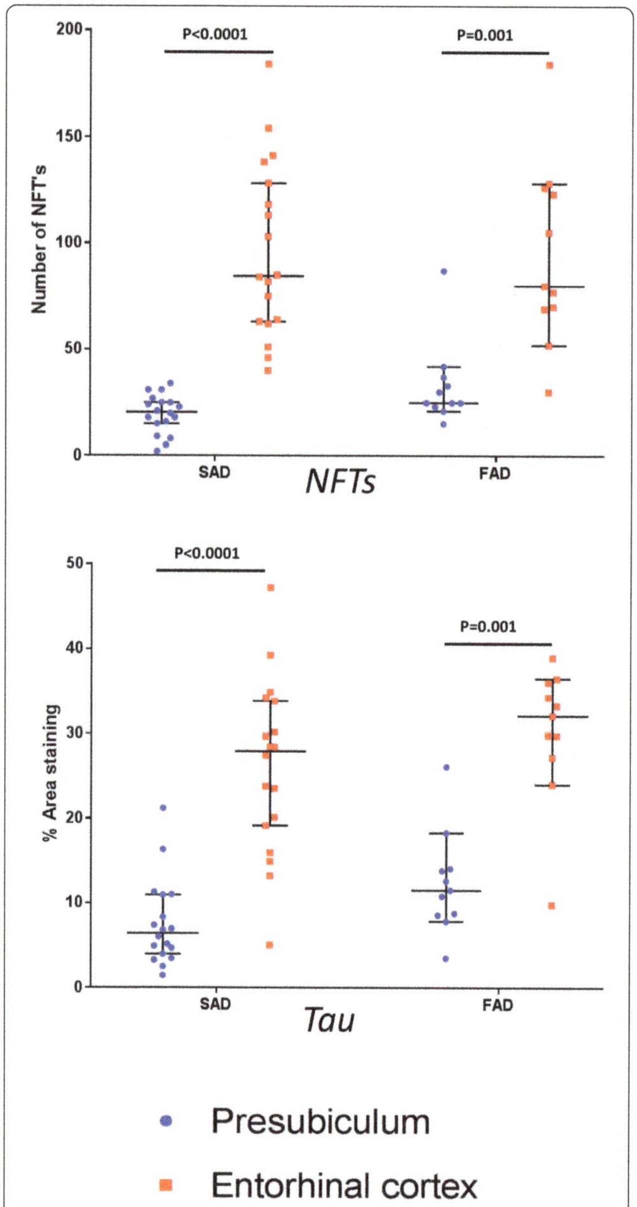

Fig. 3 Quantification of microglial immunohistochemistry in the presubiculum and entorhinal cortex. The overall numbers of microglia were similar in the two anatomical areas as shown by the Iba1. However the presubiculum had significantly less activated microglia, positive for CD68 and CR3-43, than the entorhinal cortex in both sporadic and familial AD cases. FAD; Familial Alzheimer's disease: SAD; Sporadic Alzheimer's disease. Bars represent medians with 95% confidence intervals. Wilcoxon paired rank test was performed in each case and *p* values are shown

species specific antibodies might show some minor cross-reactivity with other Aβ species (e.g. unmodified Aβ3–42) [85].

Proteomic expression in the presubiculum in FAD and SAD

We investigated alterations in protein expression in the presubiculum compared to the entorhinal cortex using MS^e label free proteomics. Samples were analysed as soluble protein supernatant and insoluble protein pellet fractions with a total of 561 proteins detected in the supernatant and 1824 proteins in the pellet. Some proteins were detected in both fractions (303 proteins) or only in one (supernatant 254 proteins, pellet 1488 proteins). SAD cases were pooled into one sample and FAD cases pooled into another. Due to pooling the samples, statistics could not be undertaken, instead fold change between regions was determined to highlight the greatest changes occurring. The fold change expression was calculated for each protein for the presubiculum compared to the entorhinal cortex. SAD and FAD cases were analysed separately and additionally, an average fold change between both was calculated. When analysing the average fold change between SAD and FAD, a total of 112 proteins had an increased fold change of 1.5 or greater in the presubiculum compared to the entorhinal cortex in the supernatant and 313 in the pellet (Additional file 1: Table S1 and Additional file 2: Table S2). Proteins were also found to be decreased in the presubiculum compared to the entorhinal cortex in the supernatant (130 proteins) and the pellet (703 proteins) (Additional file 3: Table S3 and Additional file 4: Table S4). Several proteins were markedly increased in the presubiculum or entorhinal cortex at a level above 1.5-fold, highlighting proteomic differences between the two regions. Webgestalt gene ontology analysis of the proteins with > 1.5-fold change in expression highlighted the top biological processes enriched at a level of $p < 0.05$ (Additional file 5: Table S5 and Additional file 6: Table S6). The proteins that were shown to increase in the presubiculum compared to the entorhinal cortex were enriched for biosynthetic and biogenetic processes as well as metabolic changes. However, the proteins that were shown to decrease in the presubiculum compared to the entorhinal cortex were enriched for cell organisation and cell signalling.

Among the proteins identified as altered between the two brain regions, we found a proportion previously reported as AD-associated proteins. These included proteins associated with amyloid processing and fibrillisation, tau accumulation, and inflammation such as SNX6 and RAB21 which were only detected in the entorhinal cortex and S100A8 and OTUB1 were decreased in the presubiculum (14.8-fold and 2-fold respectively). SNX6 negatively regulates BACE1 cleavage of APP [54]. RAB21 overexpression results in greater Aβ production, whereas silencing of this gene reduces the Aβ levels [70]. S100A8 is thought to aggregate itself prior to Aβ plaque formation and treatment of a neuronal cell line with S100A8 leads to increased Aβ1–42 but decreased levels of Aβ1–40 [45]. Furthermore, S100A8 forms a heterodimeric complex with S100A9 molecules which then elicits an inflammatory response. S100A9 is increased in the presubiculum in this data set, whereas S100A8 was decreased [19, 29]. Therefore we can

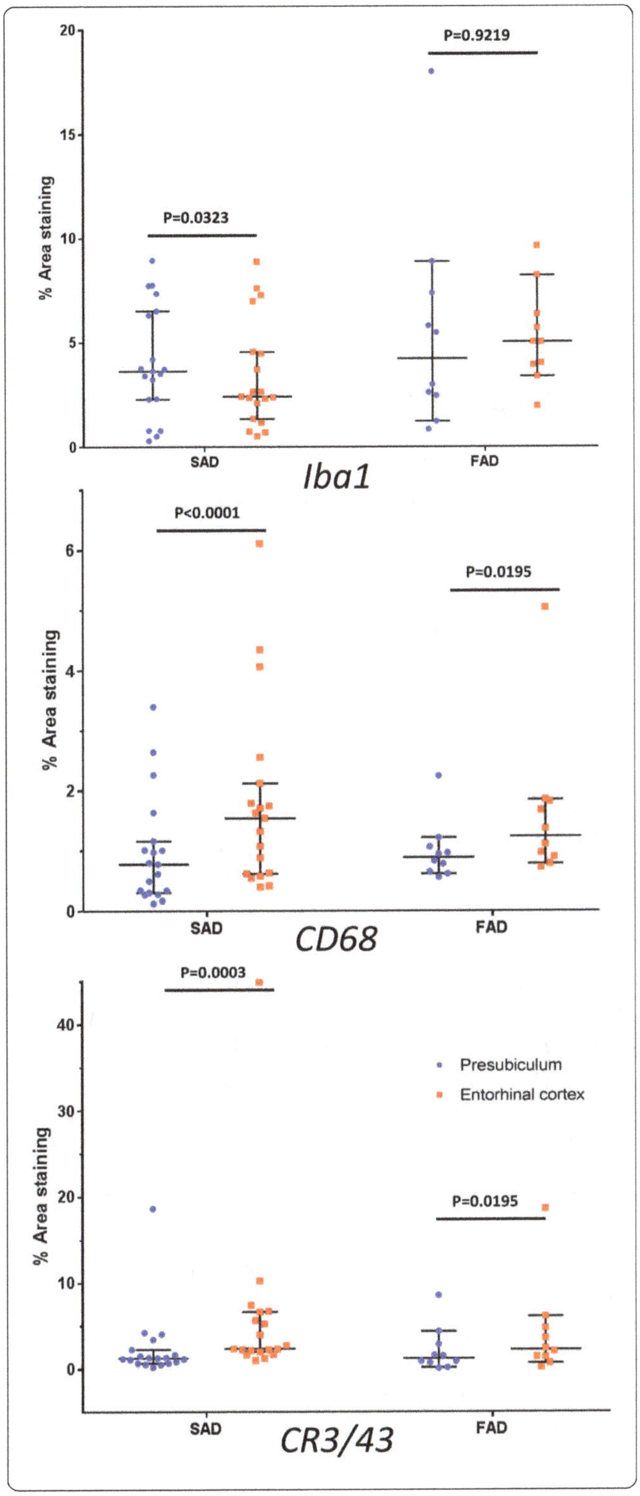

Fig. 4 Quantification of tau immunohistochemistry in the presubiculum and entorhinal cortex. The density of the tau immunohistochemistry observed in the entorhinal cortex and presubiculum was quantitated. The overall density included NFTs and neuropil threads was significantly higher in the entorhinal cortex compared to the presubiculum. The number of NFTs was also significantly higher in the entorhinal cortex compared to the presubiculum. FAD; Familial Alzheimer's disease: SAD; Sporadic Alzheimer's disease. Bars represent medians with 95% confidence intervals. Wilcoxon paired rank test was performed in each case and *p* values are shown.

hypothesis that this complex is not active in the presubiculum [36, 37]. OTUB1 (OTU Deubiquitinase, Ubiquitin Aldehyde Binding 1), a tau deubiquitinating enzyme, has been shown to increase AT8 positive tau accumulation and to increase tau-seeded tau aggregation [82].

Inflammatory proteins detected included DOCK2, decreased 9.4 fold in the presubiculum and INPP5D, increased 2.2-fold in the presubiculum. DOCK2 is part of the prostaglandin pathway and has been shown to modulate microglial cytokine secretion and phagocytosis [12]. INPP5D is a negative regulator of the innate immune system. It has been linked to AD in GWAS studies [18, 24, 49]. Additionally, multiple annexins showed protein expression changes between regions. ANXA4 (329.9 fold, pellet), ANXA7 (4.3 fold, pellet), ANXA1 (2 fold, pellet), ANXA6 (1.7 fold, pellet), ANXA5 (1.4 fold, pellet, 1.2 supernatent), ANXA11 (1.4 fold, pellet) and ANXA2 (1.03 fold, pellet) were found to be decreased in the presubiculum. The annexins are a multigene family that are Ca^{2+} and phospholipid binding proteins. They have a range of roles including involvement in inflammation. Annexin A1 promotes resolution of inflammation by supressing microglial activation and inhibiting secretion of their pro-inflammatory cytokines [59]. Annexin A2 has been shown to modulate pro-inflammmtory cytokines and reactive oxygen species [26]. Annexin A5 inhibits phagocytosis and also regulates cytokine secretion and Annexin A6 has a role in T cell proliferation [14, 62].

Immunohistochemical analysis of candidate proteins in AD

To validate the proteins of interest detected by MS^e label free proteomics, immunohistochemical analysis was performed on the hippocampal sections containing the presubiculum and entorhinal cortex. Proteins to validate were chosen based on the proteomic data, published literature and commercially available antibodies previously used with paraffin embedded tissue. To assess the effect on inflammation in the presubiculum one protein that was increased in the presubiculum (DOCK2), one protein that was decreased in the presubiculum (INPP5D). The annexin protein family were also significantly changes between the two brain regions and two annexins (ANXA1 and ANXA2) were investigated using commercially available antibodies. DOCK2, and INPP5D did not show any

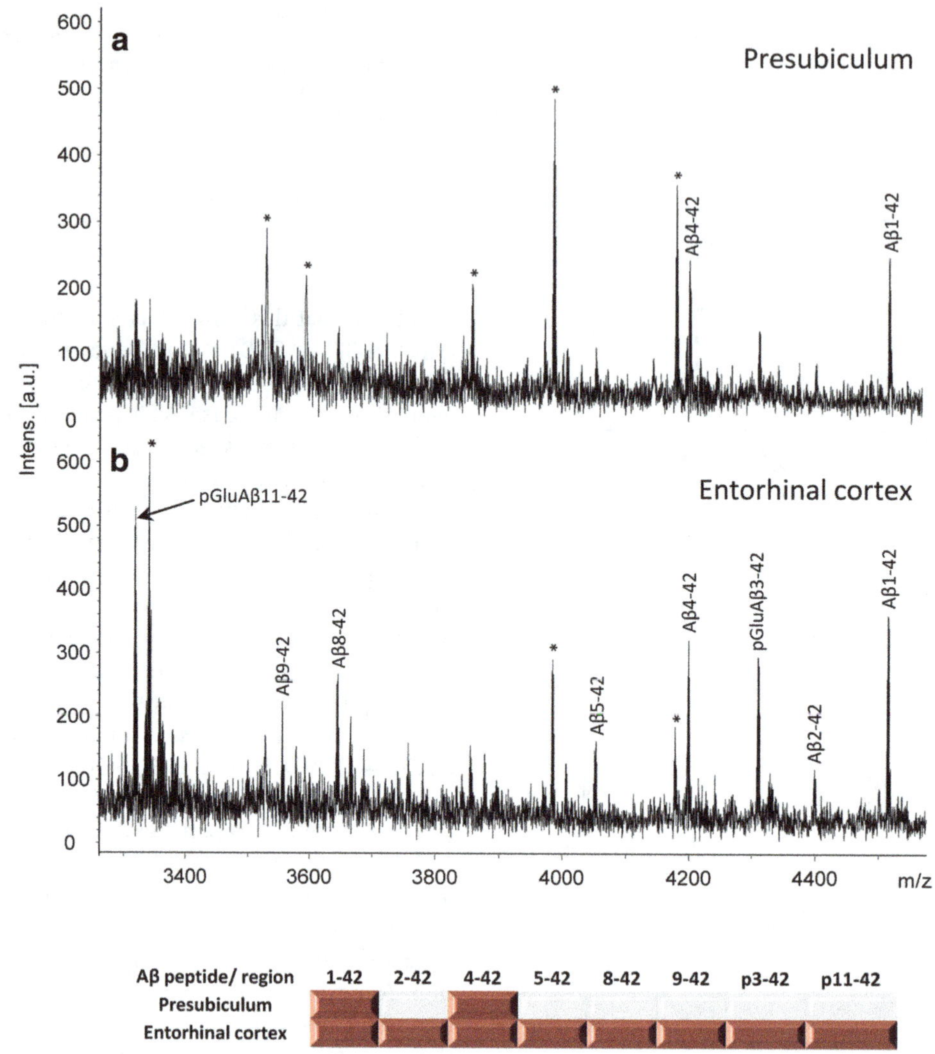

Fig. 5 Mass spectra of the Aβ peptide pattern from the presubiculum and entorhinal cortex. Representative mass spectra from case 3 highlights the differences between the full length Aβ species identified in the presubiculum (**a**) compared to the truncated and post-translationally modified Aβ species identified in the entorhinal cortex (**b**).The table shows the Aβ isoforms present in the presubiculum and entorhinal cortex from six Alzheimer's disease cases. * represent unidentified non-Aβ related peaks. A peak was considered as identified if the signal-to-noise was > 2

positive staining in the presubiculum or the entorhinal cortex. However ANXA1 and ANXA2 antibodies stained astrocytes and astrocytic processes in the entorhinal cortex. However there was no staining in the presubiculum (Fig. 7), validating the proteomic results obtained in the pellet by mass spectrometry.

Discussion

This study aimed to investigate the pathological features in the morphologically diverse presubiculum and entorhinal cortex in three cerebral amyloidosis. We have shown that, regardless of the amino acid sequence of the three amyloid peptides Aβ, ABri and ADan they form similar diffuse, 'lake-like' structures in the presubiculum in AD, FBD and FDD respectively. This observation underpins the notion that this morphological phenomenon of the presubiculum is not a unique feature of the Aβ peptide of AD, but is also seen in FBD and FDD. The lack of binding to β-pleated sheet ligands, such as Thioflavin-S, implies that the large diffuse 'lake-like' deposits seen in the presubiculum of the three cerebral amyloid diseases are primarily composed of non-fibrillar peptide aggregates [2, 30, 31, 84]. A recent study on binding of amyloid tracers to Aβ aggregates showed no binding of the PiB PET ligand in the presubiculum of AD patients, also indicating that the Aβ deposits found in the presubiculum are not in amyloid conformation [36].

It has been suggested that diffuse plaques with non-fibrillar Aβ undergo fibrillization and become amyloid/neuritic plaques [13, 33, 46, 55, 57]. However, the large

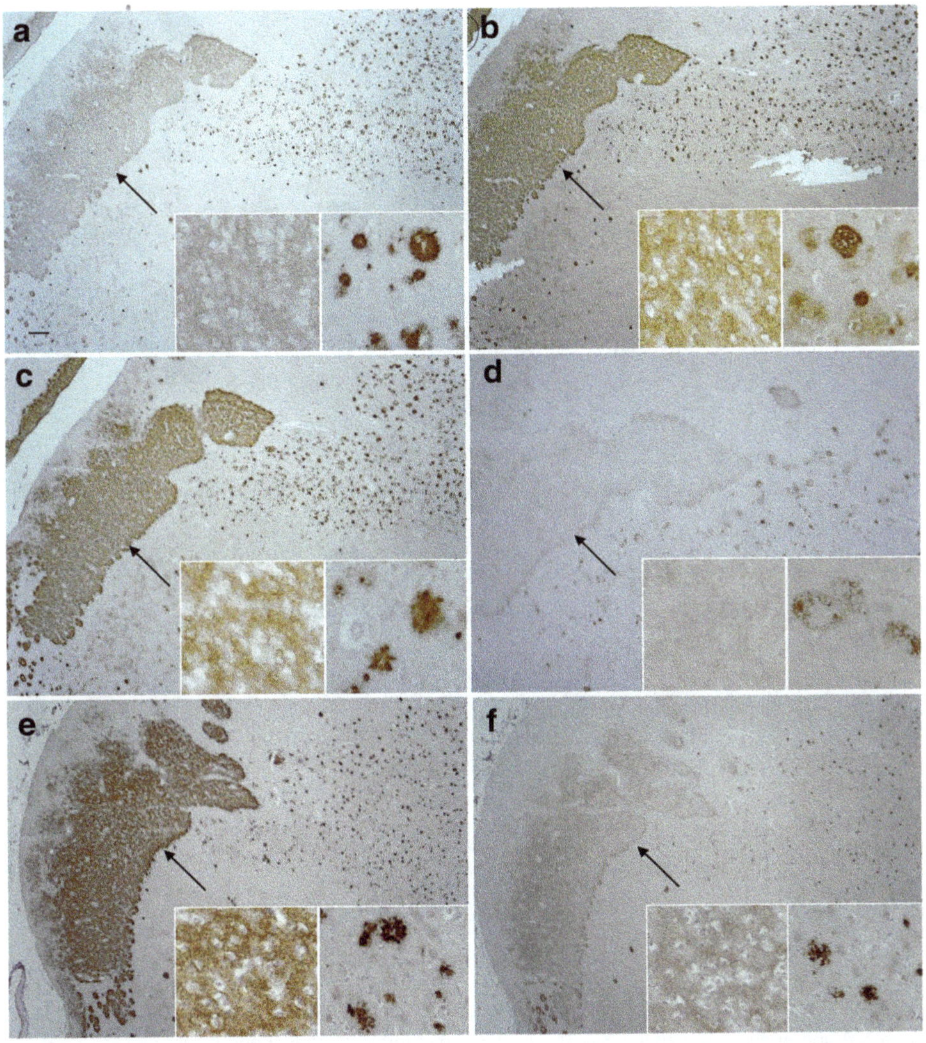

Fig. 6 pGlu-Aβ immunohistochemistry in the presubiculum and entorhinal cortexImmunohistochemical analysis of pGlu truncated Aβ species was carried out with four antibodies Aβ-pE3 (**a**; Synaptic systems 218,311; clone 1–57); Aβ-pE3 (**b**; Synaptic systems 218,011; clone 2–48); Aβ-pE3 (**c**; Synaptic systems 218,003); Aβ-pE11 (**d**; Synaptic systems 218,811; clone 173D8); Aβ4-x (**e**; [83]; Aβ1–5 (**f**; Synaptic systems 218,231). All antibodies showed a degree of positive staining in both the presubiculum and the entorhinal cortex. Bar in A represents 250 μm in a, b, c and d and 20 μm in the inserts

diffuse, 'lake-like' Aβ deposits of the presubiculum do not progress into mature amyloid plaques. Considering the phases of Aβ deposition in AD, diffuse plaques appear in the presubiculum in Thal phase 2 in around one third of the cases to be present in all cases by Thal phase 3. The morphology of such 'lake-like' deposits remains unaltered during progression of the amyloid pathology from Thal phase 3 to Thal phase 5 indicating that these large Aβ deposits do not fibrillise into amyloid [74].

In this study further biochemical and proteomic analysis was carried out in the AD cases to understand the morphological differences between the presubiculum and the entorhinal cortex. Biochemical analysis was carried out in a limited number of cases, however the results were conclusive for each case and the proteomic investigations were carried out as preliminary investigations to understand difference in molecular pathways between the two brain regions. In this study we identified $A\beta_{1-42}$ and $A\beta_{4-42}$ in the presubiculum and no Aβ peptides terminating at residue 40 with mass spectrometry, whereas plaques isolated from the entorhinal cortex contained a mixture of Aβ peptides of various lengths with pyroglutamate modifications at positions 3 and 11. The Aβ peptides are generated by proteolytic cleavage of the larger amyloid precursor protein (APP) by β- and γ-secretase [22, 27, 67]. While a single protein BACE1 is responsible for the β-secretase activity, γ-secretase is composed of four essential subunits: presenilin 1 (PS1) or presenilin 2 (PS2), together with nicastrin, APH-1 and PEN-2 [53, 76]. The γ-secretase complex cleaves at multiple sites within the transmembrane domain

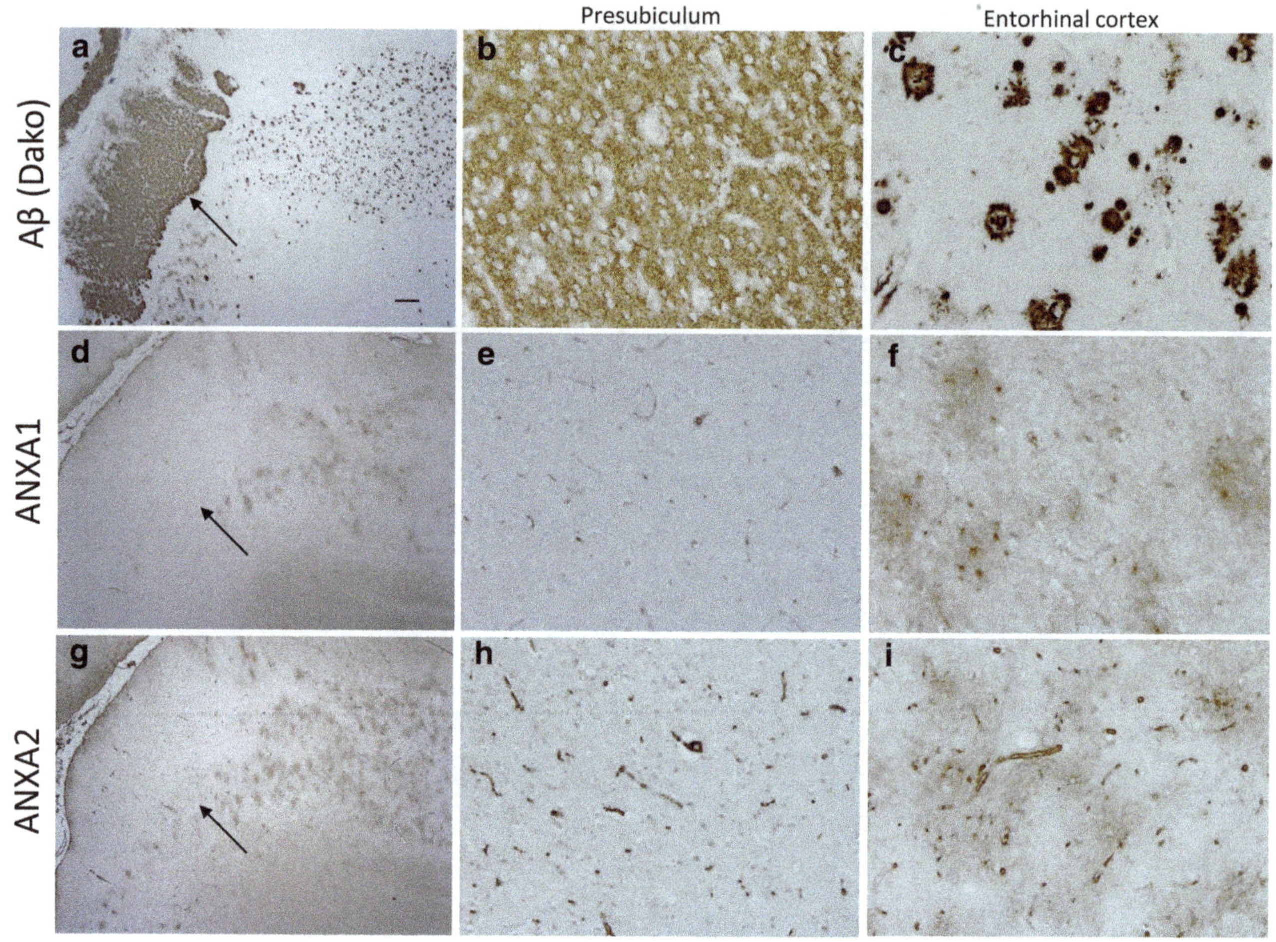

Fig. 7 Immunohistochemical analysis of annexins in the presubiculum and entorhinal cortex. Immunohistochemical analysis of Annexin A1 (**d-f**) and Annnexin A2 (**g-i**) compared with Aβ deposition (**a-c**). Serial sections were immunostained for Aβ to identify the 'lake-like' Aβ deposit found in the presubiculum (arrows), with image of higher magnification showing the different Aβ morphologies in the presubiculum (**b**) and entorhinal cortex (**c**). Positive Annexin A1 and Annexin A2 staining was observed in the entorhinal cortex (**f** and **i**) compared to a lack of positive staining in the presubiculum (**e** and **h**). Bar in A represents 250 μm in **a**, **d** and **g** and 50 μm in rest of panels

of APP, generating Aβ peptides ranging in length [66]. It is known that the distribution of these species varies among different pathological lesions. Parenchymal deposits consist of $A\beta_{42}$ as the major component, whereas Aβ deposits within vessels are mainly $A\beta_{40}$ [61]. The reasons and relevance of this selectivity remains unclear. The biophysical and biochemical properties of Aβ vary immensely with its length, the longer $A\beta_{42}$ has a much greater tendency to aggregate than the shorter $A\beta_{40}$ [34, 35]. Furthermore the relative ratio of $A\beta_{40}$ to $A\beta_{42}$ influences the biological effects of the Aβ mixture in vivo and in vitro even when total amounts of Aβ are kept equal [40] suggesting that the ratio of $A\beta_{40}/A\beta_{42}$ is more important than the absolute amounts of $A\beta_{42}$ [72]. The ratio also influences the morphological phenotype of the underlying pathology; by increasing the amount of $A\beta_{42}$ the pathology shifts from predominantly CAA to parenchymal plaques [28]. Post-translational modifications of Aβ result in N-terminally truncated Aβ with pyroglutamate modifications at position 3 ($A\beta_{N3pE}$) or 11 ($A\beta_{N11pE}$). Pyroglutamate modification is associated with enhanced aggregation into oligomers and fibrils. Biochemically, $A\beta_{42}$ is the first Aβ species to accumulate in the human brain [33, 44]. $A\beta_{40}$ is detected subsequently, followed by N-terminal truncated and pyroglutamate-modified $A\beta_{N3pE}$ and/or $A\beta_{N11pE}$. These modified forms of Aβ are frequently detected in plaques of all AD cases [33, 44, 60]. The Aβ species detected by mass spectrometry in the presubiculum showed no pyroglutamate modifications, suggesting that the Aβ peptides found in the presubiculum are not modified overtime. However, we could detect pyroglutamate modified peptides when using pGlu specific antibodies. This may indicate that relatively small concentrations of these peptides are found in the presubiculum. It is also of note that the FAD cases investigated in this study carried mutations in the *APP* and *PSEN1* genes, both mutations resulting in the production of different amounts of the Aβ variants. Yet all cases regardless of mutation status have the same characteristic morphology, and mass spectrometry profile of Aβ in the presubiculum. N-terminally truncated and pyroglutamate-modified Aβ peptides have previously been shown in dense amyloid plaques, so lower quantities in the presubiculum may suggest that these modifications of Aβ are required for amyloid fibrils to form.

Although the contribution of the canonical α-, β- and γ-secretases to APP processing have been studied in depth, the proteolytic cleavage of APP may be more complex. An increasing number of additional secretases have been identified that also proteolytically process APP [3]. However, further investigations on the underlying secretases involved in the processing and cleavage of Aβ are needed to determine whether other secretases or related proteins are found in the presubiculum compared to the entorhinal cortex [11, 71]. This though would not account for the large diffuse protein deposit composed of ABri or ADan in FBD and FDD as these proteins are not cleaved by secretases [41]. A link between BRI2 and APP has been demonstrated; where BRI2 has been shown to specifically interact with APP. As a result of this interaction BRI2 masks the cleavage sites of β- and α-secretase on APP and the γ-secretase docking site on the APP C-terminal fragment C99. Thus, BRI2 modulates APP processing by inhibiting Aβ formation and its deposition properties [20, 47, 48]. FBD and FDD are due to mutations in the *BRI2* gene, and both mutations cause the precursor protein to be extended and through a furin-like processing two 34 amino acid peptides are generated (ABri and ADan respectively). ABri molecules have a higher tendency to form ordered oligomeric assembles than $A\beta_{42}$ [63]. Therefore the morphological phenomenon observed in the presubiculum of three neurodegenerative diseases caused by the deposition of three different proteins would suggest that the observed phenomenon would likely be due to local tissue factors in the presubiculum rather than the processing of the different proteins.

It has previously been shown that despite the accumulation of Aβ in the presubiculum, neurofibrillary degeneration is minimal [2, 7, 21, 37], whereas the neighbouring entorhinal cortex and subiculum had considerable numbers of NFTs [7]. We have quantitated these findings in this study and found significantly more NFTs in the entorhinal cortex compared to the minimal number of NFTs found in the presubiculum. Previous studies have demonstrated that there is no neuronal loss in the presubiculum in AD compared to normal controls [21], showing that although neurons are present significantly fewer NFTs form in the presubiculum.

In the healthy brain microglia actively support neurons through the release of nerve growth factors [15, 50, 78] and have been shown to carry out many activities including synaptic pruning [1, 65]. The classification of microglia into pro-inflammatory or anti-inflammatory forms is based on the phenotypes of peripheral macrophages [38, 51, 58]. Pro-inflammatory are characterised by increased expression of pro-inflammatory mediators and cytokines [58] that retract their processes and adopt an amoeboid morphology often migrating closer to the site of injury [16]. Anti-inflammatory microglia are characterised by increased cytokine expression and associated with increased ramification of processes [58]. In the AD brain activated pro-inflammatory microglia are typically located in brain regions affected by disease and surround Aβ amyloid plaques [32]. However, the involvement of microglia in the neuroinflammatory processes is now understood to be a complex continuum rather than the originally proposed pro-inflammatory and anti-inflammatory polarised states [86]. In this study we showed a significant increase in the presence of CD68 and CR3–43 positive microglia in the entorhinal cortex compared to the presubiculum. Even though the number of microglia within the presubiculum and entorhinal cortex, as demonstrated by Iba1 staining, were not significantly different. Microglia have been proposed to assist in the clearance of Aβ from the brain [73], however this clearance by microglia is reduced in AD [43]. The lack of reactive microglia in the presubiculum would suggest that these cells are not engaged in pre-amyloid removal and are able to undertake their non-inflammatory functions specifically relating to maintenance of the central nervous system [1, 65]. Recently, Sosna et al. demonstrated that when microglia are ablated via CSF1R (Colony-stimulating factor 1 receptor) inhibition, there is a significant reduction of neuritic plaque formation and pre-fibrillar amyloid present in 5xFAD Tg mice [68], suggesting that microglia are instrumental in the formation of neuritic plaques.

We investigated alterations in protein expression in the presubiculum compared to the entorhinal cortex to assess whether a local difference in protein expression could contribute to the morphological and biochemical differences in the two brain regions. We demonstrated that 429 proteins had an increased expression in the presubiculum compared to the entorhinal cortex in both soluble and insoluble fractions whereas 850 proteins were shown to be decreased in the presubiculum. The proteins identified spanned many different biological processes from phospholipase activity and enzyme inhibitor activity being increased to neurotransmitter transport and synaptic transmission being decreased. We selected proteins for further validation based on the most prominent biological functions represented, the greatest fold change and the availability of commercially available antibodies. From the proteins selected, ANXA1 and ANXA2 both differed in staining pattern showing positive staining in the entorhinal cortex and was negative in the presubiculum. Further investigation into the annexin pathways and inflammatory mechanisms may identify why this region appears to be protected from neurodegeneration compared to its neighbouring regions.

We found that the 'lake-like' pre-amyloid deposits found in the presubiculum are not a unique feature in AD but is also found in other cerebral amyloidosis. Significant quantitative differences were found in the amount of tau, number of NFTs and the amount of microglial activation in the presubiculum compared to the entorhinal cortex. Proteomic differences were found in the Aβ species and the whole proteome between the two brain regions. In summary, understanding why the presubiculum has a different morphological appearance, biochemical and proteomic makeup compared to surrounding brain regions severely affected by neurodegeneration could lead us to understanding protective mechanisms in neurodegenerative diseases.

Additional files

Additional file 1: Table S1. Proteins identified in supernatant with increased expression in the presubiculum compared to the entorhinal cortex in Alzheimer's disease post-mortem brain tissue. (DOCX 24 kb)

Additional file 2: Table S2. Proteins identified in the pellet with increased expression in the presubiculum compared to the entorhinal cortex in Alzheimer's disease post-mortem brain tissue. (DOCX 38 kb)

Additional file 3: Table S3. Proteins identified in supernatant with decreased expression in the presubiculum compared to the entorhinal cortex in Alzheimer's disease post-mortem brain tissue. (DOCX 24 kb)

Additional file 4: Table S4. Proteins identified in the pellet with decreased expression in the presubiculum compared to the entorhinal cortex in Alzheimer's disease post-mortem brain tissue. (DOCX 86 kb)

Additional file 5: Table S5. Webgestalt GO ontology terms showing increased expression in the presubiculum compared to the entorhinal cortex in Alzheimer's disease post-mortem brain tissue. (DOCX 18 kb)

Additional file 6: Table S6. Webgestalt GO ontology terms showing decreased expression in the presubiculum compared to the entorhinal cortex in Alzheimer's disease post-mortem brain tissue. (DOCX 18 kb)

Acknowledgements and funding

Tammaryn Lashley is supported by an Alzheimer's Research UK senior fellowship. Christina Murray was supported by an Alzheimer's Research UK PhD Studentship and is now supported by the UK Dementia Research Institute at UCL. Priya Gami-Patel and Henrik Zetterberg are supported by the Leonard Wolfson Centre for Experimental Neurology. Tamas Revesz is supported by a grant from CBD Solutions. The Queen Square Brain Bank is supported by the Reta Lila Weston Institute for Neurological Studies, the Progressive Supranuclear Palsy Association and the Medical Research Council. Janice Holton is supported by the Multiple System Atrophy Trust; the Multiple System Atrophy Coalition; Fund Sophia, managed by the King Baudouin Foundation; Alzheimer's Research UK and CBD Solutions. This research was partly supported by the UK Dementia Research Institute at UCL and the National Institute for Health Research (NIHR) Queen Square Biomedical Research Unit in Dementia based at University College London Hospitals (UCLH), University College London (UCL). The views expressed are those of the author(s) and not necessarily those of the NHS, the NIHR or the Department of Health. The Clinical Neurochemistry Laboratory is supported by the Swedish and European Research Councils, the Knut and Alice Wallenberg Foundation, the Swedish Brain Foundation, the Torsten Söderberg Foundation and Alzheimerfonden. FDD samples were provided by Neuropathology Department, Århus Kommunehospital, Århus, Denmark and FBD samples provided by Department of Neuropathology, UCL Institute of Neurology. We would like to thank the Peto Foundation for their kind donations to the UCL mass spectrometry research group.

Authors' contributions

TL and TR drafted the study design, CM and PGP undertook the wet lab work and analysis. JG and OW provided the antibodies. EG, GB, EP, WH, KB, KM and HZ provided support and expertise for the mass spectrometry. All authors read and contributed to the final manuscript.

Author details

[1]The Queen Square Brain Bank for Neurological Disorders, Department of Molecular Neuroscience, UCL Institute of Neurology, London WC1N 3BG, UK. [2]Institute of Neuroscience and Physiology, Department of Psychiatry and Neurochemistry, The Sahlgrenska Academy at the University of Gothenburg, Mölndal, Sweden. [3]Clinical Neurochemistry Laboratory, Sahlgrenska University Hospital, Mölndal, Sweden. [4]Department of Psychiatry and Psychotherapy, University Medical Center (UMG), Georg-August-University, Goettingen, Germany. [5]Centre for Translational Omics, Great Ormond Street Institute of Child health, UCL, London, UK. [6]New York University, New York, NY, USA. [7]Dementia Research Institute, UCL , London, UK.

References

1. Aguzzi A, Barres BA, Bennett ML (2013) Microglia: scapegoat, saboteur, or something else? Science 339(6116):156–161. https://doi.org/10.1126/science.1227901
2. Akiyama H, Tago H, Itagaki S, McGeer PL (1990) Occurrence of diffuse amyloid deposits in the presubicular parvopyramidal layer in Alzheimer's disease. Acta Neuropathol 79(5):537–544. https://doi.org/10.1007/BF00296114
3. Andrew RJ, Kellett KAB, Thinakaran G, Hooper NM (2016) A Greek tragedy: the growing complexity of Alzheimer amyloid precursor protein proteolysis. J Biol Chem 291(37):19235–19244. https://doi.org/10.1074/jbc.R116.746032
4. Augustinack JC, Helmer K, Huber KE, Kakunoori S, Zöllei L, Fischl B (2010) Direct visualization of the perforant pathway in the human brain with ex vivo diffusion tensor imaging. Front Hum Neurosci 4(May):42. https://doi.org/10.3389/fnhum.2010.00042
5. Bland J, Regression Analysis AD (1986) Lancet:908–909
6. Bliss E, Heywood WE, Benatti M, Sebire NJ, Mills K (2016) An optimised method for the proteomic profiling of full thickness human skin. Biol Proced Biological Procedures Online 18(1):1–7. https://doi.org/10.1186/s12575-016-0045-y
7. Bobinski M, Wegiel J, Wisniewski HM, Tarnawski M, Reisberg B, Mlodzik B et al (1995) Atrophy of hippocampal formation subdivisions correlates with stage and duration of Alzheimer disease. Dementia 6(4):205–210
8. Boche D, Perry VH, Nicoll JA (2013) Review: activation patterns of microglia and their identification in the human brain. Neuropathol Appl Neurobiol 39(1):3–18. https://doi.org/10.1111/nan.12011
9. Braak H, Braak E (1991) Neuropathological stageing of Alzheimer-related changes. Acta Neuropathol 82:239–259. https://doi.org/10.1007/BF00308809
10. Caballero-Bleda M, Witter MP (1994) Projections from the presubiculum and the parasubiculum to morphologically characterized entorhinal-hippocampal projection neurons in the rat. Exp Brain Res 101(1):93–108. https://doi.org/10.1007/BF00243220
11. Chávez-Gutiérrez L, Bammens L, Benilova I, Vandersteen A, Benurwar M, Borgers M et al (2012) The mechanism of γ-secretase dysfunction in familial Alzheimer disease. EMBO J 31(10):2261–2274. https://doi.org/10.1038/emboj.2012.79
12. Cimino PJ, Sokal I, Leverenz J, Fukui Y, Montine TJ (2009 Oct) DOCK2 is a microglial specific regulator of central nervous system innate immunity

found in normal and Alzheimer's disease brain. Am J Pathol 175(4):1622–1630. https://doi.org/10.2353/ajpath.2009.090443
13. Cork L, Masters C, Beyreuther K, Price D (1990) Development of senile plaques. Relationships of neuronal abnormalities and amyloid deposits. Am J Pathol 137(6):1383–1392
14. Cornely R, Pollock AH, Rentero C, Norris SE, Alvarez-Guaita A, Grewal T et al (2016) Annexin A6 regulates interleukin-2-mediated T-cell proliferation. Immunol Cell Biol 94(6):543–553. https://doi.org/10.1038/icb.2016.15
15. Coull J a M, Beggs S, Boudreau D, Boivin D, Tsuda M, Inoue K et al (2005) BDNF from microglia causes the shift in neuronal anion gradient underlying neuropathic pain. Nature 438(7070):1017–1021. https://doi.org/10.1038/nature04223
16. Davalos D, Grutzendler J, Yang G, Kim JV, Zuo Y, Jung S et al (2005) ATP mediates rapid microglial response to local brain injury in vivo. Nat Neurosci 8(6):752–758. https://doi.org/10.1038/nn1472
17. Drexel M, Kirchmair E, Sperk G (2013) Changes in the expression of GABAA receptor subunit mRNAs in parahippocampal areas after kainic acid induced seizures. Front Neural Circuits 7:142. https://doi.org/10.3389/fncir.2013.00142
18. Efthymiou AG, Goate AM (2017) Late onset Alzheimer's disease genetics implicates microglial pathways in disease risk. Mol Neurodegener 12. https://doi.org/10.1186/s13024-017-0184-x
19. Eue I, König S, Pior J, Sorg C (2002) S100A8, S100A9 and the S100A8/A9 heterodimer complex specifically bind to human endothelial cells: identification and characterization of ligands for the myeloid-related proteins S100A9 and S100A8/A9 on human dermal microvascular endothelial cell line-1 c. Int Immunol 14(3):287–297. https://doi.org/10.1093/intimm/14.3.287
20. Fotinopoulou A, Tsachaki M, Vlavaki M, Poulopoulos A, Rostagno A, Frangione B et al (2005) BRI2 interacts with amyloid precursor protein (APP) and regulates amyloid β(Aβ) production. J Biol Chem 280(35):30768–30772. https://doi.org/10.1074/jbc.C500231200
21. Fukutani Y, Cairns N, Rossor M, Isaki K, Lantos P (1997) Cerebellar pathology in sporadic and familial Alzheimer's disease: a morphometric investigation. 149:177–184 Available from: https://onlinelibrary.wiley.com/doi/abs/10.1111/j.1750-3639.1997.tb01009.x.
22. Ghiso J, Frangione B (2002) Amyloidosis and Alzheimer's disease. Adv Drug Deliv Rev 54(12):1539–1551. https://doi.org/10.1016/S0169-409X(02)00149-7
23. Ghiso J, Rostagno A, Tomidokoro Y, Lashley T, Bojsen-Møller M, Braendgaard H et al (2006) Genetic alterations of the BRI2 gene: familial British and Danish dementias. Brain Pathol 16(1):71–79 Available from: http://www.ncbi.nlm.nih.gov/pubmed/16612984
24. Gjoneska E, Pfenning AR, Mathys H, Quon G, Kundaje A, Tsai L-H et al (2015 Feb) Conserved epigenomic signals in mice and humans reveal immune basis of Alzheimer/'s disease. Nature 518(7539):365–369. https://doi.org/10.1038/nature14252
25. Gundersen H, Bendtsen T, Korbo L, Marcussen N, Moller A, Nielsen K et al (1988) Some new, simple and efficient stereological methods and their use in pathological research and diagnosis. APMIS 96(5):379–394
26. He S, Li X, Li R, Fang L, Sun L, Wang Y et al (2016) Annexin A2 modulates ROS and Impacts inflammatory response via IL-17 signaling in Polymicrobial Sepsis mice. PLoS Pathog 12(7):1–23. https://doi.org/10.1371/journal.ppat.1005743
27. Hébert SS, Serneels L, Dejaegere T, Horré K, Dabrowski M, Baert V et al (2004) Coordinated and widespread expression of γ-secretase in vivo: evidence for size and molecular heterogeneity. Neurobiol Dis 17(2):260–272. https://doi.org/10.1016/j.nbd.2004.08.002
28. Herzig MC, Winkler DT, Burgermeister P, Pfeifer M, Kohler E, Schmidt SD et al (2004) Abeta is targeted to the vasculature in a mouse model of hereditary cerebral hemorrhage with amyloidosis. Nat Neurosci 7(9):954–960. https://doi.org/10.1038/nn1302
29. Hessian PA, Fisher L (2001) The heterodimeric complex of MRP-8 (S100A8) and MRP-14 (S100A9) antibody recognition, epitope definition and the implications for structure. Eur J Biochem 268(2):353–363. https://doi.org/10.1046/j.1432-1327.2001.01894.x
30. Holton JL, Ghiso J, Lashley T, Rostagno A, Guerin CJ, Gibb G, et al (2001) Regional distribution of amyloid-Bri deposition and its association with neurofibrillary degeneration in familial British dementia. Am J Pathol Am Soc Invest Pathol 158(2):515–526. Available from: https://www.ncbi.nlm.nih.gov/pubmed/11159188.
31. Holton JL, Lashley T, Ghiso J, Braendgaard H, Vidal R, Guerin CJ et al (2002) Familial Danish dementia: a novel form of cerebral amyloidosis associated with deposition of both amyloid-Dan and amyloid-beta. J Neuropathol Exp Neurol 61(3):254–267
32. Itagaki S, McGeer P, Akiyama H, Zhu S, Selkoe D (1989) Relationship of microglia and astrocytes to amyloid deposits of Alzheimer disease. J Neuroimmunol 24(3):173–182
33. Iwatsubo T, Saido TC, Mann DM, Lee VM, Trojanowski JQ (1996) Full-length amyloid-beta (1-42(43)) and amino-terminally modified and truncated amyloid-beta 42(43) deposit in diffuse plaques. Am. J Pathol 149(6):1823–1830. https://doi.org/10.1002/ejoc.201001502
34. Jarrett J, Berger E, Lansbury P (1993) The carboxy terminus of the beta amyloid protein is critical for the seeding of amyloid formation: implications for the pathogenesis of Alzheimer's disease. Biochemistry 32(18):4693–4697
35. Jarrett JT, Lansburry PT (1993) Seeding "one dimensional cristallization" of amyloid: a pathogenic mechanism in Alzheimer's disease and scrapie? Cell 73:1055–1058. https://doi.org/10.1016/0092-8674(93)90635-4
36. Ji B, Chen CJ, Bando K, Ashino H, Shiraishi H, Sano H et al (2015) Distinct binding of amyloid imaging ligands to unique amyloid-β deposited in the presubiculum of Alzheimer's disease. J Neurochem 135(5):859–866. https://doi.org/10.1111/jnc.13293
37. Kalus P, Braak H, Braak E, Bohl J (1989) The presubicular region in Alzheimer's disease: topography of amyloid deposits and neurofibrillary changes. Brain Res 494(1):198–203. https://doi.org/10.1016/0006-8993(89)90164-9
38. Kettenmann H, Hanisch U-K, Noda M, Verkhratsky A (2011) Physiology of microglia. Physiol Rev 91(2):461–553. https://doi.org/10.1152/physrev.00011.2010
39. Korzhevskii DE, Kirik OV (2016) Brain microglia and microglial markers. Neurosci Behav Physiol 46(3):284–290. https://doi.org/10.1007/s11055-016-0231-z
40. Kuperstein I, Broersen K, Benilova I, Rozenski J, Jonckheere W, Debulpaep M et al (2010) Neurotoxicity of Alzheimer's disease Aβ peptides is induced by small changes in the Aβ42 to Aβ40 ratio. EMBO J 29(19):3408–3420. https://doi.org/10.1038/emboj.2010.211
41. Lashley T, Revesz T, Plant G, Bandopadhyay R, Lees A, Frangione B et al (2008) Expression of BRI2 mRNA and protein in normal human brain and familial British dementia:its relevance to the pathogenesis of disease. Neuropathol Appl Neurobiol 34(5):492–505. https://doi.org/10.1111/j.1365-2990.2008.00935.x.Expression
42. Lashley T, Rohrer JD, Bandopadhyay R, Fry C, Ahmed Z, Isaacs AM et al (2011 Sep) A comparative clinical, pathological, biochemical and genetic study of fused in sarcoma proteinopathies. Brain 134(Pt 9):2548–2564. https://doi.org/10.1093/brain/awr160
43. Lee CYD, Landreth GE (2010) The role of microglia in amyloid clearance from the AD brain. J Neural Transm 117(8):949–960. https://doi.org/10.1007/s00702-010-0433-4
44. Lemere CA, Blusztajn JK, Yamaguchi H, Wisniewski TM, Saido TC, Selkoe DJ (1996) Sequence of deposition of heterogeneous amyloid beta-peptides and APO E in Down syndrome: implications for initial events in amyloid plaque formation. Neurobiol Dis 3(1):16–32. https://doi.org/10.1006/nbdi.1996.0003
45. Lodeiro M, Puerta E, Ismail M-A-M, Rodriguez-Rodriguez P, Rönnbäck A, Codita A et al (2017) Aggregation of the Inflammatory S100A8 Precedes Aβ Plaque Formation in Transgenic APP Mice: Positive Feedback for S100A8 and Aβ Productions. J Gerontol A Biol Sci Med Sci 72(3):319–328. https://doi.org/10.1093/gerona/glw073
46. Mann D, JOnes D, South P, Snowden J, Neary D (1992) Deposition of amyloid beta protein in non-Alzheimer dementias: evidence for a neuronal origin of parenchymal deposits of beta protein in neurodegenerative disease. Acta Neruopathol 83(4):415–419
47. Matsuda S, Giliberto L, Matsuda Y, Davies P, McGowan E, Pickford F et al (2005) The familial dementia BRI2 gene binds the alzheimer gene amyloid-β precursor protein and inhibits amyloid-β production. J Biol Chem 280(32):28912–28916. https://doi.org/10.1074/jbc.C500217200
48. Matsuda S, Giliberto L, Matsuda Y, McGowan EM, D'Adamio L (2008) BRI2 inhibits amyloid -peptide precursor protein processing by interfering with the docking of secretases to the substrate. J Neurosci 28(35):8668–8676. https://doi.org/10.1523/JNEUROSCI.2094-08.2008
49. McKeever PM, Kim T, Hesketh AR, MacNair L, Miletic D, Favrin G et al (2017) Cholinergic neuron gene expression differences captured by translational profiling in a mouse model of Alzheimer's disease. Neurobiol. Aging 57(Supplement C):104–119. https://doi.org/10.1016/j.neurobiolaging.2017.05.014
50. Miao J, Ding M, Zhang A, Xiao Z, Qi W, Luo N et al (2012) Pleiotrophin promotes microglia proliferation and secretion of neurotrophic factors by activating extracellular signal-regulated kinase 1/2 pathway. Neurosci. Res. Elsevier Ireland ltd and Japan neuroscience Society 74(3–4):269–276. https://doi.org/10.1016/j.neures.2012.09.001

51. Mills C (2012) M1 and M2 macrophages: oracles of health and disease. Crit Rev Immunol 32(6):463–488
52. Montine T, Phelps C, Beach T, Bigio E, Cairns N, Dickson D et al (2012) National Institute on Aging-Alzheimer's association guidelines for the neuropathologic assessment of Alzheimer's disease: a practical approach. Acta Neuropathol 123(1):1–11. https://doi.org/10.1007/s00401-011-0910-3.National
53. Niimura M, Isoo N, Takasugi N, Tsuruoka M, Ui-Tei K, Saigo K et al (2005) Aph-1 contributes to the stabilization and trafficking of the ??-secretase complex through mechanisms involving intermolecular and intramolecular interactions. J Biol Chem 280(13):12967–12975. https://doi.org/10.1074/jbc.M409829200
54. Okada H, Zhang W, Peterhoff C, Hwang JC, Nixon RA, Ryu SH et al (2010) Proteomic identification of sorting nexin 6 as a negative regulator of BACE1-mediated APP processing. FASEB J 24(8):2783–2794. https://doi.org/10.1096/fj.09-146357
55. Pappolla MA, Omar RA, Vinters HV (1991) Image analysis microspectroscopy shows that neurons participate in the genesis of a subset of early primitive (diffuse) senile plaques. AmJPathol 139(0002–9440):599–607
56. Portelius E, Lashley T, Westerlund A, Persson R, Fox NC, Blennow K et al (2015) Brain amyloid-Beta fragment signatures in pathological ageing and Alzheimer's disease by hybrid immunoprecipitation mass spectrometry. Neurodegener Dis 15(1):50–57. https://doi.org/10.1159/000369465
57. Probst A, Langui D, Ulrich J (1991) Alzheimer's disease: a description of the structural lesions. Brain Pathol 1(4):229–239. https://doi.org/10.1111/j.1750-3639.1991.tb00666.x
58. Ransohoff RM, Perry VH (2009) Microglial physiology: unique stimuli, specialized responses. Annu Rev Immunol 27(1):119–145. https://doi.org/10.1146/annurev.immunol.021908.132528
59. Ries M, Loiola R, Shah UN, Gentleman SM, Solito E, Sastre M (2016) The anti-inflammatory Annexin A1 induces the clearance and degradation of the amyloid-β peptide. J Neuroinflammation 13(1). https://doi.org/10.1186/s12974-016-0692-6
60. Rijal Upadhaya A, Kosterin I, Kumar S, Von Arnim CAF, Yamaguchi H, Fändrich M et al (2014) Biochemical stages of amyloid-β peptide aggregation and accumulation in the human brain and their association with symptomatic and pathologically preclinical Alzheimer's disease. Brain 137(3):887–903. https://doi.org/10.1093/brain/awt362
61. Roher a E, Palmer KC, Yurewicz EC, Ball MJ, Greenberg BD. Morphological and biochemical analyses of amyloid plaque core proteins purified from Alzheimer disease brain tissue. J Neurochem 1993;61(5):1916–26. Available from: http://www.ncbi.nlm.nih.gov/pubmed/8229002
62. Rosenbaum S, Kreft S, Etich J, Frie C, Stermann J, Grskovic I et al (2011) Identification of novel binding partners (annexins) for the cell death signal phosphatidylserine and definition of their recognition motif. J Biol Chem 286(7):5708–5716. https://doi.org/10.1074/jbc.M110.193086
63. Rostagno A, Tomidokoro Y, Lashley T, Ng D, Plant G, Holton J et al (2005) Chromosome 13 dementias. Cell Mol Life Sci 62(16):1814–1825. https://doi.org/10.1007/s00018-005-5092-5
64. Russo C, Violani E, Salis S, Venezia V, Dolcini V, Damonte G et al (2002) Pyroglutamate-modified amyloid β-peptides - AβN3(pE) - strongly affect cultured neuron and astrocyte survival. J Neurochem 82(6):1480–1489. https://doi.org/10.1046/j.1471-4159.2002.01107.x
65. Schafer D, Stevens B (2013) Phagocytic glial cells: sculpting synaptic circuits in the developing nervous system. Curr Opin Neurobiol 23(6):1034–1040. https://doi.org/10.1016/j.immuni.2010.12.017.Two-stage
66. Selkoe DJ, Wolfe MS (2007) Presenilin: running with scissors in the membrane. Cell 131(2):215–221. https://doi.org/10.1016/j.cell.2007.10.012
67. Shirotani K, Edbauer D, Prokop S, Haass C, Steiner H (2004) Identification of distinct γ-secretase complexes with different APH-1 variants. J Biol Chem 279(40):41340–41345. https://doi.org/10.1074/jbc.M405768200
68. Sosna J, Philipp S, Albay RI, Reyes-Ruiz JM, Baglietto-Vargas D, LaFerla FM, et al. Early long-term administration of the CSF1R inhibitor PLX3397 ablates microglia and reduces accumulation of intraneuronal amyloid, neuritic plaque deposition and pre-fibrillar oligomers in 5XFAD mouse model of Alzheimer's disease. Mol. Neurodegener. Mol Neurodegener; 2018;13(1):1–11. doi:https://doi.org/10.1186/s13024-018-0244-x
69. Streit WJ, Braak H, Xue Q-S, Bechmann I (2009) Dystrophic (senescent) rather than activated microglial cells are associated with tau pathology and likely precede neurodegeneration in Alzheimer's disease. Acta Neuropathol 118(4):475–485. https://doi.org/10.1007/s00401-009-0556-6
70. Sun Z, Xie Y, Chen Y, Yang Q, Quan Z, Dai R et al (2017) Rab21, a novel PS1 interactor, regulates γ-secretase activity via PS1 subcellular distribution. Mol Neurobiol:1–15. https://doi.org/10.1007/s12035-017-0606-3
71. Szaruga M, Veugelen S, Benurwar M, Lismont S, Sepulveda-Falla D, Lleo A, et al. Qualitative changes in human γ-secretase underlie familial Alzheimer's disease. J. Exp. Med. 2015;(lcd):jem.20150892-. doi:https://doi.org/10.1084/jem.20150892
72. Tanzi RE, Bertram L (2005) Twenty years of the Alzheimer's disease amyloid hypothesis: a genetic perspective. Cell 120(4):545–555. https://doi.org/10.1016/j.cell.2005.02.008
73. Tarasoff-conway JM, Carare RO, Osorio RS, Glodzik L, Fieremans E, Axel L et al (2015) Clearance systems in the brain—implications for Alzheimer disease. Nat Rev Neurol 11(8):457–470. https://doi.org/10.1038/nrneurol.2015.119.Clearance
74. Thal DR, Rüb U, Orantes M, Braak H (2002) Phases of Aβ-deposition in the human brain and its relevance for the development of AD. Neurology 58(12):1791–1800. https://doi.org/10.1212/WNL.58.12.1791
75. Thal DR, Rüb U, Schultz C, Sassin I, Ghebremedhin E, Del Tredici K et al (2000 Aug) Sequence of Abeta -protein deposition in the human medial temporal lobe. J Neuropathol Exp Neurol 59(8):733–748. https://doi.org/10.1093/jnen/59.8.733
76. Thinakaran G, Koo EH (2008) Amyloid precursor protein trafficking, processing, and function. J Biol Chem 283(44):29615–29619. https://doi.org/10.1074/jbc.R800019200
77. Tomidokoro Y, Lashley T, Rostagno A, Neubert TA, Bojsen-Møller M, Braendgaard H et al (2005) Familial Danish dementia - co-existence of Danish and Alzheimer amyloid subunits (ADan and a beta) in the absence of compact plaques. J Biol Chem 280(44):36883–36894 Available from: https://www.ncbi.nlm.nih.gov/pubmed/16091362
78. Ueno M, Fujita Y, Tanaka T, Nakamura Y, Kikuta J, Ishii M et al (2013) Layer V cortical neurons require microglial support for survival during postnatal development. Nat Neurosci Nature Publishing Group 16(5):543–551. https://doi.org/10.1038/nn.3358
79. van Strien NM, Cappaert NLM, Witter MP (2009) The anatomy of memory: an interactive overview of the parahippocampal-hippocampal network. Nat Rev Neurosci 10(4):272–282. https://doi.org/10.1038/nrn2614
80. Vidal R, Frangione B, Rostagno A, Mead S, Révész T, Plant G et al (1999) A stop-codon mutation in the BRI gene associated with familial British dementia. Nature 399(6738):776–781. https://doi.org/10.1038/21637
81. Vidal R, Revesz T, Rostagno A, Kim E, Holton JL, Bek T et al (2000) A decamer duplication in the 3′ region of the BRI gene originates an amyloid peptide that is associated with dementia in a Danish kindred. Proc Natl Acad Sci U S A 97(9):4920–4925. https://doi.org/10.1073/pnas.080076097
82. Wang P, Joberty G, Buist A, Vanoosthuyse A, Stancu I-C, Vasconcelos B et al (2017) Tau interactome mapping based identification of Otub1 as tau deubiquitinase involved in accumulation of pathological tau forms in vitro and in vivo. Acta Neuropathol 133(5):731–749. https://doi.org/10.1007/s00401-016-1663-9
83. Wirths O, Walter S, Kraus I, Klafki HW, Stazi M, Oberstein TJ et al (2017) N-truncated Aβ4–x peptides in sporadic Alzheimer's disease cases and transgenic Alzheimer mouse models. Alzheimers. Res. Ther. Alzheimers Res Ther 9(1):80. https://doi.org/10.1186/s13195-017-0309-z
84. Wisniewski HM, Sadowski M, Jakubowska-Sadowska K, Tarnawski M, Weigiel J (1998) Diffuse, Lake-like amyloid-Beta deposits in the Parvopyramidal layer of the Presubiculum in Alzheimer disease. J Neuropathol Exp Neurol 57(7): 674–683
85. Wittnam JL, Portelius E, Zetterberg H, Gustavsson MK, Schilling S, Koch B et al (2012) Pyroglutamate amyloid β(aβ) aggravates behavioral deficits in transgenic amyloid mouse model for Alzheimer disease. J Biol Chem 287(11):8154–8162. https://doi.org/10.1074/jbc.M111.308601
86. Xue J, Dong JH, Huang GD, Qu XF, Wu G, Dong XR (2014) NF-κB signaling modulates radiation-induced microglial activation. Oncol Rep 31(6):2555–2560. https://doi.org/10.3892/or.2014.3144
87. Zhang XHF, Leslie CS, Chasin LA (2005) Computational searches for splicing signals. Methods 37(4):292–305. https://doi.org/10.1016/j.ymeth.2005.07.011

7

Doublecortin-expressing cell types in temporal lobe epilepsy

Joan Y. W. Liu[1,2,7], Mar Matarin[1], Cheryl Reeves[1,2], Andrew W. McEvoy[1,5], Anna Miserocchi[5], Pamela Thompson[1,4,6], Sanjay M. Sisodiya[1,3,6] and Maria Thom[1,2*]

Abstract

Doublecortin (DCX) is widely regarded as a marker of immature and migrating neurons during development. While DCX expression persists in adults, particularly in the temporal lobe and neurogenic regions, it is unknown how seizures influence its expression. The aim of the present study was to explore the distribution and characteristics of DCX-expressing cells in surgical and postmortem samples from 40 adult and paediatric patients, with epilepsy and with or without hippocampal sclerosis (HS), compared to post mortem controls. The hippocampus (pes and body), parahippocampal gyrus, amygdala, temporal pole and temporal cortex were examined with DCX immunohistochemistry using four commercially-available DCX antibodies, labelled cells were quantified in different regions of interest as well as their co-expression with cell type specific markers (CD68, Iba1, GFAP, GFAP∂, nestin, SOX2, CD34, OLIG2, PDGFRβ, NeuN) and cell cycle marker (MCM2). Histological findings were compared with clinical data, as well as gene expression data obtained from the temporal cortex of 83 temporal lobe epilepsy cases with HS. DCX immunohistochemistry identified immature (Nestin^{-}/NeuN^{-}) neurons in layer II of the temporal neocortex in patients with and without epilepsy. Their number declined significantly with age but was not associated with the presence of hippocampal sclerosis, seizure semiology or memory dysfunction. DCX^{+} cells were prominent in the paralaminar nuclei and periamygdalar cortex and these declined with age but were not significantly associated with epilepsy history. DCX expressing cells with ramified processes were prominent in all regions, particularly in the hippocampal subgranular zone, where significantly increased numbers were observed in epilepsy samples compared to controls. DCX ramified cells co-expressed Iba1, CD68 and PDGFRβ, and less frequently MCM2, OLIG2 and SOX2, but no co-localization was observed with CD34, nestin or GFAP/GFAP ∂. Gene expression data from neocortical samples in patients with TLE and HS supported ongoing DCX expression in adults. We conclude that DCX identifies a range of morphological cell types in temporal lobe epilepsy, including immature populations, glial and microglial cell types. Their clinical relevance and biological function requires further study but we show some evidence for alteration with age and in epilepsy.

Keywords: Doublecortin, Temporal lobe epilepsy, Hippocampus, Memory, Microglia

Introduction

Doublecortin (DCX) is a microtubule-associated protein critical for normal neuronal migration during development. It has been widely used as a reliable marker to study post-mitotic, immature neurons in the adult mammalian brain [11, 14, 33, 37] as well as responses of these cell types to brain insults [9, 25, 51]. There is anatomically restricted expression in the normal mature mammalian brain, with DCX^{+} multipolar and 'tangled' neurons reported in cortical layer II, mainly in the temporal lobe, in a variety of species [36, 49] and in the peri-amygdala association cortex and amygdala [52]. The physiological function of persisting DCX^{+} neurons is unknown: roles in olfactory processing and memory have been postulated [6]. DCX^{+} neurons remain relatively unexplored in humans and their clinical significance is uncertain. DCX^{+} populations diminish with age in animals [6] but studies have suggested seizure-enhanced maturation and proliferation of DCX^{+} cell types occurs in temporal lobe epilepsy (TLE) [9, 28, 40] indicative of their underlying plasticity

* Correspondence: M.Thom@ucl.ac.uk
[1]Department of Clinical and Experimental Epilepsy, UCL Institute of Neurology, Queen Square, London WCN1BG, UK
[2]Department of Neuropathology, National Hospital for Neurology and Neurosurgery, UCL Institute of Neurology, Queen Square, London WC1N 3BG, UK
Full list of author information is available at the end of the article

and responsiveness. In addition, reports have noted DCX expression in non-neuronal cell types, including in relation to cortical pathology and brain injury and repair [25, 46].

The aim of this study was to further explore the morphology, phenotype, distribution and density of DCX$^+$ cells in TLE. We included surgical samples from a wide age range both with and without hippocampal sclerosis (HS), the commonest pathology in TLE [4]. We compared this to findings in post-mortem (PM) samples from patients with epilepsy and HS and non-epilepsy controls to explore any differences in the morphology and number of DCX $^+$ cells between these groups. In addition we compared the neuropathological findings to available gene-expression data from a parallel study of the temporal lobe cortex from a large series of TLE patients. Neuropathology findings were also correlated with clinical epilepsy history, including type of seizures, aura and any memory dysfunction, to explore pathophysiological roles of these cell types.

Methods

Case selection

Fifty-two cases were included in the histological study (Table 1). Adult temporal lobe epilepsy (TLE) cases from patients undergoing elective surgery for the treatment of refractory epilepsy ($n = 19$) were selected from the databases of the Epilepsy Society Brain and Tissue Bank at UCL Institute of Neurology and pediatric TLE surgical cases ($n = 5$) were obtained from Great Ormond Street Hospital NHS Trust. Adult post mortem (PM) tissue from patients with ($n = 16$) or without ($n = 12$) epilepsy during life (healthy controls) was obtained from the Epilepsy Society and MRC sudden death brain banks respectively; none of these patients had undergone neurosurgical treatments during life. The study has ethical approval and all cases were consented for use in research (Ethics committee approval NRES17/SC/0573). In 18/24 surgical cases and 8/16 of the epilepsy PM cases, hippocampal sclerosis (HS) ILAE type 1 [5] was present. None of these cases had additional temporal lobe sclerosis/cortical dysplasia [43] or other lesion.

Tissue was examined from six regions of the temporal lobe in the majority of adult surgical cases, including: (i) temporal neocortex (superior temporal gyrus to fusiform gyrus at 1 cm rostral to temporal pole) (Fig. 1a), (ii) temporal pole, (iii) mid-hippocampus body, (iii) pes hippocampus, (iv) parahippocampal gyrus (PHG) and (v) amygdala. As a standard anterior temporal lobectomy procedure was performed and a routine tissue handling and processing protocol was followed, the regions selected were anatomically comparable between cases. In surgical cases, the amygdala tissue was typically fragmented which limited identification of all subnuclei. In PM cases, coronal sections of the mid hippocampal body, adjacent temporal cortex and/or sections through the entire mid to caudal amygdala, including the paralaminar nuclei, were examined (Fig. 2a, Additional file 1: Table S1 for details).

Immunohistochemistry

Immunochemistry for DCX was carried out on 5 μm thick formalin-fixed, paraffin-embedded sections. We trialed four DCX commercially-available antibodies on selected

Table 1 Clinical and pathology details of cases and control groups (Further detail of each case is available in Additional file 1: Table S1)

Group	Tissue type	NUMBER	Predominant pattern of HS in body	Age (at surgery or death); mean (range, years)	Gender	Regions examined/study
Adult epilepsy TLE/HS (S1–13)	Surgical Fixed	13	ILAE Type 1 HS	41.3 (22–54)	7F: 6 M	HB,PES,PHG,TPole, TLobe, Amyg / qIHC
Paediatric epilepsy TLE/HS (S1–5)	Surgical Fixed	5	ILAE type 1 HS only	12.2 (8–15)	2F: 3 M	HB, TLobe / q IHC
Adult epilepsy TLE/NO HS (S19–24)	Surgical Fixed	6	NO HS	28.6 (24–35)	2F: 4 M	HB,PES,PHG,TPole, TLobe, Amyg / q IHC
Adult epilepsy (EPM1–16)	Post Mortem	16	ILAE type 1 HS in 8 CASES	48.7 (18–75)	8F: 8 M	HB, PHG, Amyg, Temporal Cortex (Both hemispheres included in 4 cases) / q IHC
Adult non-epilepsy controls (C1–12)	Post mortem	12	No HS	56.4 (28–85)	5F: 7 M	HB, PHG, Amyg, Temporal Cortex / q IHC
Adult epilepsy TLE/HS	Fresh	83 77[a]	All HS (16 with TLS) All HS (15 with TLS)	36.3 (16–63) 35.6 (16–57)	45F-38M 39F-38M	Middle temporal gyrus (cortex) / RNA
Adult non-epilepsy controls	Fresh	73[b] 59[a]	No HS No HS	50.8 (20–79) 28.8 (13–55)	14F–53F 30F-29M	Middle temporal gyrus (cortex)/ RNA A1C, inferior and superior TC

S surgical epilepsy case, *EPM* adult epilepsy post-mortem, *C* Post-mortem control, *HB* Hippocampal body, *PES* pes hippocampus, *PHG* parahippocampal gyrus, *TPole* temporal pole, *TLobe* temporal lobe, *TLS* temporal lobe sclerosis, *Amyg* amygdala, *HS* hippocampal sclerosis, *qIHC* qualitative and quantitative immunohistochemistry, *RNAseq* RNA sequencing and expression analysis, *ILAE* International League against epilepsy, *TLE* temporal lobe epilepsy.

[a]Only samples from adolescence and young and middle adulthood period. Controls from Kang et al.

[b]Samples obtained from the MRC brain bank, Edinburgh. A1C = Primary auditory cortex

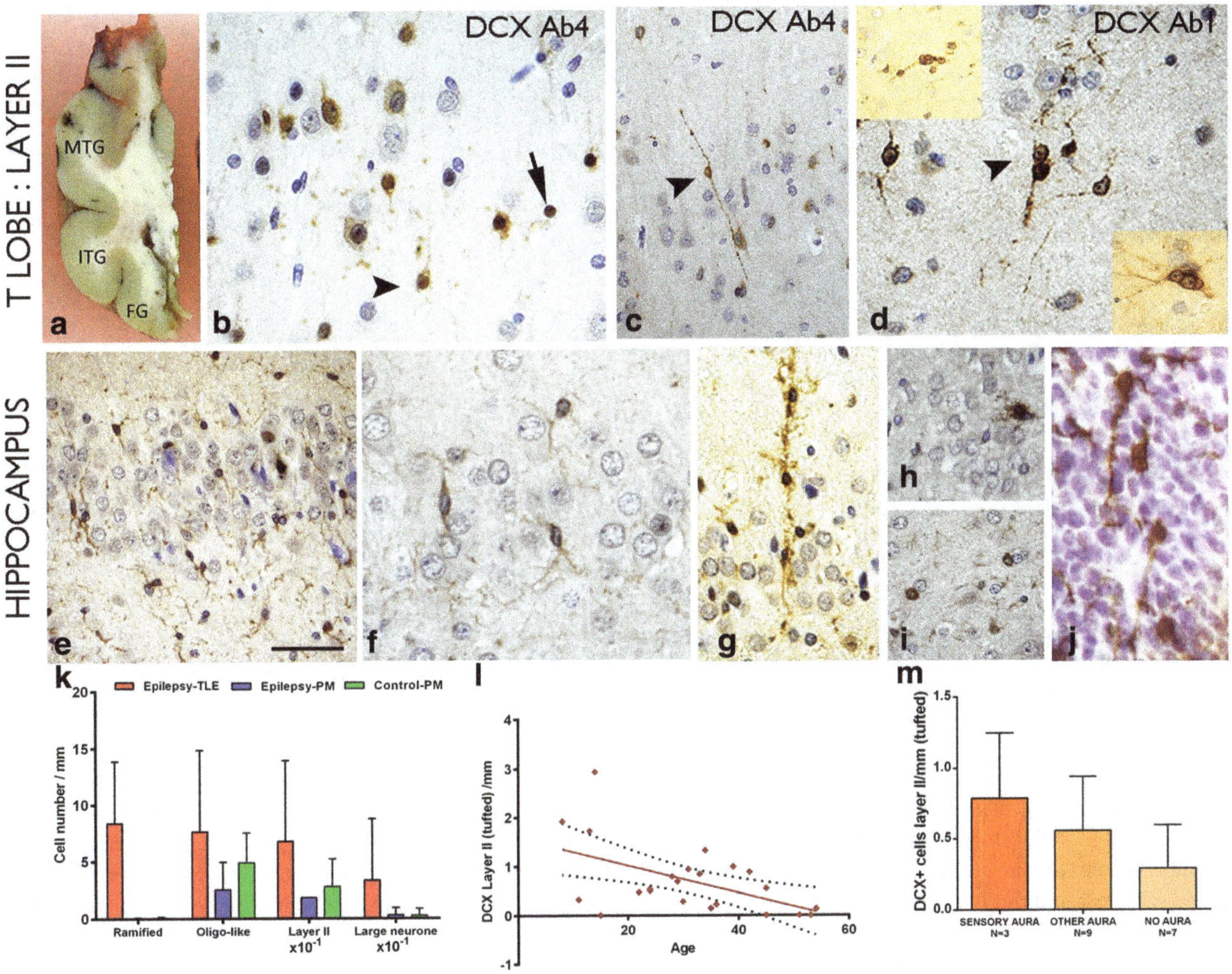

Fig. 1 Doublecortin (DCX) in the cortex and hippocampus. **a** Section though a temporal lobe indicating the regions studies (MTG = middle temporal gyrus, ITG, inferior temporal gyrus, FG = fusiform gyrus) **b** Layer II DCX positive cells (DCX$^+$) using DCX Ab 4 (see Table 2). Cells of different size, including some with more neuronal features and radial perpendicular processes (arrowhead) as well as dense nuclear labelling of small cells without processes (arrow) were observed. **C.** A bipolar cell in cortical layer II with DCX labelling with long beaded processes extending perpendicularly into layer I. **d** Clusters of small, intensely labelled DCX+ cells at interface of layer II and I labelled using DCX Ab1 (see Table 2). Top insert shows clusters of DCX$^+$ cells; the bottom insert shows prominent nucleoli and neuronal appearance of DCX$^+$ cells. **e** In the hippocampus granule cell layer (GCL) small DCX$^+$ cells with ramified, multiple processes were observed; **f** In another case, the delicate branching processes of the ramified cells are shown. **g** A column of DCX$^+$ cells extending though the GCL was observed in another case. **h** Granule cell neurons showed occasional DCX expression. **i** Small round DCX$^+$ oligo-like cells were noted in the hippocampus in satellite location to neurons. **j**.DCX expression, in the periventricular germinal matrix of the lateral ventricle, in a developmental human control of 13 weeks, showing small cells with extended processes. **k** Bar chart showing greater linear densities for all morphological DCX$^+$ cell types in surgical epilepsy cases compared to post mortem (PM) epilepsy controls and controls with statistically significant differences noted for ramified cell types only ($p < 0.0001$). **l** The linear density of layer II tufted DCX$^+$ cell types showed an inverse correlation with age for all cases (surgical and PM) ($p = 0.001$) as well as for surgical cases alone ($p = 0.016$; not shown on graph). **m** Although greater DCX$^+$ linear densities of tufted cells were present in patients with sensory aura of abnormal taste and smell compared to other aura types or no auras but these differences were not significant. Bar = 1 cm in A; B, D, F, G-J = 20 μm approx. (original magnification × 400) and C and E = 50 μm approx

surgical and PM cases. All four antibodies were previously validated in publications on human tissues [9, 28, 34, 40, 46] (Table 2; DCX Ab1 to 4). All DCX antibodies showed immunopositive labelling, but DCX Ab1 (clone 4604, Cell signaling, Boston, USA) labelled a greater diversity of cell types, and more intense labelling was observed in both surgical and PM human brain tissues. Consequently, DCX Ab1 was used across all cases for the descriptive and quantitative analysis. Double label immunofluorescent studies were performed on all anatomical regions of five selected surgical cases (Additional file 1: Table S1); combinations included DCX Ab1 with different DCX antibodies, and DCX Ab1 with astroglial (GFAP, GFAP-∂), microglial (Iba1, HLA-DR, CD68), mature neuronal (NeuN), immature/stem cells

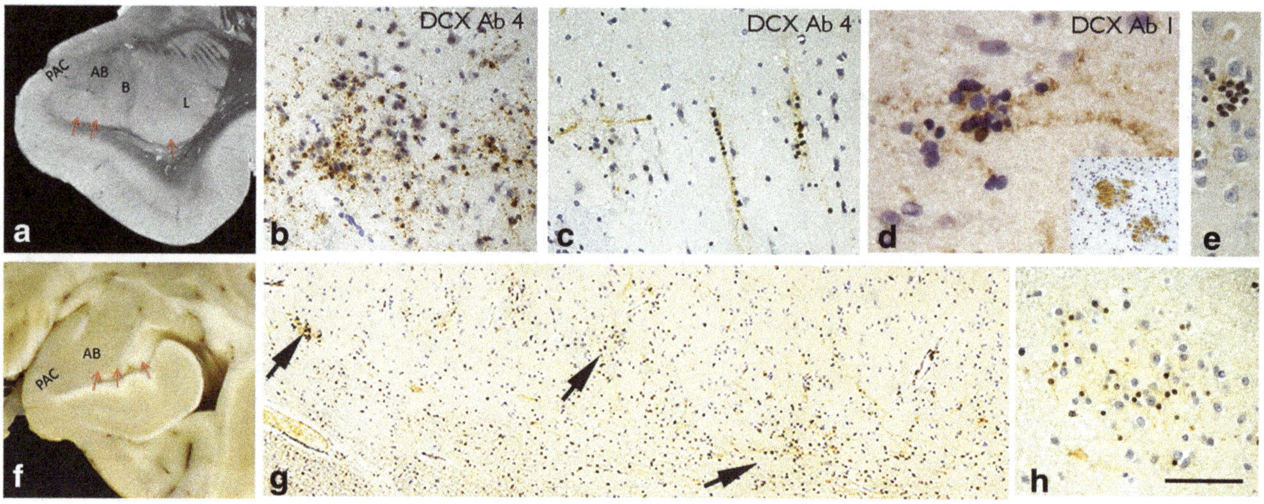

Fig. 2 Amygdala and DCX expression. **a** Coronal level though caudal amygdala in a post mortem case indicating the location of the paralaminar nucleus with red arrows. PAC = peri-amygdala cortex, AB = accessory basal, B = basal and L = lateral nuclei. **b** DCX positive cells clusters and beaded fibres in the PAC of a surgical patient with TLE/HS; **c** In a further case, columns of DCX+ cells were seen in the PAC as well as horizontal processes. **d** Further surgical TLE/HS case with DCX Ab1 (see Table 2) with clusters of small immature cells with beaded processes and some with nuclear labelling (inset: shows coarser DCX+ bundles traversing the amygdala in a surgical case). **e** Clusters of small densely labelled immature DCX+ cells and processes in the amygdala in post mortem samples of paralaminar nucleus. **f** Post mortem caudal amygdala indicating the location of the paralaminar nucleus above the ventricle. **g** The paralaminar nucleus shown at low magnification in DCX labelled section, with nests of positive cells and clusters of processes indicated (arrows) running along the border. **h** At higher magnification these clusters correspond to small DCX$^+$ cells intermingled with DCX immunonegative-negative mature neurons. Bar in A, F = 800 μm approx.; G = 100 μm approx.; in B, C, E, H = 50 μm approx.; in D = 20 μm approx

(nestin, CD34, SOX2), oligodendroglia (OLIG2), NG2-cells and pericytes (PDGFRβ) [11, 16] and cell cycle markers (MCM2). Details of the immunostaining protocols are included in Table 2 and the Additional file 2.

Quantitative and qualitative analysis

DCX-immuno-labelled cells (DCX$^+$) at the boundaries of cortical layer I/II in the temporal lobe of all cases were quantified using Image pro plus (Media Cybernetics, Cambridge, UK). Sequential images were captured at × 40 using a Leica DBMR microscope along the entire length of layer I and II from the gyrus to the sulcus of the most inferior-mesial gyrus (fusiform gyrus (FG) or inferior temporal gyrus (ITG))(Fig. 1a). DCX$^+$ cells of different morphologies were counted and expressed as cells per mm of gyrus length. DCX$^+$ cell types in other anatomical regions were semi-quantified as: (0) absent, (+) rare/occasional, (++) moderate numbers, (+++) many cells. In PM cases where the entire coronal cross-section of the paralaminar nucleus was present, the presence of DCX$^+$ cells was evaluated as: (0) absent, (+) single cluster, (++) 2–3 clusters, and (+++) > 4 clusters. In the adjacent peri-amygdala cortex (PAC; Fig. 2a) DCX in the superficial cortex was assessed as: (+) occasional single DCX$^+$ cell, (++) several single cells or one cluster, (+++) 2–3 clusters, (++++) > 4 clusters.

Qualitative examinations of double-labelled sections were carried out with a Zeiss Axio Imager Z2, and confocal laser scanning microscope (LSM-Meta 710, Zeiss, Göttingen, Germany). The software, Zen 2012 blue lite version (Zeiss, Göttingen, Germany), was used to view z-stacks of confocal images, and to compose three-dimensional orthogonal projections.

DCX mRNA analysis

Histology data was compared to DCX mRNA expression analyses from 83 surgical TLE cases (Table 1); in 16 of these cases there was evidence of temporal neocortical sclerosis (layer II/III neuronal loss and gliosis) in addition to hippocampal sclerosis [43]. TLE samples were obtained from the UCL Epilepsy Society Brain and tissue bank and compared to 73 PM non-epilepsy control tissues samples from the MRC Sudden Death Brain and Tissue Bank (Table 1). This data formed part of a separate study (Matarin et al., in preparation). We also compared this data to pre-existing expression array data; specifically DCX mRNA expression in ten different brain regions of non-epilepsy control cases including occipital, temporal, frontal, hippocampus, putamen, thalamus, substantia nigra, white matter, medulla and cerebellum as well as different life periods from embryonic to late adulthood [21].

For temporal lobe cases (patients and controls), RNA was isolated from the middle temporal gyrus (MTG) cortex and samples were randomly placed and hybridized to Affymetrix Exon 1.0 ST arrays as previously described [22]. Control tissue from other brain regions and different

Table 2 Immunohistochemistry panel

Antibody	Product code, Supplier	Dilution (method)	Target Epitope
DCX Ab1	4606, Cell Signaling Tech. Boston, US. *Used in [28]	1:250 (IHC, IF)	Amino acid sequence 40–70 and 350–410 of human DCX
DCX Ab2	AB18723, Abcam, Cambridge, UK. *Used in [34, 40]	1:4000 (IF)	AA 300 to the C-terminus of synthetic human DCX
DCX Ab3	SC-8066, Santa Cruz Biotech. Heidelberg, Germany. *Used in [11, 24, 27]	1:400 (IF)	C-terminus 365–402 of human DCX
DCX Ab4	AB2253, EMD Millipore, Watford UK. *Used in [45, 46]	1:1000 (IHC, IF)	C-terminus 350–365
Nestin	AB22035, Abcam, Cambridge, UK.	1:1000 (IHC, IF)	150 aa recombinant fragment from human nestin conjugated to GST
Nestin	AB105389, Abcam, Cambridge, UK.	1:100 (IF)	Synthetic peptide corresponding to the C terminus of Human Nestin.
Sox 2	AB5603, EMD Millipore, Hertfordshire, UK.	1:400 (IF)	KLH-conjugated linear peptide corresponding to a C-terminal region sequence of human Sox2
GFAP-∂	AB93251, Abcam, Cambridge, UK,	1:4000 (IF)	Synthetic peptide conjugated to KLH derived from within residues 350 to the C-terminus of Mouse GFAP ∂
GFAP	Z0334, DAKO, Cambridgeshire, UK.	1:1500 (IF)	GFAP
NeuN	MAB377, EMD Millipore, Hertfordshire, UK.	1:100 (IF)	Purified neuronal nuclei
Iba1	019–19,741, WAKO, Osaka, Japan.	1:6000 (IF)	Synthetic peptide corresponding to C-terminus of Iba1
CD68	AB783, Abcam, Cambridge, UK.	1:50 (IF)	Macrophages, microglia
CD34	IR632, DAKO, Cambridgeshire, UK.	1:25 (IF)	Endothelial cells
Olig 2	AB9610, EMD Millipore Hertfordshire, UK	1:200 (IF)	Recombinant mouse Olig-2
PDGFR-beta	AB32570, Abcam, Cambridge, UK.	1:1000 (IF)	Synthetic peptide within Human PDGF Receptor beta aa 1050 to the C-terminus
MCM2	610,700, BD biosciences, Oxford, UK.	1:900 (IF)	Human BM28 aa. 725–888

For all antibodies, sections were pre-treated in sodium citrate solution (pH 6.0) microwaved at 800 W for twelve minutes. All primary antibodies were incubated overnight at 4 °C, except for anti-Iba1, CD68 and GFAP which were incubated for an hour at room temperature, and anti-GFAP ∂ which was incubated for 48 h at 4 °C. *Previous studies using DCX in human tissue studies.
Abbreviations: *IHC* immunohistochemistry, *IF* immunofluorescence

life periods were also originally analysed with Affymetrix Exon 1.0 ST arrays [21] and data files were downloaded from the NCBI Gene Expression Omnibus (accession GSE25219 and GSE46706). Quality control analyses included background correction, quantile normalization, log2 transformation and median polishing probe-set summarization. The effects of several methodological and biological covariates were tested for significance and was included in the linear regression or MANOVA models when significant. All gene expression data was analyzed with Affymetrix Power Tools software package and Partek Genomics Suite (Partek Incorporated, St. Louis, MO, USA) and R software.

Clinical data

The age of onset of seizures, age at surgery, seizure types, laterality and outcomes at two years following surgery were obtained from the clinical records of epilepsy patients (Table 1 and Additional file 1: Table S1). Pre-operative memory function tests were carried out as part of the routine clinical assessment as previously described [44] and detailed in Additional file 2: Methods. Data on memory function was available in 15 adult surgical patients (Additional file 1: Table S1). Statistical analysis was carried out between pathology and clinical groups using non-parametric tests (including Kruskal-Wallis with post-hoc corrections and Spearman correlation) SPSS (IBM, California, version 22); p values of ≤0.05 were regarded as significant.

Results

Qualitative findings

DCX⁺ neuronal cell types

Neuronal-appearing unipolar (Fig. 1b), bipolar (Fig. 1c) and multipolar DCX^+ cells (Fig. 1d) were identified mainly at the interface between layer I and II of the temporal cortex as single cells or more rarely in clusters or rows (Fig. 1d); they were observed in 18 of the 22 surgical cases studied and henceforth are collectively referred to as 'layer II DCX^+ cells'. The processes of multipolar tufted cells extended mainly perpendicularly to the cortical surface, projecting into layer I, where rarer horizontally-orientated DCX^+ cells and processes could be observed. In all cases, layer II DCX+ cells intermingled with other small, intensely labelled DCX$^+$ cells without processes in layer II (Fig. 1b) and occasionally with larger DCX$^+$ cells with more overt neuronal morphology (Fig. 1b). Layer II DCX$^+$ cells appeared more frequent along the ITG and FG compared to MTG in surgical TLE cases. Layer II DCX$^+$ cells were also observed in the temporal pole of over half of the cases studied, but less frequently in the resected parahippocampal gyrus (PHG) and PM TLE and control cases. Rare large DCX$^+$ neuronal cells were noted in the granule cell layer of the hippocampus in surgical cases (Fig. 1h).

DCX$^+$ glial cell types

Ramified DCX$^+$ cells with multiple, branching processes were visualized mainly with the DCX antibody DCX Ab1 (Fig. 1e). Ramified DCX$^+$ cells were present in all regions of all TLE cases, with and without HS, and all PM cases and noted in the gray and white matter. In the hippocampus, ramified DCX$^+$ cells were particularly prominent in the hilus and subgranular zone of the dentate gyrus, extending through the granule cell layer. Occasional clusters or columns of DCX$^+$ cells were seen (Fig. 1g) and proximity to CA1 pyramidal neurones. There were also present in the pes hippocampus and PHG in all cortical layers and white matter. Ramified cells were morphologically reminiscent of microglia and NG2$^+$ cells as well as immature migrating neurons in the developing fetal brain in the periventricular zone (Fig. 1j). Occasional cells were also noted alongside vessels. In addition, a population of small round DCX$^+$ oligo-like cells, without cytoplasmic processes, were scattered in white matter and cortex, visualized with all DCX antibodies; similar cells were often seen in a satellite position adjacent to neurons (Fig. 1i), particularly in deep cortical layers, as previously reported [40].

DCX$^+$ cells in amygdala

Surgical cases The peri-amygdala cortex (PAC) and paralaminar/periventricular nuclei could be anatomically identified in surgical cases, but were incompletely represented. All DCX antibodies labelled clusters of small DCX$^+$ cells, mainly in the superficial cortex of the PAC (Fig. 2b-d). These DCX$^+$ cells were sometimes arranged in horizontal or vertical columns, with beaded linear processes (Fig. 2c). Fragments of amygdalar nuclei with a ventricular border (paralaminar nuclei) showed aggregates of small, intensely-labelled DCX$^+$ cells and fibres intermingled with DCX-negative, mature neurons. Coarse fibre tracts and bundles of DCX$^+$ processes were also occasionally noted in the amygdala of all surgical cases (Fig. 2d, inset). In addition, ramified DCX$^+$ cells with cytoplasmic labelling, as observed in other regions, were widespread. **PM cases:** Variable labelling of small DCX$^+$ cell aggregates in the paralaminar nucleus of the amygdala was noted, particularly along the ventricle wall in the caudal amygdala (Fig. 2f, g). In these regions, clusters of small immature DCX$^+$ nuclei were intermingled with larger and intermediate-sized DCX-negative neurones. (Fig. 2h). Some DCX$^+$ cells were associated with fine beaded bipolar processes Fig. 2e). In the PAC, scattered small immature DCX$^+$ cells with processes were noted, occasionally in clusters, mainly at the interface between layer I and II in either horizontal or perpendicular arrangements, as in the surgical cases.

Double labelling studies and comparison of different DCX antibody labelling

DCX antibodies DCX Ab1 showed the most extensive labelling of cells and processes in different regions but co-localization was confirmed in a proportion of small cells with the three other different DCX antibodies (Table 2, Fig. 3a). **Temporal neocortex:** In layer II of the temporal lobe, DCX$^+$ tufted cells showed only rare co-localisation with mature neuronal marker NeuN (Fig. 3b, c). There was no cellular co-expression of DCX with mature glial marker GFAP, immature stem cell markers nestin or GFAP∂, which both showed labelling of the sub-pial band of astrocytes (Fig. 3e). There were a few DCX$^+$/Sox2$^+$ cells noted. There were no CD34$^+$ neuroglial cells in any of the surgical epilepsy cases. A minor proportion of small oligo-like DCX+ cells in the white matter co-expressed OLIG2 (Fig. 3d); in contrast, MCM2/DCX$^+$ cells were not observed (Fig. 3d inset). There was extensive co-localisation between ramified DCX$^+$ cells and Iba1, CD68 and, to a lesser extent, PDGFRβ. **Hippocampus body and pes:** Very rare DCX$^+$/NeuN$^+$ cells were observed in the granule cell layer (Fig. 3f). We did not observe any co-expression between GFAP, GFAP∂ and nestin with DCX and these markers highlighted distinct cell populations in all regions (Fig. 3g). There was, however, prominent co-localization of ramified, multipolar DCX+ cells with Iba1 (Fig. 3h) and CD68 (Fig. 3i), particularly in the granule cell layer region. In addition, co-expression of DCX with PDGFRβ was evident in some small branching cells as well as MCM2 (Fig. 3j). Occasional double-labelling of small oligo-like cells with DCX and OLIG2 as well as SOX2 was noted in hippocampal regions but not with CD34. **Amygdala:** Although DCX$^+$ and nestin-expressing cells were observed in similar anatomical regions, particularly in the paralaminar nucleus, they highlighted distinct cell populations and processes (Fig. 3k, l). Multipolar, ramified DCX$^+$ cells showed co-expression with Iba1 (Fig. 3m) and occasionally with PDGFRβ (Fig. 3n), but only in a proportion of cells. Cellular co-expression of DCX with NeuN, CD34, GFAP or MCM2 (fig. 3o) was not observed in the amygdala of the cases examined and there was rare co-expression of DCX with OLIG2 or SOX2.

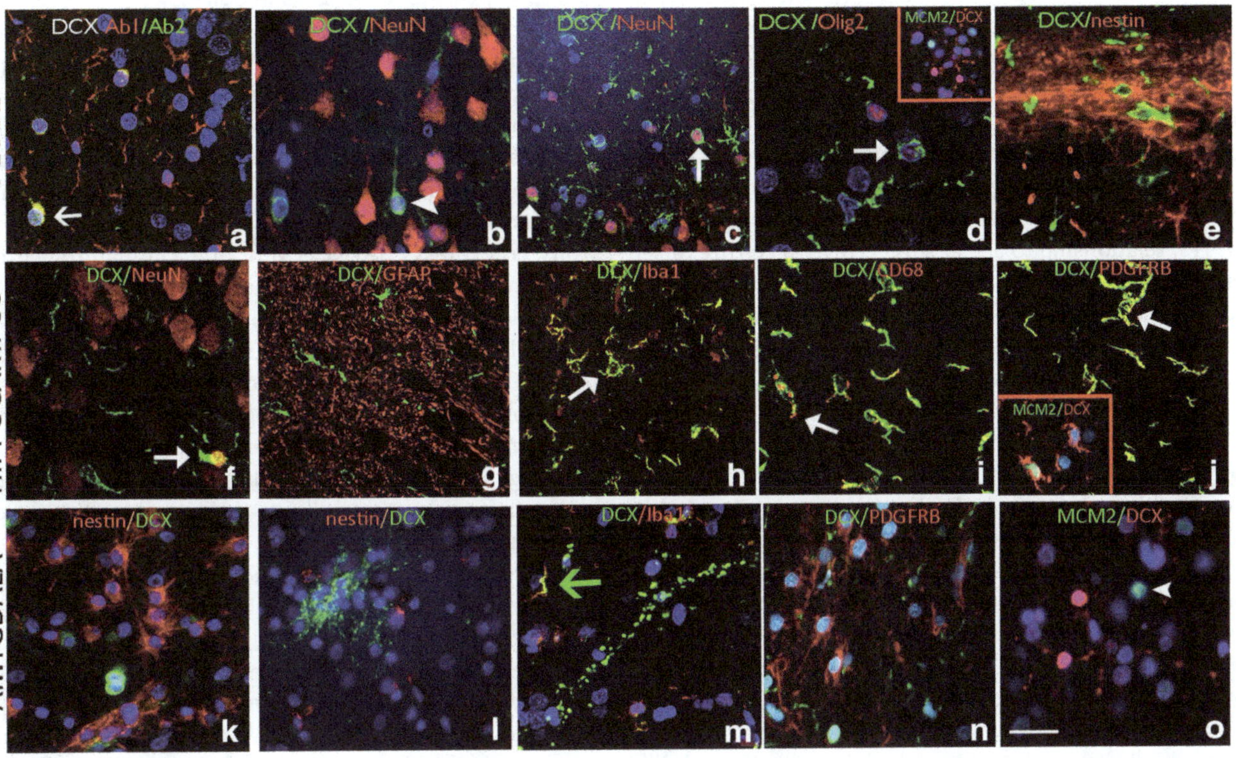

Fig. 3 Characterizing DCX positive cells in the temporal cortex, hippocampus and amygdala of surgical patients with epilepsy, and comparison of commercial antibodies. In all panels, the arrowheads indicate single labelled cells, while arrows point to double labelled cells. Confocal images are merged projections of 5 to 7 images acquired in a z-stack. **a**. The immunoreactivity of two different commercially-available anti-Dcx antibodies. Both DCX Ab2 AB18723 (Abcam, Cambridgeshire, UK) and DCX Ab 1 #4606 (Cell Signaling Technology, Inc. MA, USA) labelled small cells in the hippocampal granule cell layer (GCL) of a patient with epilepsy and HS Type 1 (arrow) (Table 2). DCX Ab1 labelled more cells overall than DCX Ab2. ***DCX+ positive cells in the remaining figures were labelled using DCX Ab1.*** **Temporal Cortex Layer I/II: b**. NeuN expression was not frequently observed in small DCX+ cells located in layer II of the temporal lobe cortex (arrowhead). **c**. In another case, DCX/NeuN positive cells were more frequently observed in the superficial temporal cortex than in the temporal pole (arrows). **d**. DCX positive cells expressing Olig2 in the nucleus (arrow) were noted in layer 1 of an epilepsy case (arrow), but MCM2/DCX+ cells were not observed (inset). **e**. Nestin+ glial fibres were observed in the subpial layer and layer I and II, but did not co-localise with DCX expression. **Hippocampus: f**. In general there were rare DCX/NeuN colocalised cells in the dentate gyrus; in this image there is a rare co-localised cell (arrow). **g**. GFAP showed dense labelling of astroglial process in hippocampal regions but no co-localisation with DCX was noted. **h**. Labelling with Iba1 highlighted mature microglial cell types, with ramified processes, particularly in the subgranular zone as shown, and many co-expressed DCX (arrow); **i** Co-labelled CD68/DCX+ cells were also observed (arrow). **j**. PDGFRβ was expressed in multipolar cells in the hippocampus and temporal lobe in addition to pericytes; focal co-labelling with DCX was noted in some cells (arrow); Inset show a DCX+ ramified cell expressing MCM2 in the nucleus. **Amygdala. k**. Distinct populations or clusters of nestin+ or DCX+ cells in the amygdala periventricular nuclei; **l**. In another area, nests of DCX+ processes were also distinct from nestin-expressing cells. **m**. In the amygdala, although DCX+ processes were largely Iba1 negative, Iba1/DCX+ ramified DCX+ cells were observed (arrow). **n**. PDGFRβ and DCX in the amygdala showing distinct populations of small cells. **o**. DCX in the amygdala were mainly MCM2 negative. Bar is equivalent to 20 μm. Individual channels for immunofluorescence images are shown in Additional file 4: Figure S2

Quantitative analysis

Based on the above findings our hypothesis was that quantitative analysis would confirm greater densities in the number of DCX$^+$ cells in epilepsy than control groups. In the **temporal lobe** we confirmed higher linear densities for all morphological DCX$^+$ cell types in surgical epilepsy cases compared to PM epilepsy cases and non-epilepsy controls (Fig. 1k) with statistically significant differences noted for ramified DCX$^+$ cell populations ($p < 0.0001$). We also investigated their relationship with patient age and cortical region. The linear density of layer II cells compared to other DCX$^+$ cell types showed an inverse correlation with age for all cases (surgical and PM) ($p = 0.001$) (Fig. 1l) as well as for surgical cases alone ($p = 0.016$) and for age of seizure onset ($p = 0.035$). There were significantly higher linear densities of tufted DCX$^+$ cells in the FG compared to the ITG ($p = 0.004$) but not for other DCX$^+$ cells types. We also hypothesized if there was a relationship between DCX$^+$ linear densities and the presence of HS but did not confirm this. Similarly, we considered if DCX cell densities related to clinical parameters; there was no significant difference in DCX$^+$ cells in relation to seizure types (focal or generalized seizures), history of aura (Fig. 1m) or if patients were seizure free (or not) two years following surgery. We noted an association for increased ramified DCX$^+$ in cortical layer II in patients with severe verbal pre-operative memory deficit (Additional file 3: Figure S1; $p = 0.027$). In other regions **(hippocampus, pes hippocampus, PHG and temporal pole and amygdala),** semi-quantitative analysis of DCX$^+$ ramified and small cell types in surgical cases did not show any significant differences between cases with HS or without HS, relationship to age at surgery, age of seizure onset, seizure types or outcome at 2 years. In PM cases, there were no significant differences in DCX populations in amygdala and PAC between epilepsy controls and controls; there was a negative correlation between DCX$^+$ cells in the PAC and age over all PM cases ($p = 0.04$).

mRNA expression

From published data [21] *DCX* mRNA was expressed in all brain regions tested and exhibited temporal and regional significant differential expression (False Discovery Rate 5%). There was higher *DCX* mRNA expression in temporal, frontal and occipital regions and lower in cerebellum. DCX expression in the temporal cortex was higher in periods before and early birth (embryonic, fetal and early infancy) than in periods following the early infancy (late infancy, childhood, adolescence and adulthood) (Fig. 4a). We observed no significant differences in *DCX* expression in the temporal cortex between left and right hemispheres in controls [21] or TLE patients (adolescence and young and middle adulthood periods) (Fig. 4b). We did not find significant differences between patients with and without temporal lobe sclerosis and neither between patients with epilepsy and the 2 PM control groups (Fig. 4c) (For all p values > 0.05 and fold change < 1.2).

Discussion

DCX is currently widely used as developmental marker for post-mitotic, immature neurons in the brain and for persistent neurogenesis in adulthood [14, 37]. Our study highlights the varied morphologies of DCX$^+$ cells in adult TLE with ongoing expression supported by a parallel gene expression study. Tangled DCX$^+$ cells in layer II of the temporal cortex did not express nestin, NeuN or MCM2, declined in numbers with age and did not significantly associate with clinical seizure semiology, memory dysfunction or the presence of HS. Amygdala DCX+ immature neuronal populations were primarily located in the paralaminar nucleus, but their number and morphology were not different between cases and controls. We also identified a subset of ramified and small cells with DCX antibodies, representing a range of glial cell types and supporting non-neuronal DCX expression; these were increased in number in the neocortex in epilepsy, associated with memory impairment and may represent reactive populations.

Temporal cortical DCX$^+$ cells in epilepsy

The presence of persistent, immature, DCX$^+$ neocortical cells in layer II, primarily in the temporal lobe and piriform cortex, has been recognized in a range of adult mammalian species since 2001 (reviewed in [6]). They are less studied in humans and their precise physiological function remains elusive. They have been variable termed 'tangled and tufted' cells or 'semilunar/transitional' neurons, co-express PSA-NCAM or other immature neuronal markers but reported to be mainly negative with mature neuronal marker NeuN. Although the number of DCX$^+$ cortical cells decline with age, they are considered to endow the cortex with enhanced synaptic plasticity [23] and roles in olfactory learning and memory have been postulated [6]. In mammals they are not considered to be newly generated in adulthood, but to arise during development from migrating cells of the lateral cortical stream [2]. A persistent *temporal lobe migratory stream* has also been recently described in adult mammals, extending from the temporal pole of the lateral ventricle to the piriform cortex and amygdala [14] and we have also recently reported evidence for vestiges of a similar migratory stream in the human adult mesial temporal lobe [27]. In TLE an increased plexus of PSA-NCAM-positive neurons was reported in layer II of the entorhinal cortex [30] and increased DCX$^+$ cells were noted in the temporal neocortex in epilepsy compared to controls with evidence for some maturation with NeuN expression, yet maintaining a persistent immature phenotype (98% co-expressing PSA-NCAM and 82% Tuj1) [28]. Similar tangled DCX$^+$ cells in layer II were also prominent in young patients with FCD type Ia [40].

In the current series, layer II DCX+ temporal neocortical cells showed infrequent NeuN expression, in keeping with some previous studies [15, 40]; the additional lack of expression of the stem cell marker nestin could support their intermediate differentiation between progenitor cells and mature neurons [27]. We confirmed their anatomical distribution, with increased density in more mesial temporal neocortex, as suggested in previous reports [6, 28]. They were not prominent in the parahippocampal gyrus cortex however and we also observed a significant decline in the number of tangled cells with age. In our recent study of TLE/HS patients aged over 50 years with early Alzheimer-like pathology in temporal lobe resections, we reported a lack of tau accumulation in layer II DCX+ cells, suggesting their resistance to age-related neurodegeneration [42], as also supported by experimental models [52]. We have shown in this study that the number of tangled neurons is not increased in epilepsy patients compared to controls, nor is the number related to clinical olfactory/sensory auras, memory dysfunction the presence of hippocampal sclerosis or post-surgical outcome. In a parallel gene expression study from patients with TLE/HS there

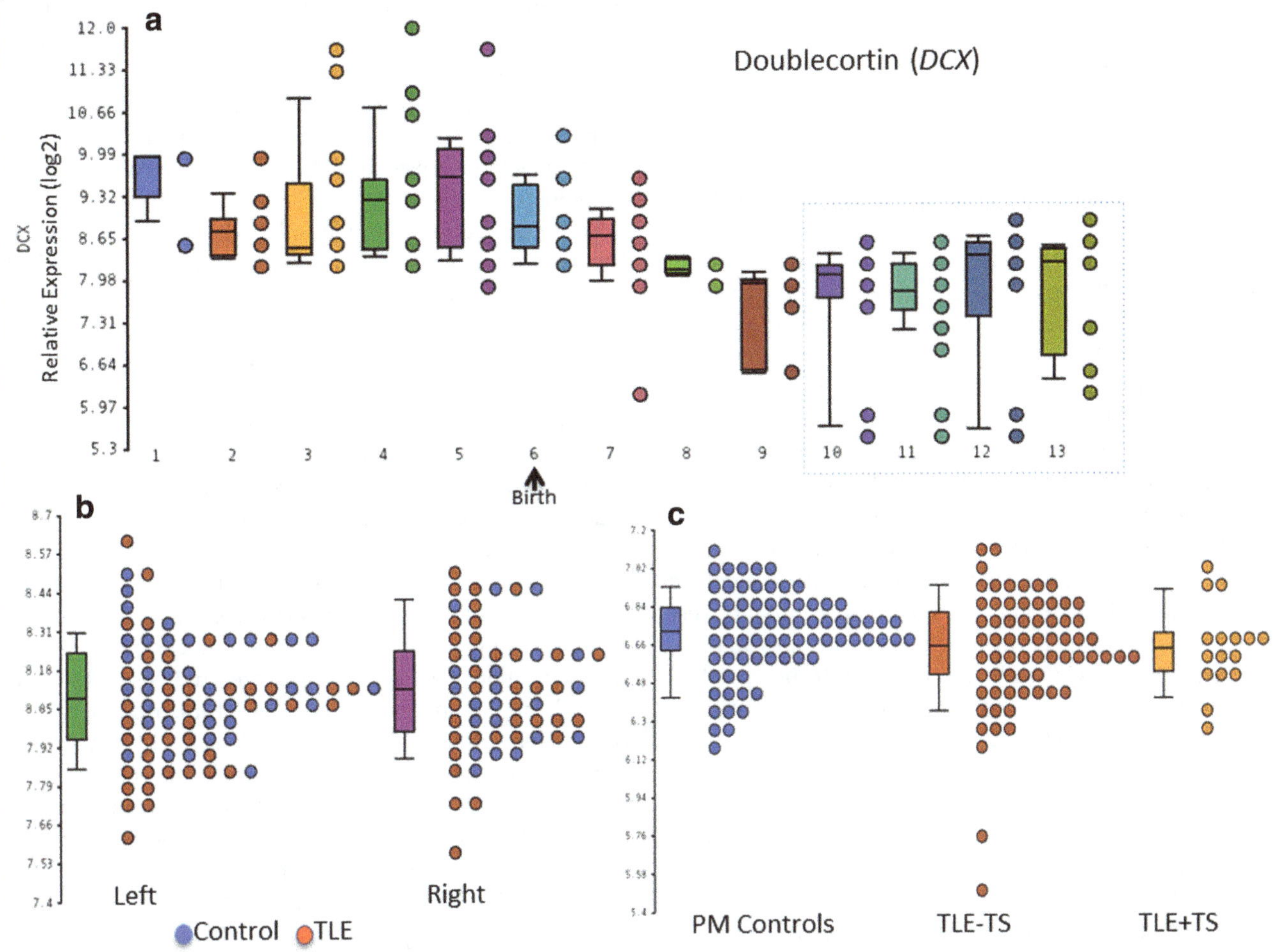

Fig. 4 DCX mRNA expression data. **a** Significant DCX temporally differential expression between periods on temporal cortex (*p* value: 4.5e-[113]) [21]. Periods 1: Embryonic, 2: Early Fetal, 3: Early midfetal 4: Late midfetal- 5 Late fetal 6 Neonatal and early Infancy 7 Late infancy 8 Early childhood 9 Middle and Late adulthood 10:Adolescence 11: Young adulthood 12: Middle adulthood 13: Late adulthood **b** DCX expression on right (R) and left (L) temporal cortex on patients with temporal lobe epilepsy (TLE) [22] and controls [21] after correcting for batch differences. Periods 10, 11 and 12 **c)** DCX mRNA expression data from 83 TLE (divided into cases with or without temporal lobe sclerosis (TS) (neuronal loss from the superficial neocortex in addition to hippocampal sclerosis [43]) and controls from the MRC brain bank, Edinburgh, after correcting for batch, age, gender and RIN differences. Periods 10 to 13

were no significant differences in patients with additional temporal lobe superficial cortical neuronal loss and gliosis (also called temporal lobe sclerosis) [43] from those with normal/preserved neocortex. These findings could suggest that layer II DCX+ cell types are unlikely to be clinical or pathologically relevant to functional and acquired pathologies in temporal lobe epilepsy.

Amygdala and DCX+ populations

The amygdala can initiate seizures in TLE and volume changes, including enlargement are recognized in TLE in addition to gliosis [3]. During development, migrating DCX+ cells in the lateral cortical stream give rise to neuronal and glial populations in the amygdala [2]; persisting DCX+ cells in adulthood have been reported in the primate amygdala and PAC, forming chains of cells, a proportion of which co-express NeuN, their number declining with age [52]. Similar cell types were also confirmed in the human amygdala [29], in particular the paralaminar nucleus of the amygdala, where abundant rests of immature DCX+ neurons were shown in one study [10]. The paralaminar nucleus, which sits along the ventricle wall, is composed of nodules of small primitive appearing cells, and is interconnected with other amygdala nuclei receiving high serotonergic input. Its precise functions are uncertain [10]. In the current study, DCX^+ immature cells, primarily in the paralaminar nucleus and PAC, were confirmed to exist in the amygdala, in both surgical tissue as well as PM cases. Diminished populations were associated with increasing age but the cells did not show atypical morphology or altered numbers in epilepsy or associate with the presence of hippocampal sclerosis. Nevertheless, application of DCX+ may be helpful in clinical practice to enable their anatomical identification and avoid over-interpretation as small malformations or hamartias, described in surgical resections in TLE [17].

DCX – A reliable marker of neurogenesis in the mature human brain?

There is increasing awareness of DCX expression in non-neuronal cells types. DCX-expressing astroglial cells have been noted in adult post mortem tissues in patients with epilepsy and controls [46], in balloon cells in FCD IIB and multipolar astroglial like cells in temporal lobe sclerosis [40]. DCX+ stellate cells have been reported in the vicinity of acute infarcts with co-expression of astroglial lineage markers (GFAP, S100) rather than microglial or mature neuronal markers as NeuN [25]. In another study however, DCX+ 'rod' cells in the infant hippocampal subgranular zone region, that morphologically resembled microglia, lacked CD68 and HLADR expression and were argued to represent neural progenitor cell types [34]. In adult mammals, DCX+ cells are reported to be enriched in the subgranular zone of the hippocampus, and are described as 'ramified', although exhibiting more overt neuronal morphology with apical dendrites [14, 36]. Experimental tracing studies of DCX+ cell fate during temporal lobe development show that 95% give rise to TBR1-positive pyramidal neurons but a small proportion differentiate to GFAP astrocytes (3.4%) and a further population of small bipolar cells with sparsely branching processes are of uncertain lineage (1.7%) [2]. Single cell transcriptomics of isolated DCX+ populations has also provided evidence of cell subsets enriched for divergent pathways, including astrocytic and myelinating oligodendroglial fates [15]. Identification of DCX expression in oligodendroglial precursor cells (OPC) was proposed to reflect cell migration rather than neuronal differentiation [7] and DCX expression is also speculated to have a role in glioblastoma infiltration [1].

Our current study adds further support to DCX expression in non-neuronal cell types. We noted frequent ramified, multipolar DCX+ cells and oligo-like cells without processes in many regions, including the SGZ, and these were significantly increased in surgical TLE compared to controls. These were observed mainly with one DCX antibody although overlap of expression was noted in a proportion of small cells with other commercial DCX antibodies, suggesting different sensitivities. Although DCX+ ramified cells in the dentate gyrus resembled cells in the developing human sub-ventricular zone, they lacked the typical unipolar or bipolar morphology [36]. Furthermore, we confirmed that a proportion of ramified DCX+ cells co-expressed microglial markers, as well as PDGFRβ, supporting non-neuronal lineages. Significantly more ramified DCX+ cells were noted in surgical epilepsy cases in the temporal cortex compared to controls. However there were no differences between epilepsy cases with or without hippocampal sclerosis. These different observations suggest enhanced DCX expression in reactive glial cells types in epilepsy could be independent of underlying pathology.

The observation of DCX in microglia was an unexpected finding. Microglial cells are dynamic, motile cells which show changes in morphology in response to brain activity and injury, with increasingly recognized diverse and complex roles [8, 32] including neurodevelopment as well as epilepsy [13]. Understanding of these cells has advanced with proteomic and transcriptomic analysis of isolated microglia, aiming to identify specific proteins more abundantly expressed, as candidate lineage and activation markers [12, 38, 48, 53] (see https://omictools.com/glia-open-access-database-tool). Although proteomics and gene expression studies have suggested that DCX is not expressed in microglia at significant levels [18–20, 38, 50, 53], differential gene expression studies do show DCX is dependent on their activation state. For example, one study using laser single cell capture and gene expression of microglial cell types of different morphology showed that DCX was highly enriched in activated amoeboid microglia and confirmed by immunohistochemistry and PCR of a murine microglial cell line [35]. Recent studies have also highlighted expression of putative immature neuronal markers in reactive cell types, including microglia in human slice cultures [47].

Intriguingly we also noted PDGFRβ+ co-expression in some of the ramified DCX+ cells in TLE tissues; DCX expression has been previously shown in pericytes [53]. Although PDGFRβ+ is widely recognized as a CNS pericyte marker [41] it is also expressed in OPC/NG2 parenchymal glial cell types, which are reactive to seizures [16, 26, 31, 39]. We also noted occasional DCX+ small cells to co-express OLIG2 in keeping with reported low DCX expression in OPC lineages [7, 53]. In our parallel gene expression study from TLE cortex, DCX expression was confirmed in adult temporal cortex and, although expression was not significantly increased in TLE compared to controls, more detailed single cell analysis is warranted to further investigate differential cellular expression in epilepsy. Our findings therefore support ongoing DCX expression in adults; expression in non-neuronal cells, particularly in adults undergoing surgery for refractory epilepsy, may suggest aberrant upregulation under pathological conditions, including seizures.

Study limitations

There are several limitations to the study. The ages in the epilepsy and control groups for the histology were not precisely matched as in the mRNA study and although ramified DCX+ cell densities did not show a relationship with age, we cannot exclude that this may have had an effect. The PM cases with epilepsy and HS did not all have syndromic TLE and limited memory tests were available. The gene expression data on MTG was obtained on homogenized cortex from all cases rather than micro dissected cortical layers or cells and was not carried out on the ITG or FG where greater numbers of DCX^{+} cells are observed. We did not have complete representation of the FG in the surgical specimens, compared to the PM cases in the analysis of Layer II DCX^{+} cells and in the amygdala surgical specimens were fragmentation which limits analysis of the entire nucleus.

Conclusions

DCX identifies a range of morphological cell types in temporal lobe epilepsy, including immature populations in the superficial cortex and amygdala that decline with age but may not be specifically relevant to the epilepsy or local pathology. We observed DCX^{+} reactive glial cell types, including microglial lineages with some evidence for increased numbers in epilepsy tissue. This suggests that DCX not only is expressed in residual immature neuronal cell types, but may have a role in brain responses to seizure injury.

Additional files

Additional file 1: Table S1. Detail of each case used in the study including clinical and psychometric data and the type of study carried out (DOCX 29 kb)

Additional file 2: Supplementary Methods (DOCX 18 kb)

Additional file 3: Figure S1. Bar graphs of the relationship between pre-operative memory function and DCX+ cells in the superficial temporal lobe. **A**. There was an association between severe memory deficit and increased ramified type DCX+ cells ($p = 0.027$). However the number of patients in this series is small and requires validation with a larger cohort. **B**. There was no association between the number of tufted DCX+ neuronal cells in layer II of the temporal cortex and pre-operative memory function. (JPG 181 kb)

Additional file 4: Figure S2. Split channels for DCX double labelling as indicated in temporal lobe, hippocampus and amygdala for images shown in Fig. 3. (TIF 15727 kb)

Abbreviations

DCX: Doublecortin; FG: Fusiform gyrus; HS: Hippocampal sclerosis; ILAE: International league against epilepsy; ITG: Inferior temporal gyrus; MTG: Middle temporal gyrus; OPC: Oligodendroglial precursor cells; PAC: Perimagydala cortex; PHG: Parahippocampal gyrus; PM: Post mortem; TLE: Temporal lobe epilepsy

Acknowledgements

We are grateful to the MRC sudden death brain bank in Edinburgh for the provision of control cases, to the Human Developmental Biology Resource for paediatric and fetal brain specimens and to Simon Paine and Tom Jacques for the provision of cases from Great Ormond Street Hospital.

Funding

This work is supported by a grant from the MRC MR/J01270X/1. MM is supported by Marie Curie International Re-integration Grant (FP7-PEOPLE-2009-RG grant No 256545) and Epilepsy Research UK (F1206). JL is currently supported by EPITARGET. This work was undertaken at UCLH/UCL, which received a proportion of funding from the Department of Health's NIHR Biomedical Research Centres funding scheme. The UCL Epilepsy Brain and Tissue Bank is supported by the Katy Baggott Foundation through the Epilepsy Society.

Authors' contributions

JL and MT prepared the manuscript and figures and carried out all the data analysis. JL carried out the double labelling studies. CR carried out the single labelling studies. MM carried out all the gene expression data and analysis. AM, AM, SS and PT provided all the clinical data. All authors have been involved in final manuscript approval.

Competing interests

All co-authors have no personal, professional or financial relationships that could potentially be construed as a conflict of interest.

Author details

[1]Department of Clinical and Experimental Epilepsy, UCL Institute of Neurology, Queen Square, London WCN1BG, UK. [2]Department of Neuropathology, National Hospital for Neurology and Neurosurgery, UCL Institute of Neurology, Queen Square, London WC1N 3BG, UK. [3]Department of Neurology, National Hospital for Neurology and Neurosurgery, London, UK. [4]Department of Neuropsychology, National Hospital for Neurology and Neurosurgery, London, UK. [5]Department of Neurosurgery, National Hospital for Neurology and Neurosurgery, London, UK. [6]Chalfont Centre for Epilepsy, Chesham Lane, Chalfont St Peter, Buckinghamshire SL9 0RJ, UK. [7]Department of Biomedical Sciences, University of Westminster, W1W6UW, London, UK.

References

1. Ayanlaja AA, Xiong Y, Gao Y, Ji G, Tang C, Abdikani Abdullah Z, Gao D (2017) Distinct features of Doublecortin as a marker of neuronal migration and its implications in Cancer cell mobility. Front Mol Neurosci 10:199. https://doi.org/10.3389/fnmol.2017.00199
2. Bai J, Ramos RL, Paramasivam M, Siddiqi F, Ackman JB, LoTurco JJ (2008) The role of DCX and LIS1 in migration through the lateral cortical stream of developing forebrain. Dev Neurosci 30:144–156. https://doi.org/10.1159/000109859
3. Beh SMJ, Cook MJ, D'Souza WJ (2016) Isolated amygdala enlargement in temporal lobe epilepsy: a systematic review. Epilepsy & behavior: E&B 60:33–41. https://doi.org/10.1016/j.yebeh.2016.04.015
4. Blumcke I, Spreafico R, Haaker G, Coras R, Kobow K, Bien CG, Pfafflin M, Elger C, Widman G, Schramm J et al (2017) Histopathological findings in brain tissue obtained during epilepsy surgery. N. Engl. J. Med. 377:1648–1656. https://doi.org/10.1056/NEJMoa1703784
5. Blumcke I, Thom M, Aronica E, Armstrong DD, Bartolomei F, Bernasconi A, Bernasconi N, Bien CG, Cendes F, Coras R et al (2013) International consensus classification of hippocampal sclerosis in temporal lobe epilepsy: a Task Force report from the ILAE Commission on Diagnostic Methods. Epilepsia 54:1315–1329. https://doi.org/10.1111/epi.12220
6. Bonfanti L, Nacher J (2012) New scenarios for neuronal structural plasticity in non-neurogenic brain parenchyma: the case of cortical layer II immature neurons. Prog Neurobiol 98:1–15. https://doi.org/10.1016/j.pneurobio.2012.05.002
7. Boulanger JJ, Messier C (2017) Doublecortin in oligodendrocyte precursor cells in the adult mouse brain. Front Neurosci 11:143. https://doi.org/10.3389/fnins.2017.00143
8. Cartier N, Lewis CA, Zhang R, Rossi FM (2014) The role of microglia in human disease: therapeutic tool or target? Acta Neuropathol 128:363–380. https://doi.org/10.1007/s00401-014-1330-y
9. D'Alessio L, Konopka H, Lopez EM, Seoane E, Consalvo D, Oddo S, Kochen S, Lopez-Costa JJ (2010) Doublecortin (DCX) immunoreactivity in hippocampus

of chronic refractory temporal lobe epilepsy patients with hippocampal sclerosis. Seizure 19:567–572. https://doi.org/10.1016/j.seizure.2010.09.004
10. deCampo DM, Fudge JL (2012) Where and what is the paralaminar nucleus? A review on a unique and frequently overlooked area of the primate amygdala. Neurosci Biobehav Rev 36:520–535. https://doi.org/10.1016/j.neubiorev.2011.08.007
11. Dennis CV, Suh LS, Rodriguez ML, Kril JJ, Sutherland GT (2016) Human adult neurogenesis across the ages: an immunohistochemical study. Neuropathol Appl Neurobiol 42:621–638. https://doi.org/10.1111/nan.12337
12. Dong X, You Y, Wu JQ (2016) Building an RNA sequencing transcriptome of the central nervous system. The Neuroscientist: a review journal bringing neurobiology, neurology and psychiatry 22:579–592. https://doi.org/10.1177/1073858415610541
13. Eyo UB, Murugan M, Wu LJ (2017) Microglia-neuron communication in epilepsy. Glia 65:5–18. https://doi.org/10.1002/glia.23006
14. Fasemore TM, Patzke N, Kaswera-Kyamakya C, Gilissen E, Manger PR, Ihunwo AO (2018) The distribution of Ki-67 and Doublecortin-Immunopositive cells in the brains of three Strepsirrhine Primates: Galago demidoff, Perodicticus potto, and Lemur catta. Neuroscience 372:46–57. https://doi.org/10.1016/j.neuroscience.2017.12.037
15. Gao Y, Wang F, Eisinger BE, Kelnhofer LE, Jobe EM, Zhao X (2016) Integrative single-cell transcriptomics reveals molecular networks defining neuronal maturation during postnatal neurogenesis. Cereb Cortex. https://doi.org/10.1093/cercor/bhw040
16. Garbelli R, de Bock F, Medici V, Rousset MC, Villani F, Boussadia B, Arango-Lievano M, Jeanneteau F, Daneman R, al BF (2015) PDGFRbeta(+) cells in human and experimental neuro-vascular dysplasia and seizures. Neuroscience 306:18–27. https://doi.org/10.1016/j.neuroscience.2015.07.090
17. Gawelek KL, Gales JM, Prayson RA (2018) Hamartia in hippocampal sclerosis associated mesial temporal lobe epilepsy. Ann Diagn Pathol 32:63–66. https://doi.org/10.1016/j.anndiagpath.2017.08.004
18. Han D, Moon S, Kim Y, Kim J, Jin J, Kim Y (2013) In-depth proteomic analysis of mouse microglia using a combination of FASP and StageTip-based, high pH, reversed-phase fractionation. Proteomics 13:2984–2988. https://doi.org/10.1002/pmic.201300091
19. Hickman SE, Kingery ND, Ohsumi TK, Borowsky ML, Wang LC, Means TK, El Khoury J (2013) The microglial sensome revealed by direct RNA sequencing. Nat Neurosci 16:1896–1905. https://doi.org/10.1038/nn.3554
20. Ji P, Schachtschneider KM, Schook LB, Walker FR, Johnson RW (2016) Peripheral viral infection induced microglial sensome genes and enhanced microglial cell activity in the hippocampus of neonatal piglets. Brain Behav Immun 54:243–251. https://doi.org/10.1016/j.bbi.2016.02.010
21. Kang HJ, Kawasawa YI, Cheng F, Zhu Y, Xu X, Li M, Sousa AM, Pletikos M, Meyer KA, al SG (2011) Spatio-temporal transcriptome of the human brain. Nature 478:483–489. https://doi.org/10.1038/nature10523
22. Kasperaviciute D, Catarino CB, Matarin M, Leu C, Novy J, Tostevin A, Leal B, Hessel EV, Hallmann K, al HMS (2013) Epilepsy, hippocampal sclerosis and febrile seizures linked by common genetic variation around SCN1A. Brain: a journal of neurology 136:3140–3150. https://doi.org/10.1093/brain/awt233
23. Klempin F, Kronenberg G, Cheung G, Kettenmann H, Kempermann G (2011) Properties of doublecortin-(DCX)-expressing cells in the piriform cortex compared to the neurogenic dentate gyrus of adult mice. PLoS One 6:e25760. https://doi.org/10.1371/journal.pone.0025760
24. Knoth R, Singec I, Ditter M, Pantazis G, Capetian P, Meyer RP, Horvat V, Volk B, Kempermann G (2010) Murine features of neurogenesis in the human hippocampus across the lifespan from 0 to 100 years. PLoS One 5:e8809. https://doi.org/10.1371/journal.pone.0008809
25. Kunze A, Achilles A, Keiner S, Witte OW, Redecker C (2015) Two distinct populations of doublecortin-positive cells in the perilesional zone of cortical infarcts. BMC Neurosci 16:20. https://doi.org/10.1186/s12868-015-0160-8
26. Kyyriainen J, Ekolle Ndode-Ekane X, Pitkanen A (2017) Dynamics of PDGFRbeta expression in different cell types after brain injury. Glia 65:322–341. https://doi.org/10.1002/glia.23094
27. Liu J, Reeves C, Jacques T, McEvoy A, Miserocchi A, Thompson P, Sisodiya S, Thom M (2018) Nestin-expressing cell types in the temporal lobe and hippocampus: morphology, differentiation, and proliferative capacity. Glia 66:62 77. https://doi.org/10.1002/glia.23211
28. Liu YW, Curtis MA, Gibbons HM, Mee EW, Bergin PS, Teoh HH, Connor B, Dragunow M, Faull RL (2008) Doublecortin expression in the normal and epileptic adult human brain. Eur J Neurosci 28:2254–2265. https://doi.org/10.1111/j.1460-9568.2008.06518.x
29. Marti-Mengual U, Varea E, Crespo C, Blasco-Ibanez JM, Nacher J (2013) Cells expressing markers of immature neurons in the amygdala of adult humans. Eur J Neurosci 37:10–22. https://doi.org/10.1111/ejn.12016
30. Mikkonen M, Soininen H, Kalvianen R, Tapiola T, Ylinen A, Vapalahti M, Paljarvi L, Pitkanen A (1998) Remodeling of neuronal circuitries in human temporal lobe epilepsy: increased expression of highly polysialylated neural cell adhesion molecule in the hippocampus and the entorhinal cortex. Ann Neurol 44:923–934. https://doi.org/10.1002/ana.410440611
31. Milesi S, Boussadia B, Plaud C, Catteau M, Rousset MC, De Bock F, Schaeffer M, Lerner-Natoli M, Rigau V, Marchi N (2014) Redistribution of PDGFRbeta cells and NG2DsRed pericytes at the cerebrovasculature after status epilepticus. Neurobiol Dis 71:151–158. https://doi.org/10.1016/j.nbd.2014.07.010
32. Nayak D, Roth TL, McGavern DB (2014) Microglia development and function. Annu Rev Immunol 32:367–402. https://doi.org/10.1146/annurev-immunol-032713-120240
33. Nogueira AB, Sogayar MC, Colquhoun A, Siqueira SA, Marchiori PE, Teixeira MJ (2014) Existence of a potential neurogenic system in the adult human brain. J Transl Med 12:75. https://doi.org/10.1186/1479-5876-12-75
34. Paine SM, Willsher AR, Nicholson SL, Sebire NJ, Jacques TS (2014) Characterization of a population of neural progenitor cells in the infant hippocampus. Neuropathol Appl Neurobiol 40:544–550. https://doi.org/10.1111/nan.12065
35. Parakalan R, Jiang B, Nimmi B, Janani M, Jayapal M, Lu J, Tay SS, Ling EA, Dheen ST (2012) Transcriptome analysis of amoeboid and ramified microglia isolated from the corpus callosum of rat brain. BMC Neurosci 13:64. https://doi.org/10.1186/1471-2202-13-64
36. Patzke N, LeRoy A, Ngubane NW, Bennett NC, Medger K, Gravett N, Kaswera-Kyamakya C, Gilissen E, Chawana R, Manger PR (2014) The distribution of doublecortin-immunopositive cells in the brains of four afrotherian mammals: the Hottentot golden mole (Amblysomus hottentotus), the rock hyrax (Procavia capensis), the eastern rock sengi (Elephantulus myurus) and the four-toed sengi (Petrodromus tetradactylus). Brain Behav Evol 84:227–241. https://doi.org/10.1159/000367934
37. Shahsavani M, Pronk RJ, Falk R, Lam M, Moslem M, Linker SB, Salma J, Day K, Schuster J, al ABM (2017) An in vitro model of lissencephaly: expanding the role of DCX during neurogenesis. Mol Psychiatry. https://doi.org/10.1038/mp.2017.175
38. Sharma K, Schmitt S, Bergner CG, Tyanova S, Kannaiyan N, Manrique-Hoyos N, Kongi K, Cantuti L, Hanisch UK (1819) Philips MAet al (2015) cell type- and brain region-resolved mouse brain proteome. Nat Neurosci 18:–1831. https://doi.org/10.1038/nn.4160
39. Shepherd C, Liu J, Goc J, Martinian L, Jacques TS, Sisodiya SM, Thom M (2013) A quantitative study of white matter hypomyelination and oligodendroglial maturation in focal cortical dysplasia type II. Epilepsia 54:898–908. https://doi.org/10.1111/epi.12143
40. Srikandarajah N, Martinian L, Sisodiya SM, Squier W, Blumcke I, Aronica E, Thom M (2009) Doublecortin expression in focal cortical dysplasia in epilepsy. Epilepsia 50:2619–2628. https://doi.org/10.1111/j.1528-1167.2009.02194.x
41. Sweeney MD, Ayyadurai S, Zlokovic BV (2016) Pericytes of the neurovascular unit: key functions and signaling pathways. Nat Neurosci 19:771–783. https://doi.org/10.1038/nn.4288
42. Tai XY, Koepp M, Duncan JS, Fox N, Thompson P, Baxendale S, Liu JY, Reeves C, Michalak Z, Thom M (2016) Hyperphosphorylated tau in patients with refractory epilepsy correlates with cognitive decline: a study of temporal lobe resections. Brain J Neurol 139:2441–2455. https://doi.org/10.1093/brain/aww187
43. Thom M, Eriksson S, Martinian L, Caboclo LO, McEvoy AW, Duncan JS, Sisodiya SM (2009) Temporal lobe sclerosis associated with hippocampal sclerosis in temporal lobe epilepsy: neuropathological features. J Neuropathol Exp Neurol 68:928–938. https://doi.org/10.1097/NEN.0b013e3181b05d67
44. Thompson PJ, Baxendale SA, McEvoy AW, Duncan JS (2015) Cognitive outcomes of temporal lobe epilepsy surgery in older patients. Seizure 29:41–45. https://doi.org/10.1016/j.seizure.2015.03.017

45. Verwer RW, Sluiter AA, Balesar RA, Baaijen JC, de Witt Hamer PC, Speijer D, Li Y, Swaab DF (2015) Injury response of resected human brain tissue in vitro. Brain Pathol 25:454–468. https://doi.org/10.1111/bpa.12189
46. Verwer RW, Sluiter AA, Balesar RA, Baayen JC, Noske DP, Dirven CM, Wouda J, van Dam AM, Lucassen PJ, Swaab DF (2007) Mature astrocytes in the adult human neocortex express the early neuronal marker doublecortin. Brain J Neurol 130:3321–3335. https://doi.org/10.1093/brain/awm264
47. Verwer RW, Sluiter AA, Balesar RA, Baayen JC, Speijer D, Idema S, Swaab DF (2016) Altered loyalties of neuronal markers in cultured slices of resected human brain tissue. Brain Pathol 26:523–532. https://doi.org/10.1111/bpa.12330
48. Wes PD, Holtman IR, Boddeke EW, Moller T, Eggen BJ (2016) Next generation transcriptomics and genomics elucidate biological complexity of microglia in health and disease. Glia 64:197–213. https://doi.org/10.1002/glia.22866
49. Xiong K, Luo DW, Patrylo PR, Luo XG, Struble RG, Clough RW, Yan XX (2008) Doublecortin-expressing cells are present in layer II across the adult Guinea pig cerebral cortex: partial colocalization with mature interneuron markers. Exp Neurol 211:271–282. https://doi.org/10.1016/j.expneurol.2008.02.003
50. Yoo Y, Byun K, Kang T, Bayarsaikhan D, Kim JY, Oh S, Kim YH, Kim SY, Chung WI, Kim SU et al (2015) Amyloid-beta-activated human microglial cells through ER-resident proteins. J. Proteome Res 14:214–223. https://doi.org/10.1021/pr500926r
51. Zhang L, Hernandez VS, Estrada FS, Lujan R (2014) Hippocampal CA field neurogenesis after pilocarpine insult: the hippocampal fissure as a neurogenic niche. J Chem Neuroanat 56:45–57. https://doi.org/10.1016/j.jchemneu.2014.02.002
52. Zhang XM, Cai Y, Chu Y, Chen EY, Feng JC, Luo XG, Xiong K, Struble RG, Clough RW, Patrylo PR et al (2009) Doublecortin-expressing cells persist in the associative Cereb Cortex and amygdala in aged nonhuman Primates. Front Neuroanat 3:17. https://doi.org/10.3389/neuro.05.017.2009
53. Zhang Y, Chen K, Sloan SA, Bennett ML, Scholze AR, O'Keeffe S, Phatnani HP, Guarnieri P, Caneda C, al RN (2014) An RNA-sequencing transcriptome and splicing database of glia, neurons, and vascular cells of the Cereb Cortex. J Neurosci Off J Soc Neurosci 34:11929–11947. https://doi.org/10.1523/JNEUROSCI.1860-14.2014

8

Endothelial damage, vascular bagging and remodeling of the microvascular bed in human microangiopathy with deep white matter lesions

Karin M. E. Forsberg[1†], Yingshuang Zhang[2†], Johanna Reiners[3], Martina Ander[3], Alexandra Niedermayer[3], Lubin Fang[3], Hermann Neugebauer[4], Jan Kassubek[4], Istvan Katona[5], Joachim Weis[5], Albert C. Ludolph[4], Kelly Del Tredici[3], Heiko Braak[3] and Deniz Yilmazer-Hanke[3*†]

Abstract

White matter lesions (WMLs) are a common manifestation of small vessel disease (SVD) in the elderly population. They are associated with an enhanced risk of developing gait abnormalities, poor executive function, dementia, and stroke with high mortality. Hypoperfusion and the resulting endothelial damage are thought to contribute to the development of WMLs. The focus of the present study was the analysis of the microvascular bed in SVD patients with deep WMLs (DWMLs) by using double- and triple-label immunohistochemistry and immunofluorescence. Simultaneous visualization of collagen IV (COLL4)-positive membranes and the endothelial glycocalyx in thick sections allowed us to identify endothelial recession in different types of string vessels, and two new forms of small vessel/capillary pathology, which we called vascular bagging and ghost string vessels. Vascular bags were pouches and tubes that were attached to vessel walls and were formed by multiple layers of COLL4-positive membranes. Vascular bagging was most severe in the DWMLs of cases with pure SVD (no additional vascular brain injury, VBI). Quantification of vascular bagging, string vessels, and the density/size of CD68-positive cells further showed widespread pathological changes in the frontoparietal and/or temporal white matter in SVD, including pure SVD and SVD with VBI, as well as a significant effect of the covariate age. Plasma protein leakage into vascular bags and the white matter parenchyma pointed to endothelial damage and basement membrane permeability. Hypertrophic IBA1-positive microglial cells and CD68-positive macrophages were found in white matter areas covered with networks of ghost vessels in SVD, suggesting phagocytosis of remnants of string vessels. However, the overall vessel density was not altered in our SVD cohort, which might result from continuous replacement of vessels. Our findings support the view that SVD is a progressive and generalized disease process, in which endothelial damage and vascular bagging drive remodeling of the microvasculature.

Keywords: Leukoaraiosis, Binswanger's disease, Endothelial glycocalyx, Basement membrane, Blood brain barrier, Microglia activation, String vessel

* Correspondence: deniz.yilmazer-hanke@uni-ulm.de
†Karin M. E. Forsberg, Yingshuang Zhang and Deniz Yilmazer-Hanke contributed equally to this work.
[3]Clinical Neuroanatomy Section, Neurology, School of Medicine, Ulm University, Helmholtzstr. 8/1, 89081 Ulm, Germany
Full list of author information is available at the end of the article

Introduction

Cerebral small vessel disease (SVD) or cerebral microangiopathy are overarching terms for a group of heterogeneous disorders with different etiologies and pathogeneses, which compromise the cerebral microcirculation [75]. SVD encompasses atherosclerosis and lipohyalinosis of small arteries and arterioles, cerebral amyloid angiopathy (CAA), hereditary forms of non-CAA microangiopathies (e.g., CADASIL), inflammatory angiitis, venous collagenosis, and miscellaneous forms, e.g., SVD that results from radiation or non-CAA-related vessel degeneration in Alzheimer's disease. Pathologic alterations caused by sporadic and hereditary forms of SVD include white matter lesions (WMLs), lacunar infarcts, microinfarcts, and microbleeds [64].

WMLs, also referred to as leukoaraiosis, are large areas of pallor in the subcortical deep white matter and in periventricular areas with ill-defined margins that show hyperintense signals in T2-weighted magnetic resonance images [61]. They are frequently found in the healthy, elderly population, and their prevalence increases from 11 to 21% in adults around the age of 64 to 94% in those around 82 years of age [34, 62, 87]. WMLs are largely considered a clinically silent brain injury, but their presence increases the risk of developing stroke and vascular mortality [28, 46, 47, 82]. WMLs are also commonly associated with cognitive decline and dementia [33, 74], general brain atrophy [5], and gait disorders [26, 81], often leading to the diagnosis of Binswanger's disease, particularly in the presence of lacunar infarctions [43]. The pathogenesis of WMLs has not been fully established yet, but the prevailing view is that they result from white matter ischemia owing to hypertension or chronic hypoperfusion [10, 64, 70].

Pathological changes found in WMLs such as hyalinosis of small arterioles, arteriolosclerosis, and arterial tortuosity are widespread in the elderly population and in hypertension, probably contributing to disturbances in the perfusion of deep white matter areas [17, 32, 58, 65]. Nevertheless, in some stroke patients with WMLs no subcortical arteriosclerotic changes have been detected [48]. In the human brain, deep white matter areas that are particularly vulnerable to injury from hypoperfusion are the so-called watershed areas, which are located at the border between territories supplied by terminal branches of leptomeningeal and perforating arteries [57, 64]. In experimental models, the predominant microvascular pathology in chronically hypoperfused white matter areas is endothelial cell damage [42, 78]. Reduced expression of endothelial markers and leakage of plasma proteins into arteriole walls and the white matter have also been reported in human WMLs [15, 84, 89]. Further histopathological features of human WMLs include dilated perivascular Virchow-Robin spaces, loss of oligodendrocytes leading to demyelination, axonal damage and vacuolization (spongiosis) of the white matter, and potentially alterations in the density of so-called string vessels, which are collagenous tubes connecting two vessels and are regarded as remnants of basement membranes in regressing vessels [18, 19, 21, 61].

The aim of this study was to investigate markers and mechanisms that may be involved in remodeling of vessels in SVD patients with WMLs. Vascular bagging, defined here as the space between the vessel wall and external collagenous membranes of small vessels, as well as string vessels were analyzed at lesion sites and in control regions using double-labeling for endothelial and basement membrane markers. Using Z-stack imaging, different types of string vessels as well as the relationship of activated IBA1- and CD68-positive cells to the cerebral microvasculature were studied in thick sections. Widened perivascular spaces, also called état criblé or status cribrosus, and plasma protein leakage to the vessel walls or brain parenchyma were examined in thin paraffin sections. Hereby, we focused on deep WMLs (DWMLs), because periventricular WMLs that are often associated with prominent fibrosis in the wall of periventricular veins, also called venous collagenosis [58], might be assignable to a different pathological entity [35]. Particular attention was also paid to excluding concomitant pathologies related to Alzheimer's and Parkinson's disease or other tauopathies and alpha-synucleinopathies, which can affect the microvascular bed [19, 86]. Moreover, SVD cases with vascular brain injury (VBI) were studied separately from "pure" SVD cases without VBI, because especially in the acute/subacute phase cerebral infarctions can lead to the infiltration of the brain with peripheral blood cells [9], potentially confounding findings related to chronic alterations in SVD.

Material and methods

Study population and neuropathological evaluation of the brain

The study cohort consisted of brain tissue from 14 human subjects (7 females, 7 males) with an average age of 64.1 ± 10.2 years (mean ± standard deviation, SD). Demographics and relevant data for the patient cohort are provided in (Additional file 1: Table S1). The patients were divided into 3 groups: "pure" SVD cases with DWMLs but without additional VBI ($n = 5$), SVD + VBI cases with DWMLs and remote cerebrovascular incidents ($n = 5$), and control cases without SVD (NoSVD) or history of neurological disorders ($n = 4$). NoSVD controls died from myocardial infarction, ovarian cancer, esophageal cancer, and pulmonary edema due to left heart failure. Among cases with pure SVD, one case suffering from chronic hypertension and generalized arteriosclerosis died following aortic valve replacement surgery (24 h blood pressure levels of 149/70 mmHg under a combination therapy with the diuretic hydrochlorothiazide, the beta-blocker metoprolol, the calcium channel blocker amlodipine, and the angiotensin receptor 1 blocker valsartan). A second case had advanced peripheral artery disease at Fontaine stage IIb to III and died from a gastrointestinal infarct due to occlusion of the pelvic artery. The other three pure SVD cases were diagnosed with pulmonary embolism, highly malignant non-hodgkin lymphoma and renal cancer, respectively. In three SVD + VBI cases, pontine bleeding and a contralateral (sub)acute ischemic stroke (MCA-l) with/without thalamic infarction was the cause of death. An SVD + VBI case with ischemic stroke in the contralateral internal capsule died from breast cancer and the other case with a chronic ischemic cerebral infarct (2 years old) from sudden cardiovascular arrest. All autopsied subjects underwent routine neuropathological examination and were screened for tauopathies, alpha-synucleinopathies and beta-amyloid (Aβ) deposition. Inclusion criteria for entering the study were: No history of neurodegenerative disorders; i.e., no Alzheimer-related tau pathology exceeding neurofibrillary stage II [13] or other tauopathy, as well as no Parkinson's disease [14], multisystem atrophy or other alpha-synuclein-related pathology. Furthermore, all cases included to the study had Aβ phases II or less [76]. This retrospective study was performed in compliance with the university ethics committee guidelines as well as German federal and state law governing human tissue usage. Informed written permission was obtained from all patients and/or their next of kin for autopsy.

Histology

Brains fixed in a 4% solution of formaldehyde were cut in approximately 1 cm thick coronal slices. Tissue blocks containing frontoparietal and temporal lobe areas that were devoid of macroscopically visible small or large infarcts or cysts in the white matter were embedded in polyethylene glycol (PEG 1000, Merck, Carl Roth Ltd., Karlsruhe, Germany). Multiple 100 µm thick consecutive sections were obtained using a sliding microtome (Jung, Heidelberg, Germany). For histological orientation, sections were stained for lipofuscin pigment and the Nissl substance using aldehyde fuchsine and Darrow red [12]. For neuropathological evaluation and the identification of DWMLs, thick coronal sections were stained with a modified hematoxylin eosin (H&E) procedure by replacing eosin with acid fuchsine, which allowed examination of entire hemisphere sections [60]. Paraffin embedding was performed on tissue blocks dissected out of deep white matter areas neighboring the regions that have been analyzed in thick coronal sections. From paraffin embedded blocks, 7 µm thick sections were cut with a microtome (Slee Medical GmbH, Mainz, Germany). Myelin staining was performed with a modified Heidenhain procedure using 2.5% ammonium iron(III) sulfate (30 min) and a solution containing 9% hematoxylin and 0.03% lithium carbonate (60 min) [44].

Upon neuropathological evaluation, arteriolosclerotic changes were found in the basal ganglia of the case with hypertension (pure SVD), which showed prominent concentric hyaline thickening of vessel walls and stenosis of the vessel lumen, and two other cases also showed minor hyalinosis (NoSVD control; SVD + VBI). However, vessels with an "onion-skin" pattern and Charcot-Bouchard microaneurysms were not observed. SVD cases with VBI also presented subcortical microbleeds (4 out of 5 cases). Particularly enlarged perivascular spaces were found in the basal ganglia and thalamus of 4 SVD cases around vessels of various calibers (2 pure SVD; 2 SVD + VBI), although the NoSVD controls and other SVD cases also showed some widening of perivascular spaces.

Immunohistochemistry in thick sections

Free-floating 100 µm thick sections were treated for 30 min with a mixture of 10% methanol and 3% concentrated H_2O_2 in Tris-buffered saline (TBS) to inhibit endogenous peroxidase activity. Bovine serum albumin (BSA) was applied for 30 min for blocking non-specific binding sites. Antigen retrieval was performed using Tris-EDTA buffer at pH 9.0 or citrate buffer at pH 6.0 for 1/2 h at 100 °C or pretreatment with 1.3 µg/ml proteinase K for 10–15 min at 37 °C (Invitrogen/Life Technologies, Darmstadt, Germany). For single labeling, sections were incubated at 4 °C with the primary antibody for a duration of 12–48 h (depending on the antibody). The three primary antibodies used were directed against collagen IV (COLL4; 1:5000, rabbit, Abcam, Cambridge, UK), the microglia/macrophage marker ionized calcium binding adapter molecule 1 (IBA1; 1:5000, rabbit, Abcam, Cambridge, UK) or the macrophage marker from the lysosomal/endosomal-associated membrane glycoprotein (LAMP) family CD68 (1:200, mouse, DAKO, Glostrup, Denmark). Sections were transferred for 2 h to a solution containing the corresponding secondary biotinylated antibody (1:200; Vector Laboratories, Burlingame, CA, USA). Alternatively, sections were incubated for 48 h with *Ulex europaeus* lectin (UEA-l; 1: 800, biotin-coupled, GeneTex, Irvine, CA, USA). Immunohistochemical reactions or lectin binding were visualized by incubating the sections for 2 h with an avidin-biotin-peroxidase complex (ABC Vectastain, Vector Laboratories, Burlingame, CA, USA). The reaction product of the peroxidase was visualized with the chromogen 3,3′-diaminobenzidine tetrahydrochloride (DAB; Sigma Taufkirchen, Germany). For double-label immunohistochemistry, sections were washed with TBS at 95 °C for 5 min, and the immunohistochemical procedure was repeated using the next primary and secondary antibodies. Subsequently, a blue chromogen (Vector SK-4700 peroxidase substrate kit, Linaris, Doffenheim; Germany) was used to visualize the reaction product. Omission of the primary antibody resulted in non-staining.

Immunohistochemistry and immunofluorescence in paraffin sections

Thin paraffin sections were treated with 10% methanol and 3% H_2O_2 in TBS for 30 min and/or with BSA for 30–60 min. For antigen retrieval, Tris-EDTA or citrate buffer were used at 100 °C for 10–20 min or proteinase K was applied for 10–15 min as described above. For immunohistochemistry (IHC) and immunofluorescence (IF), sections were incubated with primary antibodies against COLL4 (IHC: 1:5000, IF 1:4000, rabbit, Abcam), alkaline phosphatase (ALPL; IHC 1:1000, rabbit, Atlas Antibodies, Sweden), fibrinogen (FIBR; IHC 1:200, rabbit, DAKO), human IgG (IHC/IF 1:200, Vector Laboratories) or myelin basic protein (MBP; IHC 1:1000, rat, BioRad, Puchheim, Germany). For IHC, sections were treated with a biotinylated secondary antibody (1:200 for 2 h, Vector Laboratories, Burlingame, CA, USA) or UEA-l (1:800 for 48 h, GeneTex) and transferred to a ABC Vectastain solution for 2 h. The reaction product was visualized with DAB, SK-4700 or SK-4800 (Vector Laboratories), and the sections were coverslipped. For IF, binding of UEA-l (1:100, biotin-coupled, overnight) or primary antibody was visualized by incubating sections with streptavidin coupled to Alexa 532 (1:1000, Invitrogen/Life Technologies) or with a secondary antibody (Abcam) coupled to Alexa 594 (1:200, anti-rabbit) or Alexa 647 (1:300, anti-goat). Sections were coverslipped with Moviol (Polysciences Europe, Hirschberg an der Bergstrasse, Germany). Omission of primary antibodies resulted in absence of IHC and IF.

Image acquisition and processing

Alterations in the microvascular bed and microglia activation were assessed qualitatively and quantitatively with the aid of a AX10 microscope (Zeiss, Jena, Germany). Digital micrographs were taken with a Jenoptik Progres Gryphax® Prokyon camera using the Progres Gryphax® microscope camera software (Jena, Thüringen, Germany). In IHC-stained sections, either single images were taken or z-stacks were obtained. For documentation of tortuous vessels and pathological alterations, multiple single images and z-stacks were combined using manual construction with Adobe Photoshop, version 10.0 for qualitative analyses as needed. Microscope and camera settings (exposure, gain, and hue) were held constant when taking images for quantitative analyses. For IF applications, sections were imaged with a LED fluorescence lamp and narrow band filter sets (AHF Analysetechnik, Tübingen, Germany). Consistency of immunohistochemical staining throughout 100 µm thick sections was verified by confirming staining at different focus levels (see Additional files 2 and 3: Videos S1 and S2 showing videos of vessels and microglia). For video-documentation, an Eclipse LV100ND microscope was used that was equipped with a digital DS-Fi3 camera and the NIS-Elements software (NIKON GmbH, Düsseldorf, Germany) and with a motorized object table (Märzhäuser Wetzlar, Wetzlar, Germany).

Quantification of vessel densities, vessel diameters and microglia

Quantitative analyses were performed in 100 µm thick sections using the Image J software version v1.51 k (NIH, Bethesda, Maryland, MD, USA). The density and diameter of vessels were quantified in thick sections double-labeled for UEA-l and COLL4, and the density of central nervous system (CNS) macrophages in sections double-labeled for CD68 and COLL4 by a blind investigator. The boundaries of DWMLs and in-case control areas (approx. 1 cm^2) were marked on the immunostained sections after identifying pale white matter areas in adjacent sections stained for modified H&E. Depending on the localization of the lesion site, in-case control areas were positioned in the medial or lateral frontoparietal region, and an additional remote control area in the lateral temporal lobe was included. All areas studied were located in the subcortical deep white matter proximal to U-fibers.

Vessel densities were measured within the marked white matter area in images taken with the 5x objective. After transforming each image into an 8-bit gray image, the distribution of gray values and the standard deviation (SD) were determined. From these 8-bit gray images, binary images were obtained using an established pipeline by first subtracting the background (mean gray value minus 2x SD) and then by median filtering (1.5 px range). After superimposing a grid on the binary image, the vessel density was measured in every second grid box (area 0.3025 mm^2) by selecting the grid boxes in a checkerboard pattern. Grid boxes containing arteries or veins were skipped by moving to the next available grid box. Altogether, 35 grids were analyzed in NoSVD controls, 74 grids in pure SVD, and 70 grids in SVD + VBI. In addition, string vessels with different morphologies were counted by screening the white matter with the 10x objective. The number of string vessels counted was divided by the size of the area screened to calculate the density of string vessels. Overall, the density of string vessels was determined in an area of 8.905 mm^2 in NoSVD control cases, of 9.577 mm^2 in pure SVD cases and of 7.603 mm^2 in SVD + VBI cases. For quantification of vessel diameters, images of vessels were taken with the 20x objective at a distance of 1 mm in both the x- and y-axes. In these images, vessel diameters were measured by selecting vessel segments that were in focus (all vessel components sharp and clearly discernable). The regular diameter of the vessels (UEA-l- and COLL4-labeled) and the maximum outer diameter (at the COLL4-labeled outer vascular bag membrane) were measured. In addition, the length of each vessel segment was determined, in which the two vessel diameters were recorded. The calculated difference between the maximum outer diameter and corresponding actual vessel diameter was used as an indicator of vascular bagging. Overall, vessel diameters were analyzed in 2709 vessel segments with an average length of 93.45 ± 75.8 μm (SD) per vessel segment, thereby resulting in a total vessel length of 253,152 μm.

CD68-positive cells (macrophages) were quantified in sections double-labeled for COLL4. Lesion and control white matter areas were marked on the sections by using neighboring sections stained for modified H&E to identify the DWML. Z-stack images were taken with the 20x objective throughout the entire section. The images covered an area of 0.495 μm^2 in the xy-plane and had a distance of 1 mm in the x- and y-axes. The area of the cell body was measured manually for each CD68-positive cell in the z-stack images. Crests/cups of cell bodies cut at the surface or bottom of the section (< 20 μm^2 area) were excluded from analyses. The number of cells and the area of cell bodies were quantified in the parenchyma as well as at perivascular sites by identifying cells attached to the outer wall of COLL4-positive vessels. Cell densities (cell counts / image area) were calculated for each image taken. The number of images analyzed was 128 in the NoSVD controls, 153 in the pure SVD group, and 122 in the SVD + VBI group.

Statistical analysis

Statistical analyses were performed with the software IBM SPSS Statistics Version 25. Small vessels included in the statistical analyses were identified by determining large vessels with extreme values using explorative descriptive statistics, thereby permitting the exclusion of outliers with a vessel diameter above the 95th percentile. For comparing two groups, a t-test was performed (Welch test with Satterthwaite's approximation to compute the degrees of freedom). Multiple groups were compared using generalized linear models for the main factors vascular disease (NoSVD control, pure SVD or SVD + VBI), presence of DWMLs (NoSVD control, in-case control or DWMLs) and white matter location (frontoparietal or temporal) and covariate age with the aid of a three-way ANOVA or one-way ANOVA followed by the posthoc Games-Howell test. Data were presented as mean ± S.E.M. and outcomes were deemed significant at a two-tailed level of $p < 0.05$.

Results

DWMLs showed pallor, spongiosis and reduced oligodendrocyte densities

The DWMLs analyzed in the present study were situated in the frontoparietal region, with some lesions extending into the dorsal portion of the internal capsule except for a single DWML area that was located in the temporal lobe. In thick coronal sections stained with modified H&E, DWMLs could be identified as pale areas separated from the apparently normal surrounding tissue (Fig. 1a). At higher magnification, pale areas within DWMLs showed a patchy staining pattern, and contained a variable density of putative oligodendrocytes with small, round and heterochromatin-rich nuclei. However, cavitation and tissue loss were not evident in the white matter areas studied (Fig. 1b-c). In thin paraffin sections, IHC for MBP and myelin staining revealed loosening of the white matter architecture with spongiosis and a reduced density of oligodendrocytes in DWML areas. In contrast, NoSVD controls exhibited dense bundles of fiber tracts with clear boundaries that ran in various directions and had a high density of oligodendrocytes (Additional file 4: Figure S1).

Vascular bagging was revealed as a hallmark of white matter pathology in SVD

Double-labeling for UEA-l and COLL4 studied allowed the visualization of the endothelial cell layer and basement membrane of vessels, respectively. Analyses of large white matter areas in thick sections revealed pouches formed by COLL4-positive membranes around many vessels, which we designated as 'vascular bagging' (Fig. 2). The endothelium occasionally showed indentations in the absence of abnormalities in the basement membrane (Fig. 2b). However, vascular bags with irregular expansions of COLL4-positive outer membranes were more common. They often formed multiple layers attached to the vessel surface, suggesting duplication or

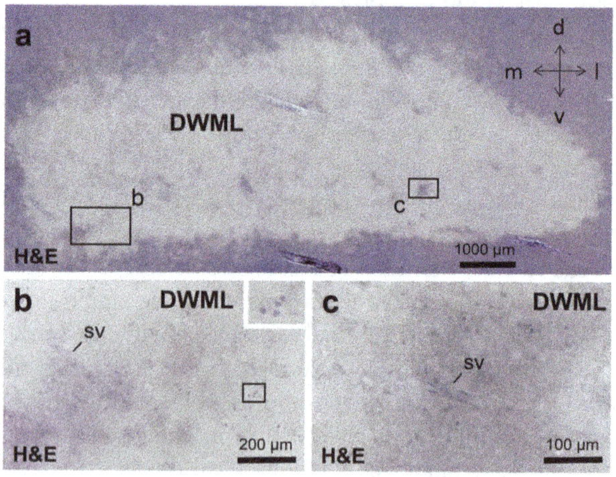

Fig. 1 Example of deep white matter lesion (DWML) in a case with small vessel disease (SVD) in thick sections (**a-c**). **a** Pale DWML with unclear boundaries and islands with less pale areas. **b-c** Insets from (**a**) show more oligodendrocytes in relatively well-preserved less pale areas compared to severely affected pale areas, and also small vessels (sv). Case 6 (non-hodgkin lymphoma) with "pure" SVD, i.e., this case has only SVD, but no additional vascular brain injury (VBI) resulting from a ischemic or hemorrhagic cerebral infarct. Scale bars: 1000 μm in (**a**), 200 μm in (**b**), 100 μm in (**c**)

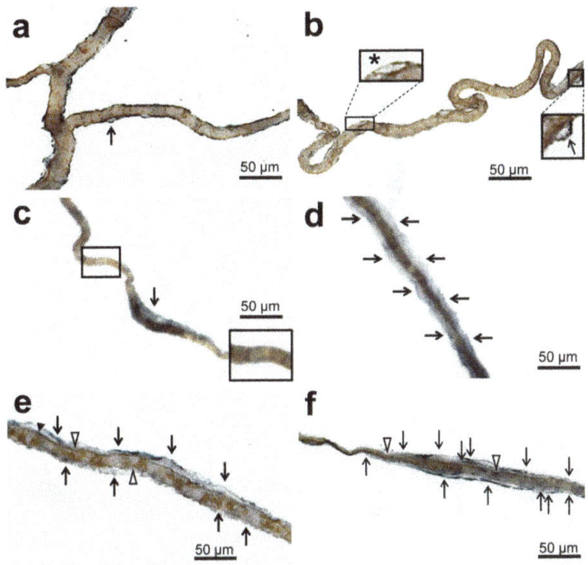

Fig. 2 Z-stack images of vessels double-labeled for the endothelial marker *Ulex europaeus* lectin (UEA-I, brown) and collagen IV (COLL4, blue) in 100 µm thick sections. **a-b** In healthy vessels (type 1), COLL4-positive membranes are only visible in areas with bubble-shaped expansions (arrows) as seen in a control case without SVD (NoSVD). Small endothelial indentations are also found in healthy vessels (star; type 2a), which have COLL4-positive basement membranes with smooth contours (see Fig. 6b for comparison with type 2b vessel). **c-d** COLL4- positive basement membranes of small vessels are often barely distinguishable from the staining of the endothelium (labeled with UEA-I) in healthy vessels (inset in **c**) in thick sections except in vessel segments with vascular bags. Vascular bags (arrows) are formed by external COLL4-positive membranes detached from the vessel wall. In NoSVD controls they are usually limited to short vessel segments (type 3a, see **c**), whereas in SVD they can cover long distances (type 3b, see **d**). **e-f** Severely diseased vessels (type 4) show both endothelial irregularities (open arrow heads) and vascular bagging with thickened basement membranes (small black arrow head). Vascular bagging can extend over considerable distances in type 4 vessels with various diameters (arrows) in SVD. Double arrows indicate multiple layers of collagenous membranes. Images obtained from Case 1 (myocardial infarction, NoSVD) (**a-b**), Case 2 (ovarian cancer, NoSVD) (**c-d**), and Case 6 (non-hodgkin lymphoma, pure SVD) (**e-f**). For viewing vascular bags, also see Additional file 2: Video S1 of Vessels. Scale bars 50 µm

multiplication of the basement membrane. Such external vascular bags largely differed in their size and extent, and some vascular bags accompanied the affected vessels for distances in excess of several hundred micrometers in DWMLs (Fig. 2c-d and Fig. 6b).

Based on these observations, four types of morphologies were identified in small vessels or vessel segments (Additional file 5: Figure S2). Type 1 normal vessels had an intact endothelium labeled with UEA-1 and a smooth COLL4-positive basement membrane lying directly underneath the endothelium and tightly attached to it. These vessels were the most common type in our study population. Type 2 vessels, which showed an intact basement membrane but indentations or irregularities of various degrees in their endothelial layer, were comparatively rare. Type 3 vessels had COLL4-positive bags attached to the vessel wall that were formed by external collagenous membranes and resembled small pouches or long tubes. However, the vessel wall was smooth and the endothelium with its underlying basement membrane appeared intact. Type 4 vessels displayed irregularities in both the endothelial layer and external collagenous membranes (bagging), which sometimes consisted of multiple layers or were discontinuous.

Vascular bagging was more prominent in DWMLs and age-dependent in control areas

Vascular bags consisting of the space between the basement membrane of the UEA-1 labeled endothelium and the external COLL4-positive membranes forming the outermost vessel boundaries were quantified in small vessels using thick sections. Large vessels with diameters above 95th percentile (> 22.7 µm) were excluded from analyses (Additional file 6: Figure S3). The effect of vascular disease, presence of DWML, and white matter location on vessel diameters, the outer membrane diameters and vascular bagging (difference between the two diameters) were analyzed with the aid of three-way ANOVA (Fig. 3). Results indicated that vascular disease had a significant effect on the vessel diameters ($F_{2,2700} = 17.927$, $p < 0.001$) and outer membrane diameters of small vessels ($F_{2,2700} = 16.056$, $p < 0.001$). In addition, the presence of a DWML had a significant effect on vascular bagging ($F_{2,2700} = 5.836$, $p < 0.05$). Posthoc analyses revealed that the vessel diameters in the frontoparietal white matter were significantly reduced in SVD + VBI cases when compared to NoSVD controls (Fig. 3a). In contrast, the outer membrane diameters were significantly increased in the DWMLs in pure SVD compared to white matter areas of all other groups (Fig. 3b). Vascular bagging was also increased significantly in the frontoparietal white matter of both SVD groups (pure SVD, SVD + VBI) compared to NoSVD controls, and this was not confined to DWMLs and included in-case control areas, indicating a generalized disease process in widespread white matter areas in SVD. Moreover, in pure SVD vascular bagging was more prominent in the DWMLs than in in-case control sites, compatible with a more advanced disease state in DWMLs in this vascular disease group (Fig. 3c).

Three-way ANOVA further showed that the white matter location (frontoparietal versus temporal) had a significant effect on the vessel diameters ($F_{2,2700} = 4.247$, $p < 0.05$), outer membrane diameters ($F_{2,2700} = 11.085$, $p = 0.001$), and vascular bagging ($F_{2,2700} = 7.551$, $p < 0.01$), combined with a significant interaction between presence of DWML and white matter location for the vessel

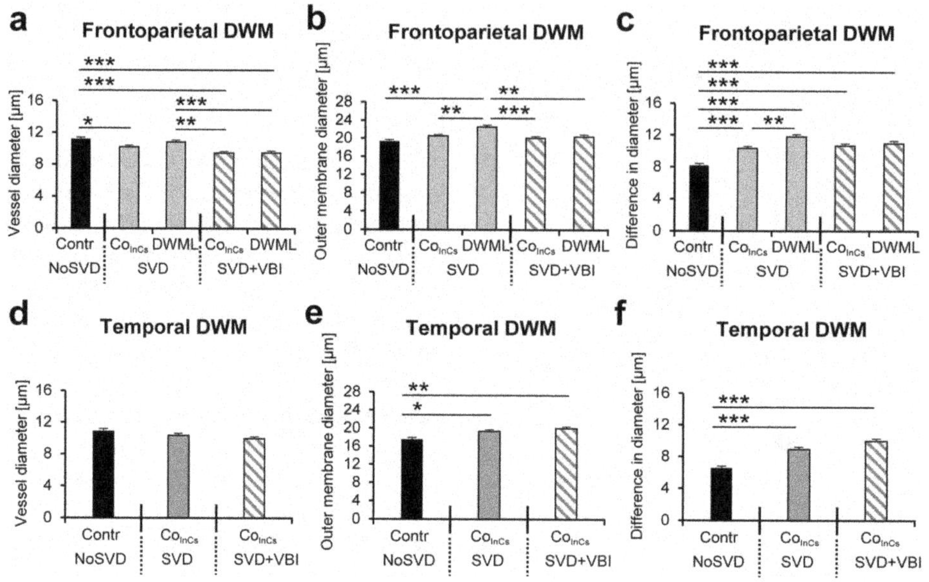

Fig. 3 Quantification of vascular bagging (**c** and **f**), which was defined as the difference between the diameter of the vessel lumen (**a** and **d**) and outer COLL4-positive bag membrane (**b** and **e**). In general, vessel diameters are larger and vascular bagging is more severe in the deep white matter (DWM) of frontoparietal areas than in the temporal lobe. **a** and **d** Vessel calibers are slightly smaller in the in-case control area of "pure" SVD cases and all white matter areas of SVD + VBI cases in the frontoparietal region compared to NoSVD controls (**a**), but no differences are seen in the temporal lobe (**d**). **b** and **e** In the frontoparietal region, the outer membrane diameters (measured at the outer border of bags) are significantly higher in DWMLs of "pure" SVD cases than in all other groups studied. In the temporal lobe, the in-case control areas exhibit significantly increased outer membrane diameters in both "pure" SVD and SVD + VBI cases when compared to NoSVD controls (**b**). **c** and **f** In the frontoparietal region, vascular bagging is more severe in SVD (both pure SVD and SVD + VBI) in all regions studied (DWML and in-case control) than in NoSVD cases. Furthermore, in "pure" SVD cases vascular bagging is significantly increased in DWMLs when compared to in-case control areas (**c**). In the temporal lobe, in-case control areas of SVD cases show a significant increase in vascular bagging when compared to NoSVD control cases, indicating a generalized disease process (**f**). The "pure" SVD cases were referred to as SVD in the diagrams. * $p < 0.05$, ** $p < 0.01$, *** $p < 0.001$

diameters ($F_{2,2700} = 7.069$, $p < 0.01$). However, posthoc analyses only confirmed significantly smaller outer membrane diameters and less vascular bagging in the temporal lobe when compared to frontoparietal areas of NoSVD controls and SVD cases. Nonetheless, outer membrane diameters and vascular bagging were also increased significantly in the temporal lobe of SVD cases compared to NoSVD controls (Fig. 3e-f), whereas the actual vessel diameters were not affected (Fig. 3d). In the three-way ANOVA (vascular disease x presence of DWML x white matter location), the covariate age had a significant effect specifically on outer membrane diameters ($F_{1,2700} = 101.374$, $p < 0.001$) and vascular bagging ($F_{2,11} = 166.641$, $p < 0.001$), although the individuals from the different vascular disease groups did not significantly differ in their age as confirmed by one-way ANOVA ($F_{2,11} = 0.33$, $p > 0.10$).

Vascular bags contained leaked plasma proteins

Multiple-label IHC and IF were employed in thin paraffin sections to investigate vascular bagging in more detail (Figs 4 and 5). In the H&E stain, the eosinophilic collagenous membranes forming the wall of bags and their eosinophilic contents were not distinguishable from the adjacent white matter. However, IHC combined with H&E showed that COLL4-positive basement membranes tightly covered the UEA-I labeled endothelium of capillary-size small vessels in the white matter of NoSVD controls (Fig. 4a), whereas vessels in DWMLs had vascular bags with multiple layers of external COLL4-positive membranes filled with eosinophilic material (Fig. 4b). Further analyses showed that the vascular bags contained the plasma proteins FIBR and IgG, whereas pericyte nuclei and enlarged perivascular spaces were situated outside the bags (Fig. 4c-f). Double-label IHC for plasma proteins and ALPL, an endothelial marker highly expressed in arteries and arterioles [59], showed strong IgG and FIBR accumulation in the vascular bags around capillaries and ALPL-positive pre-capillary arterioles, from where the plasma proteins spilled to the white matter parenchyma. In contrast, IgG and FIBR levels were low in the media of larger arterioles (Fig. 4g-h). Triple-label IF confirmed the presence of a basement membrane at the inner (endothelial) side of vascular bags (Fig. 5). The basement membrane lying directly underneath the endothelium was clearly separable from the UEA-I labeled glycocalyx expressed on the endothelial surface (Fig. 5d). The outer collagenous membranes of vascular bags were directly attached to the basement

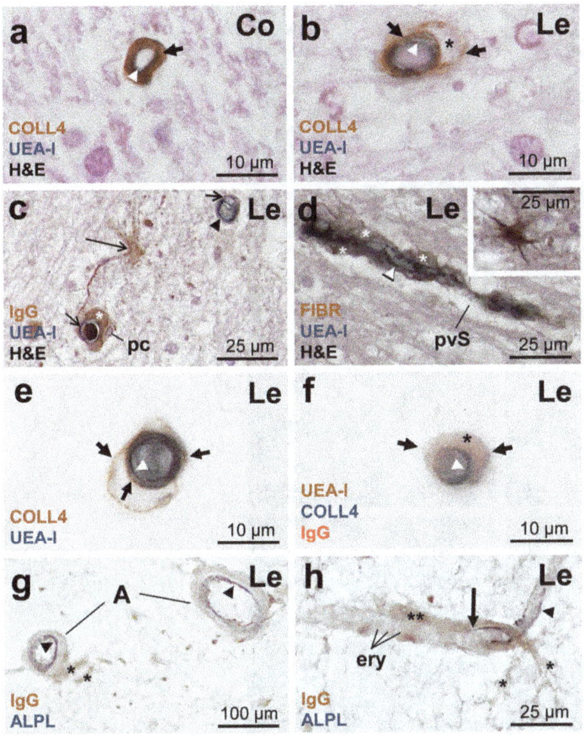

Fig. 4 Double- and triple-label immunohistochemistry (IHC) for UEA-I, COLL4, the plasma proteins fibrinogen (FIBR) or immunoglobulin G fraction (IgG) and the endothelial marker alkaline phosphatase protein (ALPL) in 7 µm thick paraffin sections. **a-b** The healthy capillary in the control white matter (Co) of a NoSVD case does not have vascular bags (**a**). Vascular bag (short thick arrow) in a SVD case with multiple layers of COLL4-positive membranes around the UEA-I-labeled endothelium (white arrowhead) of a small vessel (< 10 µm diameter) at a lesion (Le) site. Hematoxylin eosin (H&E) counterstaining reveals eosinophilic material (star) in the vascular bag (**b**). **c-d** Capillaries with a UEA-I positive endothelium (white arrowhead) and endothelial cell nuclei (short thin arrows) are surrounded by pericytes (pc) and a sharply delineated area filled with plasma proteins IgG or FIBR (star) suggestive of vascular bagging. Plasma proteins also leak to the white matter parenchyma (large thin arrow), but the widened perivascular space (pvS) outside the vascular bag appears empty. **e-f** Vascular bags with COLL4-positive walls around the UEA-I positive endothelium are filled with IgG protein (star). **g-h** ALPL expression is found in the endothelium of small arteries (**a**) and arterioles (black arrowheads), but is lost at the transition from the pre-capillary arteriole to the capillary (large thick arrow). IgG accumulation found around the pre-capillary arteriole and capillary with erythrocytes (ery) extends into the nearby white matter (stars). Images obtained from Case 2 (ovarian cancer, NoSVD) (**a**), Case 13 (contralateral subacute ischemic stroke in the territory of the medial cerebral artery (MCA) with thalamic infarction, SVD + VBI) (**b-e**), and Case 6 (non-hodgkin lymphoma, pure SVD) (**f-h**). The list of (immuno)histochemical markers is provided on the lower left corner of each image (color-coded for the chromogen used). Uppermost marker: brown (Diaminobenzidine, DAB); Middle (or lower in double-label IHC) marker: blue (SK-4700, Vector Laboratories); Lower stain/marker: H&E or red (SK-4800, Vector Laboratories); ery erythrocyte

membrane, suggesting a splitting or duplication of the membrane (Fig. 5c). While vascular bags with COLL4-positive walls were loaded with plasma proteins, no IgG or FIBR accumulation could be detected in the subendothelial space on the luminal side of the basement membrane (Fig. 5i).

White matter regions showed four types of string vessels - S1-S4

In thick sections, we could identify four types (S1-S4) of string vessels with COLL4-immunoreactive walls (Fig. 6). The first type exhibited focal loss of the UEA-I-positive endothelial glycocalyx (S1 in Fig. 6a), but string-like vessel segments with irregularities in the endothelial layer were also observed (Fig. 6b). The second type of string vessels were formed by wide collagenous tubes (S2 in Fig. 6c), and the third type by collapsed tubes (partial constrictions in wide string vessels or fully collapsed, S3 in Fig. 6d, e), whereas the fourth type consisted of discontinuous remnants of string vessels that still connected vessels, but were broken up into individual segments. The latter string vessels were named ghost string vessels, or briefly string ghosts (S4 in Fig. 6f).

String vessel density is increased in SVD but the overall vessel density is not altered

After characterizing the morphology of string vessels, the different types of string vessel (S2-S4) were quantified in the frontoparietal white matter except the rare S1 type vessels (Fig. 7a). Two-way ANOVA (vascular disease x presence of DWML) showed that only the total density of string vessels was significantly increased by vascular disease ($F_{1,24} = 4.924$, $p = 0.036$), but the presence of DWMLs had no effect on the string vessel density, and there was no interaction between the two main factors. Since no differences were detected between pure SVD and SVD + VBI in posthoc comparisons, the two groups were pooled for further analyses. A comparison of string vessel densities between NoSVD controls and all SVD cases (both pure SVD and SVD + VBI) showed a significant increase in SVD for the density of all types of string vessels ($t = -3.63$, df = 26.8, $p = 0.001$), the S2 string tubes ($t = -2.879$, df = 26.9, $p = 0.008$) and the S4 string ghosts ($t = -2.624$, df = 20.4, $p = 0.016$), but not the S3 type collapsed string vessels ($t = -1.042$, df = 27, n.s.).

Next, we studied whether the overall density of small vessels was altered in SVD (Fig. 7b), but the percentage of white matter area covered by microvessels was not affected by vascular disease ($F_{2,170} = 0.043$, $p > 0.10$) and presence of DWMLs ($F_{2,170} = 1.071$, $p > 0.10$), and did not differ between the frontoparietal and temporal white matter ($F_{2,170} = 1.663$, $p > 0.10$) as shown by three-way ANOVA. In addition, no differences were found in vessel densities when comparing all SVD cases with NoSVD controls using a t-test ($t = -1.826$, df = 25, $p = 0.08$).

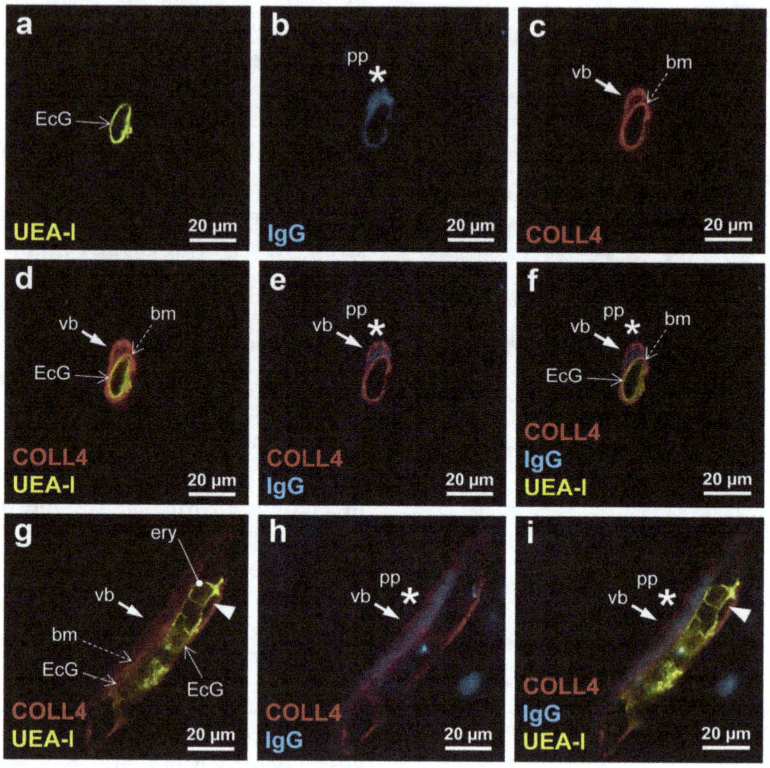

Fig. 5 Triple-label immunofluorescence showing the location of the plasma protein (pp) IgG in relation to the endothelial cell glycocalyx (EcG) labeled with UEA-I, and COLL4-positive basement membrane (bm) and wall of vascular bag (vb). **a-f** Transverse or oblique section through small vessel with a smooth endothelial cell layer (continuous open arrow) and vascular bag (closed arrow), which is attached to the basement membrane (broken open arrow) and contains IgG (star). **g-i** Longitudinal section through a capillary-size small vessel shows the UEA-I-labeled EcG (open arrows) and erythrocytes (ery). The tubular vascular bag (closed arrow) around the vessel, which is filled with IgG (star), is formed by a COLL4-positive external membrane and the basement membrane (broken open arrow). An endothelial indentation with detachment from the basement membrane (arrow head) is also seen, but there is no IgG deposition between the endothelial layer and basement membrane. Case 12 (pontine bleeding, SVD + VBI)

Density and size of CNS macrophages was significantly increased in SVD

White matter regions of NoSVD controls displayed mainly IBA1- and CD68-positive thin cellular processes and relatively few labeled cell bodies. In contrast, IBA1-positive microglial cells were highly branched and had hypertrophic cell bodies in SVD. Round and ameboid cells suggesting a phagocytic phenotype showed both IBA1 and CD68 immunoreactivity and appeared to be more numerous in SVD (Fig. 8). Therefore, CD68-positive cells were quantified in the white matter parenchyma (Fig. 9) and at perivascular sites (see Additional file 7: Figure S4 showing perivascular analyses). Three-way ANOVA (vascular disease x presence of DWML x white matter location) indicated that the density of parenchymal microglial cells was significantly increased by vascular disease $F_{2,394} = 9.230$, $p = 0.003$) and presence of DWML ($F_{2,394} = 11.068$, $p = 0.001$), and was also influenced by the white matter location ($F_{1,394} = 5.882$, $p = 0.016$) and the covariate age ($F_{1,394} = 99.371$, $p < 0.001$). Posthoc analyses showed an increased density of parenchymal macrophages in SVD (pure or with VBI) in frontoparietal areas (DWMLs and/or in-case control) when compared to NoSVD controls. However, the two SVD groups did not show differences in cell densities between the DWML site and in-case control areas, suggesting a generalized microglial activation).

As the size of macrophages can be an indicator of their functional status, next the cell body area of parenchymal CD68-positive cells was analyzed with three-way ANOVA (Fig. 9; vascular disease x presence of DWML x white matter location). Results indicated that the size of parenchymal CD68-positive cells was significantly increased by vascular disease ($F_{2,2210} = 248.516$, $p < 0.001$), which showed an interaction with presence of DWMLs ($F_{1,2210} = 10.744$, $p = 0.001$) and the white matter location ($F_{1,2210} = 43.811$, $p < 0.001$). Posthoc analyses revealed that parenchymal CD68-positive cells were larger in DWMLs and the temporal white matter in SVD + VBI compared to both pure SVD and/or NoSVD. In addition, the covariate age had a significant effect on the density ($F_{1,394} = 99.371$, $p < 0.001$) and size ($F_{2,2210} = 43.867$, $p < 0.001$) of parenchymal microglial cells as indicated by three-way ANOVA (vascular disease x presence of DWML x white matter location).

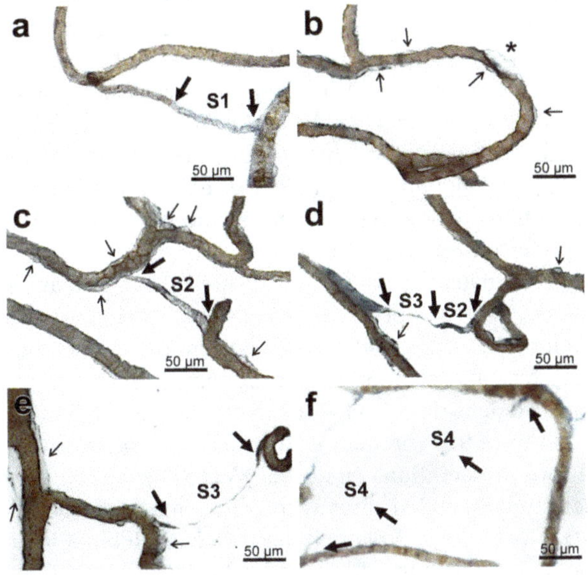

Fig. 6 Z-stack images obtained from 100 µm thick sections double-labeled for the endothelial marker UEA-I (brown) and COLL4 (blue) showing endothelial damage and various stages of string vessels. **a** Gradual loss of the endothelium in an early string vessel (S1 type) that connects two other vessels. **b** Focal endothelial damage with a large COLL4-positive bag (star) in the vicinity of areas with vascular bagging (thin black arrows). **c** Early string vessel of the S2 type with an empty collagenous tube that connects two vessels but completely lacks endothelial lining. **d** String vessel with a tube section (S2 type) and with a thin collapsed collagenous section classified as S3 type. **e** Fully collapsed string vessel (S3 type) between two vessels. **f** Segmented string vessel with extremely thin or broken sections (S4 type), which was called here a ghost string vessel or briefly string ghost. Images obtained from Case 1 (myocardial infarction, NoSVD) (**a**, **c** and **d**), Case 6 (non-hodgkin lymphoma, "pure" SVD) (**b** and **e**), and Case 9 (chronic hypertension, "pure" SVD) (**f**). For viewing tubular and ghost string vessels, also see Additional file 2: Video S1 of Vessels. Thin black arrows: vascular bags; thick black arrows: origin or segment of string vessel. Scale bars: 50 µm

CNS macrophages were found in white matter zones with ghost vessels

To pursue the hypothesis that activated CNS macrophages are involved in the removal of pathologically altered vessels, vessels traveling over large areas were analyzed in z-stack images obtained from 100 µm thick sections. The z-stacks revealed large areas with networks of COLL4-positive ghost vessels in DWMLs (Fig. 10a), which resembled the string ghosts described above (Fig. 6). Further evaluation of the same white matter locations used for quantitative analyses revealed several areas with networks of string ghosts in SVD, some of which were large (*40% of pure SVD cases*: 3 in DWMLs as well as 2 in frontoparietal and 1 temporal in-case control area; *40% of SVD + VBI cases*: 3 DWMLs as well as 2 frontoparietal and 1 temporal in-case control area), whereas in NoSVD controls areas containing a higher density of string ghosts were rather small and often barely detectable (*75% of controls*: 2 frontoparietal and 2 temporal). Moreover, double-label IHC showed a high density of CD68-positive cells with a phagocytic phenotype in white matter areas, which were covered with networks of string ghosts (Fig. 10b).

Discussion

This study sought to characterize vascular abnormalities and microglial changes in SVD patients. We discovered collagenous pouches and tubes around small vessels, now referred to as vascular bagging, which we suggest to use as a marker of SVD. Key outcomes were the identification of (i) multiple layers of collagenous vascular bags supporting a chronic disease process, (ii) plasma proteins within the vascular bags indicating a porous endothelium and basement membrane, (iii) four types of string vessels suggesting different stages of string vessel formation, and (iv) an enhanced density of COLL4-positive string vessels and ghost vessels that resembled remnants of string vessels.

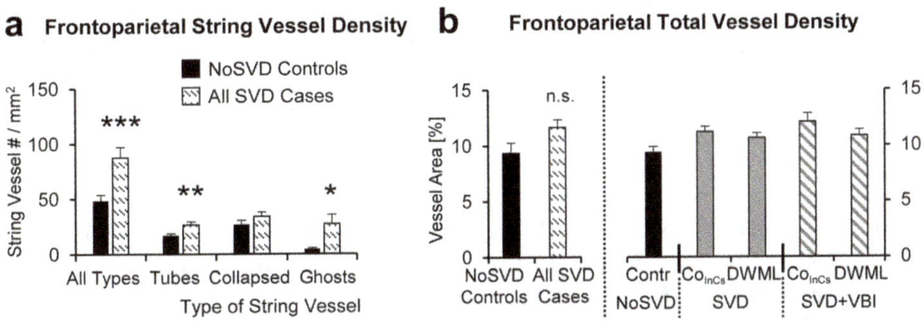

Fig. 7 Quantitative analyses of the density of string vessels and of the overall vessel density in the frontoparietal white matter. **a** The density of all types of string vessels as well as the density of string vessel tubes (S2 type) and string vessel ghosts (S4 type) is significantly increased in all SVD cases (pure SVD and SVD + VBI) when compared to NoSVD controls, whereas the density of collapsed/constricted string vessels (S3 type) is not affected (see Fig. 6 for morphology of S2 to S4 type string vessels quantified). **b** In contrast, the overall density of frontoparietal small vessels is not altered when all SVD cases are compared to NoSVD controls (left) or if a more detailed analysis is performed, in which DWMLs are compared to in-case control areas in the two SVD groups or to control areas in NoSVD cases (right). The "pure" SVD cases were referred to as SVD in the diagrams. * $p < 0.05$, ** $p < 0.01$, *** $p < 0.001$, n.s. not significant

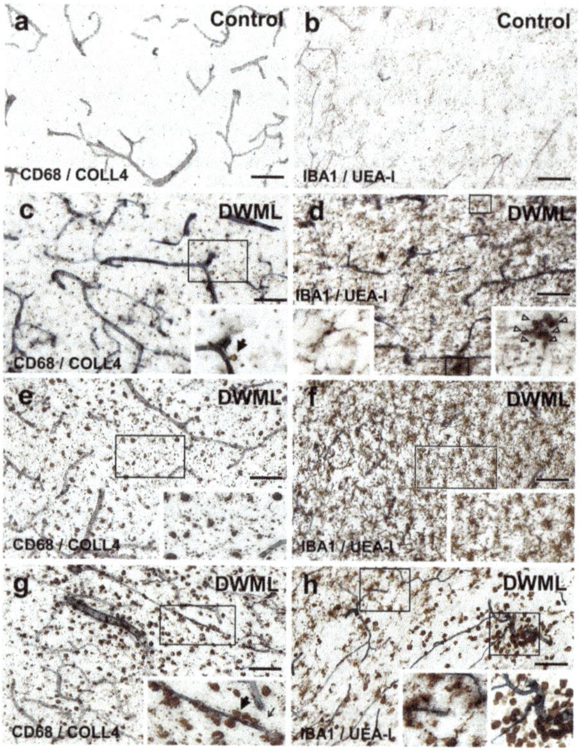

Fig. 8 Parenchymal and perivascular CD68-positive macrophages and IBA1-positive microglial cells in white matter areas in thick sections double-labeled for COLL4 and UEA-I, respectively. **11a-b** In NoSVD controls, IBA1- and CD68-positive cellular processes are observed in the subcortical white matter, but the density of labeled cell bodies is rather low compared to SVD cases. **c-d** In "pure" SVD, more IBA1- and CD68-positive cells with thicker processes are found in the white matter parenchyma compared to NoSVD. Some CD68 positive cells have a close relationship to the wall of vessels. Many IBA1-labeled cells have complex morphologies and clusters with IBA1-labeled cells somata are seen. **e-h** In cases with SVD + VBI, DWMLs exhibit numerous enlarged CD68-positive macrophages with a phagocytic phenotype, and COLL4-positive dots are found among CD68-positive cells (thin arrow in inset of **g**). The density of IBA1-positive microglial cells is also high in the DWMLs, and their morphology indicates an activated (hypertrophic) or a phagocytic (round) state. Thick arrows (insets in **c** and **g**) show examples of CD68-positive cells quantified at perivascular sites with a direct association to the wall of COLL4-positive vessels. Images were obtained from Case 2 (ovarian cancer, NoSVD) (**a-b**), Case 5 (pulmonary embolism, pure SVD) (**c-d**), and Case 12 (pontine bleeding, SVD + VBI) (**e-h**). For a more detailed morphology of IBA1-positive cells, also see Additional file 3: Video S2 of Microglia. Scale bars: 100 μm (**a**, **c**, **e** and **g**) and 50 μm (**b**, **d**, **f** and **h**)

Infiltration of areas with networks of ghost vessels by CD68-positive CNS macrophages further supported the phagocytic removal of vessel fragments. The fact that the overall density of small vessels in the white matter was not altered pointed to a continuous replacement of vessels.

Generalized white matter involvement and role of aging in SVD

One indication that the changes in our SVD cases are of a chronic nature was the presence of vascular bagging formed by multiple layers of collagen around vessels. Ultrastructural studies have found splitting, branching and thickening of the capillary basement membrane and perivascular deposition of collagen, also called microvascular fibrosis, in the brains of aged rats [24, 40] and rhesus monkeys [51, 67] as well as in aged individuals or Alzheimer's disease patients [22, 29, 30, 79]. Our current analyses extend these previous observations to vascular bagging in the frontoparietal and temporal control deep white matter.

Quantitative analyses further showed that vascular bagging in SVD is not restricted to small vessels located within the DWMLs, but extends beyond the visible lesions to neighboring frontoparietal white matter areas. Likewise, enhanced densities of activated microglia and CNS macrophages were not confined to the DWMLs consistent with previous observations made in SVD [89], although the prior study included cases with concomitant neurodegenerative pathology. Enlarged perivascular Robin-Virchow spaces also occur in widespread subcortical areas in SVD as shown in previous histopathological investigations [50, 56] and imaging studies, which have confirmed a statistical association between enlarged MRI-visible perivascular spaces and white matter hyperintensities [6, 68].

Therefore, vascular bagging may develop in the frontoparietal and temporal white matter before manifestation of further parenchymal damage, especially in "pure" SVD (without additional VBI), where this pathology was more severe in the DWMLs than in-case control regions. Nevertheless, vascular bagging was comparatively mild in the temporal lobe, compatible with the relative resistance of this region to the development of DWMLs [88]. The progressive character of SVD is also supported by deterioration of astrocytic function at late stages of white matter hyperintensities as shown in a recent clinicopathological study [21]. Similarly, MRI studies provide hints that reversible changes in the normal-appearing white matter such as altered interstitial fluid mobility and water content may precede permanent late-stage changes including demyelination and axonal damage [85]. Altogether these findings support the view that SVD is an age-related generalized and progressive white matter disease fueled by a chronic disease process that globally affects the white matter rather than only the lesion site.

Vascular bagging is a common feature of SVD with DWMLs

Atrial fibrillation, hypertension and left ventricular hypertrophy are commonly associated with white matter hyperintensities in SVD patients [11, 36, 72, 73]. Studies matching white matter hyperintensities to histological sections have shown that the hyperintensities reflect myelin pallor and dilatation of perivascular spaces and only rarely represent lacunar infarcts [31, 55, 56, 69]. Although subcortical lacunar infarctions are common in patients with WMLs and their presence is a requirement

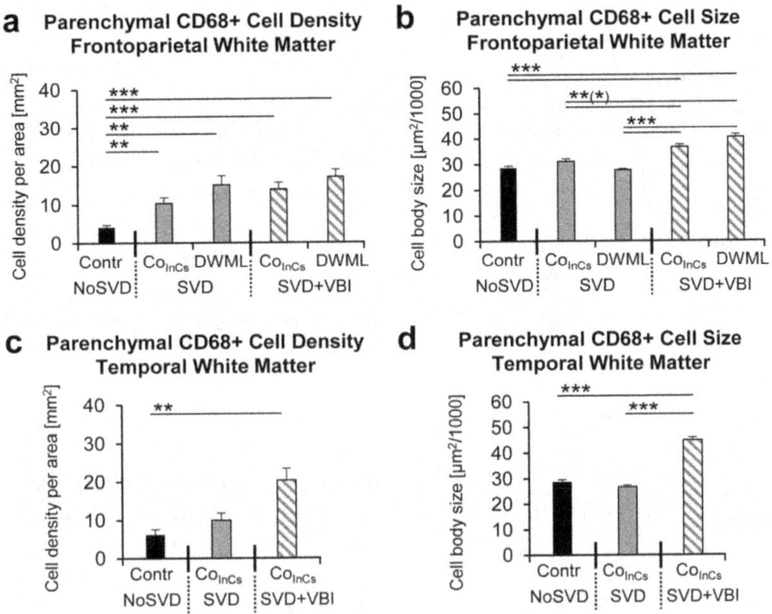

Fig. 9 Quantitative analyses of CD68-positive cells. **a-b** In pure SVD, the density of parenchymal and perivascular cells is higher in DWMLs compared to the frontoparietal control region, and the same is also true for parenchymal cells quantified in the frontoparietal in-case control area. In SVD associated with VBI, there is a prominent increase in the density of parenchymal and perivascular cells in all white matter areas compared to corresponding control tissue except for perivascular cells in DWMLs. **c-d** CD68-positive parenchymal cells are significantly enlarged in all areas in SVD + VBI, whereas these changes are less prominent for perivascular cells. Notably, the size of perivascular cells is also significantly higher in DWMLs of SVD + VBI cases compared to DWMLs in pure SVD. * $p < 0.05$, ** $p < 0.01$, *** $p < 0.001$

for the diagnosis of Binswanger's disease [43, 80], there may be some differences in the pathogenesis of diffuse WMLs (leukoaraiosis) and SVD with lacunar infarcts [70, 75]. Especially, Binswanger's disease and lacunar infarcts have been linked to hypertension [1, 20], which causes atherosclerosis of small arteries and arteriolosclerosis [50, 52, 71]. Moreover, patients with pure lacunar infarctions showed hypercoagulability [77], and an altered haplotype of the endothelial nitric oxide gene [38]. Studies of endothelial dysfunction further showed elevated blood levels of the intercellular adhesion molecule ICAM1 in patients with lacunar infarctions [39], whereas VCAM1 and P-selectin were increased in cases with WMLs at the periventricular region but not at deep subcortical locations [27]. Therefore, further analyses are needed to study the role of our pathological markers of DWMLs/leukoaraiosis in SVD forms such as Binswanger's disease or hypertensive SVD.

Typical features of hypertensive arteriolosclerosis include hyalinosis/lipohyalinosis and fibrinoid necrosis in arterioles with calibers larger than 40 µm, which is accompanied by deposition of fibrohyaline material and blood-derived lipids in the vessel wall and narrowing of the lumen [52, 64]. The walls of sclerotic medullary arterioles with diameters > 30 µm were also shown to contain multiple layers of collagen I- and IV-positive membranes in various forms of hereditary and sporadic SVD including Binswanger's disease [23, 53]. However, only one case in our SVD cohort showed prominent hyalinosis of larger arterioles, consistent with previous observations showing manifestation of WMLs in the absence of arteriosclerotic lesions [48]. Furthermore, hypertensive arteriolosclerotic lesions are predominantly located in the basal ganglia [52], whereas this study focused on deep white matter areas. We could demonstrate here that smaller vessels including pre-capillary arterioles and capillaries exhibit vascular bags with COLL4-positive walls in SVD cases with DWMLs, including sporadic disease and SVD associated with remote VBI. Post-capillary venules may also show vascular bagging in SVD, as they cannot be distinguished from capillaries merely based on vessel diameters, deformed erythrocytes squeezing through vessels or the presence of pericytes [7].

Plasma proteins trapped in vascular bags point to blood brain barrier (BBB) disruption

Accumulation of the plasma proteins FIBR and IgG in vascular bags points to a disruption of the blood brain barrier (BBB) with a porous endothelial cell layer and basement membrane. While circular deposition of FIBR around capillaries was previously reported in the brains of Binswanger's disease patients, it was concluded that FIBR was located in the perivascular space [3]. Here, we could provide evidence that FIBR and IgG are located within the vascular bags, whereas the widened perivascular space outside the bags

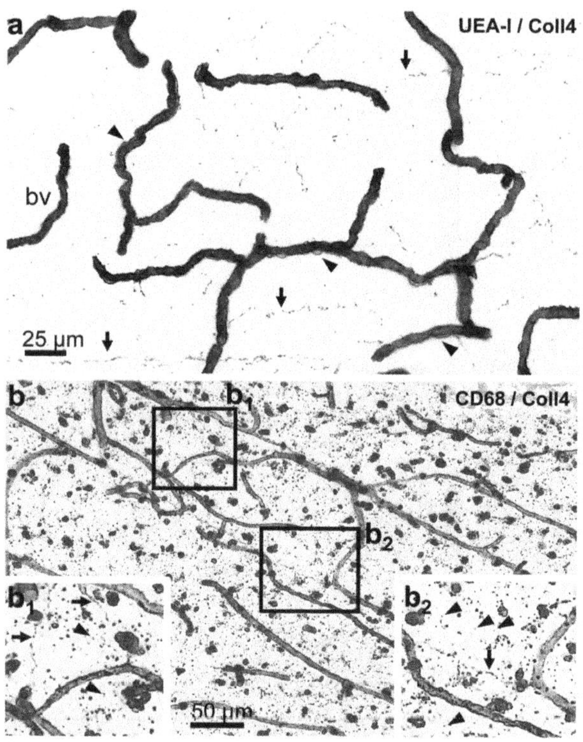

Fig. 10 Vessels and CD68-positive cells in z-stack images. **a** Image reconstructed from 57 individual images captured from a single DWML (double-labeling for UEA-I (brown) and COLL4 (blue)) shows what appears to be a network of former string vessels (arrows). Also, numerous vessels with vascular bags are seen (arrow heads) in this area. In our SVD cases, such vascular networks consisted of many ghost vessels and their branches, which had the appearance of beaded threads and dotted lines running over long distances. **b** Sections double-labeled for CD68 (brown) and COLL4 (blue) show accumulation of numerous parenchymal CD68-positive cells in areas with a high density of COLL4-positive ghost vessels (arrows) and dots (arrow heads), suggesting phagocytosis of vessel remnants by CNS macrophages. Images obtained from Case 6 (non-hodgkin lymphoma, pure SVD) (**a**) and Case 12 (pontine bleeding, SVD + VBI) (**b**). For viewing string vessels and COLL4-positive dots, also see Additional file 2: Video S1 of Vessels. Scale bars: 25 µm (**a**) and 50 µm (**b**)

did not contain plasma proteins except in areas with leakage to the white matter parenchyma. Plasma protein aggregation in the white matter has been well-established in SVD and is classically regarded as a histopathological indicator for a disrupted BBB [15, 54, 56, 89]. The outbreak of plasma proteins from vascular bags to the surrounding white matter parenchyma further indicates a discontinuity of the outer collagenous membranes of the bags.

Apart from endothelial cells and the basement membrane, astrocytic end feet and pericytes are also required for the structural integrity and maintenance of the BBB [63, 66]. In a clinicopathological study, degeneration of astrocytes with clasmatodendrocytic morphologies and aberrant subcellular expression of aquaporin 4 pointed to a breakage of the BBB in areas with white matter hyperintensities [21]. Loss of pericytes can also lead to a BBB breakdown and exudation of plasma proteins by reducing capillary perfusion as it has been shown in a mouse model of SVD with impaired PDGFR-beta signaling [8, 37]. While the pericytes found here were located outside the vascular bags, these cells and their processes are enclosed by two layers of the basement membrane [67], and therefore their degeneration might contribute to splitting of the basement membrane. The disruption of the BBB in SVD is also supported by in vivo perfusion-weighted MR imaging performed living patients [4].

Vascular bagging may be triggered by hypoperfusion

Experimental evidence favors the notion that endothelial changes are an early phenomenon of DWMLs [42], and therefore interventions that prevent endothelial damage might have a positive impact by halting SVD progression. Chronic cerebral hypoperfusion has been shown to induce the development of features of SVD including endothelial cell damage, thickening of the capillary basement membrane, gliovascular disruption and WMLs in rodents, which was associated with cognitive deficits [25, 41, 45, 78]. In patients, the impact of reduced cerebral blood flow on the development of leukoaraiosis was demonstrated in a longitudinal MRI study [10]. Glial expression of the hypoxia-inducible factors HIF1α and HIF2α was also elevated in SVD patients with DWMLs [32].

Endothelial damage is the first step in the formation of string vessels [16]. Among the four types of string vessels found here, vessels with endothelial cell recession probably represent early-stage string vessels, whereas wide open or collapsed empty collagenous tubes devoid of an endothelial cell layer correspond to late-stage string vessels. Healthy individuals also have string vessels in the CNS and other organs [16], but in SVD we found an increased density of string vessels and string ghosts that were still connected to vessels or formed extended networks. Especially the higher density of string ghosts found here suggests removal of vessel remnants from the white matter parenchyma in SVD. Alternatively, the empty basement membrane tubes left behind after the death of endothelial cells might guide regrowth of endothelial cells, which can synthetize new layers of basement membrane [49]. Thus, the multi-layered vascular bags found here may be the consequence of a chronic disease process with recurrent recanalization of empty collagenous scaffolds and repeated duplications of the basement membrane.

Role of microglia in remodeling of the white matter microvasculature

Microglia were visualized with the marker IBA1 that is expressed in both resting and activated microglial cells and phagocytic CNS macrophages were identified with

CD68 [83]. Similar to the observations by Young et al. [89], we detected activated IBA1-positive microglial cells and increased cell densities/sizes of CD68-positive macrophages in both DWMLs and the normal appearing white matter in SVD. Moreover, the increase in the density and size of macrophages was more prominent in the SVD groups with VBI compared to pure SVD. Activated microglia with truncated processes and lipid-laden macrophages immunoreactive for HLA-DR as well as clusters of microglia/macrophages labeled for leukocyte common antigen (LCA) were also described in Binswanger's disease [2]. DWML sites covered with networks of string ghosts were infiltrated by activated microglial cells and CNS macrophages suggesting that they sequestered the damaged vessels. These findings suggest chronic remodeling of vessels in SVD, because despite removal of ghost vessel networks by microglia the overall vessel densities were not altered in our SVD cases.

Conclusion

Here we report two novel findings in SVD, which are (i) vascular bags filled with leaked plasma proteins and (ii) an enhanced density of string ghosts in white matter areas that were also discovered in areas with high macrophage densities. Under the assumption that endothelial damage is the common driver of both types of lesions, the following scenario could be hypothesized for the chronic disease process in DWMLs, and to some extent, also in the normal appearing white matter in SVD. Endothelial cell damage and loss may result in the formation of empty collagenous tubes and scaffolds that can either lead to string vessel formation or persist, possibly over a long duration. Regrowth of the endothelium into persisting empty basement membrane tubes may induce the synthesis of new layers of collagenous membranes. Age-related changes in the extracellular matrix and degeneration of pericytes may also contribute to the thickening and splitting of basement membranes. This may result in the formation of the multi-layered collagenous vascular bags found in this study and leakage of plasma proteins into the bags or white matter parenchyma. When vessels are not recanalized after endothelial damage, they may eventually collapse leading to formation of various stages of string vessels. Degradation of late-stage string vessels by activated microglial cells may be related to the high density of CD68-positive cells found in areas with networks of string ghosts and their remnants.

Additional files

Additional file 1: Patient data. Demographic data and neuropathological diagnoses are shown for cases with small vessel disease (SVD) with/without vascular brain injury (VBI) and NoSVD controls included to the study. (DOCX 19.1 kb)

Additional file 2: Video of vascular bags and string vessels. The video was constructed from 116 images taken with the 20x objective at equidistant 0.7 μm steps throughout the section. Vessels are double-labeled for collagen IV (COLL4) and lectin (UEA-I) using (immuno)histochemistry. Vessel pathology is shown in the deep white matter lesion (DWML) of a case with SVD and a contralateral subacute ischemic cerebral infarct (Case 14). Vascular bags formed by collagenous membranes around vessels are attached to the vessel walls. A string vessel with a short constricted segment becomes discontinuous. Therefore, the latter types of vessel remnants were called ghost string vessels or briefly string ghosts. In addition, an empty collagenous tube without an endothelial layer is seen that may correspond to an early non-collapsed string vessel. Please also note the multiple COLL4-positive dots in the white matter parenchyma, which form vessel-like shaped rows in z-stack images. (AVI 16324 kb)

Additional file 3: Video of IBA1-positive microglia. The video was constructed from 100 images taken with the 20x objective at equidistant 0.7 μm steps throughout the section. The section double-labeled for the IBA1 and lectin shows complex microglia morphologies in the in-case control region of a SVD case with an ischemic cerebral infarct in the contralateral internal capsule (Case 10). (AVI 16671 kb)

Additional file 4: White matter spongiosis in SVD. Images show immunohistochemical demonstration of myelin basic protein (MBP) and myelin staining performed with a modified Heidenhain procedure. **a** and **c**: Deep white matter lesions (DWMLs) show a loosening of the white matter resulting in spongiosis and a crisscross pattern of remaining axons due to loss of MBP-positive/myelinated fiber tracts (Case 6, SVD). **b** and **d**: In contrast, the control white matter (Case 2, NoSVD) contains well-organized fiber tracts with bundles of longitudinal axons (LAx) and horizontal axons (HAx). Scale bars: 50 μm. (TIF 19818 kb)

Additional file 5: Drawing of vascular bagging. The drawing gives an overview of the vessel types and their proportion (%) among all vessel segments analyzed. Brown color represents labeling of the endothelium with UEA-I and blue color COLL4-positive membranes. Type 1 vessels with an intact endothelium and basement membrane are the most common type in the study population, whereas type 2 vessels with irregularities restricted to the endothelium are rare. DWMLs express a high proportion of type 3 vessels with vascular bags. Likewise type 4 vessels with changes of both the endothelial cell layer and external collagenous membranes are common. (TIF 12345 kb)

Additional file 6: Distribution of diameters. The diagram indicates the distribution of the diameters of small vessels (vessel calibers) (**a**) and maximum diameters at the outer membrane of the vascular bags (**b**). The diameters reported were determined in vessel segments that were in focus in images taken with the 20x objective and were used for quantitative analyses of vascular bags (see also Fig. 2). The width of the vascular bags was calculated as the difference between the two diameters (see also Fig. 3). (TIF 19068 kb)

Additional file 7: Diagram of perivascular CD68-positive macrophages showing the density (**a** and **c**) and size (**b** and **d**) of cells in the frontoparietal (**a-b**) and temporal white matter (**c-d**) analyzed with three-way ANOVA (vascular disease x presence of DWML x white matter location) and the posthoc Games-Howell test. In the three-way ANOVA, the density of perivascular macrophages was significantly increased by vascular disease ($F_{2,394} = 8.479$, $p = 0.004$) and presence of DWMLs ($F_{2,394} = 11.665$, $p = 0.001$), and also depended on the white matter location ($F_{1,394} = 9.135$, $p = 0.003$). Moreover, the size of perivascular CD68-positive cells was significantly affected by vascular disease ($F_{2,2856} = 65.003$, $p < 0.001$) in interaction with the white matter location ($F_{1,2856} = 19.668$, $p < 0.001$), and the covariate age had a significant effect on the density ($F_{1,394} = 65.231$, $p < 0.001$) and size ($F_{2,2856} = 9.527$, $p = 0.002$) of the cells. **a-b:** In the frontoparietal white matter, posthoc analyses revealed a higher density of perivascular macrophages in DWMLs of all SVD cases (pure SVD, SVD + VBI) compared to NoSVD. Also, CD68-positive cells were significantly enlarged in the DWMLs of SVD + VBI cases compared to DWMLs in pure SVD. Neither the density nor the size of CD68-positive cells was significantly altered in the in-case control areas of SVD cases compared to the control white matter in NoSVD cases. **c-d:** In the temporal white matter, posthoc analyses indicated that the density of CD68-positive cells was significantly increased in-case control areas of SVD + VBI cases but not of pure SVD cases when compared to NoSVD controls. Notably, perivascular cells were significantly larger in DWMLs of SVD + VBI cases than in DWMLs of pure SVD cases or in the control white matter of NoSVD cases. The density or size of CD68-positive cells in in-case control areas in pure SVD was not altered when compared to NoSVD. * $p < 0.05$, ** $p < 0.01$, *** $p < 0.001$. (TIF 19710 kb)

Acknowledgements
Ms. G. Ehmke and Ms. S. Baumann are acknowledged for expert technical assistance. We thank Ms. P. Häring for the quantification of vessel densities. The project was funded, in part, by the Corona Stiftung Germany, Fondation pour la Recherche sur Alzheimer, Paris, and through intramural funds.

Authors' contributions
KF and DYH have participated in the design of the study and drafted the manuscript. HB, KDT, KF and DYH have established the staining procedures in thick sections. The quantitative analyses of vascular bagging, microglial cells and string vessel densities were performed by YZ, MA and DYH, respectively. JR, AN and LF have analyzed vascular bagging and the blood-brain barrier disturbances in thin paraffin sections using immunohistochemistry (JR, AN) and immunofluorescence (JR, LF). JW, IK, HN and JK provided neuropathological expertise and contributed to collecting clinical data. DYH has conceived and coordinated the study and contributed, together with HB and ACL, to the establishment of investigations on cerebral microangiopathies in thick brain sections. All authors have read and approved the final manuscript.

Competing interests
The authors declare that they have no competing interests.

Author details
[1]Department of Medical Biosciences & Pathology, Umeå Universitet, Umeå, Sweden. [2]Department of Neurology, Peking University Third Hospital, Beijing, China. [3]Clinical Neuroanatomy Section, Neurology, School of Medicine, Ulm University, Helmholtzstr. 8/1, 89081 Ulm, Germany. [4]Department of Neurology, Ulm University Hospital, Ulm University, Ulm, Germany. [5]Institute of Neuropathology, School of Medicine, RTWH Aachen University Hospital, Aachen, Aachen, Germany.

References

1. Akiguchi I, Budka H, Shirakashi Y, Woehrer A, Watanabe T, al SA (2014) MRI features of Binswanger's disease predict prognosis and associated pathology. Ann Clin Transl Neurol 1:813–821. https://doi.org/10.1002/acn3.123
2. Akiguchi I, Tomimoto H, Suenaga T, Wakita H, Budka H (1997) Alterations in glia and axons in the brains of Binswanger's disease patients. Stroke 28: 1423–1429
3. Akiguchi I, Tomimoto H, Suenaga T, Wakita H, Budka H (1998) Blood-brain barrier dysfunction in Binswanger's disease; an immunohistochemical study. Acta Neuropathol 95:78–84
4. Arba F, Leigh R, Inzitari D, Warach SJ, Luby M, Lees KR et al (2017) Blood-brain barrier leakage increases with small vessel disease in acute ischemic stroke. Neurology 89:2143–2150. https://doi.org/10.1212/WNL.0000000000004677
5. Aribisala BS, Valdes Hernandez MC, Royle NA, Morris Z, Munoz Maniega S, Bastin ME et al (2013) Brain atrophy associations with white matter lesions in the ageing brain: the Lothian birth cohort 1936. Eur Radiol 23:1084–1092. https://doi.org/10.1007/s00330-012-2677-x
6. Aribisala BS, Wiseman S, Morris Z, Valdes-Hernandez MC, Royle NA, Maniega SM et al (2014) Circulating inflammatory markers are associated with magnetic resonance imaging-visible perivascular spaces but not directly with white matter hyperintensities. Stroke 45:605–607. https://doi.org/10.1161/STROKEAHA.113.004059
7. Attwell D, Mishra A, Hall CN, O'Farrell FM, Dalkara T (2016) What is a pericyte? J Cereb Blood Flow Metab 36:451–455. https://doi.org/10.1177/0271678X15610340
8. Bell RD, Winkler EA, Sagare AP, Singh I, LaRue B, Deane R et al (2010) Pericytes control key neurovascular functions and neuronal phenotype in the adult brain and during brain aging. Neuron 68:409–427. https://doi.org/10.1016/j.neuron.2010.09.043
9. Benakis C, Garcia-Bonilla L, Iadecola C, Anrather J (2014) The role of microglia and myeloid immune cells in acute cerebral ischemia. Front Cell Neurosci 8:461. https://doi.org/10.3389/fncel.2014.00461
10. Bernbaum M, Menon BK, Fick G, Smith EE, Goyal M, Frayne R et al (2015) Reduced blood flow in normal white matter predicts development of leukoaraiosis. J Cereb Blood Flow Metab 35:1610–1615. https://doi.org/10.1038/jcbfm.2015.92
11. Birdsill AC, Koscik RL, Jonaitis EM, Johnson SC, Okonkwo OC, Hermann BP et al (2014) Regional white matter hyperintensities: aging, Alzheimer's disease risk, and cognitive function. Neurobiol Aging 35:769–776. https://doi.org/10.1016/j.neurobiolaging.2013.10.072
12. Braak H (1976) On the striate area of the human isocortex. A Golgi- and pigmentarchitectonic study. J Comp Neurol 166:341–364. https://doi.org/10.1002/cne.901660305
13. Braak H, Braak E (1991) Neuropathological stageing of Alzheimer-related changes. Acta Neuropathol 82:239–259
14. Braak H, Del Tredici K, Rub U, de Vos RA, Jansen Steur EN, Braak E (2003) Staging of brain pathology related to sporadic Parkinson's disease. Neurobiol Aging 24:197–211
15. Bridges LR, Andoh J, Lawrence AJ, Khoong CH, Poon WW, Esiri MM et al (2014) Blood-brain barrier dysfunction and cerebral small vessel disease (arteriolosclerosis) in brains of older people. J Neuropathol Exp Neurol 73: 1026–1033. https://doi.org/10.1097/NEN.0000000000000124
16. Brown WR (2010) A review of string vessels or collapsed, empty basement membrane tubes. J Alzheimers Dis 21:725–739. https://doi.org/10.3233/JAD-2010-100219
17. Brown WR, Moody DM, Challa VR, Thore CR, Anstrom JA (2002) Venous collagenosis and arteriolar tortuosity in leukoaraiosis. J Neurol Sci 203-204:159–163
18. Brown WR, Moody DM, Thore CR, Anstrom JA, Challa VR (2009) Microvascular changes in the white mater in dementia. J Neurol Sci 283:28–31. https://doi.org/10.1016/j.jns.2009.02.328
19. Brown WR, Thore CR (2011) Review: cerebral microvascular pathology in ageing and neurodegeneration. Neuropathol Appl Neurobiol 37:56–74. https://doi.org/10.1111/j.1365-2990.2010.01139.x
20. Caplan LR (2015) Lacunar infarction and small vessel disease: pathology and pathophysiology. J Stroke 17:2–6. https://doi.org/10.5853/jos.2015.17.1.2
21. Chen A, Akinyemi RO, Hase Y, Firbank MJ, Ndung'u MN, Foster V et al (2016) Frontal white matter hyperintensities, clasmatodendrosis and gliovascular abnormalities in ageing and post-stroke dementia. Brain 139:242–258. https://doi.org/10.1093/brain/awv328
22. Claudio L (1996) Ultrastructural features of the blood-brain barrier in biopsy tissue from Alzheimer's disease patients. Acta Neuropathol 91:6–14
23. Craggs LJ, Hagel C, Kuhlenbaeumer G, Borjesson-Hanson A, Andersen O, Viitanen M et al (2013) Quantitative vascular pathology and phenotyping familial and sporadic cerebral small vessel diseases. Brain Pathol 23:547–557. https://doi.org/10.1111/bpa.12041
24. de Jong GI, de Weerd H, Schuurman T, Traber J, Luiten PG (1990) Microvascular changes in aged rat forebrain. Effects of chronic nimodipine treatment. Neurobiol Aging 11:381–389
25. De Jong GI, Farkas E, Stienstra CM, Plass JR, Keijser JN, de la Torre JC et al (1999) Cerebral hypoperfusion yields capillary damage in the hippocampal CA1 area that correlates with spatial memory impairment. Neuroscience 91:203–210
26. de Laat KF, Tuladhar AM, van Norden AG, Norris DG, Zwiers MP, de Leeuw FE (2011) Loss of white matter integrity is associated with gait disorders in cerebral small vessel disease. Brain 134:73–83. https://doi.org/10.1093/brain/awq343
27. de Leeuw FE, de Kleine M, Frijns CJ, Fijnheer R, van Gijn J, Kappelle LJ (2002) Endothelial cell activation is associated with cerebral white matter lesions in patients with cerebrovascular disease. Ann N Y Acad Sci 977:306–314
28. Debette S, Markus HS (2010) The clinical importance of white matter hyperintensities on brain magnetic resonance imaging: systematic review and meta-analysis. BMJ 341:c3666. https://doi.org/10.1136/bmj.c3666

29. Farkas E, de Vos RA, Donka G, Jansen Steur EN, Mihaly A, Luiten PG (2006) Age-related microvascular degeneration in the human cerebral periventricular white matter. Acta Neuropathol 111:150–157. https://doi.org/10.1007/s00401-005-0007-y
30. Farkas E, Luiten PG (2001) Cerebral microvascular pathology in aging and Alzheimer's disease. Prog Neurobiol 64:575–611
31. Fernando MS, O'Brien JT, Perry RH, English P, Forster G, McMeekin W et al (2004) Comparison of the pathology of cerebral white matter with post-mortem magnetic resonance imaging (MRI) in the elderly brain. Neuropathol Appl Neurobiol 30:385–395. https://doi.org/10.1111/j.1365-2990.2004.00550.x
32. Fernando MS, Simpson JE, Matthews F, Brayne C, Lewis CE, Barber R et al (2006) White matter lesions in an unselected cohort of the elderly: molecular pathology suggests origin from chronic hypoperfusion injury. Stroke 37:1391–1398. https://doi.org/10.1161/01.STR.0000221308.94473.14
33. Garde E, Lykke Mortensen E, Rostrup E, Paulson OB (2005) Decline in intelligence is associated with progression in white matter hyperintensity volume. J Neurol Neurosurg Psychiatry 76:1289–1291. https://doi.org/10.1136/jnnp.2004.055905
34. Garde E, Mortensen EL, Krabbe K, Rostrup E, Larsson HB (2000) Relation between age-related decline in intelligence and cerebral white-matter hyperintensities in healthy octogenarians: a longitudinal study. Lancet 356: 628–634. https://doi.org/10.1016/s0140-6736(00)02604-0
35. Griffanti L, Jenkinson M, Suri S, Zsoldos E, Mahmood A, Filippini N et al (2018) Classification and characterization of periventricular and deep white matter hyperintensities on MRI: A study in older adults. Neuroimage 170: 174–181. https://doi.org/10.1016/j.neuroimage.2017.03.024
36. Hajjar I, Quach L, Yang F, Chaves PH, Newman AB, Mukamal K et al (2011) Hypertension, white matter hyperintensities, and concurrent impairments in mobility, cognition, and mood: the Cardiovascular Health Study. Circulation 123:858–865. https://doi.org/10.1161/circulationaha.110.978114
37. Hall CN, Reynell C, Gesslein B, Hamilton NB, Mishra A, Sutherland BA et al (2014) Capillary pericytes regulate cerebral blood flow in health and disease. Nature 508:55–60. https://doi.org/10.1038/nature13165
38. Hassan A, Gormley K, O'Sullivan M, Knight J, Sham P, Vallance P et al (2004) Endothelial nitric oxide gene haplotypes and risk of cerebral small-vessel disease. Stroke 35:654–659. https://doi.org/10.1161/01.str.0000117238.75736.53
39. Hassan A, Hunt BJ, O'Sullivan M, Parmar K, Bamford JM, Briley D et al (2003) Markers of endothelial dysfunction in lacunar infarction and ischaemic leukoaraiosis. Brain 126:424–432
40. Hicks P, Rolsten C, Brizzee D, Samorajski T (1983) Age-related changes in rat brain capillaries. Neurobiol Aging 4:69–75
41. Holland PR, Searcy JL, Salvadores N, Scullion G, Chen G, Lawson G et al (2015) Gliovascular disruption and cognitive deficits in a mouse model with features of small vessel disease. J Cereb Blood Flow Metab 35:1005–1014. https://doi.org/10.1038/jcbfm.2015.12
42. Huang Y, Zhang W, Lin L, Feng J, Chen F, Wei W et al (2010) Is endothelial dysfunction of cerebral small vessel responsible for white matter lesions after chronic cerebral hypoperfusion in rats? J Neurol Sci 299:72–80. https://doi.org/10.1016/j.jns.2010.08.035
43. Huisa BN, Rosenberg GA (2014) Binswanger's disease: toward a diagnosis agreement and therapeutic approach. Expert Rev Neurother 14:1203–1213. https://doi.org/10.1586/14737175.2014.956726
44. Hutchins B, Weber JT (1983) A rapid myelin stain for frozen sections: modification of the Heidenhain procedure. J Neurosci Methods 7:289–294
45. Ihara M, Taguchi A, Maki T, Washida K, Tomimoto H (2014) A mouse model of chronic cerebral hypoperfusion characterizing features of vascular cognitive impairment. Methods Mol Biol 1135:95–102. https://doi.org/10.1007/978-1-4939-0320-7_8
46. Imaizumi T, Inamura S, Nomura T (2014) The severities of white matter lesions possibly influence the recurrences of several stroke types. J Stroke Cerebrovasc Dis 23:1897–1902. https://doi.org/10.1016/j.jstrokecerebrovasdis.2014.02.011
47. Inzitari D, Cadelo M, Marranci ML, Pracucci G, Pantoni L (1997) Vascular deaths in elderly neurological patients with leukoaraiosis. J Neurol Neurosurg Psychiatry 62:177–181
48. Inzitari D, Mascalchi M, Giordano GP, Marini P, Sita D, Abbamondi AL (1989) Histopathological correlates of leuko-araiosis in patients with ischemic stroke. Eur Neurol 29(Suppl 2):23–26. https://doi.org/10.1159/000116461
49. Irvine AR, Wood IS (1987) Radiation retinopathy as an experimental model for ischemic proliferative retinopathy and rubeosis iridis. Am J Ophthalmol 103:790–797
50. Kalaria RN, Kenny RA, Ballard CG, Perry R, Ince P, Polvikoski T (2004) Towards defining the neuropathological substrates of vascular dementia. J Neurol Sci 226:75–80. https://doi.org/10.1016/j.jns.2004.09.019
51. Keuker JI, Luiten PG, Fuchs E (2000) Capillary changes in hippocampal CA1 and CA3 areas of the aging rhesus monkey. Acta Neuropathol 100:665–672
52. Lammie GA (2002) Hypertensive cerebral small vessel disease and stroke. Brain Pathol 12:358–370
53. Lin JX, Tomimoto H, Akiguchi I, Matsuo A, Wakita H, Shibasaki H et al (2000) Vascular cell components of the medullary arteries in Binswanger's disease brains: a morphometric and immunoelectron microscopic study. Stroke 31: 1838–1842
54. Ma KC, Lundberg PO, Lilja A, Olsson Y (1992) Binswanger's disease in the absence of chronic arterial hypertension. A case report with clinical, radiological and immunohistochemical observations on intracerebral blood vessels. Acta Neuropathol 83:434–439
55. Matsusue E, Sugihara S, Fujii S, Ohama E, Kinoshita T, Ogawa T (2006) White matter changes in elderly people: MR-pathologic correlations. Magn Reson Med Sci 5:99–104
56. McAleese KE, Alafuzoff I, Charidimou A, De Reuck J, Grinberg LT, Hainsworth AH et al (2016) Post-mortem assessment in vascular dementia: advances and aspirations. BMC Med 14:129. https://doi.org/10.1186/s12916-016-0676-5
57. Moody DM, Bell MA, Challa VR (1990) Features of the cerebral vascular pattern that predict vulnerability to perfusion or oxygenation deficiency: an anatomic study. AJNR Am J Neuroradiol 11:431–439
58. Moody DM, Brown WR, Challa VR, Ghazi-Birry HS, Reboussin DM (1997) Cerebral microvascular alterations in aging, leukoaraiosis, and Alzheimer's disease. Ann N Y Acad Sci 826:103–116
59. Moody DM, Thore CR, Anstrom JA, Challa VR, Langefeld CD, Brown WR (2004) Quantification of afferent vessels shows reduced brain vascular density in subjects with leukoaraiosis. Radiology 233:883–890. https://doi.org/10.1148/radiol.2333020981
60. Mulisch M, Welsch U (2015) Romeis - Mikroskopische Technik, 19th edn Springer Spektrum (Verlag) City
61. Munoz DG, Hastak SM, Harper B, Lee D, Hachinski VC (1993) Pathologic correlates of increased signals of the centrum ovale on magnetic resonance imaging. Arch Neurol 50:492–497
62. Nyquist PA, Bilgel M, Gottesman R, Yanek LR, Moy TF, Becker LC et al (2015) Age differences in periventricular and deep white matter lesions. Neurobiol Aging 36:1653–1658. https://doi.org/10.1016/j.neurobiolaging.2015.01.005
63. Ostergaard L, Engedal TS, Moreton F, Hansen MB, Wardlaw JM, Dalkara T et al (2016) Cerebral small vessel disease: capillary pathways to stroke and cognitive decline. J Cereb Blood Flow Metab 36:302–325. https://doi.org/10.1177/0271678X15606723
64. Pantoni L (2010) Cerebral small vessel disease: from pathogenesis and clinical characteristics to therapeutic challenges. Lancet Neurol 9:689–701. https://doi.org/10.1016/S1474-4422(10)70104-6
65. Pantoni L, Garcia JH (1997) Pathogenesis of leukoaraiosis: a review. Stroke 28:652–659
66. Persidsky Y, Ramirez SH, Haorah J, Kanmogne GD (2006) Blood-brain barrier: structural components and function under physiologic and pathologic conditions. J NeuroImmune Pharmacol 1:223–236. https://doi.org/10.1007/s11481-006-9025-3
67. Peters A, Sethares C (2012) Age-related changes in the morphology of cerebral capillaries do not correlate with cognitive decline. J Comp Neurol 520:1339–1347. https://doi.org/10.1002/cne.22809
68. Potter GM, Doubal FN, Jackson CA, Chappell FM, Sudlow CL, Dennis MS et al (2015) Enlarged perivascular spaces and cerebral small vessel disease. Int J Stroke 10:376–381. https://doi.org/10.1111/ijs.12054
69. Revesz T, Hawkins CP, du Boulay EP, Barnard RO, McDonald WI (1989) Pathological findings correlated with magnetic resonance imaging in subcortical arteriosclerotic encephalopathy (Binswanger's disease). J Neurol Neurosurg Psychiatry 52:1337–1344
70. Rosenberg GA, Wallin A, Wardlaw JM, Markus HS, Montaner J, Wolfson L et al (2016) Consensus statement for diagnosis of subcortical small vessel disease. J Cereb Blood Flow Metab 36:6–25. https://doi.org/10.1038/jcbfm.2015.172
71. Rosenblum WI (2008) Fibrinoid necrosis of small brain arteries and arterioles and miliary aneurysms as causes of hypertensive hemorrhage: a critical reappraisal. Acta Neuropathol 116:361–369. https://doi.org/10.1007/s00401-008-0416-9
72. Rostrup E, Gouw AA, Vrenken H, van Straaten EC, Ropele S, Pantoni L et al (2012) The spatial distribution of age-related white matter changes as a

function of vascular risk factors--results from the LADIS study. Neuroimage 60:1597–1607. https://doi.org/10.1016/j.neuroimage.2012.01.106
73. Ryu WS, Woo SH, Schellingerhout D, Chung MK, Kim CK, Jang MU et al (2014) Grading and interpretation of white matter hyperintensities using statistical maps. Stroke 45:3567–3575. https://doi.org/10.1161/strokeaha.114.006662
74. Schmidt R, Seiler S, Loitfelder M (2016) Longitudinal change of small-vessel disease-related brain abnormalities. J Cereb Blood Flow Metab 36:26–39. https://doi.org/10.1038/jcbfm.2015.72
75. Shi Y, Wardlaw JM (2016) Update on cerebral small vessel disease: a dynamic whole-brain disease. Stroke Vasc Neurol 1:83–92. https://doi.org/10.1136/svn-2016-000035
76. Thal DR, Rub U, Orantes M, Braak H (2002) Phases of a beta-deposition in the human brain and its relevance for the development of AD. Neurology 58:1791–1800
77. Tomimoto H, Akiguchi I, Ohtani R, Yagi H, Kanda M, Shibasaki H et al (2001) The coagulation-fibrinolysis system in patients with leukoaraiosis and Binswanger disease. Arch Neurol 58:1620–1625
78. Ueno M, Tomimoto H, Akiguchi I, Wakita H, Sakamoto H (2002) Blood-brain barrier disruption in white matter lesions in a rat model of chronic cerebral hypoperfusion. J Cereb Blood Flow Metab 22:97–104. https://doi.org/10.1097/00004647-200201000-00012
79. Uspenskaia O, Liebetrau M, Herms J, Danek A, Hamann GF (2004) Aging is associated with increased collagen type IV accumulation in the basal lamina of human cerebral microvessels. BMC Neurosci 5:37. https://doi.org/10.1186/1471-2202-5-37
80. van der Flier WM, van Straaten EC, Barkhof F, Verdelho A, Madureira S, Pantoni L et al (2005) Small vessel disease and general cognitive function in nondisabled elderly: the LADIS study. Stroke 36:2116–2120. https://doi.org/10.1161/01.STR.0000179092.59909.42
81. van der Holst HM, Tuladhar AM, Zerbi V, van Uden IWM, de Laat KF, van Leijsen EMC et al (2018) White matter changes and gait decline in cerebral small vessel disease. Neuroimage Clin 17:731–738. https://doi.org/10.1016/j.nicl.2017.12.007
82. Vermeer SE, Hollander M, van Dijk EJ, Hofman A, Koudstaal PJ, Breteler MM et al (2003) Silent brain infarcts and white matter lesions increase stroke risk in the general population: the Rotterdam Scan Study. Stroke 34:1126–1129. https://doi.org/10.1161/01.STR.0000068408.82115.D2
83. Walker DG, Lue LF (2015) Immune phenotypes of microglia in human neurodegenerative disease: challenges to detecting microglial polarization in human brains. Alzheimers Res Ther 7:56. https://doi.org/10.1186/s13195-015-0139-9
84. Wardlaw JM, Sandercock PA, Dennis MS, Starr J (2003) Is breakdown of the blood-brain barrier responsible for lacunar stroke, leukoaraiosis, and dementia? Stroke 34:806–812. https://doi.org/10.1161/01.str.0000058480.77236.b3
85. Wardlaw JM, Valdes Hernandez MC, Munoz-Maniega S (2015) What are white matter hyperintensities made of? Relevance to vascular cognitive impairment. J Am Heart Assoc 4:001140. https://doi.org/10.1161/jaha.114.001140
86. Yang P, Pavlovic D, Waldvogel H, Dragunow M, Synek B, Turner C et al (2015) String vessel formation is increased in the brain of Parkinson disease. J Parkinsons Dis 5:821–836. https://doi.org/10.3233/jpd-140454
87. Ylikoski A, Erkinjuntti T, Raininko R, Sarna S, Sulkava R, Tilvis R (1995) White matter hyperintensities on MRI in the neurologically nondiseased elderly. Analysis of cohorts of consecutive subjects aged 55 to 85 years living at home. Stroke 26:1171–1177
88. Yoshita M, Fletcher E, Harvey D, Ortega M, Martinez O, Mungas DM et al (2006) Extent and distribution of white matter hyperintensities in normal aging, MCI, and AD. Neurology 67:2192–2198. https://doi.org/10.1212/01.wnl.0000249119.95747.1f
89. Young VG, Halliday GM, Kril JJ (2008) Neuropathologic correlates of white matter hyperintensities. Neurology 71:804–811. https://doi.org/10.1212/01.wnl.0000319691.50117.54

9

Co-occurrence of chronic traumatic encephalopathy and prion disease

Satish Kumar Nemani[1†], Silvio Notari[1*†], Ignazio Cali[1], Victor E Alvarez[2,3,4], Diane Kofskey[5], Mark Cohen[1,5], Robert A. Stern[4,6], Brian Appleby[5,7], Joseph Abrams[8], Lawrence Schonberger[8], Ann McKee[2,3,4] and Pierluigi Gambetti[1*]

Abstract

Chronic traumatic encephalopathy (CTE) is a neurodegenerative disease associated with repetitive traumatic brain injury (TBI). CTE is generally found in athletes participating in contact sports and military personnel exposed to explosive blasts but can also affect civilians. Clinically and pathologically, CTE overlaps with post-traumatic stress disorder (PTSD), a term mostly used in a clinical context. The histopathology of CTE is defined by the deposition of hyperphosphorylated tau protein in neurons and astrocytes preferentially with perivascular distribution and at the depths of the cortical sulci. In addition to hyperphosphorylated tau, other pathologic proteins are deposited in CTE, including amyloid β (Aβ), transactive response (TAR) DNA-binding protein 43 kDa (TDP-43) and α-synuclein. However, the coexistence of prion disease in CTE has not been observed. We report three cases of histopathologically validated CTE with co-existing sporadic prion disease. Two were identified in a cohort of 55 pathologically verified cases of CTE submitted to the CTE Center of Boston University. One was identified among brain tissues submitted to the National Prion Disease Pathology Surveillance Center of Case Western Reserve University. The histopathological phenotype and properties of the abnormal, disease-related prion protein (PrP^D) of the three CTE cases were examined using lesion profile, immunohistochemistry, electrophoresis and conformational tests. Subjects with sporadic Creutzfeldt-Jakob disease (sCJD) matched for age, PrP genotype and PrP^D type were used as controls. The histopathology phenotype and PrP^D properties of the three CTE subjects showed no significant differences from their respective sCJD controls suggesting that recurring neurotrauma or coexisting CTE pathology did not detectably impact the prion disease phenotype and PrP^D conformational characteristics. Based on the reported incidence of sporadic prion disease, the detection of two cases with sCJD in the CTE Center series of 55 CTE cases by chance alone would be highly unlikely ($p = 8.93*10^{-6}$). Nevertheless, examination of a larger cohort of CTE is required to conclusively determine whether the risk of CJD is significantly increased in patients with CTE.

Keywords: Chronic traumatic encephalopathy, Post-traumatic stress disorder, Traumatic brain injury, Prion diseases, Sporadic Creutzfeldt-Jakob disease, Comorbidity, Tau protein, Amyloid β, Parkinson's disease

Introduction

Chronic traumatic encephalopathy (CTE) is currently defined as a distinctive neurodegenerative condition associated with repetitive, and rarely single, traumatic brain injury (TBI) [29, 30]. CTE is found among athletes practicing contact sports and military veterans but ordinary civilians with history of head trauma are equally exposed [30]. The clinical features vary but most often include combinations of cognitive, mood, behavioral and motor symptoms and signs [29]. Some individuals with pathologically verified CTE have been diagnosed with posttraumatic stress disorder (PTSD) during life as both conditions share neuropsychiatric symptoms consistent with frontal lobe dysfunction [18, 27, 30, 32, 56]. CTE is considered to be a primary tauopathy as the accumulation of hyperphosphorylated tau protein (p-tau) in neurons and astrocytes around small blood vessels, predominantly at the depths of the cerebral cortical sulci [30, 55]. However, pathologies related to the accumulation of proteins

* Correspondence: sxn194@case.edu; pxg13@case.edu
†Satish Kumar Nemani and Silvio Notari contributed equally to this work.
1Department of Pathology, Case Western Reserve University, School of Medicine, Cleveland, OH 44106, USA
Full list of author information is available at the end of the article

associated with other neurodegenerative diseases are frequently seen, particularly in the context of increased age [55]. They include amyloid β (Aβ), a hallmark of Alzheimer disease, α-synuclein, a feature of Parkinson's and Lewy body disease, and TAR DNA-binding protein 43 (TDP-43), typical of frontotemporal lobar degeneration (FTLD) and amyotrophic lateral sclerosis (ALS) [31]. Furthermore, TBI of any magnitude significantly increases the risk of dementia [2], although it is unclear whether TBI elevates the risk for Alzheimer's disease (AD) [20, 61]. Recent studies also show an increased risk for Parkinson's and Lewy body disease after TBI [1, 13] along with FTLD and motor neuron disease including ALS [28, 30]. These observations provide compelling evidence that neurotrauma creates biological conditions favoring not only CTE but also other morbidities associated with protein misfolding, the critical step shared by most neurodegenerative diseases [10].

Prion diseases are currently the archetype of protein misfolding disease. They have best exemplified the conformational basis of strain diversity and the correlation between genotype, strain characteristics and disease phenotype. Human prion diseases are characterized by a broad phenotypic heterogeneity, which is dictated not only by the various etiologies– sporadic, inherited and acquired by infection– but also by the variety of the underlying prion strains [14, 15]. In fact, the five distinct phenotypes or subtypes recognized in sporadic Creutzfeldt-Jakob disease (sCJD) are associated with diverse prion strains (Additional file 1: Table S1) [8, 11, 14, 23, 41, 47, 51]. Furthermore, human prion strains may co-occur resulting in mixed phenotypes that reflect the representation of the corresponding strain [4, 8, 47]. Evidence indicates that codon 129 of the human prion protein (PrP) gene that harbors the common methionine (M)/valine (V) polymorphism, influences the formation of a specific prion strain which encrypts the disease phenotype [14, 15, 17, 57]. The co-occurrence of prion diseases with other age-related neurodegenerative disorders has been previously reported [6, 7, 16]. However, prion disease has not been previously reported as a comorbidity in CTE nor has it been found to be associated with head trauma [27, 62].

We investigated the presence of prion disease in 55 subjects with autopsy-proven CTE and found two prion-positive cases. A third case clinically diagnosed with PTSD and prion disease had been referred to the National Prion Disease Pathology Surveillance Center (NPDPSC). Neuropathological examination confirmed that all three subjects had the unique features of severe prion disease and CTE (henceforth, they are referred to as CTE cases 1–3). In all cases, the prion histopathological phenotype showed no significant variation from the typical phenotypes of the sCJD control subjects matched to the three CTE cases by PrP genotype and the abnormal disease-related PrP (PrP^D) type. Similarly, conformational characteristics of the PrP^D also matched those of the controls pointing to the homology of the strain characteristics. To our knowledge, this is the first report demonstrating the comorbidity of sCJD in CTE.

Materials and methods

Tissues and subjects

Frozen and fixed brain tissue from two subjects (hereafter indicated as case 1 and case 2) were obtained from a 55 cohort received from the Veterans Affairs-Boston University-Concussion Legacy Foundation (VA-BU-CLF) brain bank where they received the histopathological diagnosis of CTE. One subject (case 3) was acquired from the NPDPSC of Case Western Reserve University, Cleveland, OH; this case was found serendipitously but a subsequent search revealed no additional cases. Neither cases 1 or 2 had final clinical diagnoses that included a prion disease, although case 1 had a rapid decline in his last year consistent with possible CJD and case 2 was initially suspected as having CJD. During the illness, case 1 was treated for Parkinson's disease. Case 3 was clinically diagnosed with PTSD, and, subsequently, with prion disease; thus case 3 was the only one to receive the final diagnosis of probable prion disease. Nine cases of sCJD that were matched to the study cases by sCJD subtype, sex, age at onset and disease duration were obtained from the NPDPSC (Additional file 1: Table S2). Post-mortem formalin-fixed brain tissues from the 53 additional subjects of the 55 cohort with pathologically verified CTE were also obtained from the CTE Center and examined for the presence of prion disease by immunohistochemistry (IHC).

Molecular genetics

DNA was isolated from the frozen brain tissues and genotyping of PRNP coding region was performed as previously described [40].

Antibodies

Mouse monoclonal antibodies (Abs) 3F4 to PrP residues 109–112 [21], SAF70 to PrP residues 156-162 (Cayman chemicals, Ann Arbor, MI, USA), 1E4 to PrP residues 97-108 (Cell Sciences, Canton, MA, USA) and 12B2 to PrP residues 89–93 [25]. Abs PHF-Tau (clone AT8) and α-syn (clone LB509) (Thermo Fisher Scientific Inc., Waltham, MA) as well as 4G8 (R. Kascsak at the N.Y.S. Institute for Basic Research) and TDP-43 (Cosmo Bio Co. LTD, Carlsbad, CA) were used for immunohistochemistry. Secondary Abs included the infrared Dye (IRDye) 800CW goat anti-mouse IgG (LI-COR Biosciences, Lincoln, NE, USA), and the horseradish peroxidase (HRP)-conjugated sheep anti-mouse IgG Ab (GE Healthcare, Life Sciences Piscataway, NJ, USA).

Histopathology, immunohistochemistry, Thioflavin S staining and lesion profiling

Histology and immunohistochemistry were performed essentially as earlier described with modifications [5, 6]. Histological sections from ten brain regions including frontal (FC), temporal (TC), parietal (PC), occipital (OC) and entorhinal cortices (EC), CA1 region of the hippocampus (HI), basal ganglia (BG), thalamus (TH), substantia nigra (SN) and cerebellum (CE) were examined to evaluate the severity and distribution of spongiform degeneration (SD) and gliosis. Lesion profiles were constructed from semi-quantitative scoring of SD and astrogliosis in the three CTE cases and their respective sCJD controls according to a modification of previous methods [22, 41]. Briefly, SD and astrogliosis were scored for severity in each brain region, and mean ± standard error of the mean (SEM) of the two lesions were plotted to generate a profile of brain lesion distribution for each case. IHC with the Ab 3F4 (1:1000) was carried out to determine presence, distribution and pattern of PrP deposition. In addition, IHC was carried out with Abs AT8 (1:200), 4G8 (1:3000), TDP-43 (1:7000) and α-syn (1:50) to p-tau, Aβ, TDP-43, and α-syn respectively. Thioflavin S staining was performed as previously described [6].

Western blot

Brain homogenate (BH) (10% *w*/*v*) were prepared on ice with lysis buffer (LB100) (100 mM Tris HCl pH 7.0, 100 mM NaCl, 10 mM EDTA, 0.5% Nonidet P-40 (NP-40), 0.5% sodium deoxycholate), and brought to pH 6.8 at 37 ° C [36]. When indicated, BH were treated with 54 U/ml proteinase K (PK) (Sigma-Aldrich, St. Louis, MO, USA) and incubated at 37 °C for 1 h (h). Protease digestion was stopped by adding 2 mM PMSF. Samples were mixed with equal volumes of 2× sample buffer (6% SDS, 8% 2-mercaptoethanol, 20% glycerol, 4 mM EDTA, 125 mM Tris HCl pH 6.8) and boiled for 10 min before loading. Protein samples (brain tissue equivalent 0.1–3 mg of wet tissue) were separated in 15% Criterion Tris-HCl polyacrylamide precast gels (Bio-Rad Laboratories, Hercules, CA, USA) and blotted into Immobilon-P membranes (EMD Millipore, Billerica, MA, USA) for 2 h at 60 V, blocked with 5% nonfat dry milk in TBS-T (1× TBS with 0.1% Tween 20) and probed with the indicated Abs. Immunoblots were visualized by enhanced chemiluminescence (Pierce ECL plus, Thermo Fisher Scientific, Waltham, MA, USA) on Carestream Kodak BioMax films (Carestream Health, Rochester, NY, USA) or with the Odyssey infrared imaging system (LICOR Biosciences) as described by the manufacturer.

PrP^D conformational assays

The conformational stability and solubility assay (CSSA) [45] was performed as previously described [12]. Occipital cortex was used for case 1 and the frontal cortex for cases 2 and 3. Matching brain regions were used for respective sCJD control cases [sCJDMV1-2C ($n = 3$); sCJDMV2K-C ($n = 3$); sCJDMM1 ($n = 3$)]. Briefly, aliquots of BH (20% *w*/*v*) in 1× D-PBS were mixed with an equal volume of 2× LB 100 pH 8.0 (200 mM Tris HCl pH 8.0, 200 mM NaCl, 1% NP-40, 1% sodium deoxycholate, 20 mM EDTA), incubated for 10 min at 4 °C and centrifuged at 1000 × g for 5 min at 4 °C to eliminate tissue debris. The supernatant S1 was then subjected to high speed centrifugation at 100,000 × g for 1 h and the resultant supernatant (S2) and pellet (P2) fractions were collected. The P2 were re-suspended in cold LB100 pH 8.0 and S2 stored at − 80 °C. To determine the denaturation rate of total PrP^D, aliquots of the re-suspended P2 were diluted with an equal volume of guanidine hydrochloride (GdnHCl) to obtain final concentrations of GdnHCl ranging from 0 M to 4 M, and incubated for 1 h at 37 °C under gentle shaking. The samples were then centrifuged at 16,000 × g for 20 min at 22 °C. The pellets were re-suspended in 1× sample buffer by sonication and boiled for 10 min at 100 °C. In addition, the solubility features of the PK-resistant PrP^D ($resPrP^D$), were also determined in the same manner as described above for total PrP^D with the exception that the P2 aliquots used for this procedure were digested with PK (5 U/ml) prior to incubation with GdnHCl. Finally, all samples were subjected to immunoblotting with 3F4. The automated estimation of PrP intensity at the different concentrations of GdnHCl was performed using the Odyssey application software V3.0 (LI-COR Biosciences). The curves of solubility, generated by the decreasing levels of PrP^D as a function of the increasing concentrations of GdnHCl, were best fitted to a sigmoidal dose-response equation (GraphPad Prism, 7.0). For each given curve of solubility, the $[GdnHCl]_{1/2}$, which represents concentration of GdnHCl required to solubilize 50% of PrP^D, was determined. The mean $[GdnHCl]_{1/2}$ values ± SEM were calculated and compared between groups.

The conformational stability immunoassay (CSI) was also performed according to previous procedures [4, 43, 64]. Aliquots of BH (10% *w*/*v*) in LB100 pH 8.0 were centrifuged at 1000 × g for 10 min at 4 °C to and the S1 was collected. 100 μl of S1 was diluted with an equal volume of GdnHCl to obtain a final concentrations ranging from 0 M to 4 M and incubated for 1.5 h at 22 °C. GdnHCl was subsequently removed by incubating each sample with an excess of 5-fold pre-chilled methanol overnight at − 20 °C followed by centrifugation at 17,200 × g for 30 min. Pellets were resuspended in 100 μl LB100 pH 8.0 by sonication. Each aliquot was digested with 5 U/ml PK for 1 h at 37 °C, reaction was terminated by addition of 2 mM PMSF. Samples were denatured and loaded onto 15% precast Tris HCl gels. PrP amounts at different GdnHCl concentrations were measured by Odyssey application software V3.0. The conformational stability of PrP^D, evaluated as a function of PrP^D remaining following exposure to increasing concentrations of GdnHCl was best fitted to a sigmoidal dose-response equation using Graphpad Prism. The mean $[GdnHCl]_{1/2}$ values ± SEM were calculated and compared between respective groups.

Statistical analysis

Statistical testing was performed to assess the probability of the observed outcome (two prion disease cases in the cohort of 55 CTE subjects) by chance alone. Cohort person-years were counted by sex (all subjects were male) and 10-year age categories. To calculate expected prion disease cases, we multiplied the person-years by sex- and age group-specific US prion disease rates (excluding cases with known genetic or acquired etiology) derived from national surveillance, 2003–2015 (Maddox RA et al., 2018 unpublished results). Person-years were calculated from birth until death; although the true exposure would start at the first traumatic brain injury, professional athletes would likely have started playing contact sports at a young age and rates of sporadic prion diseases below age 20 years are negligible. After determining the expected count of prion disease cases, we used a Poisson distribution to determine the probability of observing two or more prion disease cases in the cohort. Since one or possibly both of these prion disease cases might not have been ascertained in national surveillance were it not for the current investigation, we further assessed how many additional non-ascertained prion disease cases would need to exist for each ascertained prion disease case in order for the observed outcome to not significantly differ from the expected outcome. Student's T-test was used for the conformational assays.

Results

Genetic analysis

Methionine (M)/valine (V) heterozygosity at codon 129 (129MV) of the prion protein (PrP) gene was observed in cases 1 and 2, and methionine homozygosity (129MM) in case 3. No mutations or other variations in the open reading frame of the PrP gene were found.

Clinical history

Case 1: Eighty-four-year old male with no history of familial diseases nor of alcohol or substance abuse. He served as lieutenant in the US Army, but never saw combat. He played football for 4 years in high school, 4 years in college, and 1 year in the National Football League (NFL), as a defensive back and on special teams. During this period, he apparently sustained countless concussions but he only lost consciousness once and suffered a vertebral fracture. The first CTE-related clinical signs were noted at age 79 with outbursts of anger along with memory, executive function, attention, and language difficulties. He also experienced infrequent but severe headaches. Three years later, motor problems affecting dressing, walking and golf playing were also noted. The following year, he was diagnosed with Parkinson's disease, and was prescribed Levodopa. A nuclear medicine DAT scan, however, was normal. Brain MRI demonstrated generalized cerebral atrophy and small vessel white matter ischemic changes. The diagnosis of corticobasal degeneration was considered. He declined very rapidly over the last year of his life, and by the last month, he could not move or speak. He expired at the age 84 after an apparent disease duration of approximately 5 years.

Case 2: Sixty-eight-year old male with no known relevant family or military history and with no history of alcohol or substance abuse. He played football for 4 years in high school, 4 years in college, and 10 years in the NFL, an offensive lineman. At age 64, following an auto accident, he complained of cluster headaches and family members noted forgetfulness. Approximately 1 year later, he developed left sided face burning and impaired speech. Magnetic resonance imaging (MRI) performed at the time was consistent with transient ischemic attacks. With treatment, his speech improved slightly. At age 66, he showed cognitive decline and difficulty performing work-related activities. This was followed by a rapid decline in cognition, including impaired memory, attention, executive functioning and language. He also demonstrated paranoia, as well as disinhibited and impulsive behavior. Brain MRI demonstrated bilateral symmetric cortical restriction diffusion and FLAIR signal abnormality thought to be consistent with CJD. Electroencephalogram (EEG) was also abnormal but cerebrospinal fluid (CSF) examination was equivocal. At age 67, he received the diagnosis of CJD following examination at a university clinic. However, the diagnosis was considered uncertain given his borderline CSF 14-3-3 protein positivity, relatively prolonged rate of decline and absence of classic myoclonic jerks. Other possible diagnoses included autoimmune disease and paraneoplastic syndrome, but all tests were normal. Nevertheless, he was started on intravenous immunoglobulin treatment with no benefit. The diagnosis of FTLD associated with CTE was considered. In the year prior to his death, the patient developed weakness and gait disturbance. He expired at 68 years of age following an apparent disease duration of 4 years.

Case 3: Forty-eight-year-old male, premature at birth, with no history of military service. The father was affected by an unspecified psychiatric disorder and was abusive. At age 14, 6 months after parents divorced, the patient was involved in an automobile accident, which resulted in the patient's brother death, reportedly leaving the patient with feelings of guilt. At age 16 he started drinking alcohol heavily and smoking marijuana. By his mid-20s he was an alcoholic, used drugs, and was often involved in fist-fights that left facial bruises. He was involved in at least two major car accidents with evidence of head trauma; one at approximately age 29 and the other at age 47 about 1 1/2 years before death. Despite these injuries, he was able to perform his trade as carpenter. At the age of 48 years, he was noted to be confused and delirious and was diagnosed with bipolar disorder and PTSD after examination at a local hospital. Neurological examination showed ophthalmoplegia, ata xia, confusion and rigidity. He was diagnosed with Wernicke encephalopathy and possible neuroleptic malignant syndrome. Thiamine and other treatments were ineffective, and the patient was transferred to a university hospital. MRI revealed asymmetric signal hyperintensity in parietal and occipital cortices, and caudate nucleus. Sharp wave periodic complexes were found on EEG leading to the diagnosis of prion disease. The only laboratory diagnostic tests for prion disease that could be performed was, neuron specific enolase which was elevated. The patient expired at 48 years after an apparent duration of prion disease of 7 weeks.

Histopathological examination

Case 1 (CTE MV1-2C) (Additional file 1: Table S1)

Hematoxylin-eosin (HE): Severe spongiform degeneration (SD) was detected throughout most the cerebral cortex examined except for the hippocampus and insular cortex. SD was characterized by a mixture of fine and large, occasionally confluent vacuoles with severe astrogliosis and little neuronal loss. Large vacuole SD predominated in the temporal neocortex (Fig. 1a). SD with large vacuoles was also prominent in the molecular layer of cerebellum with focal distribution and enhancement in the depth of the sulci (Fig. 1b). SD was minimal in

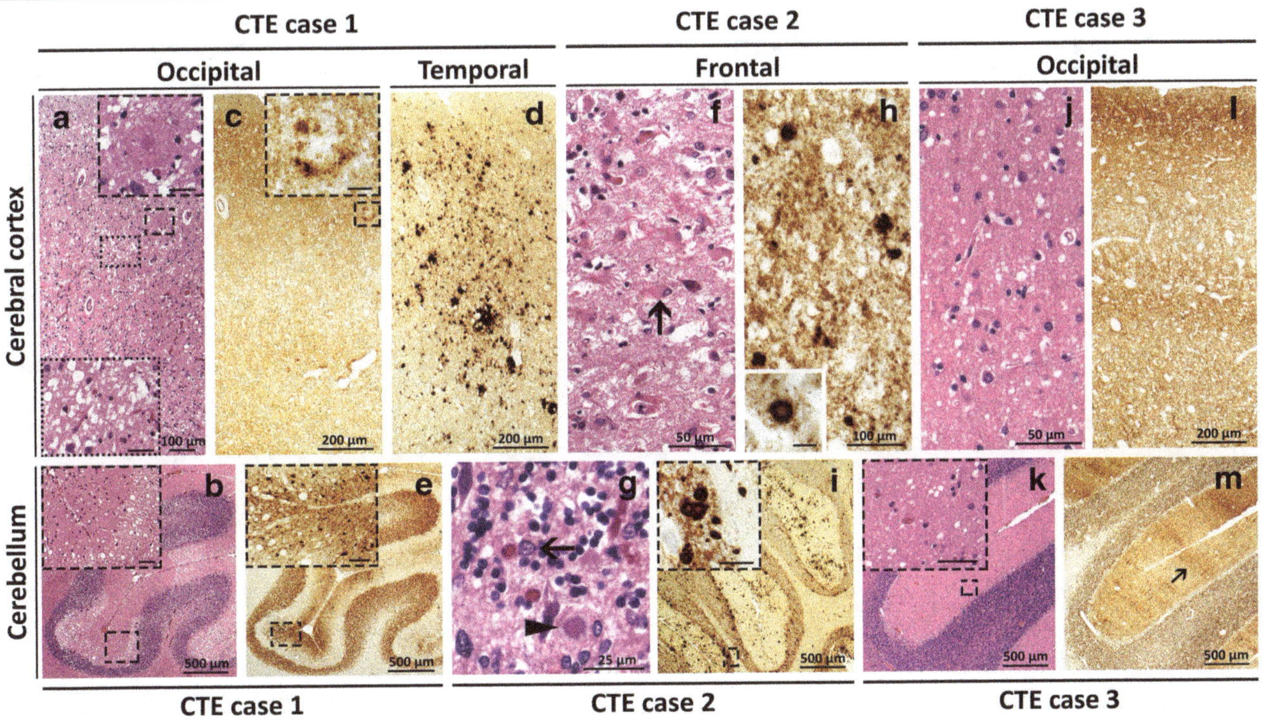

Fig. 1 Prion histopathology in CTE Cases 1–3. Hematoxylin and eosin (HE) (**a, b, f, g, j, k**) and PrP immunohistochemistry (**c-e, h, i, l, m**). **a**: Severe spongiform degeneration (SD); dashed inset: higher magnification of a core amyloid β (Aβ) plaque; dotted inset: SD with large vacuoles. **b**: Focal distribution of large vacuoles SD in the molecular layer of the cerebellum; inset: large vacuoles typically affecting the deeper region of the molecular layer. **c** and **d**: Widespread "synaptic" PrP immunostaining (**c**) along with focal coarse and perivacuolar patterns (**d**); **c**, inset: enhancement of PrP immunoreactivity around an Aβ plaque. **e**: Larger and clustered PrP granules co-distributed with small vacuoles SD in the molecular layer; inset: higher magnification in the depth of a sulcus. **f**: Severe atrophy with gliosis and neuronal loss; arrow: reactive astrocyte. **g**: Atrophy, gliosis and kuru plaques in the granular cell layer; arrow: reactive astrocyte; arrowhead: kuru plaque. **h**: Plaques and plaque-like PrP deposits in a background of coarse PrP granules; inset: PrP staining of a kuru plaque. **i**: Coarse, plaque and plaque-like PrP immunostaining patterns in molecular and granular layers, and deep white matter; inset: cluster of kuru plaques in the granular layer. **j**: Small vacuoles SD. **k**: small vacuoles SD; inset: higher magnification. **l**: "Synaptic" PrP immunostaining. **m**: Widespread PrP immunostaining with "brush stroke" pattern of PrP deposition (arrow) in molecular layer typical of sCJDMM1; Ab: 3F4. Scale bar in insets: 25 µm (**a** and **c**), 20 µm (**h**) and 50 µm (**b**, **e**, **i**, **k**)

neostriatum, thalamus and dorsal midbrain with good preservation of substantia nigra and locus coeruleus. Eosinophilic rounded structures, possibly corresponding to unstructured Aβ plaques and focal status spongiosus were present in the superficial cortex (Fig. 1a). Multiple small micro infarcts were also present in the motor cortex.

Immunohistochemistry PrP: The dominant pattern of PrP deposition in the cerebral cortex was punctate. Enhanced PrP immunoreactivity was occasionally observed around the eosinophilic structures seen on HE. (Fig. 1c). Deposits of coarse PrP were found in the temporal cortex (Fig. 1d). The subcortical white matter, neostriatum and brain stem were unstained. Coarse granular deposits and plaque-like formations in a background of fine granular deposits were common in the cerebellum where they were preferentially distributed in the superficial molecular layer, occasionally at the depths of the sulci (Fig. 1e).

P-tau: Perivascular p-tau pathology as neurofibrillary tangles (NFT), thorn-shaped astrocytes and cell processes, the pathognomonic lesion of CTE, was found throughout the motor, temporal and parietal cortices (Fig. 2a). Other neuropathological features of CTE included NFT and neuropil threads in superficial layers (II-III) of the temporal neocortex (Fig. 2b), and the glial tangles in thalamic nuclei. NFT were dense and widespread in the medial temporal lobe, including the amygdala, entorhinal cortex and hippocampus. NFT were also found in the deep nuclei, brainstem and dentate nucleus of the cerebellum.

Aβ: Subpial Aβ deposition as well diffuse and core plaques were present in the cerebral cortex (Additional file 2: Figure S1. a). Mild meningeal amyloid angiopathy was found in the occipital lobe. Small to medium size punctate Aβ deposits were present in the hippocampus and caudate; the cerebellum was unremarkable. Staining with Thioflavin S was negative. The "ABC" score ("A" = phase for Aβ plaques; "B" = Braak stage for NFT and "C" = CERAD neuritic plaque score), a score of the level of Alzheimer's disease-related neuropathology features, was

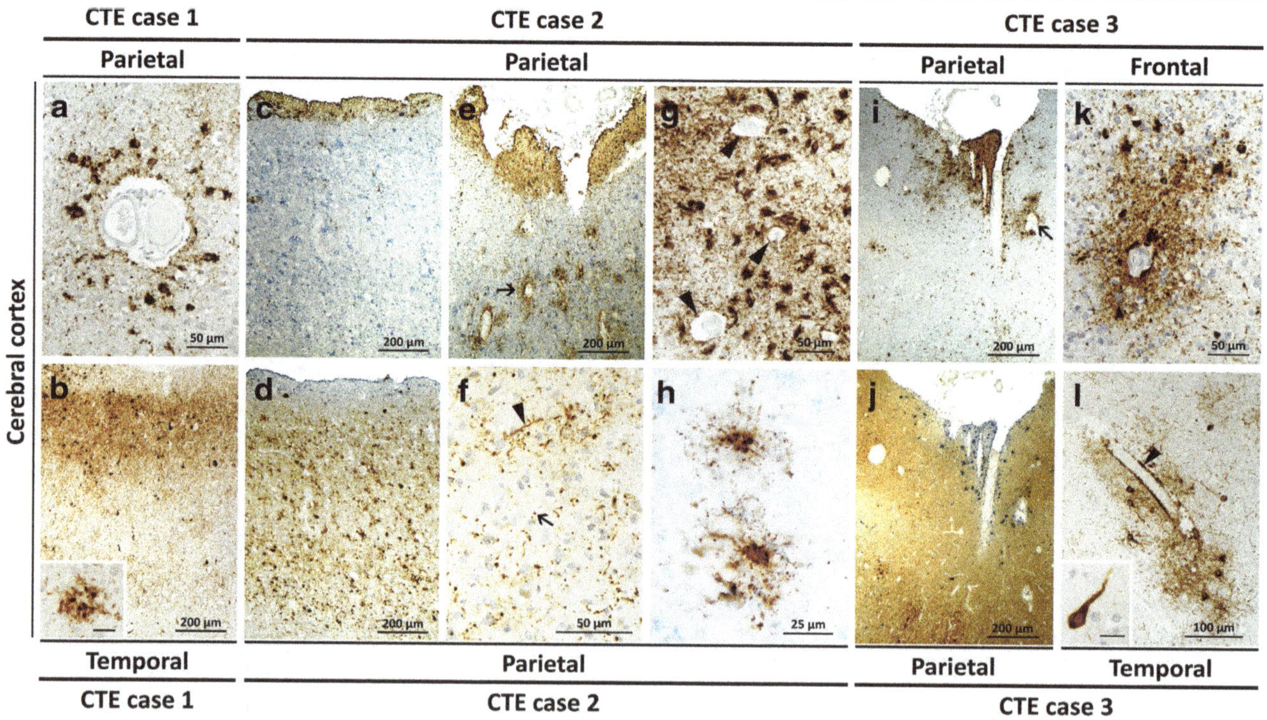

Fig. 2 Tau and PrP immunostaining in CTE Cases 1–3. **a**: Perivascular tau pathology consisting of p-tau immunoreactive neurofibrillary tangles (NFT), dotlike neurites and immunoreactive astrocytes distributed in an irregular pattern in deep cortical regions. **b**: NFT preferentially involving the superficial layers (layers II-III); inset: tau-positive dystrophic neurites associated with an Aβ plaque. **c-e** (p-tau and PrP double immunostaining): Overall, p-tau neurofibrillary pathology (brown in **c** and **e**, cyan in **d**) predominated in the superficial layers of the cerebral cortex while PrP pathology (cyan in **c** and **e**, brown in **d**) preferential affected deeper layers; **e**: arrow: perivascular p-tau pathology. **f**: P-tau immunoreactive "dot-like" structures (arrow); arrowhead: neuropil thread. **g**: Perivascular p- tau pathology with thorn-shaped astrocytes; arrowheads: blood vessels. **h**: P-tau immunoreactive astrocytes. **i** and **j** (p-tau and PrP double immunostaining): p-tau neurofibrillary pathology (brown in **i** and cyan in **j**) preferentially affecting the superficial layers of the cerebral cortex while PrP pathology (cyan in **i**, brown in **j**) predominated in deep layers; **i**: arrowhead: perivascular p-tau pathology. **k** and **l**: Perivascular p-tau NFT and dot-like neurites in a deep cortical region (**k**); subpial perivascular thorn-shaped astrocytes and NFT (**j**); **l**, inset: a NFT. Abs 3F4 (to PrP) and AT8 (to tau). Scale bar in insets: 25 µm (**b**) and 20 µm (**l**)

A2, B2, C0 corresponding to "intermediate" level of AD neuropathological change (ADNC) [33].

TDP-43 immunostaining disclosed cytoplasm inclusions and neurites in the frontal cortex, medial temporal lobe and brainstem (Additional file 2: Figure S1 b).

Alpha-synuclein immunostaining demonstrated occasional Lewy bodies and Lewy neurites in the olfactory bulbs.

In summary, the histopathological phenotype of the prion disease in this case resembled that of sCJDMV1-2C in the cerebrum and cerebellum. P-tau pathology was diagnostic for CTE, Stage IV and co-existed with diffuse and core Aβ plaques, (without neuritic plaques), consistent with intermediate ADNC, widespread TDP-43 pathology, and alpha-synuclein deposition in the olfactory bulbs.

Case 2 (CTE MV2K-C)

HE: The cerebral cortex showed widespread, severe atrophy, with prominent astrogliosis and neuronal loss. SD was scattered and comprised of medium and occasional large vacuoles; status spongiosus was present near the surface (Fig. 1f). SD was severe in neostriatum and cerebellar molecular layer (Fig. 1g). The granule cell layer of the cerebellum was atrophic and showed kuru plaques, which, to a lesser extent, were also seen in the molecular layer. The brainstem exhibited gliosis in the dorsal midbrain and SD with pigment loss in the substantia nigra.

Immunohistochemistry PrP: Immunostaining was intense in most of the brain regions; in the cerebral cortex, it was characterized by coarse and fine granular staining, mature plaques and plaque-like formations (Fig. 1h). Plaque-like formations were also seen in the neostriatum. The subcortical white matter showed a similar staining pattern suggestive of degenerating axons and glial cells (Additional file 2: Figure S1 c and d). The staining patterns in the cerebellum included kuru plaques, plaque-like and coarse granules in the molecular layer; plaques were also present in the white matter along with scattered structures probably representing degenerating axons (Fig. 1i). The dentate nucleus, substantia nigra, locus coeruleus and inferior olive were all positive.

P-Tau: NFT and thorn-shaped astrocytes populated primarily the superficial frontal, parietal and temporal cortices forming occasional perivascular clusters of NFT and glial tangles at the depths of the sulci (Fig. 2f-h), while they were present in lower density the hippocampus, entorhinal cortex and amygdala (Fig. 2c-e).

Aβ: There were granular Aβ deposits in the cortex and corpus striatum and rare Aβ core-plaques (Additional file 2: Figure S1 e). Staining with Thioflavin S was negative. The "ABC" score was A2, B1, C0 corresponding to "low" level ADNC.

TDP-43: Rare TDP-43 neurites were found in the frontal cortex and medial temporal lobe structures.

Alpha-synuclein immunostaining: negative.

In summary, the histopathological phenotype mimicked that of sCJDMV2K-C with prominent axonal degeneration in white matter. The p-tau pathology was diagnostic for CTE, Stage II while the Aβ immunostaining was of low severity and consistent with aging.

Case 3 (CTE MM1)

HE: The cerebral cortex showed fine SD and astrogliosis that were most severe in occipital than in parietal, frontal and temporal cortices (Fig. 1j). SD was also severe in the cerebellar molecular layer, moderate to minimal in neostriatum and thalamus, and absent in brainstem (Fig. 1k). The locus coeruleus and substantia nigra were well preserved. No plaques were detected.

Immunohistochemistry PrP: Intense punctate or "synaptic" staining was uniformly distributed throughout the cerebral cortex, with occasional collections of coarser granules that rarely formed noticeable aggregates (Fig. 1l). A conspicuous single plaque-like formation was present in the entorhinal region. Selective staining around the perikaryon and dendrites of neurons was seen in deep cortical regions especially the entorhinal and occipital cortices. Widespread granular staining was seen in neostriatum and brainstem but not in the locus coeruleus and substantia nigra. The cerebellum showed a "brush stroke" PrP deposition in a background of diffuse staining in molecular layer characteristic of sCJDMM (MV)1 (Fig. 1m). No immunostaining was seen in the white matter.

P-tau: Focal perivascular NFT, dot-like neurites and immunoreactive glial cells were found around small vessels at the depths of the sulci in the frontal, parietal and temporal cortices (Fig. 2i-l). No p-tau pathology was present in the medial temporal lobe structures. Pre-tangles and p-tau immunoreactive granular astrocytes were present in the thalamus and dorsal brain stem. There was no apparent regional or cellular co-localization between p-tau and PrP^D pathology.

Aβ: Diffuse plaques were scattered within the neocortex (Additional file 2: Figure S1 f). Staining with Thioflavin S was negative. The "ABC" score was A1, B1, C0 corresponding to "low" level ADNC.

TDP-43: Negative.

Alpha-synuclein: Negative.

In summary, this case showed the histopathological prion phenotype of severe sCJDMM1 associated with CTE Stage II and Aβ diffuse plaques.

Other CTE cases: Fifty-three additional cases were examined and found negative for PrP immunostaining.

Lesion profile

The lesion profiles reflecting the brain distributions and severity of SD and astrogliosis in each of the three CTE prion positive cases matched the corresponding profile of the respective controls (Fig. 3).

Detection and typing of $resPrP^D$

Immunoblot analysis of PK-digested BH demonstrated the presence of disease-related PK-resistant PrP ($resPrP^D$) in all three cases examined. Overall, the electrophoretic profiles of the three CTE cases closely resembled those of the respective controls subsets (Fig. 4). Taking advantage of four Abs, 3F4 to both $resPrP^D$ types, 12B2 and 1E4 preferentially to type 1 and 2, respectively, and SAF70 to the proximal C-terminal region, we obtained the following data for each of the three CTE cases. Case 1, CTE MV1-2C, showed the presence of type 1 in all regions except for the temporal cortex where only type 2 was present; in the frontal and entorhinal cortices types 1 and 2 co-existed in seemingly similar amounts (Fig. 4a and d) while minimal amounts of type 2 were found in all remaining regions (data not shown). Small amounts of the additional fragments 18.5 kDa, 17 kDa and CTF 13 kDa were also seen (Fig. 4a and d, and data not shown) [38, 63]. In case 2, CTE MV2K-C, $resPrP^D$ type 2 (19 kDa) was

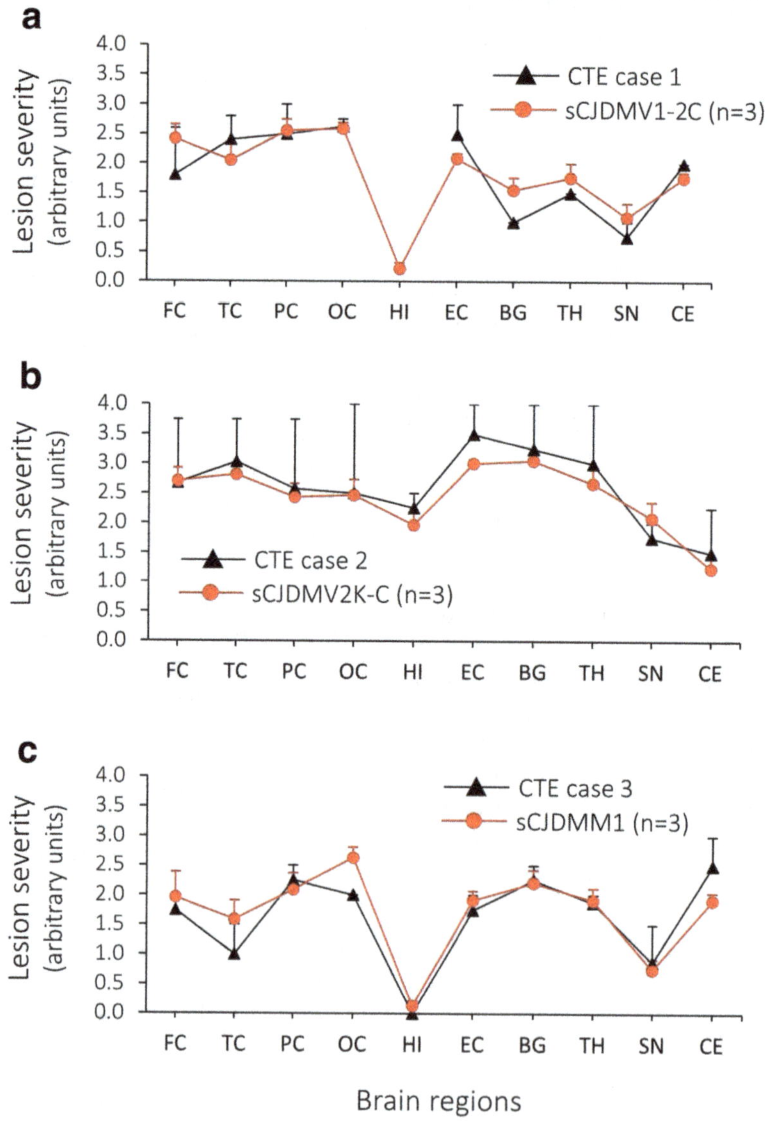

Fig. 3 Lesion profiles of CTE, and matched sCJD controls. The lesion profiles from each of the prion-positive CTE cases matched that of the respective sCJD control. **a**: CTE MV1-2C (case 1) and sCJDMV1-2C. The hippocampus from the CTE case was unavailable for lesion rating. **b**: CTE MV2K-C (case 2) and sCJDMV2K-C. **c**: CTE MM1 (case 3) and sCJDMM1. Lesion profiles were generated using the combined scores (mean ± SEM) for spongiform degeneration (SD) and gliosis for each of the 10 brain regions examined. SD was scored on a 0 to 4 scale (0, not detectable; 1, mild; 2, moderate; 3, severe). Gliosis was scored on a 0 to 4 scale (0, not detectable; 1, scattered activated nuclei; 2, moderate activated nuclei; 3, some reactive astrocytes with visible perikaryon; 4, mostly reactive astrocytes with visible perikaryon). FC: frontal cortex (cx); TC: temporal cx; PC: parietal cx; OC: occipital cx; HI: hippocampus (CA1 region); EC: entorhinal cx; BG: basal ganglia; TH: thalamus, SN: substantia nigra; CE: cerebellum

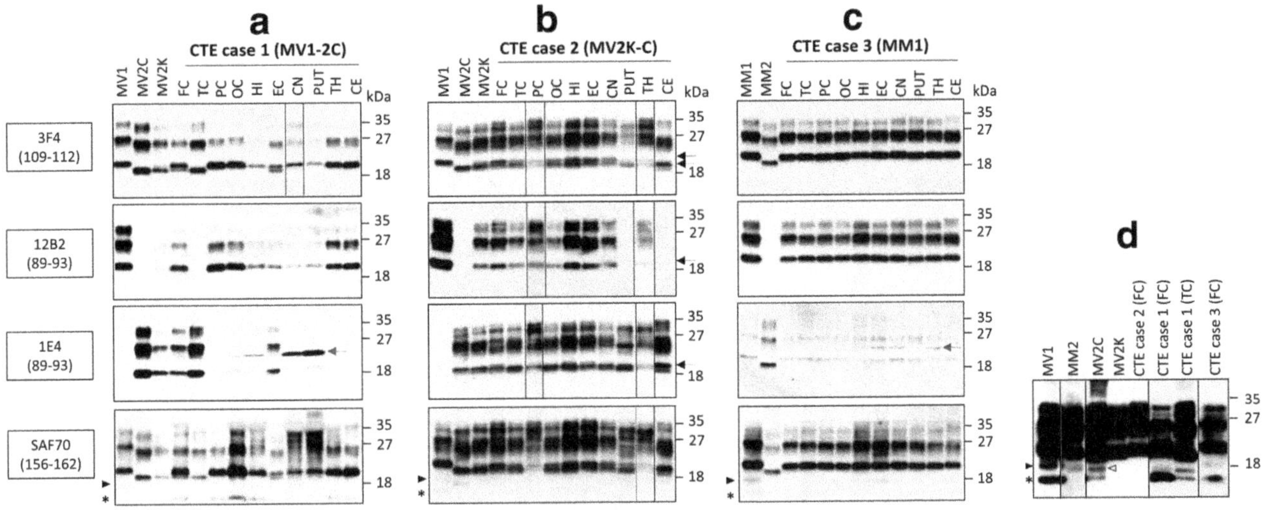

Fig. 4 Immunoblot study of PrP^D brain regional characteristics. **a-c**: Immunoblots were carried out with proteinase K (PK)-treated brain homogenates (BH) obtained from the indicated brain regions sampled from the three study cases (CTE MV1-2C, CTE MV2K-C and CTE MM1) and sCJD controls (MV1, MV2C, MV2K and MM1). Different sample volume loads or exposures were used, to obtain a comparable representation of PK-resistant PrP^D ($resPrP^D$) bands. Membranes were probed with the indicated Abs to PrP: 3F4 to both $resPrP^D$ 1 and 2, 12B2 and 1E4 preferentially to type 1 and 2, respectively; SAF70 to the proximal C-terminal region. **d**: $resPrP^D$ loaded at higher concentrations (~ 1 mg tissue equivalent) in all lanes and were probed with SAF70. **a** and **d**: In CTE MV1-2C case 1, Ab 3F4 revealed $resPrP^D$ type 1 in all brain regions either as the sole component or associated with a higher mobility band in frontal (FC) and entorhinal cortices (EC) consistent with $resPrP^D$ type 2; $resPrP^D$ type 2 only was observed in the temporal cortex (TC). This type distribution was confirmed by probing with Ab 12B2 (to PrP^D type 1) and by Ab 1E4 (preferentially to type 2). Ab SAF70, showed two fragments of 18.5 and 17 kDa commonly associated with $resPrP^D$ types 1 and 2, respectively, (solid arrowhead) and the C-terminal fragment CTF 13 kDa (asterisk). These fragments were visible, in the study case and controls BH at higher BH concentration (d). **b** and **d**: In CTE MV2K-C case 2, 3F4 showed the presence of a doublet of 19 kDa (dotted arrow) and 20 kDa (solid arrow) in all regions as typically seen in sCJDMV2K, with the exception of the cerebellum, which presented the 19 kDa band together with a fragment of about 18 kDa. Abs 12B2 and 1E4 detected the 20 kDa and 19 kDa component of the doublet, respectively. In putamen the 20 kDa fragment was detected only at the longer exposure (data not shown). SAF70 did not detect any additional fragments in the study case and sCJDMV2K control. **c** and **d**: In CTE case 3 MM1, 3F4 showed the presence of PrP^D type 1 (21 kDa) in all different brain regions, which was confirmed with 12B2 while 1E4 showed no type 2 (blue arrow: non-specific band); SAF70 demonstrated the 18.5 kDa and CTF-13 fragments, typically present in sCJDMM1(MV)1. PC: parietal cortex (cx); OC: occipital cx; HI: hippocampus; CN: caudate nucleus; PUT: putamen; TH: thalamus; CE: cerebellum

invariably present in all of the regions and it was associated with a minor 20 kDa unglycosylated fragment often referred to as "intermediate" (i) [36, 37, 41, 48] in the cerebrum but not in cerebellum. (Fig. 4b and d). An additional fragment of approximately 18 kDa was detected in the cerebellum with all Abs but 12B2 [42]. No additional fragments were detected with SAF70 (Fig. 4b and d). Case 3, CTE MM1, was straightforward featuring similar amounts of $resPrP^D$ type 1 in all ten brain regions (data not shown). The two fragments, 18.5 kDa and CTF 13 kDa, commonly associated with sCJDMM1, were detected in all regions but thalamus (Fig. 4c and d, and data not shown).

PrP^D conformational tests: Conformational stability and solubility assay (CSSA) and conformational stability immunoassay (CSI)

CSSA was performed assessing denaturation rate at increasing concentration of GdnHCl of total PrP^D ($totPrP^D$) (comprising PK-sensitive PrP^D and $resPrP^D$ isoforms) and $resPrP^D$ extracted from the three study cases and their controls. The amounts of GdnHCl needed to solubilize half of $totPrP^D$ and of $resPrP^D$ ($GdnHCl_{1/2}$ values) of cases 1–3 were similar to those of their controls (Fig. 5a-d). In contrast, and according to published results, $GdnHCl_{1/2}$ values significantly diverged when CSSA was performed on PrP^D preparations from sCJDMM1 and sCJDMM2 which harbor the distinct PrP^D strains types 1 and 2 (Fig. 5a-d).

In CSI, GdnHCl required to rendering $resPrP^D$ PK-sensitive was used as a measure of relative conformational stability [43, 44, 50]. CSI also failed to detect a difference in $resPrP^D$ stability between the three CTE cases and controls while it significantly distinguished sCJDMM1 and sCJDMM2 subtypes (Fig. 6a-b).

Prion disease incidence in CTE: Statistical analysis

The 55 CTE subjects contributed a total of 3630 person-years (mean = 66). The expected number of prion disease cases in this cohort by chance alone was 0.0042. The probability of two or more cases in this cohort occurring by chance alone was $8.93*10^{-6}$. One or both of these cases may have been undetected or not ascertained

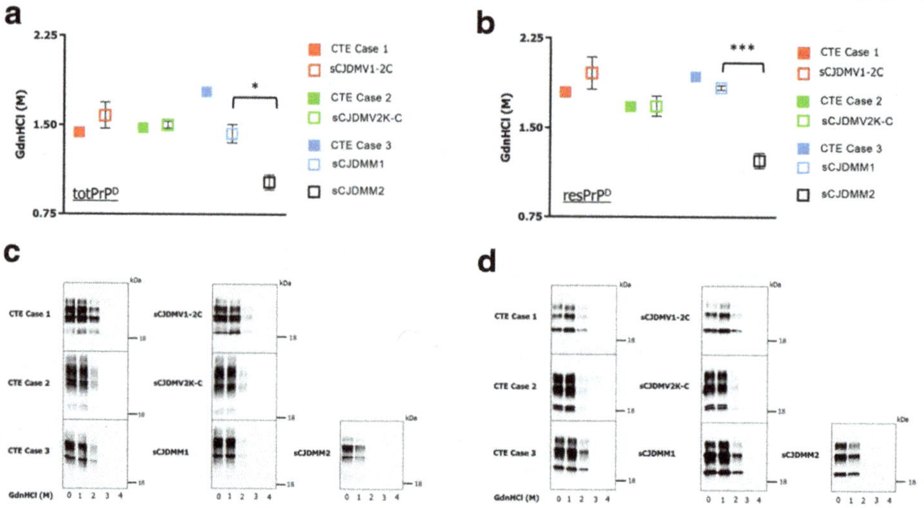

Fig. 5 Conformational stability and solubility assay (CSSA) of PrP^D species. Solubility and stability of totPrP^D (PK-) and resPrP^D (PK+) were measured as $[GdnHCl]_{1/2}$ molar values, which denotes the molar concentration competent to solubilize half of the substrate. **a** and **b**: No significant difference related to totPrP^D and resPrP^D was detected between each of the CTE cases 1–3 and their respective controls ($n = 3$). By contrast, both totPrP^D and resPrP^D values were significantly different in sCJDMM1 and sCJDMM2 as expected. Mean $[GdnHCl]_{1/2}$ molar values for totPrP^D and resPrP^D were: in CTE case 1, 1.44 and 1.8, respectively, and 1.58 ± 0.11 and 1.95 ± 0.13 in controls; in case 2, 1.49 and 1.68, with 1.5 ± 0.04 and 1.69 ± 0.14 in controls; in case 3, 1.78 and 1.93, with 1.43 ± 0.08 and 1.84 ± 0.02 in controls. Mean totPrP^D and resPrP^D values were 1.43 ± 0.08 and 1.84 ± 0.02 and 1.02 ± 0.06 and 1.22 ± 0.06 in sCJDMM1 and sCJDMM2 respectively. * $p \leq 0.05$, *** $p \leq 0.001$. **c** and **d**: Representative immunoblots of total and resPrP^D of CTE cases 1–3 and controls probed with Ab 3F4 at increasing concentrations of GdnHCl

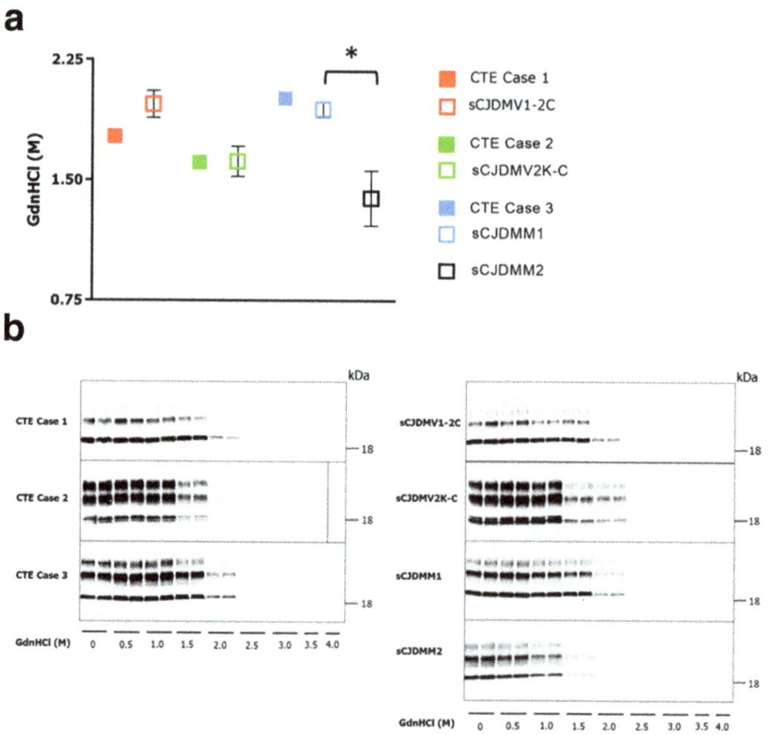

Fig. 6 Conformational stability immunoassay of resPrP^D. **a**: No significant difference was detected between each of the CTE cases 1–3 and their controls (n = 3) in PK-resistance following exposure to GdnHCl. As expected, stability of resPrP^D associated with sCJDMM1 and sCJDMM2 were both significantly different. Mean $[GdnHCl]_{1/2}$ molar values in CTE case 1–3 and controls were: 1.77 and 1.98 ± 0.08 respectively; 1.61 and 1.62 ± 0.09; and 2.01 and 1.95 ± 0.05 respectively. In sCJDMM1 and sCJDMM2 mean $[GdnHCl]_{1/2}$ molar values were 1.95 ± 0.05 and 1.39 ± 0.17, respectively. * $p \leq 0.05$. **b**: Immunoblots probed with 3F4 at increasing GdnHCl concentrations

in national surveillance except for this investigation; however, the observed number of two prion disease cases would still be significantly different from expected ($p < 0.05$) if the true incidence of prion disease (both ascertained and not ascertained) was up to 83 times the number of ascertained cases.

Discussion

We found prion disease in three subjects with neuropathologically confirmed CTE, including two subjects from a cohort of 55 CTE cases and in one subject clinically diagnosed with PTSD and probable prion disease who was found serendipitously. In all three cases, the CTE was characterized by accumulations of p-tau in neurons and astrocytes around small vessels preferentially at the depths of the cortical sulci. Two cases (ages 64 and 48 years at time of death) were diagnosed with CTE, Stage II, and the third (Case 1, age 84 years) was diagnosed with CTE, Stage IV. All three cases were associated with variable degrees of co-morbid Aβ pathology. Widespread TDP-43 deposits were found in cases 1 and 2, and alpha-synuclein deposits in the olfactory bulb of case 1.

Relatively few detailed neuropathological examinations of individuals clinically diagnosed with PTSD have been reported in the literature, primarily in military personnel exposed to blast and concussive injury [39, 52]. Of the 10 cases in the literature, seven were reported to have p-tau pathology of various severity and six were diagnosed with CTE; three cases featured only prominent astrogliosis consistent with posttraumatic scarring. The seven reported PTSD cases harboring p-tau pathology bear strong resemblance to our cases 2 and 3 with CTE Stage II. Our case 1 was diagnosed with CTE, Stage IV but was much older at the time of death compared to the other reported cases (range 22–48, mean = 37 years). All these cases underline the close correlation between PTSD and CTE [39, 52].

We evaluated the type, severity and distribution of the prion histopathology along with characteristics and conformational properties of the resPrP^D. These features, which provide a rough assessment of the PrP^D strain, did not significantly differ from corresponding features of matching sCJD subtypes used as positive controls (Additional file 1: Table S1). Specifically, prion-positive CTE case 3, which harbored the genotype MM at codon 129 of the PrP gene coupled with resPrP^D type 1 (CTE CJDMM1), showed the same phenotypic and PrP^D characteristics as the sCJDMM1 subtype. Similarly, CTE cases 1 and 2, both of whom had the MV 129 genotype, coupled with resPrP^D comprising both types 1 and 2 in case 1 (CTE CJDMV1-2C), and with PrP^D type i-2 variant in case 2 (CTE-CJDMV2K-C), matched phenotypic and PrP^D features of typical sCJDMV1-2C and sCJDMV2K-C (or sCJDMVi-2C), respectively.

Clinically, in case 3, the prion disease presented as rapidly progressive mental deterioration with motor signs as well as positive laboratory tests and MRI. CJD was suspected at disease midcourse in case 2. These clinical data combined with the severity of the prion disease pathology in all 3 cases suggest that the prion disease was superimposed on pre-existent CTE. Taken together, our findings suggest that the prion disease phenotype in CTE was not demonstrably impacted by the coexistence of CTE or the remote occurrence of neurotrauma. If prion disease were an intrinsic component of CTE, one would expect that a divergent histopathological phenotype or PrP^D characteristics [14, 34, 46, 53].

The frequent participation of two or more proteinopathies in a neurodegenerative disease is well-established and increasingly common with advanced age at death [3, 19, 27, 53, 54]. Prion proteinopathy appears to be no exception. Sporadic CJD has been reported to co-occur with AD [58, 59] and in association with the pathology of multiple system atrophy [49]. A possible pathogenic mechanism to explain multiprotein degeneration is cross-seeding, in which aggregates of misfolded proteins acting as a seed to induce the formation of misfolded aggregates of heterologous proteins [35, 60]. Experimental data have provided the proof-of-concept for cross-seeding but most of the evidence comes from in vitro experiments [35]. Cross-seeding does not exclude other mechanisms that would explain the co-occurrence of multiple pathological proteins in CTE and other neurodegenerative conditions [60] including a failure of the proteostasis network, a multisystem apparatus dedicated to assist protein folding and prevent protein aggregation. Proteostasis failure, may result from aging or local conditions as trauma and tissue stress [10, 24, 26]. Furthermore, there is accumulating evidence that the deposition of one abnormal protein creates the conditions for, or facilitates, the aggregation of other vulnerable proteins in a "cascade" sequence [19, 53, 54].

The occurrence of sCJD in 2 cases of a CTE cohort comprising 55 subjects would be statistically consistent with a sporadic prion disease incidence of over 100 cases per million people per year. This incidence is at least 83 times higher than the currently reported US incidence (Maddox RA et al., 2018, unpublished results), or a similar magnitude higher than that reported for other countries [9]. Only a rigorous population study involving many more CTE cases will conclusively establish whether the risk of CJD (or of particular subtypes thereof) is increased in patients with CTE.

Conclusions

We report for the first time the occurrence of CJD in three cases with CTE. Our results indicate that the CJD phenotype and resPrP^{D} characteristics, including conformation, in these three cases with sCJD-CTE co-occurrence show no difference from corresponding cases with sCJD occurring alone; they also provide preliminary evidence that CTE increases the risk of sCJD.

Additional files

Additional file 1: Table S1. Molecular classification of sCJD subtypes [8, 15]. **Table S2** showing sex, sCJD subtype, age at onset and death, disease duration in study cases and respective controls. (DOCX 17 kb)

Additional file 2: Figure S1. Aβ, TDP-43 and PrP immunoreactivity in CTE Cases 1–3. **a**: Widespread Aβ deposits in the subpial surface (arrow) and core dense Aβ plaques (arrowhead) in the frontal cortex. **b**: TDP-43 cytoplasmic inclusions (arrow) and "dot-like" structures (arrowhead) in the hippocampus. **c** and **d**: Plaque-like PrP deposits (arrow in **c**) and intense PrP immunoreactivity in the subcortical white matter of the temporal lobe. **e** and **f**: Granular Aβ deposits (**e**) and diffuse Aβ plaques (**f**) in the parietal (**e**) and frontal (**f**) cortices; **e**, inset: a rare core dense Aβ plaque. Abs: 4G8 (**a**, **e**, **f**), TDP-43 in (**b**), 3F4 (**c** and **d**). Scalebar inset in **e**: 20 μm. (PDF 3628 kb)

Abbreviations

Abs: antibodies; AD: Alzheimer's disease; ALS: amyotrophic lateral sclerosis; Aβ: amyloid beta; BH: brain homogenate; CENC: Chronic Effects of Neurotrauma Consortium; CJD: Creutzfeldt-Jakob disease; CSI: conformational stability immunoassay; CSSA: conformational stability and solubility assay; CTE: chronic traumatic encephalopathy; FTLD: frontotemporal lobar degeneration; GdnHCl: guanidine HCl; HE: hematoxylin-eosin; M: methionine; NFT: neurofibrillary tangles; NPDPSC: National Prion Disease Pathology Surveillance Center; PK: proteinase K; PrP: prion protein; PrP^{D}: abnormal disease-related PrP; P-tau: hyperphosphorylated tau protein; PTSD: posttraumatic stress disorder; sCJD: sporadic CJD; SD: spongiform degeneration; TBI: traumatic brain injury; TDP-43: TAR DNA binding protein 43; V: valine; VA-BU-CLF: Veterans Affairs-Boston University-Concussion Legacy Foundation; WB: Western blot; α-syn: α synuclein

Acknowledgements

We thank all the patient families, referring clinicians, The CJD Foundation, the NPDPSC technical and administrative personnel, in particular Yvonne Cohen, Miriam Warren, Katie Eppich and Janis Blevins for their invaluable assistance.

Funding

The study was supported by NIH P01AI106705, NIH 5R01NS083687 and Charles S. Britton Fund to PG, and National Institute of Neurological Disorders and Stroke (grants U01 NS086659, R01 NS078337, R56 NS078337, U01 NS093334, F32 NS096803), the National Institute on Aging (grants K23 AG046377, P30AG13846; supplement 0572063345-5, R01 AG1649, AG057902), the U.S. Department of Defense (grant W81XWH-13-2-0064), Chronic Effects of Neurotrauma Consortium (CENC) Award W81XWH-13-2-0095 and Department of Veterans Affairs CENC Award I01 CX001135, the U.S. Department of Veterans Affairs (I01 CX001038), the Veterans Affairs Biorepository (CSP 501), the Veterans Affairs Rehabilitation Research and Development Traumatic Brain Injury Center of Excellence (grant B6796-C), the Department of Defense Peer Reviewed Alzheimer's Research Program (DoD-PRARP grant 13267017), the National Operating Committee on Standards for Athletic Equipment, the Alzheimer's Association (grants NIRG-15-362697, NIRG-305779), the Concussion Legacy Foundation, Nick and Lynn Buoniconti Foundation, the Andlinger Family Foundation, WWE, and the National Football League to AMK.

Disclaimer

The findings and conclusions in this report are those of the authors and do not necessarily represent the official position of CDC and should not be construed as an official Veterans Affairs or Department of Defense position, policy or decision, unless so designated by other official documentation.

Authors' contributions

SKN, SN, IC and PG were responsible for the concept and design of the study. SKN, SN, IC, VA, DK, MC, RAS, BA JA, LS, AM and PG were responsible for data analysis and acquisition. SKN, SN, IC and PG were responsible for drafting of figures and manuscript. All authors read and approved the final manuscript.

Competing interests

The authors declare that they have no competing interests.

Author details

[1]Department of Pathology, Case Western Reserve University, School of Medicine, Cleveland, OH 44106, USA. [2]VA Boston Healthcare System, Boston, MA 02130, USA. [3]Department of Neurology and Pathology, Boston University School of Medicine, Boston, MA 02118, USA. [4]Alzheimer's Disease Center and CTE Program, Boston University School of Medicine, Boston, MA 02118, USA. [5]National Prion Disease Pathology Surveillance Center, Case Western Reserve University, Cleveland, OH 44106, USA. [6]Departments of Neurology, Neurosurgery, and Anatomy and Neurobiology, Boston University School of Medicine, Boston, MA 02118, USA. [7]Departments of Neurology and Psychiatry, Case Western Reserve University, School of Medicine, Cleveland, OH 44106, USA. [8]Division of High-Consequence Pathogens and Pathology, National Center for Emerging and Zoonotic Infectious Diseases, Center for Disease Control and Prevention, Atlanta, GA 30333, USA.

References

1. Adams JW, Alvarez VE, Mez J, Huber BR, Tripodis Y, Xia W, Meng G, Kubilus CA, Cormier K, Kiernan PT et al (2018) Lewy body pathology and chronic traumatic encephalopathy associated with contact sports. J Neuropathol Exp Neurol 77:757–768. https://doi.org/10.1093/jnen/nly065
2. Barnes DE, Byers AL, Gardner RC, Seal KH, Boscardin WJ, Yaffe K (2018) Association of Mild Traumatic Brain Injury with and without Loss of consciousness with dementia in US military veterans. JAMA Neurol 75:1055–1061. https://doi.org/10.1001/jamaneurol.2018.0815
3. Boller F, Mizutani T, Roessmann U, Gambetti P (1980) Parkinson disease, dementia, and Alzheimer disease: clinicopathological correlations. Ann Neurol 7:329–335. https://doi.org/10.1002/ana.410070408
4. Cali I, Castellani R, Alshekhlee A, Cohen Y, Blevins J, Yuan J, Langeveld JP, Parchi P, Safar JG, Zou WQ et al (2009) Co-existence of scrapie prion protein types 1 and 2 in sporadic Creutzfeldt-Jakob disease: its effect on the phenotype and prion-type characteristics. Brain 132:2643–2658. https://doi.org/10.1093/brain/awp196
5. Cali I, Castellani R, Yuan J, Al-Shekhlee A, Cohen ML, Xiao X, Moleres FJ, Parchi P, Zou WQ, Gambetti P (2006) Classification of sporadic Creutzfeldt-Jakob disease revisited. Brain 129:2266–2277. https://doi.org/10.1093/brain/awl224
6. Cali I, Cohen ML, Hasmall yi US, Parchi P, Giaccone G, Collins SJ, Kofskey D, Wang H, McLean CA, Brandel JP et al (2018) Iatrogenic Creutzfeldt-Jakob disease with amyloid-beta pathology: an international study. Acta Neuropathol Commun 6:5. https://doi.org/10.1186/s40478-017-0503-z
7. Cannon A, Bieniek KF, Lin WL, Notari S, Zou WQ, Gambetti P, Pedraza O, Graff-Radford NR, Ferman TJ, Dickson DW (2014) Concurrent variably protease-sensitive prionopathy and amyotrophic lateral sclerosis. Acta Neuropathol 128:313–315. https://doi.org/10.1007/s00401-014-1309-8
8. Cescatti M, Saverioni D, Capellari S, Tagliavini F, Kitamoto T, Ironside J, Giese A, Parchi P (2016) Analysis of conformational stability of abnormal prion protein aggregates across the Spectrum of Creutzfeldt-Jakob disease prions. J Virol 90:6244–6254. https://doi.org/10.1128/jvi.00144-16

9. Chen C, Dong XP (2016) Epidemiological characteristics of human prion diseases. Infect Dis Poverty 5:47. https://doi.org/10.1186/s40249-016-0143-8
10. Chiti F, Dobson CM (2017) Protein Misfolding, amyloid formation, and human disease: a summary of Progress over the last decade. Annu Rev Biochem 86:27–68. https://doi.org/10.1146/annurev-biochem-061516-045115
11. Collins SJ, Sanchez-Juan P, Masters CL, Klug GM, van Duijn C, Poleggi A, Pocchiari M, Almonti S, Cuadrado-Corrales N, de Pedro-Cuesta J et al (2006) Determinants of diagnostic investigation sensitivities across the clinical spectrum of sporadic Creutzfeldt-Jakob disease. Brain 129:2278–2287. https://doi.org/10.1093/brain/awl159
12. Cracco L, Notari S, Cali I, Sy MS, Chen SG, Cohen ML, Ghetti B, Appleby BS, Zou WQ, Caughey B et al (2017) Novel strain properties distinguishing sporadic prion diseases sharing prion protein genotype and prion type. Sci Rep 7:38280. https://doi.org/10.1038/srep38280
13. Crane PK, Gibbons LE, Dams-O'connor K, Trittschuh E, Leverenz JB, Keene CD, Sonnen J, Montine TJ, Bennett DA, Leurgans S et al (2016) Association of Traumatic Brain Injury With Late-Life Neurodegenerative Conditions and Neuropathologic Findings. JAMA Neurol 73:1062–1069. https://doi.org/10.1001/jamaneurol.2016.1948
14. Gambetti P, Cali I, Notari S, Kong Q, Zou WQ, Surewicz WK (2011) Molecular biology and pathology of prion strains in sporadic human prion diseases. Acta Neuropathol 121:79–90. https://doi.org/10.1007/s00401-010-0761-3
15. Gambetti P, Kong Q, Zou W, Parchi P, Chen SG (2003) Sporadic and familial CJD: classification and characterisation. Br Med Bull 66:213–239
16. Ghoshal N, Cali I, Perrin RJ, Josephson SA, Sun N, Gambetti P, Morris JC (2009) Codistribution of amyloid beta plaques and spongiform degeneration in familial Creutzfeldt-Jakob disease with the E200K-129M haplotype. Arch Neurol 66:1240–1246. https://doi.org/10.1001/archneurol.2009.224
17. Goldfarb LG, Petersen RB, Tabaton M, Brown P, LeBlanc AC, Montagna P, Cortelli P, Julien J, Vital C, Pendelbury WW et al (1992) Fatal familial insomnia and familial Creutzfeldt-Jakob disease: disease phenotype determined by a DNA polymorphism. Science 258:806–808
18. Goldstein LE, Fisher AM, Tagge CA, Zhang XL, Velisek L, Sullivan JA, Upreti C, Kracht JM, Ericsson M, Wojnarowicz MW et al (2012) Chronic traumatic encephalopathy in blast-exposed military veterans and a blast neurotrauma mouse model. Sci Transl Med 4:134ra160. https://doi.org/10.1126/scitranslmed.3003716
19. Hardy J, Selkoe DJ (2002) The amyloid hypothesis of Alzheimer's disease: progress and problems on the road to therapeutics. Science 297:353–356. https://doi.org/10.1126/science.1072994
20. Jellinger KA (2004) Head injury and dementia. Curr Opin Neurol 17:719–723
21. Kascsak RJ, Rubenstein R, Merz PA, Tonna-DeMasi M, Fersko R, Carp RI, Wisniewski HM, Diringer H (1987) Mouse polyclonal and monoclonal antibody to scrapie-associated fibril proteins. J Virol 61:3688–3693
22. Kim JI, Cali I, Surewicz K, Kong Q, Raymond GJ, Atarashi R, Race B, Qing L, Gambetti P, Caughey B et al (2010) Mammalian prions generated from bacterially expressed prion protein in the absence of any mammalian cofactors. J Biol Chem 285:14083–14087. https://doi.org/10.1074/jbc.C110.113464
23. Kobayashi A, Iwasaki Y, Otsuka H, Yamada M, Yoshida M, Matsuura Y, Mohri S, Kitamoto T (2013) Deciphering the pathogenesis of sporadic Creutzfeldt-Jakob disease with codon 129 M/V and type 2 abnormal prion protein. Acta Neuropathol Commun 1:74. https://doi.org/10.1186/2051-5960-1-74
24. Labbadia J, Morimoto RI (2015) The biology of proteostasis in aging and disease. Annu Rev Biochem 84:435–464. https://doi.org/10.1146/annurev-biochem-060614-033955
25. Langeveld JP, Jacobs JG, Erkens JH, Bossers A, van Zijderveld FG, van Keulen LJ (2006) Rapid and discriminatory diagnosis of scrapie and BSE in retro-pharyngeal lymph nodes of sheep. BMC Vet Res 2:19. https://doi.org/10.1186/1746-6148-2-19
26. Lucke-Wold BP, Turner RC, Logsdon AF, Nguyen L, Bailes JE, Lee JM, Robson MJ, Omalu BI, Huber JD, Rosen CL (2016) Endoplasmic reticulum stress implicated in chronic traumatic encephalopathy. J Neurosurg 124:687–702. https://doi.org/10.3171/2015.3.jns141802
27. McKee AC, Daneshvar DH (2015) The neuropathology of traumatic brain injury. Handb Clin Neurol 127:45–66. https://doi.org/10.1016/B978-0-444-52892-6.00004-0
28. McKee AC, Gavett BE, Stern RA, Nowinski CJ, Cantu RC, Kowall NW, Perl DP, Hedley-Whyte ET, Price B, Sullivan C et al (2010) TDP-43 proteinopathy and motor neuron disease in chronic traumatic encephalopathy. J Neuropathol Exp Neurol 69:918–929. https://doi.org/10.1097/NEN.0b013e3181ee7d85
29. McKee AC, Robinson ME (2014) Military-related traumatic brain injury and neurodegeneration. Alzheimers Dement 10:S242–S253. https://doi.org/10.1016/j.jalz.2014.04.003
30. McKee AC, Stern RA, Nowinski CJ, Stein TD, Alvarez VE, Daneshvar DH, Lee HS, Wojtowicz SM, Hall G, Baugh CM et al (2013) The spectrum of disease in chronic traumatic encephalopathy. Brain 136:43–64. https://doi.org/10.1093/brain/aws307
31. Mez J, Daneshvar DH, Kiernan PT, Abdolmohammadi B, Alvarez VE, Huber BR, Alosco ML, Solomon TM, Nowinski CJ, McHale L et al (2017) Clinicopathological Evaluation of Chronic Traumatic Encephalopathy in Players of American Football. JAMA 318:360–370. https://doi.org/10.1001/jama.2017.8334
32. Montenigro PH, Baugh CM, Daneshvar DH, Mez J, Budson AE, Au R, Katz DI, Cantu RC, Stern RA (2014) Clinical subtypes of chronic traumatic encephalopathy: literature review and proposed research diagnostic criteria for traumatic encephalopathy syndrome. Alzheimers Res Ther 6:68. https://doi.org/10.1186/s13195-014-0068-z
33. Montine TJ, Phelps CH, Beach TG, Bigio EH, Cairns NJ, Dickson DW, Duyckaerts C, Frosch MP, Masliah E, Mirra SS et al (2012) National Institute on Aging-Alzheimer's Association guidelines for the neuropathologic assessment of Alzheimer's disease: a practical approach. Acta Neuropathol 123:1–11. https://doi.org/10.1007/s00401-011-0910-3
34. Moreno JA, Telling GC (2017) Insights into mechanisms of transmission and pathogenesis from transgenic mouse models of prion diseases. Methods Mol Biol 1658:219–252. https://doi.org/10.1007/978-1-4939-7244-9_16
35. Moreno-Gonzalez I, Edwards Iii G, Salvadores N, Shahnawaz M, Diaz-Espinoza R, Soto C (2017) Molecular interaction between type 2 diabetes and Alzheimer's disease through cross-seeding of protein misfolding. Mol Psychiatry 22:1327–1334. https://doi.org/10.1038/mp.2016.230
36. Notari S, Capellari S, Giese A, Westner I, Baruzzi A, Ghetti B, Gambetti P, Kretzschmar HA, Parchi P (2004) Effects of different experimental conditions on the PrPSc core generated by protease digestion: implications for strain typing and molecular classification of CJD. J Biol Chem 279:16797–16804. https://doi.org/10.1074/jbc.M313220200
37. Notari S, Capellari S, Langeveld J, Giese A, Strammiello R, Gambetti P, Kretzschmar HA, Parchi P (2007) A refined method for molecular typing reveals that co-occurrence of PrP (Sc) types in Creutzfeldt-Jakob disease is not the rule. Lab Investig 87:1103–1112. https://doi.org/10.1038/labinvest.3700676
38. Notari S, Strammiello R, Capellari S, Giese A, Cescatti M, Grassi J, Ghetti B, Langeveld JP, Zou WQ, Gambetti P et al (2008) Characterization of truncated forms of abnormal prion protein in Creutzfeldt-Jakob disease. J Biol Chem 283:30557–30565. https://doi.org/10.1074/jbc.M801877200
39. Omalu B, Hammers JL, Bailes J, Hamilton RL, Kamboh MI, Webster G, Fitzsimmons RP (2011) Chronic traumatic encephalopathy in an Iraqi war veteran with posttraumatic stress disorder who committed suicide. Neurosurg Focus 31:E3. https://doi.org/10.3171/2011.9.focus11178
40. Parchi P, Castellani R, Capellari S, Ghetti B, Young K, Chen SG, Farlow M, Dickson DW, Sima AA, Trojanowski JQ et al (1996) Molecular basis of phenotypic variability in sporadic Creutzfeldt-Jakob disease. Ann Neurol 39:767–778. https://doi.org/10.1002/ana.410390613
41. Parchi P, Giese A, Capellari S, Brown P, Schulz-Schaeffer W, Windl O, Zerr I, Budka H, Kopp N, Piccardo P et al (1999) Classification of sporadic Creutzfeldt-Jakob disease based on molecular and phenotypic analysis of 300 subjects. Ann Neurol 46:224–233
42. Parchi P, Strammiello R, Notari S, Giese A, Langeveld JP, Ladogana A, Zerr I, Roncaroli F, Cras P, Ghetti B et al (2009) Incidence and spectrum of sporadic Creutzfeldt-Jakob disease variants with mixed phenotype and co-occurrence of PrPSc types: an updated classification. Acta Neuropathol 118:659–671. https://doi.org/10.1007/s00401-009-0585-1
43. Pastore M, Chin SS, Bell KL, Dong Z, Yang Q, Yang L, Yuan J, Chen SG, Gambetti P, Zou WQ (2005) Creutzfeldt-Jakob disease (CJD) with a mutation at codon 148 of prion protein gene: relationship with sporadic CJD. Am J Pathol 167:1729–1738. https://doi.org/10.1016/s0002-9440(10)61254-0

44. Peretz D, Scott MR, Groth D, Williamson RA, Burton DR, Cohen FE, Prusiner SB (2001) Strain-specified relative conformational stability of the scrapie prion protein. Protein Sci 10:854–863. https://doi.org/10.1110/ps.39201
45. Pirisinu L, Di Bari M, Marcon S, Vaccari G, D'Agostino C, Fazzi P, Esposito E, Galeno R, Langeveld J, Agrimi U et al (2010) A new method for the characterization of strain-specific conformational stability of protease-sensitive and protease-resistant PrPSc. PLoS One 5:e12723. https://doi.org/10.1371/journal.pone.0012723
46. Poggiolini I, Saverioni D, Parchi P (2013) Prion protein misfolding, strains, and neurotoxicity: an update from studies on mammalian prions. Int J Cell Biol 2013:910314. https://doi.org/10.1155/2013/910314
47. Puoti G, Bizzi A, Forloni G, Safar JG, Tagliavini F, Gambetti P (2012) Sporadic human prion diseases: molecular insights and diagnosis. Lancet Neurol 11: 618–628. https://doi.org/10.1016/s1474-4422(12)70063-7
48. Ritchie DL, Barria MA, Peden AH, Yull HM, Kirkpatrick J, Adlard P, Ironside JW, Head MW (2017) UK iatrogenic Creutzfeldt-Jakob disease: investigating human prion transmission across genotypic barriers using human tissue-based and molecular approaches. Acta Neuropathol 133:579–595. https://doi.org/10.1007/s00401-016-1638-x
49. Rodriguez-Diehl R, Rey MJ, Gironell A, Martinez-Saez E, Ferrer I, Sanchez-Valle R, Jague J, Nos C, Gelpi E (2012) "Preclinical" MSA in definite Creutzfeldt-Jakob disease. Neuropathology 32:158–163. https://doi.org/10.1111/j.1440-1789.2011.01232.x
50. Safar J, Prusiner SB (1998) Molecular studies of prion diseases. Prog Brain Res 117:421–434
51. Safar JG, Xiao X, Kabir ME, Chen S, Kim C, Haldiman T, Cohen Y, Chen W, Cohen ML, Surewicz WK (2015) Structural determinants of phenotypic diversity and replication rate of human prions. PLoS Pathog 11:e1004832. https://doi.org/10.1371/journal.ppat.1004832
52. Shively SB, Horkayne-Szakaly I, Jones RV, Kelly JP, Armstrong RC, Perl DP (2016) Characterisation of interface astroglial scarring in the human brain after blast exposure: a post-mortem case series. Lancet Neurol 15:944–953. https://doi.org/10.1016/s1474-4422(16)30057-6
53. Soto C, Pritzkow S (2018) Protein Misfolding, aggregation and conformational strains in neurodegenerative diseases. Nat Neurosci 21:1332–1340
54. Spires-Jones TL, Attems J, Thal DR (2017) Interactions of pathological proteins in neurodegenerative diseases. Acta Neuropathol 134:187–205. https://doi.org/10.1007/s00401-017-1709-7
55. Stein TD, Montenigro PH, Alvarez VE, Xia W, Crary JF, Tripodis Y, Daneshvar DH, Mez J, Solomon T, Meng G et al (2015) Beta-amyloid deposition in chronic traumatic encephalopathy. Acta Neuropathol 130:21–34. https://doi.org/10.1007/s00401-015-1435-y
56. Stern RA, Daneshvar DH, Baugh CM, Seichepine DR, Montenigro PH, Riley DO, Fritts NG, Stamm JM, Robbins CA, McHale L et al (2013) Clinical presentation of chronic traumatic encephalopathy. Neurology 81:1122–1129. https://doi.org/10.1212/WNL.0b013e3182a55f7f
57. Telling GC, Parchi P, DeArmond SJ, Cortelli P, Montagna P, Gabizon R, Mastrianni J, Lugaresi E, Gambetti P, Prusiner SB (1996) Evidence for the conformation of the pathologic isoform of the prion protein enciphering and propagating prion diversity. Science 274:2079–2082
58. Tousseyn T, Bajsarowicz K, Sanchez H, Gheyara A, Oehler A, Geschwind M, DeArmond B, DeArmond SJ (2015) Prion disease induces Alzheimer disease-like Neuropathologic changes. J Neuropathol Exp Neurol 74:873–888. https://doi.org/10.1097/nen.0000000000000228
59. Tsuchiya K, Yagishita S, Ikeda K, Sano M, Taki K, Hashimoto K, Watabiki S, Mizusawa H (2004) Coexistence of CJD and Alzheimer's disease: an autopsy case showing typical clinical features of CJD. Neuropathology 24:46–55
60. Vasconcelos B, Stancu IC, Buist A, Bird M, Wang P, Vanoosthuyse A, Van Kolen K, Verheyen A, Kienlen-Campard P, Octave JN et al (2016) Heterotypic seeding of tau fibrillization by pre-aggregated Abeta provides potent seeds for prion-like seeding and propagation of tau-pathology in vivo. Acta Neuropathol 131:549–569. https://doi.org/10.1007/s00401-015-1525-x
61. Weiner MW, Crane PK, Montine TJ, Bennett DA, Veitch DP (2017) Traumatic brain injury may not increase the risk of Alzheimer disease. Neurology 89: 1923–1925. https://doi.org/10.1212/wnl.0000000000004608
62. Zerr I, Brandel JP, Masullo C, Wientjens D, de Silva R, Zeidler M, Granieri E, Sampaolo S, van Duijn C, Delasnerie-Laupretre N et al (2000) European surveillance on Creutzfeldt-Jakob disease: a case-control study for medical risk factors. J Clin Epidemiol 53:747–754
63. Zou WQ, Capellari S, Parchi P, Sy MS, Gambetti P, Chen SG (2003) Identification of novel proteinase K-resistant C-terminal fragments of PrP in Creutzfeldt-Jakob disease. J Biol Chem 278:40429–40436. https://doi.org/10.1074/jbc.M308550200
64. Zou WQ, Zheng J, Gray DM, Gambetti P, Chen SG (2004) Antibody to DNA detects scrapie but not normal prion protein. Proc Natl Acad Sci U S A 101: 1380–1385. https://doi.org/10.1073/pnas.0307825100

10

Amyloid-beta and phosphorylated tau in post-mortem Alzheimer's disease retinas

Jurre den Haan[1*†], Tjado H. J. Morrema[2†], Frank D. Verbraak[3], Johannes F. de Boer[4], Philip Scheltens[1], Annemieke J. Rozemuller[2], Arthur A. B. Bergen[5,6], Femke H. Bouwman[1] and Jeroen J. Hoozemans[2]

Abstract

In-vivo labeling of retinal amyloid-beta(Aβ) and tau has potential as non-invasive biomarker for Alzheimer's disease (AD). However, literature on the presence of Aβ and phosphorylated tau (pTau) in AD retinas is inconclusive. We therefore assessed the presence of Aβ and pTau in post-mortem retinas in 6 AD and 6 control cases who donated brains and eyes to the Netherlands Brain Bank. Neuropathological diagnosis of AD was made according to NIA-AA criteria. Formalin fixed retinas were dissected in quadrants and cross-sections of medial and superior retinas were made. Immuno-histochemical stainings were performed for Aβ, amyloid precursor protein (APP) and pTau. To assess translation to an in-vivo set up using curcumin as labelling fluorophore, co-stainings with curcumin were performed. No typical Aβ-plaques and neurofibrillary tangles, like in the cerebral cortex, were observed in AD retinas. A diffuse immunoreactive signal for pTau was increased in the inner and outer plexiform layers of the retina in AD cases compared to control cases with absence of cerebral amyloid pathology. Immunostaining with anti-Aβ and anti-APP antibodies yielded signal in ganglion cells, amacrine cells, horizontal cells and Müller cells in both control and AD cases. We observed small extracellular deposits positive for anti-Aβ antibodies 12F4 and 6E10 and negative for 4G8 and curcumin. A subset of these deposits could be characterized as corpora amylacea. In conclusion we found that retinal manifestations of AD pathology appear to be different compared to cerebral AD pathology. Using a qualitative cross-sectional approach, we did not find Aβ/APP related differences in the retina between AD and control subjects. In contrast, tau related changes were found to be present in cases with cerebral AD pathology, suggesting retinal tau as a potential biomarker for AD.

Keywords: Retina, Amyloid, Tau, Post-mortem, Alzheimer's disease, Neurodegeneration

Introduction

Alzheimer's disease (AD) is the leading cause of dementia [1] and its pathology develops 15–20 years before symptom onset [19]. Key pathological hallmarks of AD are neuronal loss, extra-cellular accumulation of amyloid-plaques containing amyloid-beta (Aβ) and neurofibrillary tangles containing tau [6]. In addition, cerebral amyloid angiopathy (CAA) [33] and neuro-inflammation [13] are recognized as important events involved in AD pathology. The retina, embryologically derived from the diencephalon and sharing many features with brain tissue, is hypothesized to serve as a 'window to the brain,' as neuropathological changes in retinal neurons might mirror brain pathology [26]. Non-invasive retinal imaging is routinely performed in ophthalmology clinics with high resolution imaging (±5 μm). Fluorescent imaging of specific proteins is on the horizon and might serve as a non-invasive diagnostic tool to visualize molecular processes involved in ophthalmological and neurological disease [5, 7, 22].

Previous post-mortem studies have investigated the presence of pathological changes in human retinas in AD, however the detection of these changes was not consistent across these studies [20]. On the one hand, neuronal thinning, ganglion cell loss and tau deposition are reported [3, 30]. On the other hand, Aβ deposition was found in whole mounted retinas and cross-sections by three studies from one lab, preferentially affecting the

* Correspondence: j.denhaan1@vumc.nl
†Jurre den Haan and Tjado H. J. Morrema contributed equally to this work.
[1]Department of Neurology, Alzheimer Center Amsterdam, Amsterdam Neuroscience, Vrije Universiteit Amsterdam, Amsterdam UMC, Mailbox 7057, Amsterdam 1007 MB, The Netherlands
Full list of author information is available at the end of the article

superior retina [22–24]. Recently, results from an in-vivo study showed an increase in retinal fluorescence after curcumin supplementation in AD patients, hypothesized to reflect retinal amyloid [22]. However, Aβ presence in the retina still remains controversial as three other groups were unable to replicate this finding in AD retinas [14, 30, 34].

Possible explanations for these discrepancies are differences in methodology, as well as interpretation of findings. First, different anti-Aβ antibodies were used (including 6E10, 12F4, 6F3D and 4G8). Second, different methods of processing and dissection of retinas were applied, as some groups prepared retinal cross-sections while others generated flat mounts. A cross-sectional approach yields morphological information on layer distribution of the pathology, at the cost of sampling bias, due to the limited surface covered. In contrast, using flat mounts, a large surface of the retina is studied, yet lacking layer information. Lastly, with the predilection of pathology in the superior retina reported [22], it might be that other groups assessed parts of the retina with less pathological changes.

To better understand retinal involvement in AD pathology, we explored the presence of AD pathology with different antibodies in post-mortem retinal and brain tissue of patients with a definite post-mortem diagnosis of AD, in order to assess molecular targets for in vivo (fluorescent) retinal imaging in AD.

Materials and methods

Subjects

We assessed retinal tissue of 6 AD patients and 6 controls who donated their brain and eyes to the Dutch Brain Bank between 2010 and 2015. Neuropathological diagnosis of AD was made following NIA-AA criteria including Braak and Braak-staging for neurofibrillary tangles and amyloid, and CERAD-staging for neuritic plaques [4, 17]. We selected cases with a clinical diagnosis of AD and neuropathological staging of Braak ≥ 4. Controls were adults without cognitive decline and Braak ≤2. We excluded cases with other neurodegenerative diseases based on history or post-mortem diagnosis. Cohort characteristics are shown in Table 1.

Table 1 Cohort characteristics

#	Pathological diagnosis	Sex	Age	Braak	Amyloid
1	AD	F	73	VI	C
2	AD	M	70	VI	C
3	AD	M	56	V	C
4	AD	F	91	V	C
5	AD	F	95	IV	C
6	AD	F	89	IV	C
7	HC	F	89	II	B
8	HC	M	80	II	C
9	HC	F	76	II	O
10	HC	F	79	II	O
11	HC	F	57	0	A
12	HC	M	49	0	O

AD Alzheimer's disease, *HC* Healthy control

Tissue processing

Within 12 h post-mortem, eyes were removed. The anterior parts of the eye, including the cornea and lens, were dissected and the eyecup was filled with tissue-tek (cat# 4583, Sakura). Eyes were snap frozen using iso-pentane at − 100 °C and stored at − 80 °C. Eyes were defrosted in 4% PFA at room temperature for 48 h prior to dissection. The eye was dissected in four quadrants through the vertical and horizontal meridian resulting in naso-superior, naso-inferior, temporal-superior and temporal-inferior quadrants containing retinal tissue from macula to ora serrata (Fig. 1). Quadrants were dehydrated prior to embedding in paraffin according to the following protocol: 3 h formalin 4% at 35 °C, 1 h ethanol 70% 35 °C, 1 h ethanol 80% 35 °C, 1 h ethanol 96% 35 °C, 3 times 1 h alcohol 100% 35 °C, 3 times 1 h xylene 35 °C, 4 times 1 h paraffin 62 °C. Paraffin embedded tissue was sectioned using a microtome at 5-μm and 10-μm thickness and mounted on TOMO slides (cat# TOM-1190, Matsunami). Mounted slides were dried overnight at 37 °C prior to staining. Per patient, at least 25 sections per region were stained with APP/Aβ antibodies to overcome sampling bias.

Immunohistochemistry (IHC)

Immunohistochemistry was initially performed on 5 and 10 μm thick eye sections. As both thicknesses yielded comparable results, 10 μm sections were therefore used for the full cohort. Sections were deparaffinized and endogenous peroxidase activity was suppressed with 0.3% H_2O_2 in phosphate buffered saline (PBS) for 30 min. Antigen retrieval was performed with 10 mM/L pH 6.0 sodium citrate buffer heated by autoclave. Sections were incubated overnight at room temperature with primary antibody, diluted in antibody diluent (cat# kpxxabb500, immunologic). For primary antibodies details and dilutions, see Table 2. Omission of the primary antibodies was taken along as negative controls. Positive controls consisted of 5 μm thick paraffin sections of hippocampal regions of AD patients. Sections were incubated for 30 min with envision (cat# 5007, DAKO). 3,3′-Diaminobenzine (DAB) was used for color development. Nuclear counterstaining consisted of Mayers hematoxylin. Sections were dehydrated and cover slipped using quick-D (cat# 7281, Klinipath).

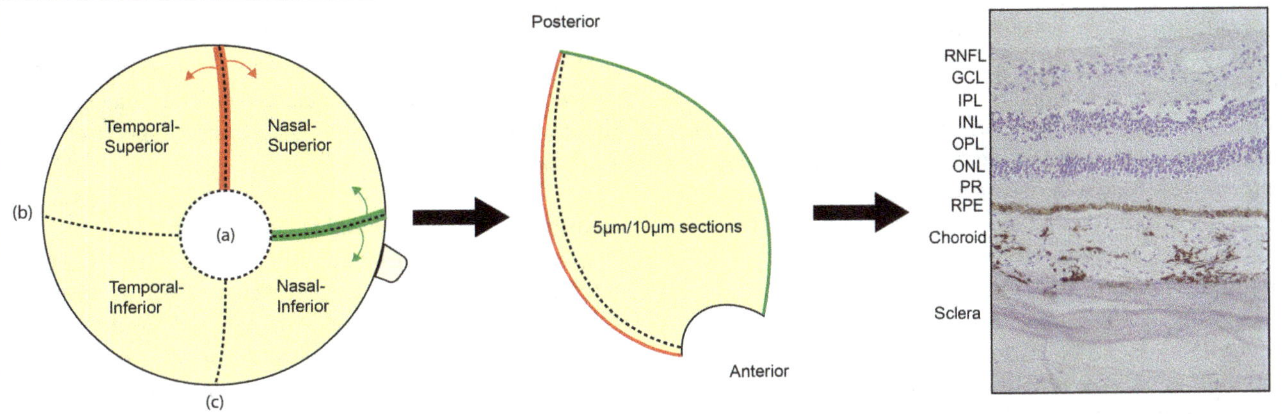

Fig. 1 Processing of post-mortem eyes. Anterior parts of eyes were removed (a). Formalin fixed eyes were dissected through the horizontal (b) and vertical meridian (c). Superior (red, arrows) and nasal (green, arrows) parts were cut in 10 µm sections from anterior to posterior. As a result, sections contained all retinal layers from ora serrata to the posterior pole: retinal nerve fiber layer (RNFL), ganglion cell layer (GCL), inner plexiform layer (IPL), inner nuclear layer (INL), outer plexiform layer (OPL), outer nuclear layer (ONL), photoreceptors (PR), retinal pigment epithelium (RPE), choroid and sclera

Alternatively, when liquid permanent red (LPR) was used as chromogen, sections were incubated for 30 min with goat anti-mouse alkaline phosphatase (AP) (1:250, cat# d0456, DAKO) at room temperature, after incubation with the primary antibody. After washing 3 times with TRIS buffered saline (TBS) sections were incubated with LPR (cat#0640, DAKO), substituted with 1 mM levamisole (to block endogenous alkaline phosphatase from blood vessels), until signal could be observed microscopically. Nuclear counterstaining was performed using Mayer's hematoxylin. Section were cover-slipped using aquatex (cat#1.08562.0050, Merck).

Curcumin

Curcumin (cat# 9386, Sigma Aldrich) was dissolved in 0.5 M NaOH to a stock concentration of 20 mg/ml and diluted to a final concentration of 0.1 mg/ml curcumin using PBS. Deparaffinized and rehydrated sections were incubated with 0.1 mg/ml curcumin for 10 min at room

Table 2 Primary antibodies used in this study

Group	Name	Epitope	Source	Concentration
APP/Aβ	12F4	Amyloid-beta$_{1-42}$	Biolegend San Diego, CA, USA	1:100
	6E10	Amyloid-beta$_{1-16}$	Covance, BioLegend, San Diego, CA, USA	1:800
	4G8	Amyloid-beta$_{17-24}$	Biolegend, San Diego, CA	1:8000
	APP	APP Y188, c-terminal (aa 750)	ABCAM, Cambridge, UK	1:6000
Tau	HT7	Tau between residue 159 and 163	Invitrogen, Thermo Fisher Scientific, MA, USA	1:8000
	AT-270	Tau phosphorylated at Thr 181	Thermo Scientific, MA, USA	1:100
	AT8	Tau phosphorylated at Ser 202, Thr205	Innogenetics, Ghent, Belgium	1:800
	AT-100	Tau phosphorylated Ser 212, Thr 214	Thermo Scientific, MA, USA	1:1000
	Anti-pS422	Tau Fibrils	ABCAM, Cambridge, UK	1:400
	MC-1	Paired helical filaments	Peter Davies, Pathology and Neuroscience, Donald and Barbara Zucker School of Medicine, Northwell, NY, USA [21]	1:1000
Other	Curcumin	Fibrillar Aβ and CAA	Sigma Aldrich, St. Louis, MO, USA	0,1 mg/ml in NaOH
	Thioflavin	Amyloid	Sigma Aldrich, St. Louis, MO, USA	1% in distilled water
	Kluver-PAS	Polysaccharides	Kluver: Luxol fast blue, BDH laboratory supplies, Avantor, PA, USA, PAS: Schiff's reagens, VWR, Avantor, PA, USA	0.1% in alcohol 96% n.a.

temperature, washed with PBS for 3 times 10 min and covered using TBS/glycerol mounting medium.

Thioflavin-S

Thioflavin-S staining was performed by incubating deparaffinized and rehydrated sections with 1% thioflavin-S (cat# T1897, Sigma Aldrich) in distilled water for 1 min, followed by removal of excess thioflavin-S using 70% alcohol. Stained sections were covered using TBS/glycerol mounting medium.

Kluver-PAS

Deparaffinized and rehydrated sections were incubated with 0.1% luxol fast blue (cat# 3404438, BDH laboratory supplies) overnight at 37 °C. Sections were subsequently rinsed in ethanol 96% and distilled water. Differentiation was performed by rinsing the slides in 0.1% lithium-carbonate, followed by 70% ethanol and distilled water. Subsequently, the sections were incubated with 0.8% periodic acid for 10 min, followed by rinsing in tap water and distilled water. Sections were incubated with Schiff's reagent (cat# 30969.261, VWR) for 30 min, followed by washing in tap water. Kluver-PAS stained sections were counterstained using Mayer's hematoxylin, quickly dehydrated using alcohol and xylene and covered using quick-D.

PAS-IHC double staining

Deparaffinized and rehydrated sections were incubated and DAB stained as described above. DAB stained sections were washed in distilled water and incubated with 0.8% periodic acid for 10 min. Subsequently, sections were incubated with Schiff's reagent for 30 min, washed with tap water and counterstained using Mayer's hematoxylin. Stained sections were quickly dehydrated using ethanol and xylene and covered using quick-D.

Fluorescent co-stainings with curcumin

Sections were deparaffinized and treated with citrate buffer as described above. Subsequently, curcumin staining was performed as described above. After curcumin staining, sections were washed 3 times for 10 min using PBS. Primary antibody was incubated overnight at room temperature. Sections were washed 3 times with PBS and incubated with fluorescently-labelled secondary antibody (1:250, alexa 594, cat# A11037, Invitrogen) for 3 h. After labelling the sections were washed in PBS and covered using DAPI containing mounting medium (cat# 0100–20, Southern Biotech).

Imaging

IHC sections were imaged by an Olympus BX41 photomicroscope using Leica Application Suite (LAS) AF lite software (Wetzlar, Germany). Fluorescently stained sections were imaged by a Leica DMi8 fluorescence microscope using LAS AF lite and ImageJ software (National Institute of Health, USA). Spectra of the Kluver-DAB double stainings were analysed using a nuance spectral imager (Perkin Elmer). Colors were assigned to binary spectra images using ImageJ.

Quantification tau immunohistochemistry

For quantitative assessment sections were photographed at four regions of interest (ROI's) from ora serrata to posterior pole of medial and superior cross-sections for each patient using an Olympus BX41 photomicroscope. Dimensions of ROI's were 316 μm × 115 μm. The DAB positive surface area (%) within the neuroretina was quantified using the color threshold plugin in ImageJ. Between group differences were assessed using a Mann-Whitney U test, using SPSS (version 22.0).

Results

Immunohistochemical detection of amyloid-beta and APP in the retina

Medial and superior retinal cross-sections were immunostained for Aβ-plaque pathology using anti-Aβ antibodies 6E10 and 12F4. Retinas stained with 6E10 showed intracellular positivity in specific retinal cell-types including ganglion cells (Fig. 2c), cells in the upper and lower portion of the inner nuclear layer (INL), most likely reflecting amacrine- and horizontal cells respectively (Fig. 2e,f), and Müller cells (Fig. 2g). In addition, staining in vessel walls (Fig. 2d) and in drusen was observed (Fig. 2h). Small extracellular deposits (5–20 μm) were incidentally seen in the ganglion cell layer (GCL) and inner plexiform layer (IPL), with a predilection for the superior retina (Fig. 2b and Fig. 3a). These deposits were small (5-20 μm), often rounded and were morphologically different from cored plaques, diffuse plaques or fibrillary plaques observed in AD brain tissue. Retinas immunostained with 12F4 showed intracellular staining of ganglion cells as well (with a granular aspect), staining in vessel walls and immunostaining of small extracellular deposits in the GCL and IPL, similar as observed with 6E10 staining (Fig. 3a). Above described immunopositive features using antibodies 6E10 and 12F4 were more apparent in the superior part of the retina then in the medial part. Global assessment of the above described features in cross-sections of 6 control and 6 AD cases did not separate AD from control cases (Fig. 3a).

In addition to Aβ, the antibody 6E10 also detects full length APP [16, 35]. Using an antibody directed against APP (C-terminal amino acid (aa) 750), similar staining as compared with 6E10 was seen in ganglion cells, amacrine cells, horizontal cells and Müller cells (Fig. 3a), but

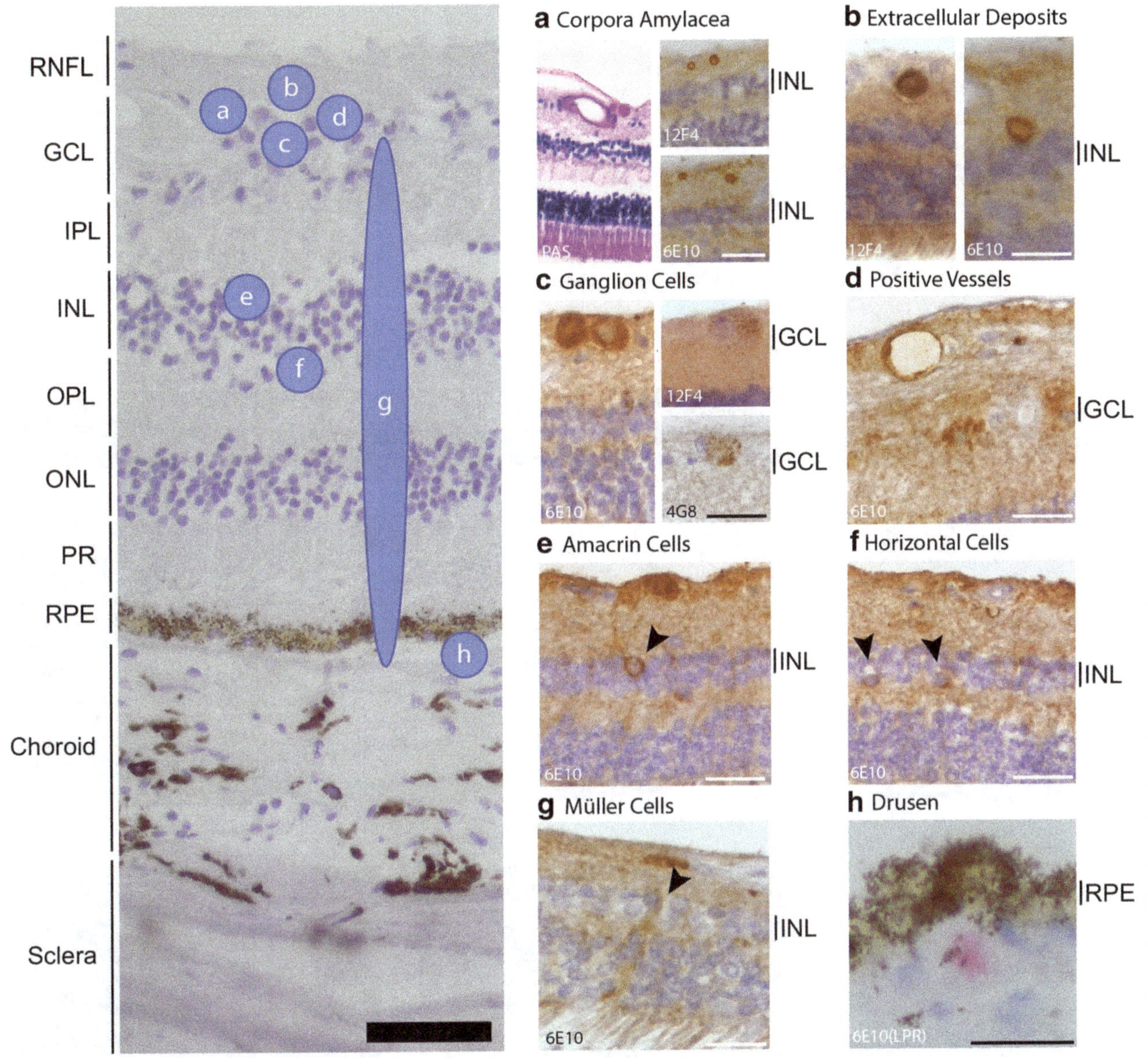

Fig. 2 Overview of different structures positive for different anti-Aβ antibodies. Overview of structures that were stained with anti-Aβ antibodies 6E10,12F4 and 4G8. Distribution of these structures over retinal layers is shown on the left (**a-h**). Abbreviations: RNFL = retinal nerve fiber layer, GCL = ganglion cell layer, IPL = inner plexiform layer, INL = inner nuclear layer, OPL = outer plexiform layer, ONL = outer nuclear layer, PR = photo receptors, RPE = retinal pigment epithelium, LPR = liquid permanent red. Scale bars 50 μm

not in extracellular and vascular deposits. Subsequently, as extracellular and vascular positivity was not observed after APP immunostaining, we expanded our stainings with anti-Aβ antibodies with less affinity for APP. Anti-Aβ antibody 4G8 showed no extracellular positivity or positivity in blood vessels in AD or control retinas (Fig. 3a). Incidentally, granular staining of ganglion cells was observed with 4G8 (Fig. 2c). Lastly, additional staining with Thioflavin-S, did not show positive staining, while plaques and tangles were observed in AD hippocampal tissue (Fig. 3a).

In summary, intracellular staining was observed with 12F4 and 6E10 and APP antibodies. In addition, 6E10 and 12F4 antibodies showed small extracellular deposits that were negative for 4G8 and APP antibodies.

Corpora amylacea are detected in AD and control retina

We investigated whether the small 6E10/12F4 positive, 4G8 negative deposits, could be related to corpora amylacea, deposits associated with aging as well as neurodegeneration [29]. We therefore assessed these deposits using a combination of 6E10 antibody and Kluver-PAS

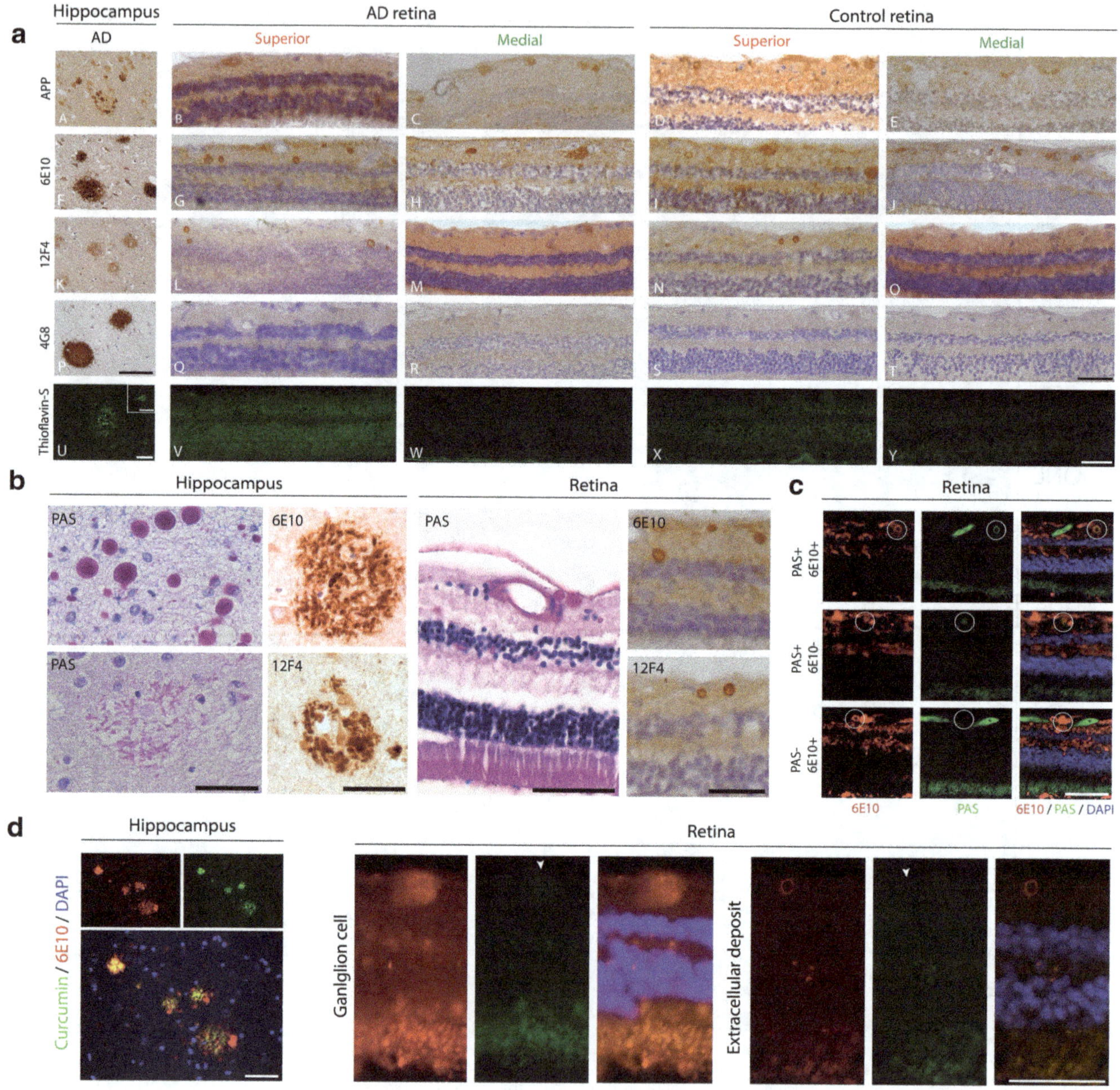

Fig. 3 APP/Aβ in the medial and superior retina. **a** Representative stainings for APP/Aβ antibodies and amyloid (Thioflavin-S) in AD hippocampus and AD and control retinas showing different staining patterns for different antibodies (superior and medial). **b** Kluver-PAS staining of corpora amylacea in hippocampus and retina compared to 6E10 and 12F4 stainings. **c** IHC co-stainings with PAS and 6E10. **d** Curcumin and 6E10 co-staining in AD hippocampus and in retinas showing a positive ganglion cell and extracellular deposit. All size bars 50 μm

staining, a histochemical staining routinely used for the detection of corpora amylacea. With the Kluver-PAS we observed staining of corpora amylacea in AD brain tissue, while plaques were not or only faintly labeled (Fig. 3b). Retinas of both AD and controls showed extracellular, rounded depositions with the Kluver-PAS staining, that were comparable in size and localization to the structures observed with the 6E10 and 12F4 antibodies in adjacent retinal cross-sections (Fig. 3b).

Next we performed double-labelling combining the Kluver-PAS staining with immunodetection with the 6E10 antibody. A subset of 6E10 positive deposits co-localized with Kluver-PAS positive deposits, while others were Kluver-PAS negative (Fig. 3c). In addition, we also observed PAS positive, 6E10 negative deposits (Fig. 3c).

To assess fibrillarity of extracellular deposits and enable translation of our findings to in-vivo imaging with curcumin, we performed Thioflavin-S and curcumin stainings of adjacent sections [8]. No extracellular deposits were detected with curcumin or Thioflavin-S (Fig. 3a and d). This finding was confirmed by fluorescent co-stainings with 6E10 and curcumin (Fig. 3d). Fluorescent co-stainings with 6E10 and curcumin did show co-localization of (faint) curcumin staining with 6E10 intracellularly (Fig. 3d).

In summary, we observed corpora amylacea in AD and control retina that explained a proportion of small 6E10 immunopositive extracellular deposits. These extracellular deposits were negative for Thioflavin or curcumin.

Tau and phosphorylated tau in AD and control retina

Next to amyloid pathology, AD is characterized by tau pathology, which encompasses accumulation of phosphorylated tau (pTau) in neuropil threads, neurofibrillary tangles (NFTs) and neuritic plaques, primarily in cortical areas of the brain [31]. We therefore assessed presence of tau and its phosphorylated isoforms in AD and control retinas. As reported previously [25], total tau assessed with antibody HT7 shows tau distribution in three distinct layers in the inner plexiform layer (IPL) and diffusely in the outer plexiform layer (OPL) (Fig. 4). Diffuse axonal positivity in IPL and OPL was observed with anti-pTau antibodies AT8, AT100 and AT270 (Fig. 4). Overall, more immunoreactivity for AT8, AT100 and AT270 was present in AD cases compared to controls (Fig. 5). However, no structures related to NFTs, neuropil threads or neuritic plaques, as observed in the cerebral cortex, were observed with these antibodies in AD or control retinas. pTau (AT8) staining was more apparent in superior than in medial parts of the retina and showed a positive gradient towards the periphery (Fig. 5). Two controls with an amyloid Braak stage B and C showed similar pTau (AT8) patterns as observed in the retina of AD cases. Table 3 shows quantification of AT8 immunoreactivity in medial and superior retinas of AD versus control cases. Mean surface of AT8 immunopositivity in medial and superior parts of the retina did not statistically differ between AD cases and controls (Mann-Whitney U test $p = 0.310$ and $p = 0.537$ respectively), as two controls with moderate to severe amyloid pathology were considerable outliers. Stratified for amyloid stage, cases with a moderate to severe amyloid stage (B,C) showed higher AT8 immunopositivity compared to cases with low amyloid stages (O, A) in medial (Mean 5.28% (±9.83) vs. 0.01%(±0.01), Mann-Whitney U test, $p = 0.004$) and superior parts of the retina (Mean 12.14%(±15.60) vs. 0.06%(±0.08), Mann-Whitney U test, $p = 0.012$). No immunostaining in control and AD retina was observed with anti-tau pS422 or antibody MC-1, which specifically detects paired helical filaments (Fig. 4).

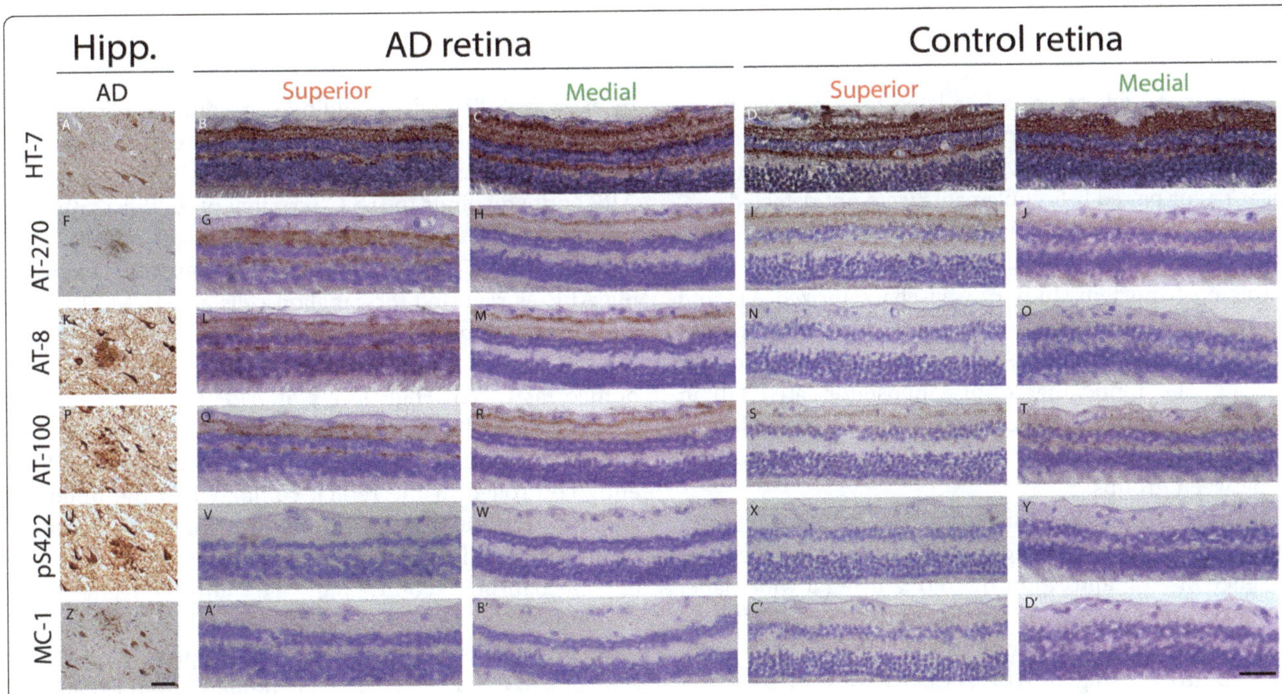

Fig. 4 (Phosphorylated) tau in AD retinas. Representative stainings of different tau antibodies in AD hippocampus and AD and control retinas (superior and medial). Antibodies are associated with total tau (HT-7), phosphorylated tau (AT-270, AT-8, AT-100), tau fibrils (anti-pS422) and paired helical filaments (MC-1). Size bars: 50 µm. Hipp. = hippocampus

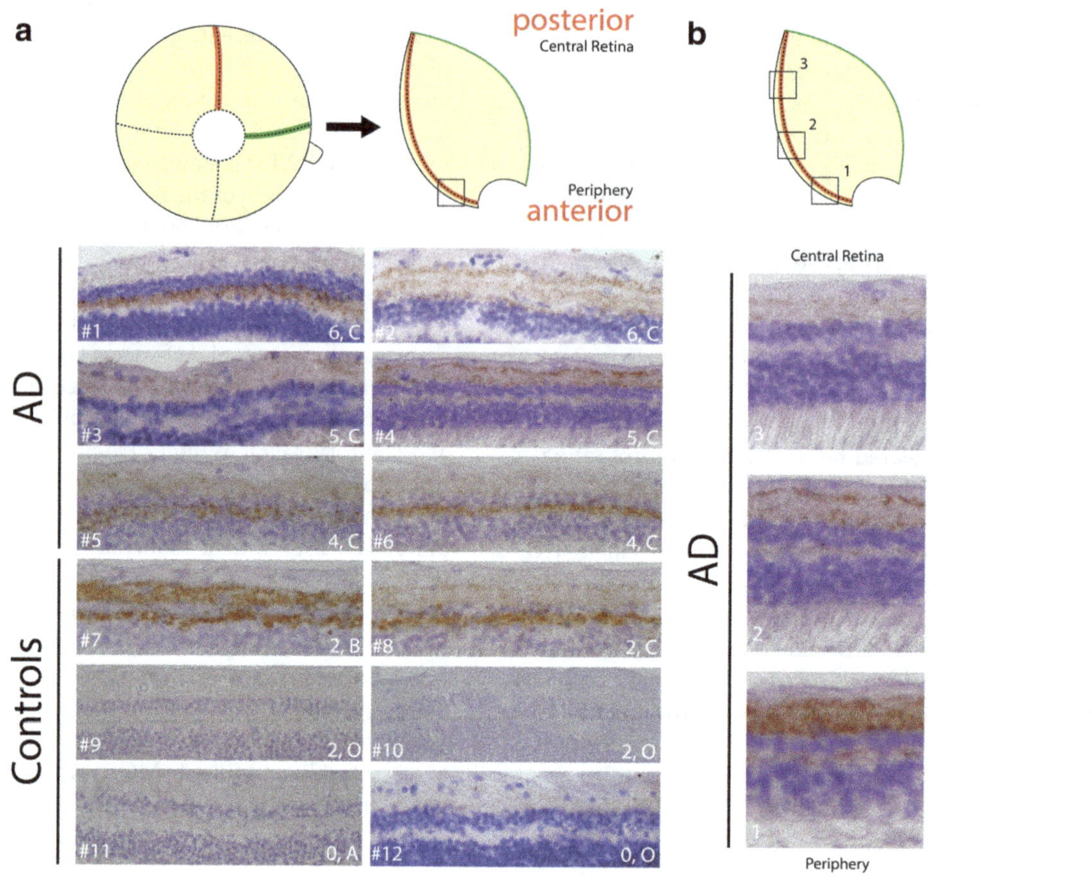

Fig. 5 Phosphorylated tau in AD and control retinas. **a** Representative pictures of phosphorylated tau (AT8) stainings of the anterior part of superior retinas for each subject. Case numbers are indicated on the left and Braak Tau and Braak Amyloid stage are indicated on the right. **b** Positive gradient of phosphorylated tau staining towards the periphery in a representative AD case (#4)

In summary, diffuse phosphorylated tau for three phosphorylation sites was observed in AD, with a predilection for the peripheral retina, while NFTs, neuritic plaques, fibrillar tau or paired helical filaments were not detected.

Discussion

In this post-mortem study of well-characterized AD and control cases, we qualitatively assessed antibody panels for APP, Aβ and tau on AD and control retinal cross-sections. We found that diffuse phosphorylated tau in the retina separated AD cases from controls while immunoreactivity for APP and Aβ in the retina did not differ between groups.

In order to resolve discrepancies between studies reporting retinal Aβ we, for the first time, assessed the presence of APP and Aβ in the retina using a wide panel of antibodies. Our results implicate that APP/Aβ pathology in the retina does not clearly separate AD cases from controls. Using an APP antibody we showed that a large proportion of immunostaining with 6E10 and 12F4 showed overlap with, and could be explained by, intracellular staining of APP in retinal cell types that are known to express APP [28]. In addition, it could also represent intraneuronal β-secretase cleaved APP β-C-terminal fragments (CTFs) including C83, C99 and AICD [11], as our APP antibody binds to the C-terminal of APP (aa750). We hypothesize that intracellular APP/Aβ might reflect metabolic activity in different retinal cell populations expressing APP, as reported for ganglion cells and INL cells [28], and (efficient) processing of APP/Aβ to the outer retina by Müller cells, cells that are responsible for retinal homeostasis [32]. High levels of APP in the absence of clear extracellular fibrillar Aβ deposits suggests that the amyloidogenic and non-amyloidogenic pathway are differently controlled in the retina, compared to the brain. In addition, the build-up of fibrillar Aβ might be confined to the intracellular compartment in the retina. Assessment of mechanisms controlling the amyloidogenic and non-amyloidogenic pathways in the retina is therefore needed to assess the precise role of Aβ processing in the retina in AD and aging. Understanding these mechanisms the role of retinal amyloid as non-invasive biomarker, but could also yield information on selective vulnerability or resilience of specific neuronal populations [9].

Table 3 Quantification of phosporylated Tau (AT8) Positivity

#	Pathological diagnosis	Braak Tau	Braak Amyloid	AT8 positivity (% surface area)			
				Superior		Medial	
				Mean	sd	Mean	sd
1	AD	VI	C	3,41	2,82	1,88	0,44
2	AD	VI	C	0,79	0,70	1,07	0,55
3	AD	V	C	1,35	0,38	0,04	0,05
4	AD	V	C	15,36	5,13	4,12	2,52
5	AD	IV	C	6,87	1,02	0,37	0,01
6	AD	IV	C	8,72	1,65	1,97	1,25
			Mean	6.08	5.50	1.57	1.47
7	HC	II	B	48,65	8,73	29,35	2,62
8	HC	II	C	11,92	1,84	3,43	1,87
9	HC	II	O	0,15	0,18	0,00	0,01
10	HC	II	O	–	–	0,01	0,01
11	HC	0	A	0,02	0,02	0,03	0,02
12	HC	0	O	0,01	0,01	0,00	0,00
			Mean	12.15	21.04	5.50	11.78

Means and standard deviations (sd) of AT8 positivity (% surface area) of four superior and medial pictures per patient. *AD* Alzheimer's disease, *HC* Healthy control

We replicated earlier findings of small extracellular deposits positive for 6E10 and 12F4 antibodies in the RNFL and GCL with a predilection to the superior retina [22]. Morphologically these deposits were different from Aβ-plaques observed in the cortex and hippocampus, smaller and also observed in control cases. Using a wide panel of anti-Aβ and APP antibodies we further characterized these deposits, considering cross-reactivity towards Aβ and APP by these antibodies [16]. Interestingly, observed deposits were negative for an anti-Aβ antibody with relatively less affinity for APP (4G8). In addition, an anti-APP antibody directed at the C-terminal (aa 750) did not show immunoreactivity towards these extracellular deposits. As 6E10 is directed to $A\beta_{3-10}$ and has affinity for APP, a possible explanation is that 6E10 recognizes an APP isoform that is not detected by the used APP antibody, for instance the soluble APPα isoform that lacks the C-terminal part of APP. Extracellular immunopositivity with the 12F4 antibody could be explained by detection of IgMs by 12F4 as described in previous literature [2]. Using IHC co-stainings with Kluver-PAS, we showed that a proportion of these deposits can be characterized as corpora amylacea, deposits previously associated with aging and neurodegeneration in the brain [29]. Finally, the absence of co-staining of these deposits with curcumin and Thioflavin suggests absence of fibrillar structures, like fibrillar Aβ [8], and questions whether these deposits can be visualized in-vivo using curcumin [22].

Secondly, we assessed the presence of tau, its phosphorylated isoforms, fibrillar tau (pS422) and paired helical filaments (MC-1). Using antibodies AT8, AT100 and AT270 directed at different phospho-epitopes of tau revealed a diffuse signal in the inner plexiform layer (IPL) and outer plexiform layer (OPL) of AD cases, while NFT's, neuropil threads and neuritic plaques were not observed. In addition, we observed no fibrillar tau or paired helical filaments. A previous report by Schön and coworkers also showed a diffuse signal of pTau with AT8, while phosphorylation sites detected by AT100, AT180 and AT270 yielded negative results [30]. In addition, similar to our study no fibrillary tau was observed, while in contrast to our findings, intracellular inclusions (NFTs) were observed in 5 out of 6 AD cases using the AT8 antibody. Discrepancies with this study may be explained by differences in antibody dilutions, retinal regions studied and differences in expression of retinal pathology between AD patients.

The diffuse signal of pTau observed in the current study was most apparent in the peripheral retina, as reported previously in tau transgenic mice [15]. This, might be of interest for in-vivo studies that currently mainly focus on imaging of the central retina. Recent developments in imaging technology make it possible to perform in-vivo peripheral imaging of the retina. This may be a promising step forward in visualizing AD pathology in the peripheral retina [27].

Interestingly, two cognitively normal controls with moderate amyloid pathology showed intense tau staining patterns similar to AD cases. This might suggest early involvement of tau-pathology in the retina in AD. Mechanistically, this could be the result of local pathology or transneuronal propagation of phosphorylated tau originating in the visual cortices [10]. Supporting the latter, both control cases had moderate to severe amyloid pathology in their visual cortices that could have already contributed to local toxicity to dendrites and subsequent tau phosphorylation [18]. On the other hand, caution is warranted for the (over)interpretation of these findings, as tau phosphorylation might also be the result of confounding (retinal) pathology, including glaucoma [12] or an aging effect. Supporting the latter, we observed that a young onset AD case (case #4, 56 years) showed little pTau immunopositivity, while two older controls (case #7 89 years, case #8 80 years) showed apparent diffuse pTau immunopositivity. Future studies in larger cohorts, including patients with a range of Braak and amyloid stages, and considering age as confounder, are needed to assess pTau as a possible AD biomarker in the retina. Studies on different tauopathies are needed to assess the specificity of these findings and the possible use of retinal tau as biomarker in other tauopathies and glaucoma. Finally, development of fluorescent labels for phosphorylated tau for human use is needed in order to translate these findings to an in-vivo set-up using targeted fluorescence. A recent proof of concept study showed the possibility of molecular imaging using targeted fluorescence, by in-vivo labeling of single-cell apoptosis in glaucoma [5].

Important strengths of this study are the use of well-characterized cases and controls, and the use of antibody panels on sequential cross-sections, permitting a qualitative assessment of retinal AD pathology and its layer distribution. Despite the fact that we aimed to address sampling bias by staining a large number of 10 μm thick sections per patient, we should note that we might have missed infrequent pathology, including the temporal and inferior retinal regions. Using flat-mounts in future studies to complement a cross-sectional approach could help overcome sampling bias. Using such an approach, inherently lacking qualitative layer information, caution should be taken that 6E10 and 12F4 positivity includes immunoreactivity towards intracellular APP, corpora amylacea and drusen. Future studies are needed to assess if (peripheral) drusen could represent an increased Aβ reservoir in aging and AD. In addition, for this study a relatively small sample size was assessed using a qualitative approach to assess neuropathological hallmarks of AD in the retina. Disease effects are typically observed in comparable cohorts. However, to further understand observed effects and study whether more subtle changes are present in the retina larger cohorts should be assessed using a quantitative approach.

Conclusion

Our findings confirm the presence of phosphorylated tau in the retina, nuance earlier findings of retinal Aβ and explain negative findings from previous studies, using antibodies with less APP affinity. Independent studies using comparable protocols for tissue processing and staining are needed to resolve discrepancies between different labs [14, 22, 30, 34]. These studies could help determine which of the observed retinal changes are age-related and which are disease related and could serve as a target for in-vivo imaging. In conclusion, neuropathological hallmarks of AD appear differently in the retina compared to the cerebral cortex. Diffuse phosphorylated tau in the peripheral retina might be a promising target for in-vivo imaging.

Abbreviations

°C: Celsius; AD: Alzheimer's disease; APP: Amyloid precursor protein; Aβ: Amyloid-beta; CAA: Cerebral amyloid angiopathy; CERAD: Consortium to establish registry for Alzheimer's disease; DAB: 3,3'-diaminobenzidine; DAPI: 4'6-diamidino-2-phenylindole; GCL: Ganglion cell layer; IHC: Immunohistochemistry; INL: Inner nuclear layer; IPL: Inner plexiform layer; LPR: Liquid permanent red; NBB: The Netherlands brain bank; NFTs: Neurofibrillary tangles; NIA-AA: National Institute of Aging and Alzheimer's Association; OPL: Outer plexiform layer; PAS: Periodic acid Schiff; PBS: Phosphate-buffered saline; PFA: Paraformaldehyde; PR: Photo receptors; pTau: Phosphorylated tau; RNFL: Retinal nerve fiber layer; RPE: Retinal pigment epithelium; TBS: Tris-buffered saline

Acknowledgements

Anti-paired helical filaments antibody (MC-1) was kindly provided by Peter Davies, Pathology and Neuroscience, Donald and Barbara Zucker School of Medicine, Northwell, NY, USA. We kindly thank the Netherlands Brain Bank, J.B. ten Brink and N.P. Smoors, for their contributions to this work.

Funding

This research was funded by Alzheimer Nederland (WE.09–2016-03) and by the Dutch Technology Foundation STW (grant number 13935), which is part of the Netherlands Organisation for Scientific Research (NWO), and which is partly funded by the Ministry of Economic Affairs.

Authors' contributions

JdH, designed the study and experiments, performed analysis, prepared figures and drafted the manuscript. THJM designed experiments, performed the experiments, performed analysis and drafted the manuscript. JJH designed the study, performed analysis and supervised the study. FHB designed and supervised the study. All authors read and approved the final manuscript.

Competing interests

The authors declare that they have no competing interests.

Author details

[1]Department of Neurology, Alzheimer Center Amsterdam, Amsterdam Neuroscience, Vrije Universiteit Amsterdam, Amsterdam UMC, Mailbox 7057, Amsterdam 1007 MB, The Netherlands. [2]Department of Pathology, Amsterdam Neuroscience, Amsterdam UMC, Vrije Universiteit Amsterdam, Amsterdam, The Netherlands. [3]Ophthalmology Department, VU University Medical Center, Amsterdam, The Netherlands. [4]Department of Physics, Bio Laser Lab Amsterdam, VU University, Amsterdam, The Netherlands. [5]Departments of Clinical genetics and Ophthalmology, Amsterdam UMC, Academic Medical Center, University of Amsterdam, Amsterdam, The Netherlands. [6]The Netherlands Institute for Neuroscience (NIN-KNAW), Amsterdam, The Netherlands.

References

1. Association As (2018) Alzheimer's disease facts and figures. https://wwwalzorg/documents_custom/2018-facts-and-figurespdf:
2. Auge E, Cabezon I, Pelegri C, Vilaplana J (2017) New perspectives on corpora amylacea in the human brain. Sci Rep 7:41807. https://doi.org/10.1038/srep41807
3. Blanks JC, Torigoe Y, Hinton DR, Blanks RH (1996) Retinal pathology in Alzheimer's disease. I. Ganglion cell loss in foveal/parafoveal retina. Neurobiol Aging 17:377–384.
4. Braak H, Braak E (1991) Neuropathological stageing of Alzheimer-related changes. Acta Neuropathol 82:239–259.
5. Cordeiro MF, Normando EM, Cardoso MJ, Miodragovic S, Jeylani S, Davis BM, Guo L, Ourselin S, A'Hern R, Bloom PA (2017) Real-time imaging of single neuronal cell apoptosis in patients with glaucoma. Brain 140:1757–1767. https://doi.org/10.1093/brain/awx088
6. Cummings JL (2004) Alzheimer's disease. N Engl J Med 351:56–67. https://doi.org/10.1056/NEJMra040223
7. Davis BM, Crawley L, Pahlitzsch M, Javaid F, Cordeiro MF (2016) Glaucoma: the retina and beyond. Acta Neuropathol 132:807–826. https://doi.org/10.1007/s00401-016-1609-2
8. den Haan J, Morrema THJ, Rozemuller AJ, Bouwman FH, Hoozemans JJM (2018) Different curcumin forms selectively bind fibrillar amyloid beta in post mortem Alzheimer's disease brains: implications for in-vivo diagnostics. Acta Neuropathol Commun 6:75. https://doi.org/10.1186/s40478-018-0577-2
9. Fu H, Hardy J, Duff KE (2018) Selective vulnerability in neurodegenerative diseases. Nature Neuroscience. https://doi.org/10.1038/s41593-018-0221-2

10. Gibbons GS, Lee VMY, Trojanowski JQ (2018) Mechanisms of cell-to-cell transmission of pathological tau: a review. JAMA Neurol. https://doi.org/10.1001/jamaneurol.2018.2505
11. Gouras GK, Tampellini D, Takahashi RH, Capetillo-Zarate E (2010) Intraneuronal beta-amyloid accumulation and synapse pathology in Alzheimer's disease. Acta Neuropathol 119:523–541.
12. Gupta N, Fong J, Ang LC, Yucel YH (2008) Retinal tau pathology in human glaucomas. Can J Ophthalmol 43:53–60. https://doi.org/10.3129/i07-185
13. Heneka MT, Carson MJ, El Khoury J, Landreth GE, Brosseron F, Feinstein DL, Jacobs AH, Wyss-Coray T, Vitorica J, Ransohoff RM et al (2015). Neuroinflammation in Alzheimer's disease. Lancet Neurol 14:388–405. https://doi.org/10.1016/s1474-4422(15)70016-5
14. Ho CY, Troncoso JC, Knox D, Stark W, Eberhart CG (2014) Beta-amyloid, phospho-tau and alpha-synuclein deposits similar to those in the brain are not identified in the eyes of Alzheimer's and Parkinson's disease patients. Brain Pathol 24:25–32. https://doi.org/10.1111/bpa.12070
15. Ho WL, Leung Y, Cheng SS, Lok CK, Ho YS, Baum L, Yang X, Chiu K, Chang RC (2015) Investigating degeneration of the retina in young and aged tau P301L mice. Life Sci 124:16–23. https://doi.org/10.1016/j.lfs.2014.12.019
16. Hunter S, Brayne C (2017) Do anti-amyloid beta protein antibody cross reactivities confound Alzheimer disease research? J Negat Results Biomed 16:1.
17. Hyman BT, Phelps CH, Beach TG, Bigio EH, Cairns NJ, Carrillo MC, Dickson DW, Duyckaerts C, Frosch MP, Masliah E et al (2012) National Institute on Aging-Alzheimer's Association guidelines for the neuropathologic. assessment of Alzheimer's disease. Alzheimers Dement 8:1–13. https://doi.org/10.1016/j.jalz.2011.10.007
18. Ittner LM, Ke YD, Delerue F, Bi M, Gladbach A, van Eersel J, Wolfing H, Chieng BC, Christie MJ, Napier IAet al (2010) Dendritic function of tau mediates amyloid-beta toxicity in Alzheimer's disease mouse models. Cell 142: 387–397 Doi https://doi.org/10.1016/j.cell.2010.06.036
19. Jack CR, Holtzman DM (2013) Biomarker modeling of alzheimer's disease. Neuron 80:1347–1358. https://doi.org/10.1016/j.neuron.2013.12.003
20. Jiang J, Wang H, Li W, Cao X, Li C (2016) Amyloid plaques in retina for diagnosis in Alzheimer's patients: a meta-analysis. Front Aging Neurosci 8:267.
21. Jicha GA, Bowser R, Kazam IG, Davies P (1997) Alz-50 and MC-1, a new monoclonal antibody raised to paired helical filaments, recognize. conformational epitopes on recombinant tau. J Neurosci Res 48:128–132
22. Koronyo Y, Biggs D, Barron E, Boyer DS, Pearlman JA, Au WJ, Kile SJ, Blanco A, Fuchs DT, Ashfaq Aet al (2017) Retinal amyloid pathology and proof-of-concept imaging trial in Alzheimer's disease. JCI Insight 2: Doi https://doi.org/10.1172/jci.insight.93621
23. Koronyo-Hamaoui M, Koronyo Y, Ljubimov AV, Ca M, Ko MK, Black KL, Schwartz M, Farkas DL (2011) Identification of amyloid plaques in retinas from Alzheimer's patients and noninvasive in vivo optical imaging of retinal plaques in a mouse model. NeuroImage 54:S204–S217. https://doi.org/10.1016/j.neuroimage.2010.06.020
24. La Morgia C, Ross-Cisneros FN, Koronyo Y, Hannibal J, Gallassi R, Cantalupo G, Sambati L, Pan BX, Tozer KR, Barboni P et al (2015) Melanopsin retinal ganglion cell loss in Alzheimer's disease. Ann Neurol. https://doi.org/10.1002/ana.24548
25. Loffler KU, Edward DP, Tso MO (1995) Immunoreactivity against tau, amyloid precursor protein, and beta-amyloid in the human retina. Invest Ophthalmol Vis Sci 36:24–31.
26. Pelak VS, Hills W (2018) Vision in Alzheimer's disease: a focus on the anterior afferent pathway. Neurodeger Dis Manag 8:49–67. https://doi.org/10.2217/nmt-2017-0030
27. Quinn N, Csincsik L, Flynn E, Curcio CA, Kiss S, Sadda SR, Hogg R, Peto T, Lengyel I (2018) The clinical relevance of visualising the peripheral retina. Prog Retin Eye Res. https://doi.org/10.1016/j.preteyeres.2018.10.001
28. Ratnayaka JA, Serpell LC, Lotery AJ (2015) Dementia of the eye: the role of amyloid beta in retinal degeneration. Eye (Lond) 29:1013–1026. https://doi.org/10.1038/eye.2015.100
29. Rohn TT (2015) Corpora Amylacea in neurodegenerative diseases: cause or effect? Int J Neurol Neurother 2(3):031. https://www.ncbi.nlm.nih.gov/pubmed/26550607.
30. Schön C, Na H, Ochs SM, Burgold S, Filser S, Steinbach S, Seeliger MW, Arzberger T, Goedert M, Kretzschmar HA et al (2012) Long-Term In Vivo Imaging of Fibrillar Tau in the Retina of P301S Transgenic Mice. PLoS ONE 7: 1–9. https://doi.org/10.1371/journal.pone.0053547
31. Spillantini MG, Goedert M (2013) Tau pathology and neurodegeneration. Lancet Neurol 12:609–622. https://doi.org/10.1016/s1474-4422(13)70090-5
32. Subirada PV, Paz MC, Ridano ME, Lorenc VE, Vaglienti MV, Barcelona PF, Luna JD, Sanchez MC (2018) A journey into the retina: Muller glia commanding survival and death. Eur J Neurosci 47:1429–1443. https://doi.org/10.1111/ejn.13965
33. Thal DR, Ghebremedhin E, Rub U, Yamaguchi H, Del Tredici K, Braak H (2002) Two types of sporadic cerebral amyloid angiopathy. J Neuropathol Exp Neurol 61:282–293.
34. Williams EA, McGuone D, Frosch MP, Hyman BT, Laver N, Stemmer-Rachamimov A (2017) Absence of Alzheimer disease Neuropathologic changes in eyes of subjects with Alzheimer disease. J Neuropathol Exp Neurol 76:376–383. https://doi.org/10.1093/jnen/nlx020
35. Youmans KL, Tai LM, Kanekiyo T, Stine WB, Jr., Michon SC, Nwabuisi-Heath E, Manelli AM, Fu Y, Riordan S, Eimer WA et al (2012) Intraneuronal Abeta detection in 5xFAD mice by a new Abeta-specific antibody. Mol Neurodegen 7: 8 Doi https://doi.org/10.1186/1750-1326-7-8

Systemic inhibition of the membrane attack complex impedes neuroinflammation in chronic relapsing experimental autoimmune encephalomyelitis

Iliana Michailidou[1,2], Aldo Jongejan[3], Jeroen P. Vreijling[2], Theodosia Georgakopoulou[1], Marit B. de Wissel[1], Ruud A. Wolterman[1], Patrick Ruizendaal[1], Ngaisah Klar-Mohamad[4], Anita E. Grootemaat[5], Daisy I. Picavet[5], Vinod Kumar[6], Cees van Kooten[4], Trent M. Woodruff[6], B. Paul Morgan[7], Nicole N. van der Wel[5], Valeria Ramaglia[1,8], Kees Fluiter[2†] and Frank Baas[2*†]

Abstract

The complement system is a key driver of neuroinflammation. Activation of complement by all pathways, results in the formation of the anaphylatoxin C5a and the membrane attack complex (MAC). Both initiate pro-inflammatory responses which can contribute to neurological disease. In this study, we delineate the specific roles of C5a receptor signaling and MAC formation during the progression of experimental autoimmune encephalomyelitis (EAE)-mediated neuroinflammation. MAC inhibition was achieved by subcutaneous administration of an antisense oligonucleotide specifically targeting murine *C6* mRNA (5 mg/kg). The C5a receptor 1 (C5aR1) was inhibited with the C5a receptor antagonist PMX205 (1.5 mg/kg). Both treatments were administered systemically and started after disease onset, at the symptomatic phase when lymphocytes are activated. We found that antisense-mediated knockdown of C6 expression outside the central nervous system prevented relapse of disease by impeding the activation of parenchymal neuroinflammatory responses, including the Nod-like receptor protein 3 (NLRP3) inflammasome. Furthermore, C6 antisense-mediated MAC inhibition protected from relapse-induced axonal and synaptic damage. In contrast, inhibition of C5aR1-mediated inflammation diminished expression of major pro-inflammatory mediators, but unlike C6 inhibition, it did not stop progression of neurological disability completely. Our study suggests that MAC is a key driver of neuroinflammation in this model, thereby MAC inhibition might be a relevant treatment for chronic neuroinflammatory diseases.

Keywords: Complement, Inflammasome, Neuroinflammation

Introduction

Neuroinflammation, or glial-cell propagated inflammation, is a broad concept describing the immune responses which are induced by inflammation or degeneration [43]. Initially considered as 'bystander damage' caused by cell injury, neuroinflammation was for a long time seen as a reaction to neuronal damage. This view was recently challenged in the light of evidence supporting a central role for neuroinflammation in neurodegenerative diseases. It is now known that the resident glial cells also have immunoprotective roles and can recruit peripheral immune cells into the central nervous system (CNS), if needed. Similar to most immune processes however, deviations from the delicate balance of homeostasis might prolong or exacerbate neuroinflammation, which in turn, promotes disease progression [14].

The complement system is a key component of innate immunity. Activation of the complement system involves various components, including C1q, mannan-binding

* Correspondence: F.Baas@lumc.nl
†Equal contributors
2Department of Clinical Genetics, Leiden University Medical Center, Einthovenweg 20, 2333, ZC, Leiden, The Netherlands
Full list of author information is available at the end of the article

lectin, C3 and C5, and has a critical role in the defense against infections, disposal of dead or dying cells, elimination of supernumerary synapses during development and response to 'danger signals' whether flagged by autoantibodies or recognized as altered-self. All pathways of complement activation lead to cleavage of the C5 molecule for generation of the anaphylatoxin C5a, and the opsonin C5b. C5b and the complement proteins C6 through C9, together form an oligomeric structure called the membrane attack complex (MAC) [66]. C5a and MAC have been shown as two major effectors of neuroinflammation and degeneration [4, 17, 47, 62, 63, 69, 85]. C5a exerts pronounced pro-inflammatory activity primarily through the G-coupled receptor for C5a (C5aR1) [81]. MAC causes cytolysis [66] or can act as an immune stimulating factor by promoting the secretion of interleukin 1 beta (IL-1β) via the Nod-like receptor protein 3 (NLRP3) inflammasome, when deposited at sub-lytic amounts [45, 78].

We propose that the terminal part of the complement system has a central role in neuroinflammation, driving degeneration. Because the individual roles of C5a and MAC in this process are not yet delineated we investigated the explicit effects of C5a and MAC on neuroinflammation using selective therapeutic inhibitors. Previous research on the role of MAC in neuroinflammation was performed under conditions in which MAC formation was inhibited already before induction of neuroinflammation [51, 83]. In these models one cannot rule out that induction of disease is affected by the deficiency of MAC. Here, we used the chronic relapsing experimental autoimmune encephalomyelitis (EAE) model of chronic neuroinflammation [35]. This model is used to study mechanisms of degeneration [44] and shows complement activation in the CNS [61]. Inhibition of the complement cascade was started after full induction of the disease, when T lymphocytes were activated. In order to discriminate between C5a- and MAC-mediated effects we selected the inhibitor PMX205, specific for the C5a receptor 1 (C5aR1), and the inhibitor RGS1104, a *C6* mRNA antisense oligonucleotide which blocks MAC formation. PMX205 is a C5aR1 antagonist with pharmacokinetics that allow inhibition in the CNS [85]. The C6 antisense oligonucleotide is an effective inhibitor of the *C6* mRNA, which is predominantly expressed in the liver [29]. Preventing production of C6 will effectively deplete the body thus, also prevent generation of MAC without affecting potential C5a-induced inflammation or upstream effects.

We show that systemic inhibition of MAC after the onset of disease prevented relapse completely in mice induced to develop chronic relapsing EAE whereas, inhibition of the C5aR1 mitigated neurological disability. Notably, MAC inhibition prevented the induction of major pro-inflammatory pathways within the mouse CNS, such as the NLRP3 inflammasome pathway. Histological examination of mouse spinal cords showed that MAC inhibition protected from relapse-induced axonal and synaptic damage or loss, two important pathological components of chronic relapsing EAE. Our data in mice suggest that MAC is a key contributor to neuroinflammation driving degeneration.

Materials and methods

Animals

Male 7 to 8-week-old Biozzi AB/H mice ($n = 52$) were obtained from Harlan (Bicester, U.K.) and housed individually in cages, at room temperature (RT), on a 12-h light: 12-h dark cycle. Animals weighed, on average, 26.93 ± 0.33 g at the beginning of the study. They were kept for at least 1 week before the start of the experiments. They were allowed free access to food and water for the entire duration of the study and provided with wetted mash as necessary. Animals were monitored for microbiological status according to the Federation of European Laboratory Animal Science Associations (FELASA) recommendations. All experiments were approved by the Academic Medical Center Animal Ethics Committee and complied with the Dutch national policy on humane care and the use of laboratory animals.

Induction and clinical scoring of chronic relapsing EAE

Disease was induced in 8–12-week-old male Biozzi AB/H mice by subcutaneous injection into the flank, at both right and left sides, of 0.3 ml of a sonicated emulsion consisting of syngeneic Biozzi AB/H spinal cord homogenate (SCH) emulsified in complete Freund's adjuvant (Sigma-Aldrich, St Louis, MO, USA), on days 0, 7, and of an emulsion consisting of SCH in incomplete Freund's adjuvant (Sigma-Aldrich) on day 24, as previously described [5, 35]. Each animal received 1 mg of SCH and 60 μg mycobacteria [*Mycobacterium tuberculosis* H37Ra, *Mycobacterium butyricum* (4:1); Difco, BD Biosciences, San Jose, CA, USA] per injection [5, 35]. Body weight and clinical signs were assessed daily, as previously described [61], using the following five-point scoring system: 0, normal; 1, loss of tail tone; 2, impaired righting reflex; 3, partial hind limb paralysis, with 1 limb affected; 4, complete hind limb paralysis, with both limbs affected; and 5, moribund. Severity of clinical disability was further analyzed by quantitative (q) PCR analysis for selected immune genes (Additional file 1: Table S1). Remission from the active disease phase was defined as the resolution of clinical paralysis, weight gain and stabilization of the neurological deficit. Relapse was defined as an increase in clinical score of at least one point, development of paresis of the lower limbs and weight loss. Results are shown as the mean clinical scores ± standard error of the mean (SEM).

Generation and administration of complement inhibitors

The C6 Locked Nucleic Acid (LNA) oligonucleotide (RGS1104, referred to as C6 antisense), blocker of the complement component C6, was synthesized with phosphorothioate backbones and methylated DNA-C (medC) by Ribotask (Odense, Denmark), on a Mermade 12, using 2 g NittoPhase (BioAutomation), as previously described [17]. Throughout the process, the oligonucleotide constitution was confirmed by MALDI-TOF mass spectrometry analysis on a Bruker Autoflex using 3-hydroxypicolinic acid as matrix. The sequence of the C6 antisense oligonucleotide is 5′-AACttgctgggAAT-3′ (LNA in capital letters, DNA in lowercase letters).

C6 antisense (5 mg/kg) was dissolved in phosphate buffered saline (PBS pH 7.4, Life technologies, Bleiswijk, The Netherlands) and delivered by osmotic pump at a rate of 0.25 μl per hour, over a period of 14 days (Alzet micro-osmotic pump, model 1002 Cupertino, CA, USA), starting on day 21 post immunization (p.i.). Phosphorothioate antisense oligonucleotides as used in these studies have a well-defined pharmacokinetic profile and biodistribution [21]. LNA wingmers like RGS1104 are efficiently taken up by the liver and mediate RNAseH-mediated mRNA cleavage. Subcutaneous dosing with an Alzet osmotic mini-pump at 5 mg/kg/day for 14 days reduced liver *C6* mRNA levels by 75%, whereas systemic C6 protein levels were reduced by 80%, as measured 10 days post-end of treatment (Additional file 2: Figure S1).

PMX205 [hydrocinnamate-(OPdChaWR)], blocker of C5aR1 [85], synthesized as previously described [47], was dissolved in distilled water and delivered by intraperitoneal injection (1.5 mg/kg), daily, starting on day 21 p.i., until the end of the experiment. The dose of PMX205 was sufficient to block C5aR1 signaling in the mouse CNS [7, 9]. A validated LC-MS/MS method was utilised for quantitative determination of PMX205 in plasma, brain and spinal cord tissue, using an API 3200 (AB SCIENX) mass spectrometer coupled with Agilent 1200 series liquid chromatographic system operated under multiple reaction mode [47]. The developed LC-MS/MS method has a limit of detection (LOD) and limit of quantification (LOQ) of 1.23 ng/ml and 3.73 ng/ml in plasma. LOD and LOQ in tissue is 1.95 ng/g and 3.28 ng/g.

Experimental groups and tissue processing

Spinal cords from non-treated SCH-immunized Biozzi AB/H mice (referred to as no drug) were harvested for histology or RNA sequencing (RNA-seq) at four time points p.i. corresponding to: i) the initial acute paralytic attack (17 days p.i., $n = 3$), ii) the first remission (25 days p.i., $n = 3$), iii) the first relapse (38 days p.i., $n = 7$), and iv) the post-relapse phase (44 days p.i., $n = 4$). Spinal cords of SCH-immunized mice were compared to adjuvant-only ($n = 9$) or naïve ($n = 3$) controls.

To study the effect of C6 antisense on chronic relapsing EAE we collected spinal cords from mice immunized with SCH and treated with the C6 antisense oligonucleotide on day 38 p.i. ($n = 7$) and day 44 p.i. ($n = 6$). Similarly, to study the effect of PMX205 on chronic relapsing EAE we collected spinal cords from mice immunized with SCH and treated with the PMX205 drug on day 38 p.i. ($n = 6$) and day 44 p.i. ($n = 4$). Spinal cords from no drug, C6 antisense- and PMX205-treated animals were compared with each other, also compared with spinal cords from healthy control mice.

Mice whose spinal columns were harvested for RNA isolation and RNA-seq, were anesthetized and intracardially perfused with PBS. The spinal columns were excised and dissected into cervical, thoracic and lumbar regions, separately snap frozen. The frozen tissue was homogenized in TRIzol reagent (Invitrogen, Life Technologies, Carlsbad, CA, USA), and RNA was purified according to the manufacturer's protocol. The concentration and quality of RNA were confirmed using a QuBit (Thermo Fisher Scientific, Waltham, MA USA) and a BioAnalyzer 2100 (Agilent, Santa Clara, CA, USA), respectively. All RNA RIN values were higher than 7.4.

Mice whose spinal columns were harvested for histology were anesthetized and intracardially perfused with PBS, followed by 4% paraformaldehyde. The spinal columns were excised and dissected into cervical, thoracic and lumbar regions; each region was further cut in two pieces and separately kept in formalin or glutaraldehyde for standard embedding in paraffin or epon, respectively.

Elisa

Blood was collected from all mice ($n = 52$) in tubes coated with ethylenediaminetetraacetic acid (EDTA, Sarstedt, Nümbrecht, Germany) to measure serum levels of C6. The serum was separated by centrifugation twice at 5000 g for 10 min at 4 °C and the supernatant was pooled and stored at -80 °C. ELISA to detect C6 in the mouse serum was performed according to a standard published protocol [40].

Quantitative (q) PCR

Liver was collected from all mice ($n = 52$) and immediately placed into RNA later, according to manufacturer's instructions (Ambion, Bleiswijk, The Netherlands), to determine mRNA levels of *C6*. Total RNA was extracted from liver tissue using TriPure (Roche Nederland BV, Woerden, The Netherlands) and chloroform for phase separation and isopropanol precipitation. For the reverse transcription reaction, 0.5 μg RNA was mixed with 125 pmol/ml OligodT12-VN and denatured for 5 min at

65 °C. cDNA was synthesized using SuperScriptIII reverse transcriptase (Invitrogen) and incubating at 50 °C for 1 h. Quantification of RNA was done on a LightCycler 480 (Roche) with the Universal probe system (Roche). Hypoxanthine phosphoribosyl transferase was used as reference gene. The primers used are indicated in (Additional file 1: Table S2). qPCR was performed according to manufacturer's instructions (Roche). Triplicates were used for each cDNA tested. Data were analyzed using the advanced relative quantification module in the LightCycler 480 software (Roche). qPCR was also performed on samples collected from homogenized spinal cords for quantification of expression levels of inflammasome or other immune genes (Additional file 1: Table S1; Additional file 2: Figure S2).

RNA sequencing

Tissue was lysed in a MagNA Lyser using TriPure (Sigma-Aldrich) and MagNA Lyser green beads (Roche). RNA was isolated using Qiagen QIAcube and quality check was done with a BioAnalyzer RNA Nano Chip (Agilent). cDNA synthesis was performed using NuGEN Ovation RNA-Seq System V2 (7102-A01; NuGEN, San Carlos, CA, USA) followed by purification with Qiagen MinElute Kit. DNA was sheared to 200 to 400-bp fragments. The DNA was end polished and dA tailed, and adaptors with Bioo barcodes were ligated (Life Technologies). The fragments were amplified (eight cycles) and quantified with a QuBit (Thermo Fisher Scientific). Libraries were sequenced using the HiSeq PE cluster kit v4 (Illumina Inc., San Diego, CA, USA) on the HiSeq 2500 platform (Illumina), resulting in 125-bp reads.

RNA sequencing analysis

Reads were trimmed using Trimmomatic [8] (v0.32) and subsequently aligned against the mm10 reference genome using HISAT2 [39] (v2.0.4) applying default parameters. Counts were obtained using the Ensembl GRCm38 GTF (v87) with HTSeq [1] (v0.6.1). Quality checks were performed with FastQC (https://www.bioinformatics.babraham.ac.uk/projects/fastqc/; v0.11.5). The data were analyzed using Ingenuity Pathway Analysis (IPA; QIAGEN Inc., https://www.qiagenbioinformatics.com/products/ingenuity-pathway-analysis/) [41].

Light and fluorescence microscope

Six micron-thick paraffin sections were cut and collected on Superfrost Plus glass slides (VWR international, Leuven, Belgium), dried overnight at 37 °C and subsequently deparaffinized in xylene and rehydrated through a series of ethanol. Endogenous peroxidase activity was blocked by incubation in methanol (Merck, Darmstadt, Germany) with 0.3% H_2O_2 (Merck) for 20 min at RT. Sections were then rinsed in PBS and, where appropriate, pretreated with microwave antigen retrieval (3 min at 900 W followed by 10 min at 90 W) in either 0.05 M tris buffered saline (TBS, pH 7.6) or 10 mM citric acid buffer pH 6.0 or 10 mM Tris/1 mM ethylenediaminetetraacetic acid (EDTA) buffer pH 9.0 (Additional file 1: Table S3).

Following overnight incubation at 4 °C in the appropriate primary antibody (Additional file 1: Table S3) diluted in Normal Antibody Diluent (Immunologic, Duiven, The Netherlands), sections were incubated with a donkey anti-rabbit IgG HRP-linked antibody (diluted 1:1000 in PBS, Jackson ImmunoResearch Laboratories, Inc., West Grove, PA, USA) or with a donkey anti-goat IgG HRP-linked antibody (diluted 1:1000 in PBS, Jackson ImmunoResearch Laboratories) or with a donkey anti-mouse IgG HRP-linked antibody (diluted 1:1000 in PBS, Jackson ImmunoResearch Laboratories) or with the BrightVision poly-HRP-anti-rabbit IgG biotin-free (diluted 1:1 in PBS, Immunologic) for 45 min at RT. Incubation with the Vector® M.O.M.™ Immunodetection Kit (Vector Laboratories) was applied where appropriate. The immunostaining was visualized with 3,3′-diaminobenzidinetetrahydrochloride dihydrate (DAB, Vector Laboratories, Burlingame, CA, USA) or with the EnVision detection kit, containing a high sensitivity DAB chromogenic substrate system (Dako, Glostrup, Denmark). Sections were then counterstained with hematoxylin (Sigma-Aldrich) and mounted with VectaMount (Vector Laboratories).

To control for the specificity of the antibodies mouse spinal cord sections were stained according to the protocol described above except for the primary incubation step, which was omitted. In a second experiment, the primary antibody was subjected to an adsorption test using purified protein following an established protocol [55, 70]. In both cases, no signal was observed.

For fluorescent double immunostaining, primary antibodies (Additional file 1: Table S3) were incubated simultaneously overnight followed by incubation with the donkey anti-goat or mouse fluorescein isothiocyanate (FITC)-conjugated (Sigma-Aldrich) and the donkey anti-rabbit Cy3-conjugated secondary antibodies (Sigma-Aldrich) diluted 1:200 in PBS for 45 min at RT. Nuclear staining was visualized by 4′, 6-diamidino-2-phenylindole, (DAPI, Vector Laboratories) and sections were mounted in Vectashield (Vector Laboratories).

Images were acquired with a digital camera (DP25; Olympus, Zoeterwoude, The Netherlands) attached to a light microscope (Olympus, BX41, The Netherlands) for colorimetric staining or with a digital camera (DFC345FX, Olympus, The Netherlands) attached to a Leica-2 DM IRBE confocal microscope (Leica Microsystems BV, Rijswijk, The Netherlands) for immunofluorescent staining. Confocal image stacks were processed with Leica Application Suite (LAS) AF microscope software V2.3.5 (Leica Microsystems BV).

Electron microscope

After the indicated treatment, the samples were fixed in Karnovsky's glutaraldehyde (Polysciences, Inc., Warrington, PA, USA) and post-fixed with 1% osmium tetroxide (OsO_4, Electron microscopy sciences, Hatfield, PA, USA; in cacodylate buffer). Subsequently, the samples were dehydrated in an alcohol series and embedded into Epon (LX-112 resin Ladd research, Williston, VT, USA). First semi-thin (1 μm) sections were cut for overview images and stained with Richardson's staining solution [13]. Then ultrathin (80 nm) epon sections of the desired areas were cut and collected on Formvar-coated grids, counterstained with uranyl acetate and lead citrate. Sections were examined with a FEI Tecnai-12 G2 Spirit Biotwin electron microscope (Fei, Eindhoven, The Netherlands), and images were taken with a Veleta camera using Radius software (EMSIS, Münster, Germany).

Quantification of immunoreactivity

Quantification of synaptophysin (SYP) and C9 reactivity was performed in the grey matter of stereotactic paraffin sections obtained from the cervical spinal cord segment. Quantification of Luxol fast blue (LFB) signal, proteolipid protein (PLP) reactivity or ionized calcium-binding adapter molecule 1 (IBA-1) reactivity was performed in paraffin sections obtained from the cervical or the thoracic spinal cord segment. Briefly, non-overlapping images covering > 95% of the area of interest were acquired from healthy control, no drug and C6 antisense-treated mice (8–10 images/section, 3 sections/mouse, 3–6 mice/group), at a 20× magnification using an Olympus BX41 microscope (Olympus), and processed with the Cell-D software (Olympus). Quantitative analysis of immunostaining was performed using the 'measurement' function of the Image J software (Image Pro Plus 5.1, National Institutes of Health, Bethesda, USA). Briefly, for each picture, the immunoreactive area was measured and divided to the total area of measurement. For measurement of the immunoreactive area a threshold was set and applied to all images in the same staining group. The percentage of immunoreactive area over the total area assessed was then calculated for each section. Average measurements per mouse were finally plotted for each group. Data were represented as mean ± SEM.

Quantification of axonal damage

Quantification of axonal damage was performed in the ventrolateral column of Richardson-stained epoxy resin sections obtained from the cervical and thoracic spinal cord segments. Non-overlapping images covering > 95% of the ventrolateral column were acquired from the C4 and T4 level of healthy control, no drug and C6 antisense-treated mice (10–12 images/section, 2 sections/mouse, 4–6 mice/group). Images were captured at a 100× magnification using a Olympus BX41 microscope (Olympus). All animals were analyzed in a blinded fashion by two individual observers. Quantification of the damaged axons was performed using the Image J software (Image Pro Plus 5.1, National Institutes of Health, Bethesda, USA). Briefly, for each section an approximate number of 1000 axons was counted manually, using the 'Cell Counter' option of the 'Plugins' function. A second counter was then used for the quantification of damaged axons only. The percentage of damaged axons over the total number of counted axons was then calculated for each section. Damaged axons showed signs of demyelination and/or degeneration. Data were represented as mean ± SEM.

Statistical analysis

Statistical tests were performed using Prism software (v7; GraphPad software, San Diego, CA, USA). The variable distribution was assessed by the Shapiro-Wilk test. When the test distribution was not normal, a non-parametric Kruskal–Wallis test was used followed by a Dunn's multiple comparison test to assess intergroup differences. When the test distribution was normal, a One-Way Analysis of Variance (ANOVA) test was applied followed by Bonferroni correction for multiple comparisons. Data were represented as a mean ± SEM. The results were considered significant when p value < 0.05 at a 95% confidence level.

Results

Systemic inhibition of MAC or C5aR1 limits relapse

To study the specific effect of MAC on neuroinflammation we used an antisense oligonucleotide (5 mg/kg) targeting the mRNA of complement component C6. The majority of C6 produced in the body is synthesized in the liver [29] and this oligonucleotide strongly reduces liver mRNA levels (Additional file 2: Figure S1). By reducing the *C6* mRNA levels in the liver the body is depleted of C6 (Additional file 2: Figure S1) and this prevents MAC assembly. We compared the effect of C6 antisense on clinical scores of mice with chronic relapsing EAE to that of PMX205 (1.5 mg/kg), an antagonist of C5aR1, thereby blocking C5aR1-mediated inflammation [47] (Fig. 1a). Unlike the C6 antisense oligonucleotide which cannot permeate the CNS, PMX205 enters the intact CNS (Additional file 2: Figure S3). Both drugs were systemically administered. Treatments started after disease onset, on day 21 p.i., between first disease episode and first relapse, when T lymphocytes were activated and disease-related damage was present.

Treatment with the C6 antisense oligonucleotide prevented relapse (clinical scores at day 38 p.i., C6 antisense vs no drug, 0.17 ± 0.16 vs 2.32 ± 0.34, mean ± SEM, $^{***}p < 0.001$) and all the C6 antisense-treated

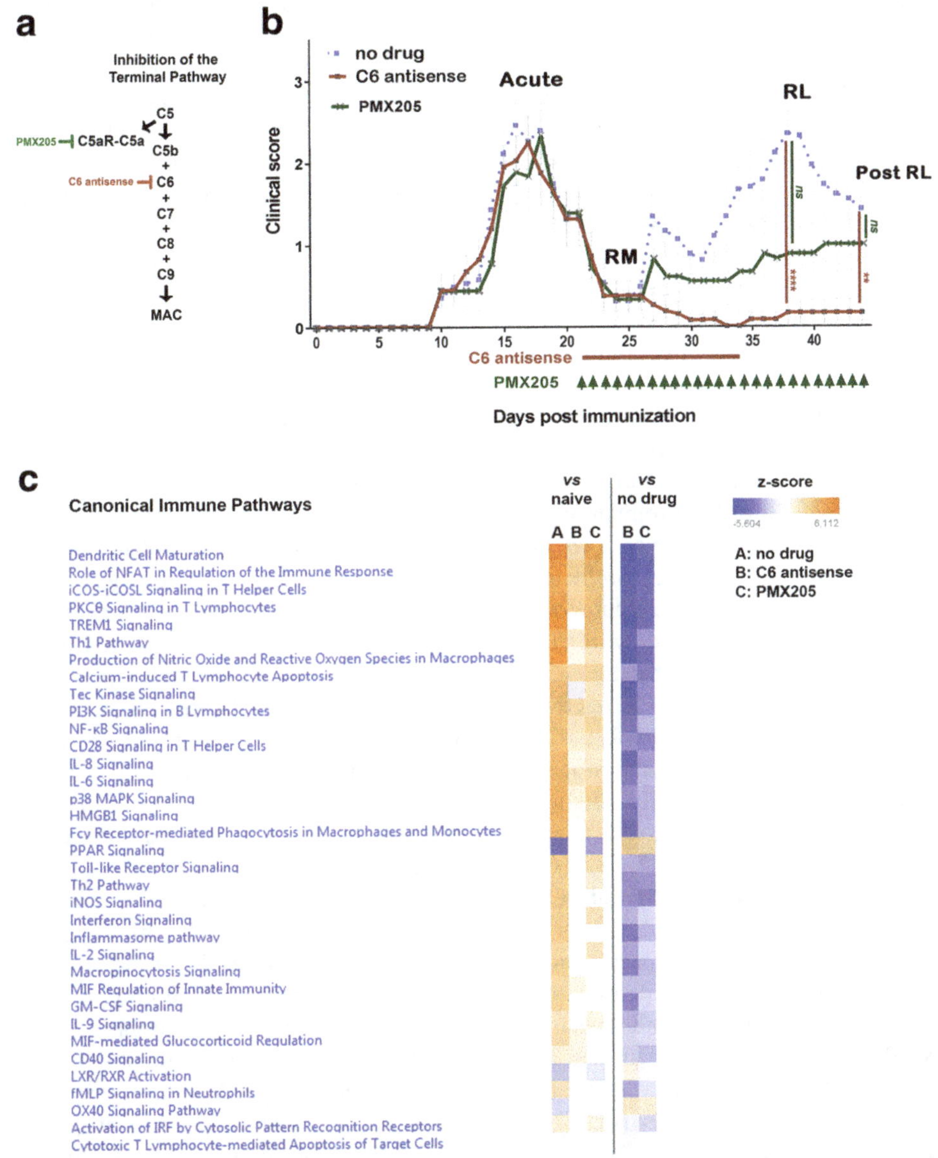

Fig. 1 MAC inhibitor prevents relapse whereas, inhibitor of C5aR1-mediated inflammation ameliorates disability. Scheme illustrating inhibition of the terminal complement pathway **a**. at the level of C5b-C9 (MAC) by antisense targeting of complement *C6* mRNA (C6 antisense, 5 mg/kg), **b**. at the level of C5aR-mediated inflammation by an antagonist of C5aR1 (PMX205, 1.5 mg/kg) (**a**). Clinical scores of mice with chronic relapsing EAE receiving C6 antisense ($n = 13$, in red) or PMX205 ($n = 10$, in green) or no drug ($n = 17$, in blue). The C6 antisense-treated mice did not show relapse or neurological deterioration post-relapse phase. In contrast, PMX205 did not stop progression of neurological disability completely. Differences between groups were analyzed by using the Kruskal-Wallis test by ranks. Data represent the average clinical scores (mean) ± SEM. Statistical differences are indicated (**$p < 0.01$, ****$p < 0.0001$). RL, relapse; RM, remission; *ns*, not significant (**b**). Heatmap showing Ingenuity Pathway Analysis (IPA) canonical immune pathways induced by EAE and significantly affected by treatment with the C6 antisense or the PMX205 inhibitor. Pathways are ranked according to the z-score that predicts activation (orange) /suppression (blue). PMX205 is a less efficient inhibitor of neuroinflammation compared with the C6 antisense. Data were obtained from RNA-seq of mouse spinal cords collected at relapse (3 mice/group) (**c**)

mice showed a stable phenotype post-relapse phase (clinical scores at day 44 p.i., C6 antisense vs no drug, 0.17 ± 0.16 vs 1.41 ± 0.33, mean ± SEM, **$p < 0.01$). Clinical scores in the PMX205-treated mice were lower but not significantly different compared to the no drug littermates (day 38 p.i., PMX205 vs no drug, 0.89 ± 0.35 vs 2.32 ± 0.34, mean ± SEM, $p = 0.06$; day 44 p.i., PMX205 vs no drug, 1.00 ± 0.33 vs 1.41 ± 0.33, mean ± SEM, $p > 0.99$; Fig. 1b).

To understand the mechanisms responsible for the C6 antisense- and PMX205-mediated effects on chronic relapsing EAE we analyzed the RNA expression profiles of spinal cords from C6 antisense-treated chronic relapsing EAE ($n = 3$) and PMX205-treated chronic relapsing EAE

($n = 3$) at relapse, at the point where there was the largest difference in clinical severity (day 38 p.i), and compared them with cords from no drug chronic relapsing EAE ($n = 3$) mice or cords from healthy controls ($n = 3$) to perform pathway analysis using IPA [41]. Focusing on canonical pathways we found that key inflammatory pathways were activated in the no drug mice when compared to healthy controls (colored orange, z-score > 0), while these pathways were partially activated or not altered (blank, z-score = 0) in the two treatment groups. Interestingly, the Tec kinase signaling was slightly downregulated in the C6 antisense-treated mice, but upregulated in the PMX205-treated mice. Comparison between each of the two treatments with the no drug mice showed a general downregulation of neuroinflammation-related pathways (colored blue, z-score < 0). Notably, PMX205 is a less efficient inhibitor of neuroinflammation compared with the C6 antisense. Moreover, two anti-inflammatory pathways, the peroxisome proliferator-activated receptor (PPAR) and the liver X receptor/retinoid X receptor (LXR/RXR) pathway, were downregulated in the no drug mice, but upregulated after treatment with the C6 antisense. Treatment with the PMX205 activated only the PPAR pathway, not the LXR/RXR pathway (Fig. 1c). This suggests that the treatments not only reduce inflammation but also specifically affect inflammation inhibitory pathways.

Systemic MAC inhibition prevents upregulation of NLRP3 components in contrast to C5aR1 inhibition

Previous studies have shown that MAC activates the inflammasome [45, 78], initiating signaling pathways that drive inflammatory responses as shown for endothelial cells [38] and fibroblasts [80]. Activation of the inflammasome is critical for the induction of EAE since mice deficient in various inflammasome components are at least partially, resistant to the disease [19, 22, 28, 31–33, 36, 67, 74].

Analysis of RNA-seq data from spinal cords collected at relapse (day 38 p.i) showed that MAC-induced inflammasome activation occurred in chronic relapsing EAE. We found that the no drug mice showed upregulation of most genes related to the NLRP3 inflammasome pathway; in contrast, the C6 antisense-treated mice had no NLRP3 inflammasome gene expression. The PMX205-treated mice had reduced inflammasome gene expression compared to no drug mice, but still showed higher expression levels of genes linked to the NLRP3 inflammasome compared to the controls (Fig. 2a-c; for log fold change values of genes see Additional file 1: Table S4).

Because inflammasome activation leads to cleavage of the precursor pro-IL-1β and release of the pro-inflammatory cytokine IL-1β [24] we performed immunostaining for IL-1β/pro-IL-1β on paraffin-embedded spinal cord tissue from C6 antisense-treated ($n = 4$), PMX205-treated ($n = 3$), and no drug ($n = 4$) mice, collected at relapse (day 38 p.i.). In line with our RNA-seq data, we found strong IL-1β/pro-IL-1β reactivity in the no drug mice, on glial cells, and sparse IL-1β/pro-IL-1β reactivity in the PMX205-treated mice. No IL-1β/pro-IL-1β immunoreactivity was ever observed in any of the C6 antisense-treated mice examined (Fig. 3a-e).

Systemic MAC inhibition protects from axonal and synaptic damage

Since the C6 antisense MAC-blocking treatment has a protective effect on chronic relapsing EAE, we studied the role of MAC on the pathology of the mouse spinal cord. To this end, formalin-fixed, paraffin embedded spinal cord tissue, collected post-relapse (day 44 p.i.) from no drug chronic relapsing EAE ($n = 4$), C6 antisense-treated chronic relapsing EAE ($n = 6$) or healthy control ($n = 6$) mice was analyzed. As expected, the no drug mice had severe lesions within the ventrolateral columns. Lesions were demyelinated as they showed loss of LFB (Fig. 4a, c) and PLP signal (Fig. 4d, f), and inflammatory as they showed abundant eosinophilic cell infiltrates, CD3+ lymphocytes within the meninges (Additional file 2: Figure S4), and strong reactivity for IBA-1, a marker of microglia/macrophages (Fig. 4g, j). Immunostaining for C9, a marker for MAC deposition, revealed abundant reactivity within the ventral horns (Fig. 4k, l, n), the areas composed of motor neurons, suggesting a link between MAC and motor disability. In contrast, none of the C6 antisense-treated mice had demyelinated lesions (Fig. 4b, e). Quantification of LFB and PLP signal showed a trend towards decrease in the C6 antisense-treated mice compared to controls which is likely a result of acute disease (Fig. 4c, f). All the C6 antisense-treated mice showed IBA-1+ microglia of a resting morphology (Fig. 4h, i), amounts of IBA-1 reactivity similar to those found in controls (Fig. 4j) and lack of CD3+ lymphocytes in the parenchyma or the meninges (Additional file 2: Figure S4). Reactivity for C9 was sparse (Fig. 4m), consistent with a drastic reduction of MAC formation by the C6 antisense (~ 70%, $^{***}p < 0.001$; Fig. 4n).

Next, we quantified axonal damage on osmium-fixed, epon-embedded spinal cord tissue, collected post-relapse (day 44 p.i.) from no drug chronic relapsing EAE ($n = 4$), C6 antisense-treated chronic relapsing EAE ($n = 6$) or healthy control ($n = 6$) mice. We report that all the no drug mice showed wide zones of axonal damage corresponding to the lesioned areas (Fig. 5a). Electron microscopy demonstrated various types of axonal damage that we detected and quantified; 1: destruction of the myelin sheath, 2: deformation of the myelin sheath with gaps between tangent layers, 3: infoldings of the myelin sheath within the axoplasmic area, and 4: onion bulbs (Fig. 5b). In contrast, the C6 antisense-treated mice examined had only a few damaged axons (arrows in Fig. 5c, d and arrows

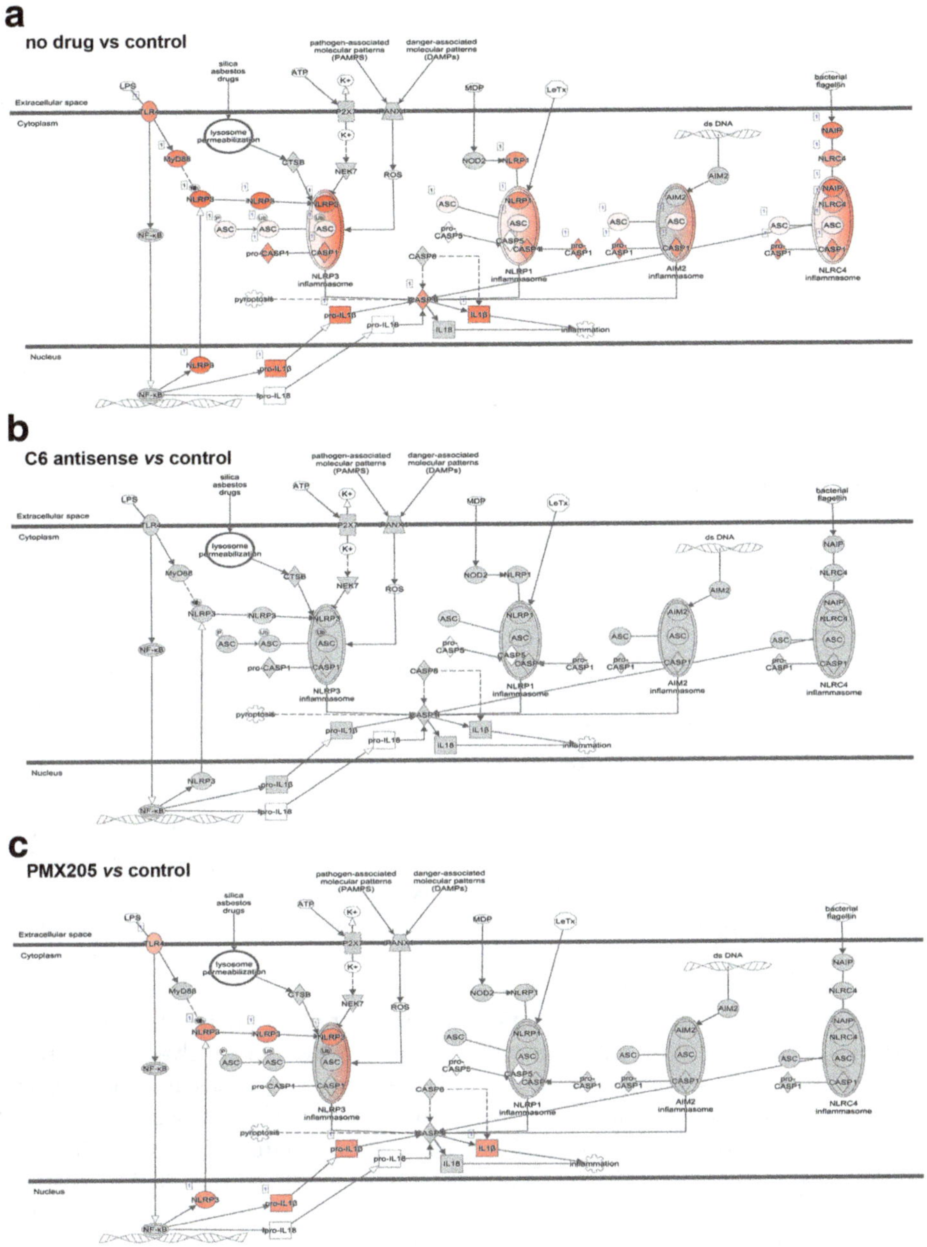

Fig. 2 MAC inhibitor completely blocks NLRP3 inflammasome components while, in contrast, C5aR1 inhibition only partially decreases expression. The inflammasome pathway was modeled by Ingenuity Pathway Analysis (IPA) after analyses of gene expression data from mouse spinal cords collected at relapse (3 mice/group). Genes showing higher expression levels in the first compared to the second group of each comparison are colored red. The grey color indicates no changes of expression levels. Note that genes linked to NLRP3 inflammasome activation show no changes of expression levels in the C6 antisense group (MAC inhibitor, genes colored grey), but increased levels in the PMX205 group (inhibitor of C5aR1-mediated inflammation, genes colored red) when compared with healthy controls at relapse (**a-c**). Log fold change values of genes are shown in Additional file 1: Table S4

in Fig. 5e) and an average percentage of axonal damage that was significantly smaller than that found in the no drug littermates (C6 antisense vs no drug, 4.23 ± 0.44 vs 31.56 ± 2.67, mean ± SEM, $^{***}p < 0.001$; Fig. 5f). Control mice contained intact axons only (Fig. 5g, h).

Finally, we quantified the number of synapses and neurons in the grey matter of stereotactic sections of formalin-fixed spinal cords collected post-relapse (day 44 p.i.) from no drug chronic relapsing EAE ($n = 4$), C6 antisense-treated chronic relapsing EAE ($n = 6$) or healthy control ($n = 6$) mice. All the C6 antisense-treated mice showed higher levels of reactivity for SYP, a marker of synapses, compared with the no drug mice (C6 antisense vs no drug, 66.59 ± 3.49 vs 55.75 ± 2.06, mean ±

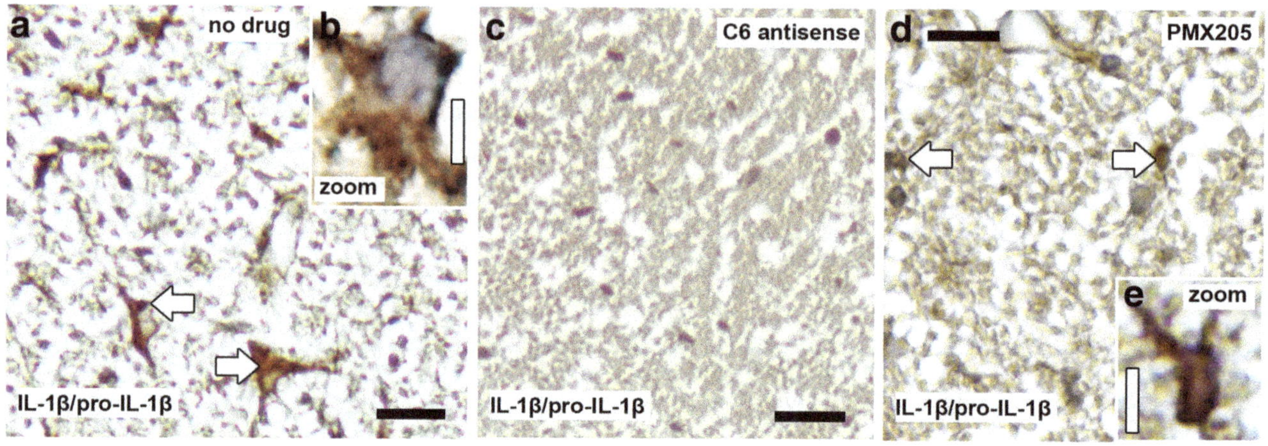

Fig. 3 MAC inhibitor completely inhibits IL-1β synthesis while, in contrast, C5aR1 inhibition only partially decreases expression. Immunostaining for interleukin 1 beta (IL-1β)/pro-IL-1β, indicator of NLRP3 inflammasome activation, shows reactivity within the spinal cord of no drug mice (n = 4, arrows in **a**), on cells with a glial morphology (**a, b**). IL-1β/pro-IL-1β was never detected in the cords of C6 antisense-treated mice (n = 4) (**c**), while PMX205-treated mice showed sparse reactivity (n = 3) (arrows in **d, e**). Tissue was collected at relapse. Scale bars (**a, c, d**) 25 μm, (**b, e**) 5 μm. Hematoxylin was used as counterstain in (**a-e**)

SEM, $^{*}p < 0.05$). Comparison with the controls indicated that the no drug mice had an average 23% decrease of SYP+ punctae (no drug vs control, 55.75 ± 2.06 vs 79.00 ± 2.60, mean ± SEM, $^{***}p < 0.001$), while in contrast, the C6 antisense-treated mice had a smaller 12% decrease (C6 antisense vs control, 66.59 ± 3.49 vs 79.00 ± 2.60, mean ± SEM, $^{*}p < 0.05$) (Fig. 6a). Neuron counts showed no significant differences between the groups (*data not shown*), suggesting that any loss of SYP reactivity was not related to neuronal loss. Correlation analysis indicated a significant negative correlation between C9 and SYP (coefficient, $r = -0.74$, $^{***}p < 0.0001$) (Fig. 6b), supporting a link between MAC deposition and synaptic changes. Histological examination of the ventral horns of no drug mice showed a punctate staining pattern for C9, indicative of a synaptic localization (Fig. 6d) that was further confirmed by the co-localization of the C9 and SYP markers (Additional file 2: Figure S5). Notably, deposition of C9 within the ventral horns of no drug mice was associated with the presence of abundant microglia or macrophages (Fig. 6e) and NLRP3 immunoreactivity (Additional file 2: Figure S6). Examination of the ventral horns of C6 antisense-treated mice showed abundant SYP+ punctae, few microglia of a resting phenotype and absence of NLRP3 reactivity (Fig. 6f-h and Additional file 2: Figure S6).

Discussion

This study demonstrates that systemic knockdown of complement *C6* mRNA, when applied after the disease induction, prevents relapse in chronic relapsing EAE. Inhibition of MAC formation is the most likely mechanism of action of the C6 antisense oligonucleotide. Reduced amounts of MAC in the CNS are associated with lack of activation of local parenchymal inflammatory pathways known to induce or maintain neuroinflammation, such as the NLRP3 inflammasome. Protection against clinical disability conferred by MAC inhibition is exerted through the prevention of axonal and synaptic damage. Overall, these data suggest that even in the presence of activated T lymphocytes, MAC is a key contributor to neuroinflammation driving degeneration. Inhibition of C5aR1-mediated inflammation also affected disease severity but only ameliorated progressive neurological disability.

The complement system, a major component of innate immunity, is a sensor of immune homeostasis and a versatile effector of host defense. The classical pathway of complement activation involves recognition of pathogen- or danger-associated molecular patterns by C1q, induction of pro-inflammatory responses by cleaved C3 and C5, and elimination of targeted cells by MAC. While complement proteins are rapidly recruited to protect the human body against intruders, this pathway may also transform to an unwanted self-attacking mechanism that perpetuates injury if uncontrolled [66].

Because of the central role of complement in immunity, the interest in anti-complement therapeutics has increased over the last decades. Multiple agents targeting different components of the complement system have been developed [57]. The terminal pathway of complement is undoubtedly an interesting signaling branch for intervention. Inhibition at this level prevents potentially deleterious inflammatory responses without affecting upstream complement functions that are beneficial [75]. Eculizumab (Soliris; Alexion Pharmaceuticals) is an inhibitor of the C5 component and the only terminal pathway-specific drug that has so far received approval for clinical use. Soliris is prescribed in patients with

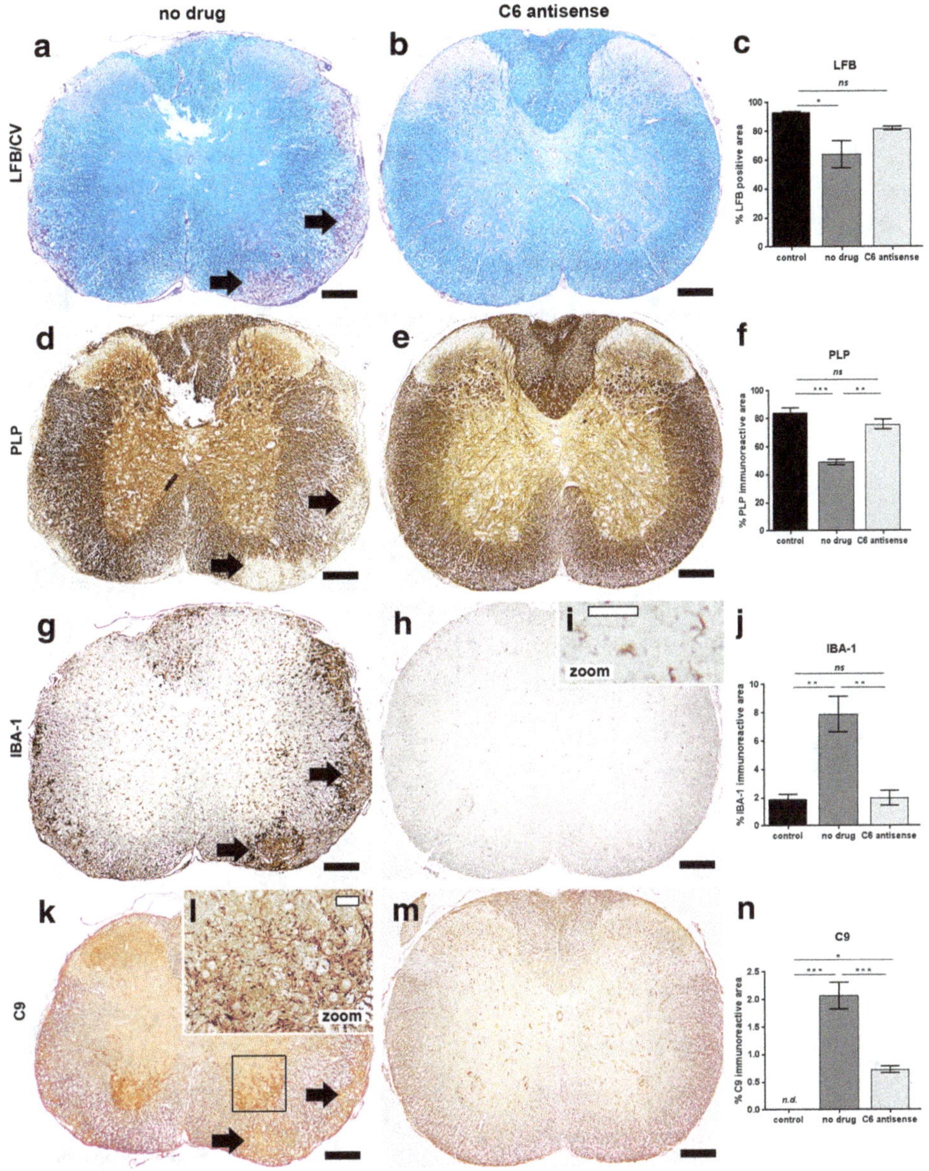

Fig. 4 C6 antisense-mediated MAC inhibition prevents demyelination and microglia/macrophage activation in chronic relapsing EAE. Histological analysis of semi-serial paraffin sections of the mouse cervical spinal cord segment showed lesions in the no drug mice ($n = 4$) but no signs of active disease in the C6 antisense-treated mice ($n = 6$). Tissue was collected post-relapse phase. Staining for Luxol fast blue (LFB) and quantification of the signal (**a-c**) as well as staining for proteolipid protein (PLP) and quantification of the reactivity (**d-f**) indicated demyelination in the no drug mice (demyelinated lesions pointed by arrows in **a** and **d**), but no significant myelin loss in the C6 antisense-treated mice (**c**, **f**). Immunostaining for ionized calcium-binding adapter molecule 1 (IBA-1) (**g-j**) revealed microglia/macrophages within the lesions (arrows in **g**) and at the peri-lesional area of the no drug mice with a morphology consistent with an activated status. In contrast, all the C6 antisense-treated mice showed amounts of IBA-1+ reactivity similar to the ones found in controls and morphology of IBA-1+ microglia consistent with a resting status (**h-j**). Moreover, the no drug mice had abundant reactivity for C9, a marker of MAC deposition, within the ventral horns of the spinal cord. In contrast, the C6 antisense-treated mice showed only small amounts of MAC (**k-n**). Scale bars: (**a**, **b**, **d**, **e**, **g**, **h**, **k**, **m**) 200 μm, (**i, l**) 50 μm. Cresyl violet (CV) was used as counterstain in (**a**, **b**). Hematoxylin was used as counterstain in (**d, e, g-i, k-m**)

paroxysmal nocturnal hemoglobinuria (PNH) or atypical hemolytic uremic syndrome (aHUS) [27, 84] and is currently undergoing phase III of a clinical trial for the prevention of neuromyelitis optica (NMO) relapses (https://clinicaltrials.gov/ct2/show/NCT01892345). It targets C5, blocking both MAC assembly and the formation of C5a [27, 84].

MAC is the end product of complement activation and the most inflammatory component of the terminal complement pathway [66]. Lytic levels of MAC can directly destroy infected or damaged cells, by disrupting plasma membranes, which are then cleared by recruited phagocytes [20, 30]. Moreover, sub-lytic amounts of MAC can trigger the activation of NLRP3 inflammasome

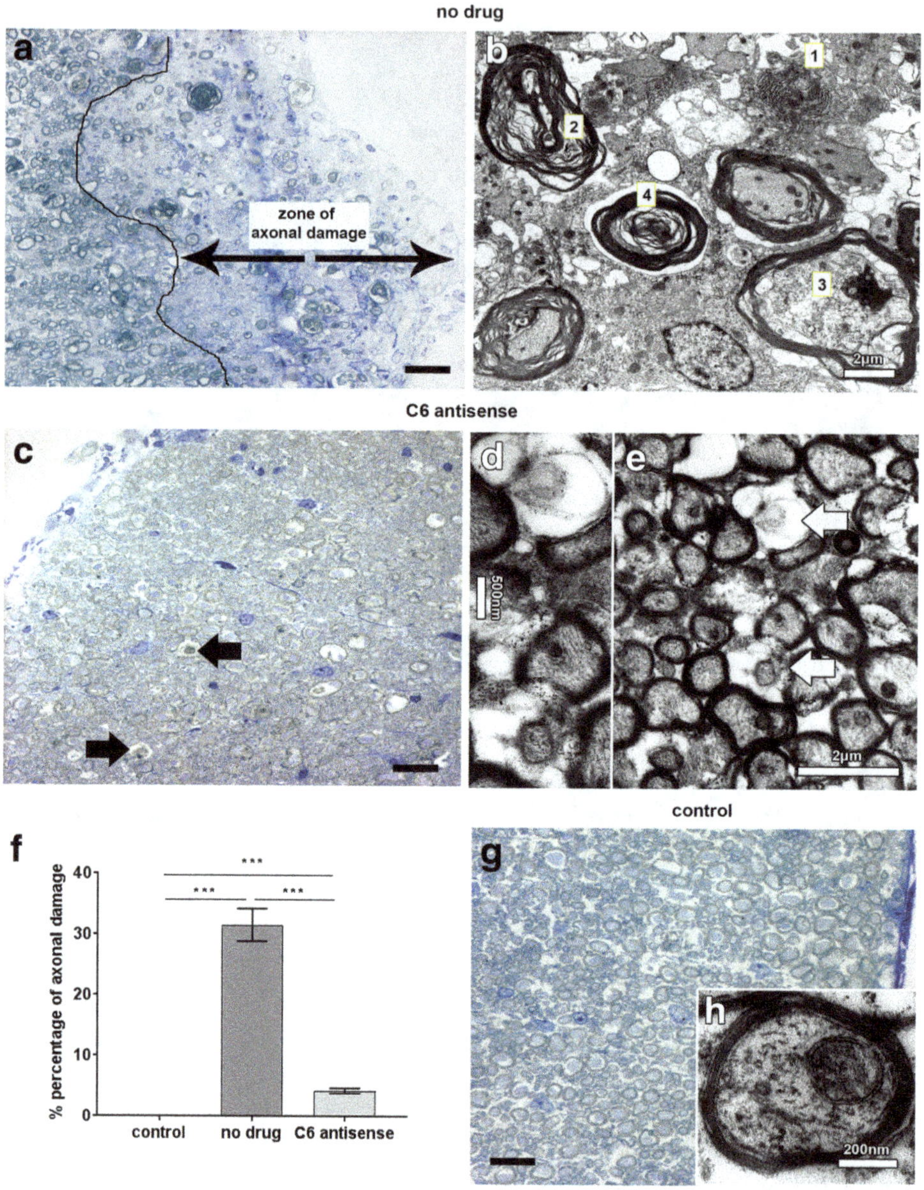

Fig. 5 C6 antisense-mediated MAC inhibition protects from axonal damage. Richardson's staining on spinal cord tissue from no drug mice showed wide areas of axonal damage corresponding to the lesioned areas (**a**). Electron microscopy micrograph indicates the types of axonal damage detected and quantified: 1. destruction of the myelin sheathe, 2. deformation of the myelin sheathe with gaps between tangent layers, 3. infoldings of the myelin sheathe within the axoplasmic area, and 4. onion bulbs (**b**). Picture of Richardson's stained spinal cord section and electron microscopy micrograph from C6 antisense-treated mice (**c**-**e**) showing rarely detected damaged axons (arrows in **c, d** and arrows in **e**). Graph shows the percentage of axonal damage as quantified in the ventral and lateral column of the cervical and thoracic spinal cord segments from control ($n = 6$), no drug ($n = 4$) or C6 antisense-treated ($n = 6$) mice, collected post-relapse. Comparisons between groups were performed using the Kruskal-Wallis test by ranks. Data are expressed as the average (mean) ± SEM. Statistical differences are indicated (***$p < 0.001$) (**f**). Pictures from control mice showed intact axons only (**g**, **h**). Scale bars: (**a**, **c**, **g**) 25 μm, (**b**, **e**) 2 μm, (**d**) 500 nm (**h**) 200 nm

in the target cells, promoting clinical disease and primary or secondary tissue damage [45, 78].

On the other hand, C5a is known to have both pro-and anti-inflammatory properties depending on the receptor-ligand interaction and disease studied [9, 47]. More specifically, C5a can bind to one of the two competing receptors, C5aR1 (CD88) and C5aR2 (C5L2), and the balance in C5a occupancy determines whether the response is pro- or anti-inflammatory [81, 87]. Pro-inflammatory responses include G-protein-dependent cell signaling leading to intracellular Ca^{+2} production, chemotaxis and oxidative stress. Anti-inflammatory responses include non G-protein-dependent signaling that alters pro-inflammatory cytokine production, limiting inflammation [46, 81].

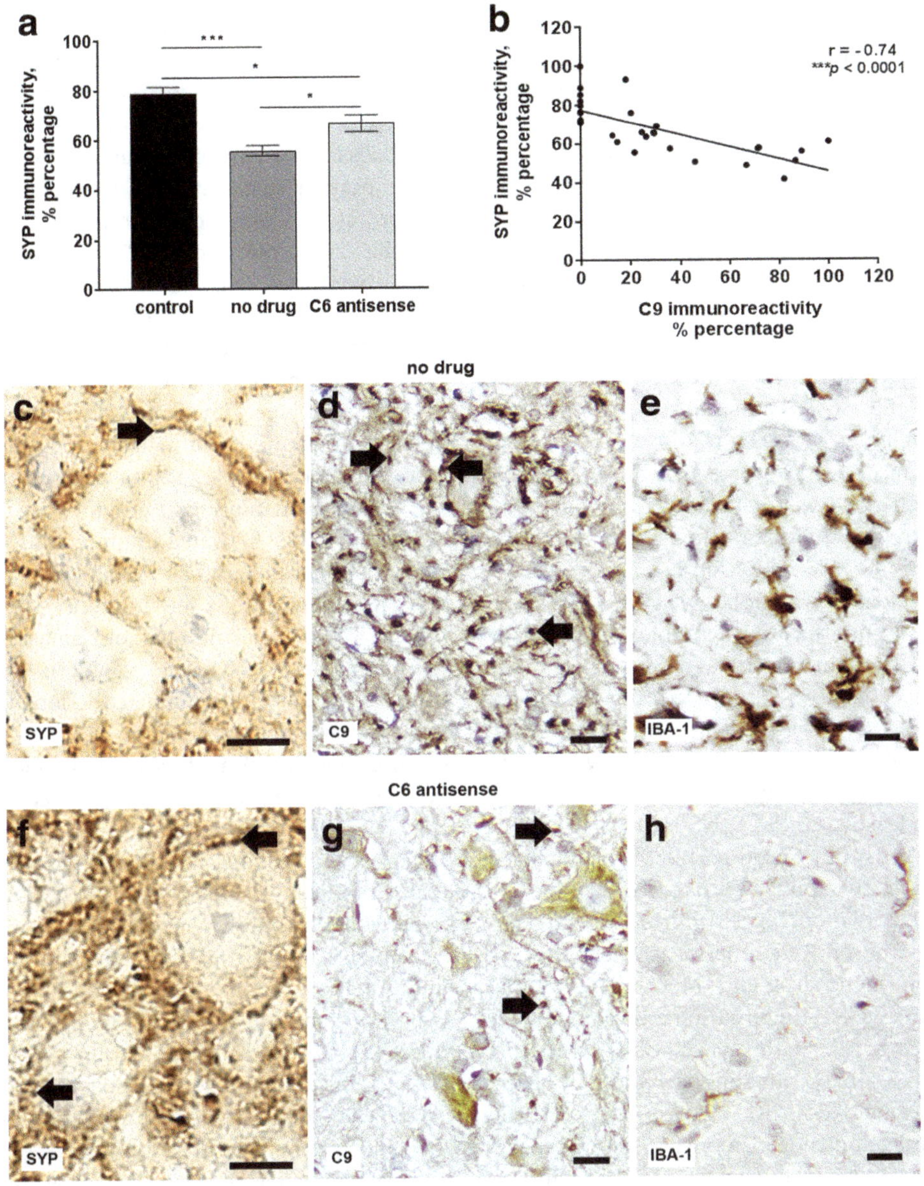

Fig. 6 C6 antisense-mediated MAC inhibition protects from synaptic alterations. Quantification of synaptophysin (SYP) positive punctae showed a significant decrease of synaptic densities (*$p < 0.05$) in the no drug ($n = 4$) compared to the C6 antisense-treated mice ($n = 6$), post-relapse phase. Differences between groups were analyzed by using the One-Way Analysis of Variance test. Data are expressed as the average (mean) ± SEM. Statistical differences are indicated (*$p < 0.05$, ***$p < 0.001$). Controls are healthy mice injected with adjuvant only ($n = 6$) (**a**). Pearson's correlation coefficient showed a significant negative correlation between SYP and the C9 marker of MAC (coefficient, $r = -0.74$, ***$p < 0.0001$), in the mouse spinal cord ($n = 29$ corresponding fields plotted) (**b**). Histological analysis of paraffin spinal cord sections from no drug mice showed low densities of SYP+ punctae (arrow pointing to a synapse), sign of synaptic alterations or loss (**c**), abundant C9 reactivity (arrows) (**d**), and ionized calcium-binding adapter molecule 1 (IBA-1) positive microglia/macrophages with a morphology consistent with an activated status (**e**). In contrast, histological analysis of spinal cords from C6 antisense-treated mice showed abundant SYP+ punctae (arrows) (**f**), sparse C9 reactivity (arrows) (**g**), and IBA-1+ microglia with a morphology consistent with a resting status (**h**). Scale bars: (**c-h**) 10 μm. Hematoxylin was used as counterstain in (**c-h**)

Thus far, there is no complete understanding of the role of the terminal complement pathway on neuroinflammation. A number of studies showing deletion or pharmacological inhibition of complement components, related fragments or complement receptors have been published reporting controversies. More specifically, deficiency or blockade of C5a receptors failed to protect against acute EAE, while expression of C5a in the brain did not exacerbate EAE [56, 64, 65]. Moreover, deficiency of C5 reduced remyelination in chronic EAE possibly due to an effect of MAC on oligodendrocyte apoptosis [58, 83]. In contrast, deficiency of C6 in a rat model of acute EAE protected against demyelination and immune cell infiltration [51, 77]. Notably, reconstitution of C6 in these rats restored EAE [51].

In this study, we aimed to define the role of MAC on neuroinflammation by delineating its effect from that induced by C5aR1, and compare the effect of a MAC inhibitor, being a knockdown of C6, to that of a C5aR1 antagonist. We found that systemic administration of the MAC inhibitor after disease onset prevented relapse in mice with chronic relapsing EAE by suppressing key pro-inflammatory pathways within the CNS. In contrast, administration of the C5aR1 antagonist only mitigated neurological disability.

Which factor determines the molecular and/or clinical differences between the two treatment groups? Expression profiling of the spinal cords of the chronic relapsing EAE animals shows that C6 inhibition has a major effect on the NLRP3 inflammasome pathway. The NLRP3 inflammasome is a multiprotein complex abundantly expressed in the CNS that is activated by a wide range of endogenous or exogenous signals to potentiate neuroinflammatory responses with the release of IL-1β and IL-18 [79]. Activation of the inflammasome was previously linked to MAC deposition [45, 78]. MAC precursor proteins can leak into the CNS during transient openings of the blood–spinal cord barrier (BSCB) caused by immunization with spinal cord antigens in the chronic relapsing EAE model [71]. Our RNA-seq data demonstrated that the NLRP3 inflammasome pathways are 'switched on' in the no drug and the C5aR1-inhibited mice, but not in the MAC-inhibited mice in comparison with controls. Moreover, pathway analysis with IPA showed that the Tec kinase signaling, a regulator of the NLRP3 inflammasome [34], was upregulated in the C5aR1-inhibited mice, but not in the MAC-inhibited littermates. These data were consistent with our finding that all the no drug and the C5aR1-inhibited mice showed IL-1β/pro-IL-1β + glial cells while, none of the C6 antisense-treated mice showed any IL-1β/pro-IL-1β immunostaining. Our data confirm previous reports of a specific effect of MAC on the activation of NLRP3 inflammasome [45, 78] and further suggest that MAC formation stimulates immune responses in glial cells to initiate or boost neuroinflammation in this model.

Indeed, examination of spinal cords from no drug mice showed MAC deposition associated with abundant microglia/macrophages, sign of local immune reaction to MAC. MAC was deposited on synapses and its reactivity was negatively correlated to synaptic densities. In contrast, spinal cords of MAC-inhibited mice showed a few microglia of a resting phenotype and higher synaptic densities. These data together with our observation that MAC deposits are restricted to the ventral horns, the area of motor neurons, and are linked to local NLRP3 expression suggest a link between MAC, accumulation and/or activation of microglia and neurological disability in chronic relapsing EAE. It is possible that deposition of MAC on synapses leads to synaptic damage due to pore formation. Pores may in turn, promote the release of ATP [59], an important messenger that can be sensed by the neighboring glia via the purinoceptor 7 (P2X7) receptor [49], to induce bystander NLRP3 inflammasome activation for release of IL-1β. IL-1β can then exacerbate disease by triggering the opening of the BSCB and promoting the infiltration of immune cells in the CNS [73].

Once peripheral immune cells enter the CNS parenchyma, complement can regulate their differentiation, in the case of lymphocytes [2, 12], or promote their activation by the release of anaphylatoxins, in the case of macrophages or neutrophils [25]. Activated immune cells are important mediators of neuroinflammation and lesion formation. Importantly, we found only a few immune cells, no demyelinated lesions and a small number of damaged axons in all the MAC-inhibited mice tested while, in contrast, all the no drug mice showed demyelinated lesions with abundant cell infiltrates and damaged axons. These data are in line with our previous finding that MAC inhibition reduces the numbers of infiltrating macrophages, impeding degeneration in the CNS after brain trauma [17, 69]. In addition, C6 deficient rats (rats genetically unable to form MAC) showed reduced numbers of CD68+ and CD11b + cells at the site of injury after crush nerve injury [63].

Comparison of RNA-seq data from MAC-inhibited mice to those from no drug mice showed activation of two important anti-inflammatory pathways, the PPAR and the LXR/RXR pathway [15, 37, 76]. It is known that the C6 antisense oligonucleotide does not penetrate the CNS. Therefore, we speculate that activation of these protective mechanisms in the MAC-inhibited mice might be an intra-parenchymal response that is related either to blockade of immune cell infiltration or to another unknown function of the C6 antisense oligonucleotide. In contrast, the C5aR1-inhibited mice showed activation of the PPAR pathway only. This is an interesting observation since the C5aR1 antagonist enters the CNS and may therefore act both in the periphery and the CNS.

MAC has been involved in the pathology of a wide range of acute and chronic neuroinflammatory diseases. Acute multiple sclerosis, stroke, traumatic brain injury (TBI) and NMO are major examples of acute or recurrent neuroinflammatory brain conditions in which MAC may have an important pathological contribution [6, 17, 48, 54]. Moreover, MAC, detected by an antibody against a neo-epitope in C9 (C9neo), was found in brains from donors with the chronic course of multiple sclerosis, in the absence of fulminate inflammation [82], in Alzheimer's disease brains on senile plaques [50, 55], and in amyotrophic lateral sclerosis (ALS) brains on still innervated motor endplates, suggesting a role as a modifier of disease progression [3]. Although chronic diseases are far less inflammatory than acute, their pathology does include inflammatory responses, but of a type different than the acute ones, and this might explain the failure of current treatments to halt disease progression [42]. Our finding in mice that MAC is linked to NLRP3 inflammasome activation and IL-1β production might have implications for the diagnosis and therapy of neuroinflammation-related diseases in humans, especially in the view of accumulating evidence pointing towards a pathogenic role of IL-1β. IL-1β transcript or protein was detected in the cerebrospinal fluid, blood or lesions of patients with multiple sclerosis [11, 26, 60] and was linked to the extent of cortical demyelination or to disease severity [68, 72]. Interestingly, treatment of multiple sclerosis patients with the FDA-approved therapeutic agents type-I IFN, glatiramer acetate or natalizumab (https://www.ncbi.nlm.nih.gov/books/NBK294198/table/introduction.t1/#__NBK294198_dtls__) was shown to affect the expression of IL-1Ra and/or the production of IL-1β [10, 23, 52, 53].

Complement inhibition, as with most immunomodulatory interventions, weakens the immune responses to pathogens, which over time, can lead to recurrent and/or severe infections in patients. Although activation of upstream complement functions suffices for protection against most infective organisms, there is one group of bacteria, the *Neisseria* species, which requires activation of the terminal pathway [16]. *Neisseria meningitides* infection leads to meningococcal sepsis or meningitis. Individuals deficient in C5 or terminal pathway components have a higher susceptibility for *Neisseria meningitides* infections. However, not all deficiencies might have similar increased risks. C6 and C7 deficiencies could be less severe [86]. For prevention of meningococcal disease it is recommended that patients receiving Soliris receive prophylactic antibiotics and are vaccinated against all meningococcal strains [18]. It remains to be demonstrated whether treatment with a C6 inhibitor will cause less risk of meningococcal infections due to the extra antimicrobial protection provided by the C5a-related anaphylactic mechanism. Therapeutic anti-C6 antibodies are now under development and in a preclinical stage [57]. These antibodies may serve to circumvent problems related to blockade of C5a-mediated inflammation.

In this study, we also show that PMX205, a C5aR1 inhibitor ameliorates disability but does not completely prevent the relapse in chronic relapsing EAE. An explanation for this difference is that MAC is a more potent pro-inflammatory molecule in this model than C5a. In addition, C5a does not have only pro-inflammatory but it also has anti-inflammatory properties [9]. Compared to the no drug mice, there is a clear effect of PMX205 however. The severity of the relapse was less. Expression profiling showed reduced expression of inflammatory pathways regulating relapse in chronic relapsing EAE. However, activation of the NLRP3 inflammasome, as measured by expression levels of related genes and by IL-1β/pro-IL-1β + glial cells, was moderately affected. It is therefore likely that MAC predominantly drives this effect in this model.

A limitation of this study is the lack of data related to the contribution of the two tested inhibitors on the mouse peripheral cell immunity. Further research is required to address impact on immune cells peripherally and in the CNS. Our findings add to previous reports of a link between the terminal complement pathway and inflammasome activation. In this study we further demonstrate that MAC is a major player in neuroinflammation that drives spinal cord degeneration, providing a rationale for the use of complement-targeting therapies to combat chronic neuroinflammatory diseases.

Conclusions

Our research demonstrates that inhibition of the terminal complement pathway at the symptomatic disease phase effectively stops neuroinflammation in the chronic relapsing EAE model. This is the first study that delineates the specific roles of C5a receptor signaling and MAC formation in vivo using selective inhibitors. Our finding that systemic inhibition of MAC prevented relapse completely in mice whereas, inhibition of the C5aR1 mitigated neurological disability reveals a key role for MAC in neuroinflammation driving degeneration. This study might represent a first step towards pre-clinical development of MAC inhibition as therapy for chronic neuroinflammatory diseases like multiple sclerosis.

Additional files

Additional file 1: Table S1. Expression levels of key immune genes in mice with chronic relapsing EAE showing mild or severe neurological disability and comparison with mice showing no disability. **Table S2.** Mouse primer sequences. **Table S3.** Primary antibodies, dilution, source. **Table S4.** Log fold change values of NLRP3 inflammasome genes in the mouse spinal cord at the relapse of chronic relapsing EAE. (PDF 215 kb)

Additional file 2: Figure S1. Systemic administration of C6 antisense knocks down C6 in mice. **Figure S2.** QPCR determination of key components of the inflammasome pathway. **Figure S3.** PMX205 concentrations in plasma, brain and spinal cord. **Figure S4.** Systemic administration of C6 antisense prevents inflammation in the spinal cord of the chronic relapsing EAE model. **Figure S5.** C9 is localized at synapses. **Figure S6.** Systemic administration of C6 antisense prevents NLRP3 inflammasome expression in the spinal cord of the chronic relapsing EAE model. (PDF 877 kb)

Acknowledgements

We would like to thank the National Multiple Sclerosis Society.

Funding
This work was funded by the National Multiple Sclerosis Society grant no. RG 4775A1/1 to F.B. and V.R.

Authors' contributions
IM performed the animal experiments, performed the histology of the mouse tissue, analyzed the data and wrote the manuscript; AJ performed the bioinformatics of RNA-seq data; JPV performed the RNA-seq; TG contributed to the histology of the mouse tissue; MBW and RAW participated in the animal experiments; PR performed the qPCR; NK-M performed the ELISA; AEG and DIP performed the electron microscopy; V.K. analyzed the biodistribution of the C5aR1 inhibitor; CK, TMW, BPM, NNW and VR participated in the conception of the study and/or contributed to the initial animal experiments; KF performed the analysis of RNA-seq data, participated in the animal experiments and participated in the conception of the study; FB performed the conception of the study, supervised and co-wrote the manuscript. All authors read and approved the final manuscript.

Competing interests
FB, KF and VR are the inventors of patents that describe the use of inhibitors of the terminal complement pathway for therapeutic purposes; they are co-founders of Regenesance BV. FB. is founder of Complement Pharma BV.

Author details
[1]Department of Genome Analysis, Academic Medical Center, Amsterdam, The Netherlands. [2]Department of Clinical Genetics, Leiden University Medical Center, Einthovenweg 20, 2333, ZC, Leiden, The Netherlands. [3]Department of Bioinformatics, Academic Medical Center, Amsterdam, The Netherlands. [4]Department of Nephrology, Leiden University Medical Center, Leiden, The Netherlands. [5]Electron Microscopy Centre Amsterdam, Department of Medical Biology, Academic Medical Center, Amsterdam, The Netherlands. [6]School of Biomedical Sciences, The University of Queensland, Brisbane, Australia. [7]Systems Immunity University Research Institute, School of Medicine, Cardiff University, Cardiff, UK. [8]Department of Immunology, University of Toronto, Toronto, Canada.

References

1. Anders S, Pyl PT, Huber W (2015) HTSeq–a Python framework to work with high-throughput sequencing data. Bioinformatics 31:166–169. https://doi.org/10.1093/bioinformatics/btu638
2. Arbore G, West EE, Spolski R, Robertson AAB, Klos A, Rheinheimer C, Dutow P, Woodruff TM, Yu ZX, O'Neill LA, Coll RC, Sher A, Leonard WJ, Kohl J, Monk P, Cooper MA, Arno M, Afzali B, Lachmann HJ, Cope AP, Mayer-Barber KD, Kemper C (2016) T helper 1 immunity requires complement-driven NLRP3 inflammasome activity in CD4(+) T cells. Science 352:aad1210. doi:https://doi.org/10.1126/science.aad1210
3. Bahia El Idrissi N, Bosch S, Ramaglia V, Aronica E, Baas F, Troost D (2016) Complement activation at the motor end-plates in amyotrophic lateral sclerosis. J Neuroinflammation 13:72. https://doi.org/10.1186/s12974-016-0538-2
4. Bahia El Idrissi N, Das PK, Fluiter K, Rosa PS, Vreijling J, Troost D, Morgan BP, Baas F, Ramaglia V (2015) M. Leprae components induce nerve damage by complement activation: identification of lipoarabinomannan as the dominant complement activator. Acta Neuropathol 129:653–667. https://doi.org/10.1007/s00401-015-1404-5
5. Baker D, O'Neill JK, Gschmeissner SE, Wilcox CE, Butter C, Turk JL (1990) Induction of chronic relapsing experimental allergic encephalomyelitis in Biozzi mice. J Neuroimmunol 28:261–270
6. Barnett MH, Parratt JD, Cho ES, Prineas JW (2009) Immunoglobulins and complement in postmortem multiple sclerosis tissue. Ann Neurol 65:32–46. https://doi.org/10.1002/ana.21524
7. Biggins PJC, Brennan FH, Taylor SM, Woodruff TM, Ruitenberg MJ (2017) The alternative receptor for complement component 5a, C5aR2, conveys neuroprotection in traumatic spinal cord injury. J Neurotrauma 34:2075–2085. https://doi.org/10.1089/neu.2016.4701
8. Bolger AM, Lohse M, Usadel B (2014) Trimmomatic: a flexible trimmer for Illumina sequence data. Bioinformatics 30:2114–2120. https://doi.org/10.1093/bioinformatics/btu170
9. Brennan FH, Gordon R, Lao HW, Biggins PJ, Taylor SM, Franklin RJ, Woodruff TM, Ruitenberg MJ (2015) The complement receptor C5aR controls acute inflammation and Astrogliosis following spinal cord injury. J Neurosci 35: 6517–6531. https://doi.org/10.1523/JNEUROSCI.5218-14.2015
10. Burger D, Molnarfi N, Weber MS, Brandt KJ, Benkhoucha M, Gruaz L, Chofflon M, Zamvil SS, Lalive PH (2009) Glatiramer acetate increases IL-1 receptor antagonist but decreases T cell-induced IL-1beta in human monocytes and multiple sclerosis. Proc Natl Acad Sci U S A 106:4355–4359. https://doi.org/10.1073/pnas.0812183106
11. Burm SM, Peferoen LA, Zuiderwijk-Sick EA, Haanstra KG, t'Hart BA, van der Valk P, Amor S, Bauer J, Bajramovic JJ (2016) Expression of IL-1beta in rhesus EAE and MS lesions is mainly induced in the CNS itself. J Neuroinflammation 13:138. https://doi.org/10.1186/s12974-016-0605-8
12. Carroll MC (2008) Complement and humoral immunity. Vaccine 26(Suppl 8):I28–I33
13. Chu AC, Smith N, MacDonald DM (1980) Evaluation of staining methods of resin embedded cutaneous tissue sections of mycosis fungoides. Br J Dermatol 103:607–613
14. Craft JM, Watterson DM, Van Eldik LJ (2005) Neuroinflammation: a potential therapeutic target. Expert Opin Ther Targets 9:887–900. https://doi.org/10.1517/14728222.9.5.887
15. Fandel D, Wasmuht D, Avila-Martin G, Taylor JS, Galan-Arriero I, Mey J (2013) Spinal cord injury induced changes of nuclear receptors PPARalpha and LXRbeta and modulation with oleic acid/albumin treatment. Brain Res 1535: 89–105. https://doi.org/10.1016/j.brainres.2013.08.022
16. Figueroa J, Andreoni J, Densen P (1993) Complement deficiency states and meningococcal disease. Immunol Res 12:295–311
17. Fluiter K, Opperhuizen AL, Morgan BP, Baas F, Ramaglia V (2014) Inhibition of the membrane attack complex of the complement system reduces secondary neuroaxonal loss and promotes neurologic recovery after traumatic brain injury in mice. J Immunol 192:2339–2348. https://doi.org/10.4049/jimmunol.1302793
18. Folaranmi T, Rubin L, Martin SW, Patel M, MacNeil JR, Centers for Disease C (2015) Use of serogroup B meningococcal vaccines in persons aged >/=10 years at increased risk for serogroup B meningococcal disease: recommendations of the advisory committee on immunization practices, 2015. MMWR Morb Mortal Wkly Rep 64:608–612
19. Furlan R, Martino G, Galbiati F, Poliani PL, Smiroldo S, Bergami A, Desina G, Comi G, Flavell R, Su MS, Adorini L (1999) Caspase-1 regulates the inflammatory process leading to autoimmune demyelination. J Immunol 163:2403–2409
20. Gasque P, Singhrao SK, Neal JW, Gotze O, Morgan BP (1997) Expression of the receptor for complement C5a (CD88) is up-regulated on reactive astrocytes, microglia, and endothelial cells in the inflamed human central nervous system. Am J Pathol 150:31–41
21. Geary RS, Norris D, Yu R, Bennett CF (2015) Pharmacokinetics, biodistribution and cell uptake of antisense oligonucleotides. Adv Drug Deliv Rev 87:46–51. https://doi.org/10.1016/j.addr.2015.01.008
22. Gris D, Ye Z, Iocca HA, Wen H, Craven RR, Gris P, Huang M, Schneider M, Miller SD, Ting JP (2010) NLRP3 plays a critical role in the development of experimental autoimmune encephalomyelitis by mediating Th1 and Th17 responses. J Immunol 185:974–981. https://doi.org/10.4049/jimmunol.0904145
23. Guarda G, Braun M, Staehli F, Tardivel A, Mattmann C, Forster I, Farlik M, Decker T, Du Pasquier RA, Romero P, Tschopp J (2011) Type I interferon inhibits interleukin-1 production and inflammasome activation. Immunity 34:213–223. https://doi.org/10.1016/j.immuni.2011.02.006
24. Guo H, Callaway JB, Ting JP (2015) Inflammasomes: mechanism of action, role in disease, and therapeutics. Nat Med 21:677–687. https://doi.org/10.1038/nm.3893
25. Guo RF, Ward PA (2005) Role of C5a in inflammatory responses. Annu Rev Immunol 23:821–852. https://doi.org/10.1146/annurev.immunol.23.021704.115835
26. Hauser SL, Doolittle TH, Lincoln R, Brown RH, Dinarello CA (1990) Cytokine accumulations in CSF of multiple sclerosis patients: frequent detection of interleukin-1 and tumor necrosis factor but not interleukin-6. Neurology 40: 1735–1739
27. Hillmen P, Young NS, Schubert J, Brodsky RA, Socie G, Muus P, Roth A, Szer J, Elebute MO, Nakamura R, Browne P, Risitano AM, Hill A, Schrezenmeier H, Fu CL, Maciejewski J, Rollins SA, Mojcik CF, Rother RP, Luzzatto L (2006) The complement inhibitor eculizumab in paroxysmal nocturnal hemoglobinuria. N Engl J Med 355:1233–1243. https://doi.org/10.1056/NEJMoa061648

28. Hisahara S, Yuan J, Momoi T, Okano H, Miura M (2001) Caspase-11 mediates oligodendrocyte cell death and pathogenesis of autoimmune-mediated demyelination. J Exp Med 193:111–122
29. Hobart MJ, Lachmann PJ, Calne RY (1977) C6: synthesis by the liver in vivo. J Exp Med 146:629–630
30. Ingram G, Loveless S, Howell OW, Hakobyan S, Dancey B, Harris CL, Robertson NP, Neal JW, Morgan BP (2014) Complement activation in multiple sclerosis plaques: an immunohistochemical analysis. Acta Neuropathol Commun 2:53. https://doi.org/10.1186/2051-5960-2-53
31. Inoue M, Chen PH, Siecinski S, Li QJ, Liu C, Steinman L, Gregory SG, Benner E, Shinohara ML (2016) An interferon-beta-resistant and NLRP3 inflammasome-independent subtype of EAE with neuronal damage. Nat Neurosci 19:1599–1609. https://doi.org/10.1038/nn.4421
32. Inoue M, Williams KL, Gunn MD, Shinohara ML (2012) NLRP3 inflammasome induces chemotactic immune cell migration to the CNS in experimental autoimmune encephalomyelitis. Proc Natl Acad Sci U S A 109:10480–10485. https://doi.org/10.1073/pnas.1201836109
33. Inoue M, Williams KL, Oliver T, Vandenabeele P, Rajan JV, Miao EA, Shinohara ML (2012) Interferon-beta therapy against EAE is effective only when development of the disease depends on the NLRP3 inflammasome. Sci signal 5:ra38. https://doi.org/10.1126/scisignal.2002767
34. Ito M, Shichita T, Okada M, Komine R, Noguchi Y, Yoshimura A, Morita R (2015) Bruton's tyrosine kinase is essential for NLRP3 inflammasome activation and contributes to ischaemic brain injury. Nat Commun 6:7360. https://doi.org/10.1038/ncomms8360
35. Jackson SJ, Lee J, Nikodemova M, Fabry Z, Duncan ID (2009) Quantification of myelin and axon pathology during relapsing progressive experimental autoimmune encephalomyelitis in the Biozzi ABH mouse. J Neuropathol Exp Neurol 68:616–625. https://doi.org/10.1097/NEN.0b013e3181a41d23
36. Jha S, Srivastava SY, Brickey WJ, Iocca H, Toews A, Morrison JP, Chen VS, Gris D, Matsushima GK, Ting JP (2010) The inflammasome sensor, NLRP3, regulates CNS inflammation and demyelination via caspase-1 and interleukin-18. J Neurosci 30:15811–15820. https://doi.org/10.1523/JNEUROSCI.4088-10.2010
37. Joseph SB, Castrillo A, Laffitte BA, Mangelsdorf DJ, Tontonoz P (2003) Reciprocal regulation of inflammation and lipid metabolism by liver X receptors. Nat Med 9:213–219. https://doi.org/10.1038/nm820
38. Kilgore KS, Schmid E, Shanley TP, Flory CM, Maheswari V, Tramontini NL, Cohen H, Ward PA, Friedl HP, Warren JS (1997) Sublytic concentrations of the membrane attack complex of complement induce endothelial interleukin-8 and monocyte chemoattractant protein-1 through nuclear factor-kappa B activation. Am J Pathol 150:2019–2031
39. Kim D, Langmead B, Salzberg SL (2015) HISAT: a fast spliced aligner with low memory requirements. Nat Methods 12:357–360. https://doi.org/10.1038/nmeth.3317
40. Kotimaa J, Klar-Mohammad N, Gueler F, Schilders G, Jansen A, Rutjes H, Daha MR, van Kooten C (2016) Sex matters: systemic complement activity of female C57BL/6J and BALB/cJ mice is limited by serum terminal pathway components. Mol Immunol 76:13–21. https://doi.org/10.1016/j.molimm.2016.06.004
41. Kramer A, Green J, Pollard J Jr, Tugendreich S (2014) Causal analysis approaches in ingenuity pathway analysis. Bioinformatics 30:523–530. https://doi.org/10.1093/bioinformatics/btt703
42. Lassmann H (2007) Multiple sclerosis: is there neurodegeneration independent from inflammation? J Neurol Sci 259:3–6. https://doi.org/10.1016/j.jns.2006.08.016
43. Lassmann H (2015) Immune response in the human central nervous system in multiple sclerosis and stroke. In: David S (ed) Neuroinflammation: new insights into beneficial and detrimental functions, 1st edn. John Wiley & Sons, Inc, Hoboken. https://doi.org/10.1002/9781118732748.ch1
44. Lassmann H, Bradl M (2017) Multiple sclerosis: experimental models and reality. Acta Neuropathol 133:223–244. https://doi.org/10.1007/s00401-016-1631-4
45. Laudisi F, Spreafico R, Evrard M, Hughes TR, Mandriani B, Kandasamy M, Morgan BP, Sivasankar B, Mortellaro A (2013) Cutting edge: the NLRP3 inflammasome links complement-mediated inflammation and IL-1beta release. J Immunol 191:1006–1010. https://doi.org/10.4049/jimmunol.1300489
46. Lee H, Whitfeld PL, Mackay CR (2008) Receptors for complement C5a. The importance of C5aR and the enigmatic role of C5L2. Immunol Cell Biol 86: 153–160. https://doi.org/10.1038/sj.icb.7100166
47. Lee JD, Kumar V, Fung JN, Ruitenberg MJ, Noakes PG, Woodruff TM (2017) Pharmacological inhibition of complement C5a-C5a1 receptor signalling ameliorates disease pathology in the hSOD1G93A mouse model of amyotrophic lateral sclerosis. Br J Pharmacol 174:689–699. https://doi.org/10.1111/bph.13730
48. Lucchinetti C, Bruck W, Parisi J, Scheithauer B, Rodriguez M, Lassmann H (2000) Heterogeneity of multiple sclerosis lesions: implications for the pathogenesis of demyelination. Ann Neurol 47:707–717
49. Mariathasan S, Weiss DS, Newton K, McBride J, O'Rourke K, Roose-Girma M, Lee WP, Weinrauch Y, Monack DM, Dixit VM (2006) Cryopyrin activates the inflammasome in response to toxins and ATP. Nature 440:228–232. https://doi.org/10.1038/nature04515
50. McGeer PL, Klegeris A, Walker DG, Yasuhara O, McGeer EG (1994) Pathological proteins in senile plaques. Tohoku J Exp Med 174:269–277
51. Mead RJ, Singhrao SK, Neal JW, Lassmann H, Morgan BP (2002) The membrane attack complex of complement causes severe demyelination associated with acute axonal injury. J Immunol 168:458–465
52. Mellergard J, Edstrom M, Vrethem M, Ernerudh J, Dahle C (2010) Natalizumab treatment in multiple sclerosis: marked decline of chemokines and cytokines in cerebrospinal fluid. Mult Scler 16:208–217. https://doi.org/10.1177/1352458509355068
53. Mellergard J, Tisell A, Dahlqvist Leinhard O, Blystad I, Landtblom AM, Blennow K, Olsson B, Dahle C, Ernerudh J, Lundberg P, Vrethem M (2012) Association between change in normal appearing white matter metabolites and intrathecal inflammation in natalizumab-treated multiple sclerosis. PLoS One 7:e44739. https://doi.org/10.1371/journal.pone.0044739
54. Michailidou I, Naessens DM, Hametner S, Guldenaar W, Kooi EJ, Geurts JJ, Baas F, Lassmann H, Ramaglia V (2017) Complement C3 on microglial clusters in multiple sclerosis occur in chronic but not acute disease: implication for disease pathogenesis. Glia 65:264–277. https://doi.org/10.1002/glia.23090
55. Michailidou I, Willems JG, Kooi EJ, van Eden C, Gold SM, Geurts JJ, Baas F, Huitinga I, Ramaglia V (2015) Complement C1q-C3-associated synaptic changes in multiple sclerosis hippocampus. Ann Neurol 77:1007–1026. https://doi.org/10.1002/ana.24398
56. Morgan BP, Griffiths M, Khanom H, Taylor SM, Neal JW (2004) Blockade of the C5a receptor fails to protect against experimental autoimmune encephalomyelitis in rats. Clin Exp Immunol 138:430–438. https://doi.org/10.1111/j.1365-2249.2004.02646.x
57. Morgan BP, Harris CL (2015) Complement, a target for therapy in inflammatory and degenerative diseases. Nat Rev Drug Discov 14:857–877. https://doi.org/10.1038/nrd4657
58. Niculescu T, Weerth S, Niculescu F, Cudrici C, Rus V, Raine CS, Shin ML, Rus H (2004) Effects of complement C5 on apoptosis in experimental autoimmune encephalomyelitis. J Immunol 172:5702–5706
59. Papadimitriou JC, Phelps PC, Shin ML, Smith MW, Trump BF (1994) Effects of Ca2+ deregulation on mitochondrial membrane potential and cell viability in nucleated cells following lytic complement attack. Cell Calcium 15:217–227
60. Peelen E, Damoiseaux J, Muris AH, Knippenberg S, Smolders J, Hupperts R, Thewissen M (2015) Increased inflammasome related gene expression profile in PBMC may facilitate T helper 17 cell induction in multiple sclerosis. Mol Immunol 63:521–529. https://doi.org/10.1016/j.molimm.2014.10.008
61. Ramaglia V, Jackson SJ, Hughes TR, Neal JW, Baker D, Morgan BP (2015) Complement activation and expression during chronic relapsing experimental autoimmune encephalomyelitis in the Biozzi ABH mouse. Clin Exp Immunol 180:432–441. https://doi.org/10.1111/cei.12595
62. Ramaglia V, King RH, Morgan BP, Baas F (2009) Deficiency of the complement regulator CD59a exacerbates Wallerian degeneration. Mol Immunol 46:1892–1896. https://doi.org/10.1016/j.molimm.2009.01.017
63. Ramaglia V, King RH, Nourallah M, Wolterman R, de Jonge R, Ramkema M, Vigar MA, van der Wetering S, Morgan BP, Troost D, Baas F (2007) The membrane attack complex of the complement system is essential for rapid Wallerian degeneration. J Neurosci 27:7663–7672. https://doi.org/10.1523/JNEUROSCI.5623-06.2007
64. Reiman R, Campos Torres A, Martin BK, Ting JP, Campbell IL, Barnum SR (2005) Expression of C5a in the brain does not exacerbate experimental autoimmune encephalomyelitis. Neurosci Lett 390:134–138. https://doi.org/10.1016/j.neulet.2005.08.022
65. Reiman R, Gerard C, Campbell IL, Barnum SR (2002) Disruption of the C5a receptor gene fails to protect against experimental allergic encephalomyelitis. Eur J Immunol 32:1157–1163. https://doi.org/10.1002/1521-4141(200204). 32:4<1157::AID-IMMU1157>3.0.CO;2-M

66. Ricklin D, Hajishengallis G, Yang K, Lambris JD (2010) Complement: a key system for immune surveillance and homeostasis. Nat Immunol 11:785–797. https://doi.org/10.1038/ni.1923
67. Ronchi F, Basso C, Preite S, Reboldi A, Baumjohann D, Perlini L, Lanzavecchia A, Sallusto F (2016) Experimental priming of encephalitogenic Th1/Th17 cells requires pertussis toxin-driven IL-1beta production by myeloid cells. Nat Commun 7:11541. https://doi.org/10.1038/ncomms11541
68. Rossi S, Studer V, Motta C, Germani G, Macchiarulo G, Buttari F, Mancino R, Castelli M, De Chiara V, Weiss S, Martino G, Furlan R, Centonze D (2014) Cerebrospinal fluid detection of interleukin-1beta in phase of remission predicts disease progression in multiple sclerosis. J Neuroinflammation 11: 32. https://doi.org/10.1186/1742-2094-11-32
69. Ruseva MM, Ramaglia V, Morgan BP, Harris CL (2015) An anticomplement agent that homes to the damaged brain and promotes recovery after traumatic brain injury in mice. Proc Natl Acad Sci U S A 112:14319–14324. https://doi.org/10.1073/pnas.1513698112
70. Saper CB, Sawchenko PE (2003) Magic peptides, magic antibodies: guidelines for appropriate controls for immunohistochemistry. J Comp Neurol 465:161–163. https://doi.org/10.1002/cne.10858
71. Schellenberg AE, Buist R, Yong VW, Del Bigio MR, Peeling J (2007) Magnetic resonance imaging of blood-spinal cord barrier disruption in mice with experimental autoimmune encephalomyelitis. Magn Reson Med 58:298–305. https://doi.org/10.1002/mrm.21289
72. Seppi D, Puthenparampil M, Federle L, Ruggero S, Toffanin E, Rinaldi F, Perini P, Gallo P (2014) Cerebrospinal fluid IL-1beta correlates with cortical pathology load in multiple sclerosis at clinical onset. J Neuroimmunol 270: 56–60. https://doi.org/10.1016/j.jneuroim.2014.02.014
73. Shaftel SS, Carlson TJ, Olschowka JA, Kyrkanides S, Matousek SB, O'Banion MK (2007) Chronic interleukin-1beta expression in mouse brain leads to leukocyte infiltration and neutrophil-independent blood brain barrier permeability without overt neurodegeneration. J Neurosci 27:9301–9309. https://doi.org/10.1523/JNEUROSCI.1418-07.2007
74. Shaw PJ, Lukens JR, Burns S, Chi H, McGargill MA, Kanneganti TD (2010) Cutting edge: critical role for PYCARD/ASC in the development of experimental autoimmune encephalomyelitis. J Immunol 184:4610–4614. https://doi.org/10.4049/jimmunol.1000217
75. Stokowska A, Atkins AL, Moran J, Pekny T, Bulmer L, Pascoe MC, Barnum SR, Wetsel RA, Nilsson JA, Dragunow M, Pekna M (2017) Complement peptide C3a stimulates neural plasticity after experimental brain ischaemia. Brain 140:353–369. https://doi.org/10.1093/brain/aww314
76. Straus DS, Glass CK (2007) Anti-inflammatory actions of PPAR ligands: new insights on cellular and molecular mechanisms. Trends Immunol 28:551–558. https://doi.org/10.1016/j.it.2007.09.003
77. Tran GT, Hodgkinson SJ, Carter N, Killingsworth M, Spicer ST, Hall BM (2002) Attenuation of experimental allergic encephalomyelitis in complement component 6-deficient rats is associated with reduced complement C9 deposition, P-selectin expression, and cellular infiltrate in spinal cords. J Immunol 168:4293–4300
78. Triantafilou K, Hughes TR, Triantafilou M, Morgan BP (2013) The complement membrane attack complex triggers intracellular Ca2+ fluxes leading to NLRP3 inflammasome activation. J Cell Sci 126:2903–2913. https://doi.org/10.1242/jcs.124388
79. Triantafilou M, Hughes TR, Morgan BP, Triantafilou K (2016) Complementing the inflammasome. Immunology 147:152–164. https://doi.org/10.1111/imm.12556
80. Wang Q, Rozelle AL, Lepus CM, Scanzello CR, Song JJ, Larsen DM, Crish JF, Bebek G, Ritter SY, Lindstrom TM, Hwang I, Wong HH, Punzi L, Encarnacion A, Shamloo M, Goodman SB, Wyss-Coray T, Goldring SR, Banda NK, Thurman JM, Gobezie R, Crow MK, Holers VM, Lee DM, Robinson WH (2011) Identification of a central role for complement in osteoarthritis. Nat Med 17: 1674–1679. https://doi.org/10.1038/nm.2543
81. Ward PA (2009) Functions of C5a receptors. J Mol Med (Berl) 87:375–378. https://doi.org/10.1007/s00109-009-0442-7
82. Watkins LM, Neal JW, Loveless S, Michailidou I, Ramaglia V, Rees MI, Reynolds R, Robertson NP, Morgan BP, Howell OW (2016) Complement is activated in progressive multiple sclerosis cortical grey matter lesions. J Neuroinflammation 13:161. https://doi.org/10.1186/s12974-016-0611-x
83. Weerth SH, Rus H, Shin ML, Raine CS (2003) Complement C5 in experimental autoimmune encephalomyelitis (EAE) facilitates remyelination and prevents gliosis. Am J Pathol 163:1069–1080. https://doi.org/10.1016/S0002-9440(10)63466-9
84. Wong EK, Kavanagh D (2015) Anticomplement C5 therapy with eculizumab for the treatment of paroxysmal nocturnal hemoglobinuria and atypical hemolytic uremic syndrome. Transl Res 165:306–320. https://doi.org/10.1016/j.trsl.2014.10.010
85. Woodruff TM, Crane JW, Proctor LM, Buller KM, Shek AB, de Vos K, Pollitt S, Williams HM, Shiels IA, Monk PN, Taylor SM (2006) Therapeutic activity of C5a receptor antagonists in a rat model of neurodegeneration. FASEB J 20: 1407–1417. https://doi.org/10.1096/fj.05-5814com
86. Wurzner R, Orren A, Potter P, Morgan BP, Ponard D, Spath P, Brai M, Schulze M, Happe L, Gotze O (1991) Functionally active complement proteins C6 and C7 detected in C6- and C7-deficient individuals. Clin Exp Immunol 83:430–437
87. Zhang T, Garstka MA, Li K (2017) The controversial C5a receptor C5aR2: its role in health and disease. J Immunol Res 2017:8193932. https://doi.org/10.1155/2017/8193932

12

Potent prion-like behaviors of pathogenic α-synuclein and evaluation of inactivation methods

Airi Tarutani[1,2], Tetsuaki Arai[3], Shigeo Murayama[4], Shin-ichi Hisanaga[2] and Masato Hasegawa[1*]

Abstract

The concept that abnormal protein aggregates show prion-like propagation between cells has been considered to explain the onset and progression of many neurodegenerative diseases. Indeed, both synthetic amyloid-like fibrils and pathogenic proteins extracted from patients' brains induce self-templated amplification and cell-to-cell transmission in vitro and in vivo. However, it is unclear whether exposure to exogenous prion-like proteins can potentially cause these diseases in humans. Here, we investigated in detail the prion-like seeding activities of several kinds of pathogenic α-synuclein (α-syn), including synthetic fibrils and detergent-insoluble fractions extracted from brains of patients with α-synucleinopathies. Exposure to synthetic α-syn fibrils at concentrations above 100 pg/mL caused seeded aggregation of α-syn in SH-SY5Y cells, and seeded aggregation was also observed in C57BL/6 J mice after intracerebral inoculation of at least 0.1 μg/animal. α-Syn aggregates extracted from brains of multiple system atrophy (MSA) patients showed higher seeding activity than those extracted from patients with dementia with Lewy bodies (DLB), and their potency was similar to that of synthetic α-syn fibrils. We also examined the effects of various methods that have been reported to inactivate abnormal prion proteins (PrP^{Sc}), including autoclaving at various temperatures, exposure to sodium dodecyl sulfate (SDS), and combined treatments. The combination of autoclaving and 1% SDS substantially reduced the seeding activities of synthetic α-syn fibrils and α-syn aggregates extracted from MSA brains. However, single treatment with 1% SDS or generally used sterilization conditions proved insufficient to prevent accumulation of pathological α-syn. In conclusion, α-syn aggregates derived from MSA patients showed a potent prion-like seeding activity, which could be efficiently reduced by combined use of SDS and autoclaving.

Keywords: α-Synuclein, Prion-like propagation, Seeds, α-Synucleinopathy, Strains, Inactivation

Introduction

Intracellular accumulations of abnormal protein aggregates are common but defining neuropathological features of many neurodegenerative diseases. The distributions and spreading of these pathological proteins are closely correlated with clinical symptoms and progression [9, 49]. Recently, it has been suggested that the prion-like behavior of abnormal proteins may account for the onset and progression of neurodegenerative diseases [21, 62]. A growing body of evidence supports the idea that template-mediated amplification and intracerebral transmission of abnormal proteins are the main mechanisms by which pathological proteins spread along the neural circuits in the brain, although the molecular mechanisms of cell-to-cell transmission remain to be fully clarified.

α-Synucleinopathies, which include Parkinson's disease (PD), dementia with Lewy bodies (DLB) and multiple system atrophy (MSA), are characterized by accumulation of misfolded α-synuclein (α-syn) aggregates in neuronal and/or glial cells, and various pathological phenotypes and clinical symptoms are observed for each disease [22]. In PD and DLB, α-syn pathologies are mainly observed in neurons in the form of Lewy bodies (LBs) and Lewy neurites (LNs) [4, 56], whereas glial cytoplasmic inclusions (GCIs) are seen in oligodendrocytes in MSA [61]. The

* Correspondence: hasegawa-ms@igakuken.or.jp
[1]Department of Dementia and Higher Brain Function, Tokyo Metropolitan Institute of Medical Science, 2-1-6 Kamikitazawa, Setagaya-ku, Tokyo 156-8506, Japan
Full list of author information is available at the end of the article

abnormal α-syn observed in brains of patients is accumulated as fibrous or filamentous forms with cross-β structures [54, 55], existing in phosphorylated and partially ubiquitinated states [18, 24]. These abnormal α-syn species exhibit seeding activity to induce prion-like conversion, detergent-insolubility and protease-resistance of endogenous α-syn [38], being similar in these respects to the infectious forms of prion protein (PrP^{Sc}) causing Creutzfeldt-Jakob disease (CJD) and bovine spongiform encephalopathy [45].

α-Syn is a natively unfolded protein of 140 amino acid residues, which is localized in synaptic termini at relatively high concentration [33]. Although its physiological function has not been fully clarified, it appears to be involved in the regulation of SNARE complex and in dopamine production [1, 6, 12, 13]. Disease-linked missense mutations and multiplication of the *SNCA* gene encoding α-syn have been reported in familial forms of α-synucleinopathies, indicating that structural changes and overexpression of α-syn protein are involved in the development of synucleinopathies [42].

Recombinant soluble α-syn proteins purified from bacterial cells expressing α-syn form amyloid-like fibrils that are morphologically and physicochemically similar to those observed in patients' brains in vitro, upon shaking at 37 °C for a few days [14, 51]. These synthetic α-syn fibrils can act as seeds and induce seeded aggregation of α-syn in cultured cells or primary cultured neurons, as well as in rodent brains [25]. Intracerebral inoculation of synthetic α-syn fibrils induces phosphorylated and ubiqutinated α-syn pathologies not only in transgenic (Tg) mice overexpressing human α-syn, but also in wild-type (WT) mice [31, 32, 36]. In particular, Tg mice overexpressing mutant human α-syn develop lethal central nervous system (CNS) disorder after being inoculated with fibrils [37]. It has also been shown that brain homogenates or insoluble fractions extracted from brains of patients with α-synucleinopathies induce α-syn pathologies in animal brains [5, 36, 47, 63]. In addition, recent studies have suggested that α-syn strains with distinct conformations exist, which is a characteristic of prions. Synthetic α-syn fibrils formed under different physiological conditions in vitro showed distinct seeding activities and cytotoxicities in cultured cells and rat brains [8, 43]. Furthermore, MSA brain extracts exhibit distinct infectivity compared to PD or control brain extracts in human embryonic kidney (HEK) 293 cells expressing mutant A53T α-syn fused to yellow fluorescent protein and in TgM83 hemizygous mice expressing mutant A53T α-syn [46, 66].

These experimental demonstrations of prion-like propagation show that abnormal α-syn can trigger self-templated amplification of abnormal forms and spread throughout the brain. On the other hand, there is no report or evidence as yet to indicate that infection of pathogenic α-syn between individuals can occur, or that onset of α-synucleinopathy can occur following exposure to contaminated environments. It is also unclear to what extent materials contaminated with pathogenic α-syn pose a risk of secondary infection to patients, clinicians and researchers. These are clearly important issues, because iatrogenic transmission of PrP^{Sc} from human tissues derived from patients with CJD (e.g. dura mater transplants and growth hormone treatments) or from surgical instruments contaminated with PrP^{Sc} is well documented [11]. Therefore, we need to examine whether iatrogenically acquired abnormal α-syn may cause synucleinopathy or accelerate clinical symptoms. Here, we examined this question by characterizing the seeding activities of synthetic α-syn fibrils and abnormal α-syn extracted from brains of patients with MSA and DLB.

We have already established experimental models for seeded aggregation of α-syn using SH-SY5Y cells, as well as in vivo models in WT rodents and primates inoculated intracerebrally with synthetic α-syn fibrils [36, 41, 53]. Our previous study showed that the size of the amyloid-like fibrils is the key factor that determines the efficiency of seeded aggregation and propagation in these models [58]. In this study, we further investigated the seeding activities of these pathogenic α-syn species, focusing on how much pathogenic α-syn is required to seed the formation of intracellular aggregates of transiently expressed or endogenous normal α-syn beyond the capacity of maintenance mechanisms, such as lysosomal, proteasomal and autophagy-mediated protein degradation systems, to remove them. We also investigated whether the abnormal α-syn aggregates derived from MSA and DLB patients' brains show distinct prion-like properties characteristic of each disease, compared to synthetic α-syn fibrils, in our models.

It is also important to consider inactivation methodology. It has been reported that a commercially available alkaline cleanser, a hydrogen peroxide solution containing Cu^{2+} ions, and 1% sodium dodecyl sulfate (SDS) are effective for removing pathogenic α-syn adhering to surgical materials and laboratory instruments [7, 60]. In addition, BioHOCl effectively reduced the seeding activity of pathogenic α-syn derived from brains with Lewy-body pathology, as determined with a real-time quaking induced conversion (RT-QuIC) assay [26]. On the other hand, formalin fixation of tissues containing α-syn pathology derived from patients with synucleinopathies and from symptomatic Tg mice had little effect on seeding activity or infectivity [50, 65]. Notably, we found that α-syn aggregates derived from MSA patients' brains (MSA-syn) exhibited much higher seeding activity than those from DLB cases. Fortunately, however, MSA-syn and other abnormal α-syn could be efficiently reduced by combined use of SDS and autoclaving. The present findings, together with previous work, suggests that safety measures to destroy pathogenic α-syn should be mandatory in hospitals and laboratories.

Materials and methods

Expression and purification of α-syn protein

Escherichia coli BL21 (DE3) was transfected with bacterial expression plasmid pRK172, a construct containing human WT or mouse α-syn that lacks cysteine due to mutagenesis of codon 136 (TAC to TAT) [34], and the expressed protein was purified as described [39]. Protein concentrations of α-syn were determined by reverse-phase HPLC as described [35].

Preparation of recombinant α-syn fibrils

Purified recombinant α-syn proteins (5 mg/ml) containing 30 mM Tris-HCl (pH 7.5), 10 mM DTT and 0.1% sodium azide were incubated for 7 days at 37 °C in a horizontal shaker (Taitec) at 200 rpm, then ultracentrifuged at 113,000×g for 20 min at 25 °C. The pellets were washed with saline and ultracentrifuged as before. The resulting pellets were collected as α-syn fibrils and resuspended in 30 mM Tris-HCl (pH 7.5). The fibrils at a concentration of 2 mg/ml were fragmented using a cup horn sonicator (Sonifier® SFX, Branson) at 35% power for 180 s (total 240 s, 30 s on, 10 s off), then aliquoted and cryopreserved. For electron microscopy, α-syn fibrils (0.2 μg) were dropped on carbon-coated 300-mesh copper grids (Nissin EM) and incubated for 3 min. After removal of surplus material, the fibrils were negatively stained for 3 min with a drop of 2% sodium phosphotungstate and dried. Electron micrograph images were obtained with a JEOL JEM-1400 electron microscope (JEOL).

Ethics statement

Postmortem brain tissues, which had been neuropathologically confirmed as MSA or DLB, were obtained from the Brain Bank for Aging Research in Tokyo Metropolitan Geriatric Hospital & Institute of Gerontology, (Tokyo, Japan). The study protocol was approved by the ethics committees of Tokyo Metropolitan Geriatric Hospital and Tokyo Metropolitan Institute of Medical Science. All methods were performed in accordance with the relevant guidelines and regulations. All brain tissues used in this study were anonymized.

All mice were housed at the Tokyo Metropolitan Institute of Medical Science (TMiMS) in a facility in compliance with Guidelines for Proper Conduct of Animal Experiments (Science Council of Japan). Experimentation followed TMiMS Animal Care and Use Committee approved protocol #17018 in compliance with Guidelines for Proper Conduct of Animal Experiments (Science Council of Japan).

Preparation of sarkosyl-insoluble fractions from patients' brains

For each case, a brain sample (0.5 g) was homogenized in 20 volumes (*w*/*v*) of A68 buffer (10 mM Tris-HCl pH 7.5 containing 10% sucrose, 0.8 M NaCl, 1 mM EGTA) and incubated for 30 min at 37 °C, after addition of sarkosyl (final concentration: 2%). Brain homogenates were centrifuged at 9460×g for 10 min at 25 °C, then ultracentrifuged at 113,000×g for 20 min at 25 °C. The pellets were washed with saline and ultracentrifuged as before. The resulting pellets were collected as sarkosyl-insoluble fractions of patients' brains, resuspended in 30 mM Tris-HCl (pH 7.5) by sonication for 15 s, and used for introduction into cultured cells or for inactivation treatments. Resuspended fractions were centrifuged at 1000 g for 5 min. The supernatants were used for stereotaxic inoculation.

For immunoblotting analysis, sarkosyl-insoluble fractions were added to SDS-sample buffer and boiled for 3 min. The samples were separated by 12% SDS-PAGE. Immunoblotting with mouse monoclonal antibody PSer129 (1:1000) directed against α-syn phosphorylated at Ser129 [18] and other anti-α-syn antibodies, including syn131-140 (1:2000, Cosmo bio), LB509 (1:1000) and Syn102 (1:1000) was performed as described [52]. LB509 and Syn102 were kind gifts from Dr. Takeshi Iwatsubo. Phosphorylated tau was detected with monoclonal anti-Tau antibody T46 (1:1000, Thermo Fisher Scientific).

Quantification of α-syn by immunoblotting

The concentrations of α-syn in sarkosyl-insoluble fractions extracted from human brain samples were determined by immunoblotting. The standard curve was generated using serial dilutions of recombinant phosphorylated human α-syn monomer. Phosphorylated α-syn was detected with mouse monoclonal anti-PSer129 antibody. The band intensities of immunoblots were quantified using ImageQuant TL.

The concentrations of α-syn expressed in WT mice were calculated by immunoblotting as below. The standard curves were generated using recombinant mouse α-syn. C57BL/6 mouse brains were homogenized in A68 buffer and centrifuged at 10,000 g for 5 min. The supernatant were collected as A68-soluble fraction and immunoblotted with polyclonal anti-mouse α-syn antibody (1:1000, Cell Signaling Technology).

Immunoelectron microscopy

Sarkosyl-insoluble fractions extracted from MSA and DLB patients' brains were dropped onto carbon-coated nickel grids (Nissin EM). The grids were immunostained with an anti-phosphorylated α-syn rabbit monoclonal antibody EP1536Y (Abcam, 1:200) and a secondary antibody conjugated to 5 nm gold particles (BBI Solutions, 1:50) as described [23]. Electron micrograph images were recorded with a JEOL JEM-1400 electron microscope (JEOL).

Cell culture, transfection of plasmids and introduction of pathogenic proteins into cells

Human neuroblastoma SH-SY5Y cells were maintained at 37 °C in 5% CO_2 in Dulbecco's modified Eagle's medium (DMEM)/F12 medium (Sigma-Aldrich) supplemented with 10% fetal calf serum, penicillin-streptomycin glutamine (Gibco), and MEM nonessential amino acids solution (Gibco). Cells were cultured to 40–50% confluence in collagen-coated 6-well plates and transfected using X-tremeGENE 9 (Roche Life Science) with pcDNA3 encoding human WT α-syn (1.5 μg) according to the manufacturer's instructions. After transfection of plasmids, cells were incubated for 6–8 h, and pathogenic proteins (2 μl) were introduced using MultiFectam (Promega) according to the manufacturer's instructions. Transfected cells were incubated for 3 days.

Preparation of sarkosyl-insoluble fractions from transfected cells and immunoblotting

Transfected SH-SY5Y cells were collected and extracted with 1 ml of 1% sarkosyl in A68 buffer. Cell extracts were sonicated for 15 s on ice. After incubation for 30 min at 37 °C, cell extracts were ultracentrifuged at 113,000×g for 20 min at 25 °C. The supernatants were removed and collected as sarkosyl-soluble fractions, then the pellets were washed with 30 mM Tris-HCl (pH 7.5) and ultracentrifuged as before. The resulting pellets were collected as sarkosyl-insoluble fractions, resuspended in 30 mM Tris-HCl (pH 7.5) and sonicated for 15 s. Sarkosyl-insoluble and -soluble fractions were added to SDS-sample buffer and boiled for 3 min. The protein concentrations of samples were determined with a Pierce BCA Protein Assay Kit (Thermo Fisher Scientific). Immunoblotting was performed with mouse monoclonal anti-PSer129 antibody (1:1000) and polyclonal antibody syn131–140 (1:2000, Cosmo Bio). In immunoblotting, monoclonal anti-α-tubulin (1:1000, Sigma) was used to obtain a loading control. All experiments were performed at least three times. The band intensities of immunoblots were quantified using ImageQuant TL. The ID_{50} was calculated by the Spearman-Karber method based on the band intensities.

Immunofluorescence microscopy

Transfection of plasmids and introduction of pathogenic proteins were conducted as described above, using SH-SY5Y cells grown on coverslips. After incubation for 3 days, cells were fixed with 4% paraformaldehyde and treated with an anti-phosphorylated α-syn rabbit monoclonal antibody EP1536Y (1:1000, Abcam) and the secondary antibody (anti-rabbit IgG-conjugated Alexa-568, Invitrogen) as described [57]. The cells were mounted and analyzed using a BZ-X710 fluorescence microscope (Keyence).

Mice

C57BL/6 J mice were purchased from CLEA Japan, Inc.

α-Syn inoculation into mouse brains and immunohistochemistry

α-Syn samples (5 μl) were inoculated into striatum (A-P: 0.2 mm; M-L: − 2.0 mm; D-V: − 2.6 mm) as described [35]. The inoculum was injected at a rate of 5 μl per min and the needle was kept in place at the injection site for 3 min or more. At 3 months after inoculation, mice were anesthetized with isoflurane and killed by decapitation. Brains were fixed with 10% formalin neutral buffer solution (Wako) and sectioned at 50 μm with a Leica VT1200S (Leica). Immunohistochemistry with an anti-phosphorylated α-syn rabbit monoclonal antibody EP1536Y (1:1000, Abcam) was performed as described [53]. α-Syn pathologies were observed and recorded with a BZ-X710 fluorescence microscope (Keyence). Immunoreactivity for pS129 α-syn was quantified using images of coronal sections from four different regions (frontal cortex, striatum, amygdala, substantia nigra); 4–7 sections per animal for each region were used for quantification. PS129-positive cells were counted in 20× (striatum, amygdala and substantia nigra) or 10× (frontal cortex) images using BZ-H3C Hybrid Cell Count Software (Keyence).

Inactivation and protease treatments

Synthetic α-syn fibrils (2 mg/ml) and sarkosyl-insoluble fractions extracted from MSA patients' brains were incubated in saline or in 0.1% or 1% sodium dodecyl sulfate for 1 h at room temperature. Pathogenic α-syn in saline or 0.1% or 1% SDS was also incubated at 100 °C for 3 min, 120 °C for 20 min or 134 °C for 20 min. Incubations at 120 °C and 134 °C were performed using an laboratory autoclave, LSX-300 (Tomy). For protease K treatment, inactivated synthetic α-syn fibrils were treated with 5 μg/ml protease K at 37 °C for 30 min. The reaction was stopped by boiling, and samples were analyzed by immunoblotting with polyclonal antibody syn102–116 (1:2000) directed against a synthetic peptide (residues 102–116) (Cosmo Bio).

Statistical analysis

The DLB and MSA data presented in Fig. 3b were analyzed using Welch's modified t-test. All other data were analyzed using a one-way ANOVA followed by

Dunnett's post hoc test. In both cases, a P value < 0.05 was regarded as statistically significant.

Results

Seeded aggregation induced by synthetic α-syn fibrils in SH-SY5Y cells

First, we investigated the minimum amounts of pathogenic α-syn required to induce seeded aggregation and accumulation of phosphorylated α-syn in SH-SY5Y cells expressing untagged human wild-type (WT) α-syn. Serial dilutions from 10^{-1} to 10^{-7} of 1 mg/ml (70 μM) synthetic human WT α-syn fibrils (Fig. 1a) were sonicated for 3 min and then introduced into SY5Y cells as previously reported [41]. After 3 days, the sarkosyl-insoluble fraction was prepared from the transfected cells and accumulation of phospho-α-syn was analyzed by immunoblotting with PS129 antibody (Fig. 1b). The results of quantitation of the insoluble phosphorylated α-syn are shown in Fig. 1c. Accumulation of phospho-α-syn was detected in cells treated with α-syn fibrils diluted to 10^{-3}, but no increase was observed in cells treated with dilutions from 10^{-4} to 10^{-7}. The relative amounts of insoluble α-syn formed in cells were increased concentration-dependently by addition of α-syn fibrils at dilutions from 10^{-1} to 10^{-4}, but the amount was saturated at more than 10^{-1} dilution (Fig. 1c). Based on protein determination by immunoblotting, the ID_{50} (50% infectious dose or seeding activity) per 2 μL was calculated to be $10^{2.91}$ (± 0.51) by the Spearman-Karber method [64]. These results show that exposure of SH-SY5Y cells transiently expressing human α-syn to synthetic human α-syn fibrils at a concentration of above 100 pg/mL can induce seeded aggregation of the intracellular α-syn.

Characterization of insoluble α-syn extracted from brains of patients with α-synucleinopathies

Next, we investigated the prion-like properties of α-syn aggregates derived from postmortem brain tissues of patients with α-synucleinopathies. To examine whether there are structural and biochemical differences between α-syn aggregates in DLB and MSA, we performed immuno-electron microscopy and immunoblotting of sarkosyl-insoluble fractions extracted from patients'

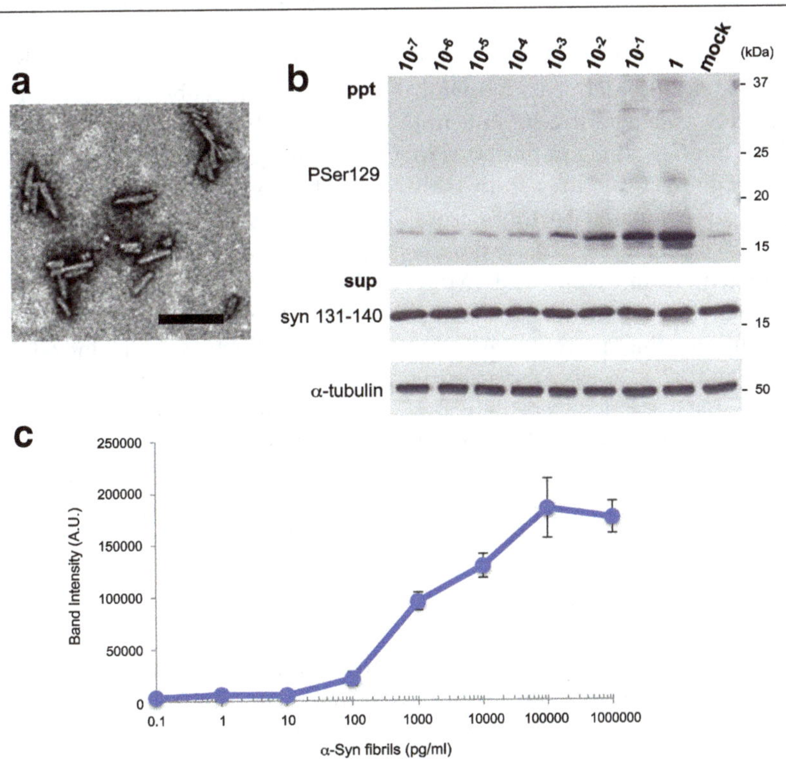

Fig. 1 Seed-dependent α-syn aggregation induced by serial dilutions of synthetic α-syn fibrils in SH-SY5Y cells. **a** Electron microscopy of human α-syn fibrils after sonication for 180 s. Negatively stained short fibrils less than 100 nm in size were observed. Scale bar, 100 nm. **b** Serial 10-fold dilutions of human α-syn fibrils (2 μl) were introduced into SH-SY5Y cells transiently expressing human WT α-syn in the presence of the transfection reagent. Immunoblot analysis of sarkosyl-insoluble fractions (ppt) and sarkosyl-soluble fractions (sup) extracted from mock-transfected cells or cells transfected with human α-syn fibrils in the range of 2 μg (1) to 0.2 pg (10^{-7}) are shown. Phosphorylated α-syn was detected with anti-phosphorylated α-syn PSer129 antibody. α-Syn was detected with anti-syn 131–140 antibody **c** Quantification of phosphorylated α-syn accumulated in SH-SY5Y cells exposed to serial dilutions of synthetic human α-syn fibrils. Band intensities from the immunoblot analyses shown in **b** were measured. The results are expressed as means ± SEM (n = 3).

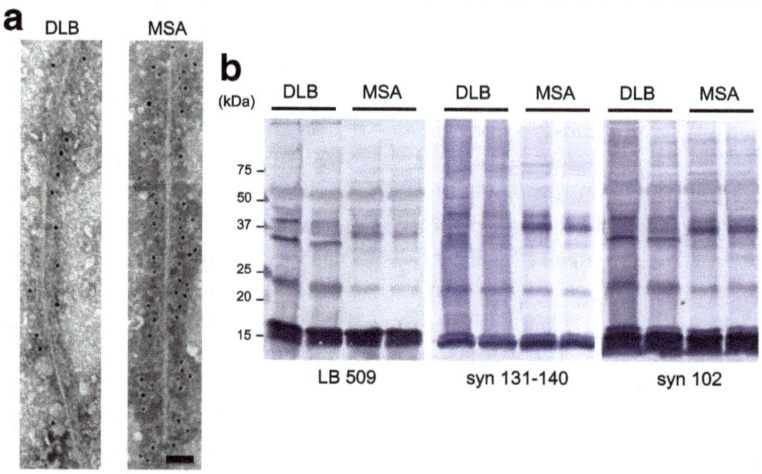

Fig. 2 Characterization of α-syn aggregates extracted from brains of synucleinopathy patients. **a** Immunoelectron microscopy of sarkosyl-insoluble fractions extracted from DLB (left) and MSA (right) patients' brains. Electron micrographs show fibrous structures positive for PSer129 antibody EP1536Y, that were labeled with secondary antibody conjugated to 5 nm gold particles. Scale bar, 50 nm. **b** Immunoblot analyses of sarkosyl-insoluble fractions prepared from brains of synucleinopathy patients. Sarkosyl-insoluble α-syn (22, 29 and 37 kDa in DLB, and 22 and 32 kDa in MSA) were detected by LB509 (left), anti-syn 131–140 (center) and Syn 102 (right) antibodies

brains. PS129-positive α-syn fibrous structures with 5–10 nm diameter and 0.1 to 1 μm length were observed in both cases, as previously reported [55] (Fig. 2a). Fibrils derived from MSA and labeled with PS129 antibody appeared slightly different from those derived from DLB. A majority of the fibrils were twisted with 80–100 nm periodicity in MSA, while thinner, straight fibrils were observed in DLB (Fig. 2a). Fibrous structures from DLB were subtle curvy and longer compared to those from MSA (Fig. 2a). Immunoblot analysis of sarkosyl-insoluble fractions extracted from DLB and MSA patients' brains with LB509, syn131–140 and Syn102 antibodies showed different banding patterns. All the antibodies detected 22, 29 and 37 kDa α-syn species in DLB, while 22 and 32 kDa α-syn species were detected in MSA (Fig. 2b). It is reported that these bands detected in DLB are ubiquitinated forms of α-syn [2, 24], suggesting that accumulated α-syn shows distinct post-translational patterns in DLB and MSA.

Prion-like properties in SH-SY5Y cells of α-syn aggregates extracted from patients' brains

To examine the seeded aggregation of α-syn in cultured cells, we prepared sarkosyl-insoluble fractions from 3 cases of MSA (cerebellum, frontal cortex and putamen), 4 cases of DLB (frontal cortex and temporal cortex), one case of Alzheimer's disease (AD) and one control, and analyzed them by immunoblotting with PS129 and anti-tau antibody T46. PS129-positive phospho-α-syn bands were detected in all the sarkosyl-insoluble fractions from both MSA and DLB (Additional file 1: Figure S1A). Pathological-tau (PHF-tau) bands at 60, 64, and 68 kDa together with C-terminal fragments were detected in AD and one case of DLB (Additional file 1: Figure S1A). Pathological tau and α-syn bands were not detected in the control case. The concentrations of phosphorylated α-syn in these sarkosyl-insoluble fractions were calculated from a calibration curve prepared with recombinant phosphorylated α-syn (Additional file 1: Figure S1B and Additional file 2: Table S1A). MSA-2 samples (frontal cortex and putamen) contained high concentrations of α-syn (3.58 and 7.72 ng/μl, respectively), but the other MSA and DLB samples contained lower amounts of α-syn in the range of 1.11~ 1.94 ng/μl (Additional file 2: Table S1A). The same amount (2 μL) of the sarkosyl-insoluble fractions was introduced into SH-SY5Y cells transiently expressing untagged human WT α-syn with Multifectam (Promega), and the cells were cultured for three days. Seeded aggregation in the cells was detected by immunoblotting of sarkosyl-insoluble phosphorylated α-syn. Little or no increase of phosphorylated α-syn was detected in cells treated with α-syn aggregates derived from DLB brains (DLB-syn from frontal and temporal cortexes) compared to those in cells treated with α-syn from control and AD brains (Fig. 3a and b). On the other hand, α-syn aggregates derived from MSA brains (MSA-syn) induced a marked increase of insoluble phosphorylated α-syn (Fig. 3a and b). Phosphorylated α-syn was not derived from the brain samples added to the cells, since no phosphorylated α-syn was detected in the insoluble fraction of SH-SY5Y cells without transient expression of α-syn after transduction with MSA-syn (data not shown). In addition, the accumulation of insoluble α-syn was correlated with the formation of PS129-positive α-syn aggregates in SH-SY5Y cells (Fig. 3c). These results are consistent with previous reports that MSA prions induced fluorescence-

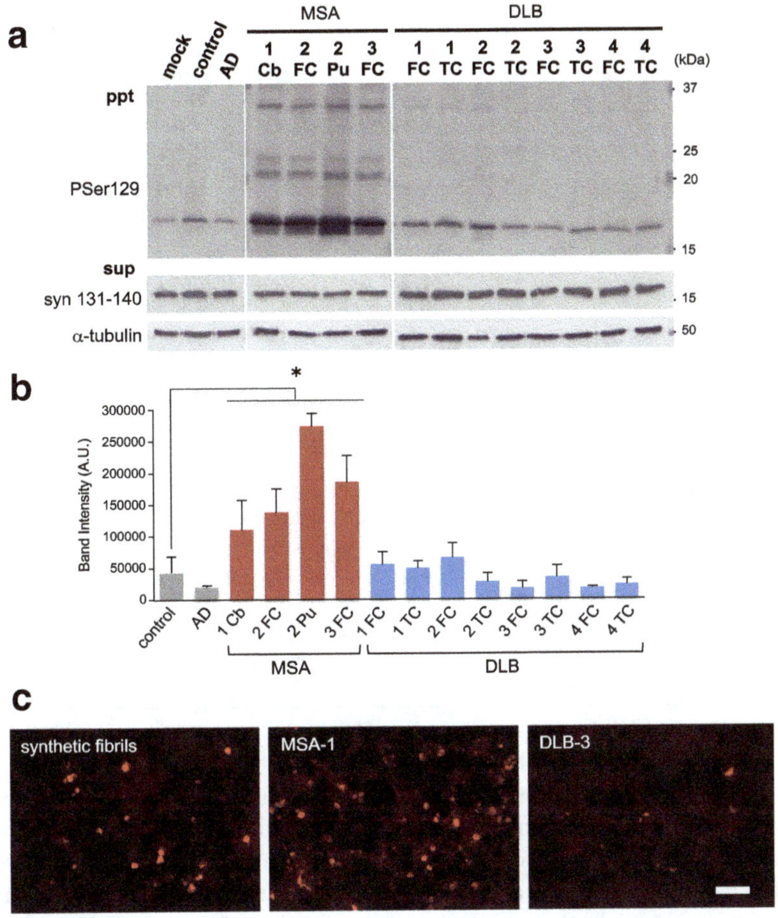

Fig. 3 Prion-like properties in SH-SY5Y cells of α-syn aggregates extracted from brains of synucleinopathy patients. **a** Sarkosyl-insoluble fractions extracted from patients' brains (2 μl) were introduced into SH-SY5Y cells transiently expressing human WT α-syn. Immunoblot analysis of sarkosyl-insoluble fractions (ppt) and sarkosyl-soluble fractions (sup) extracted from mock-transfected cells, and sarkosyl-insoluble fractions from cerebellum, frontal cortex and putamen of 3 MSA cases, frontal cortex and temporal cortex of 4 DLB cases, control brain and an AD case. Phosphorylated α-syn was detected with anti-phosphorylated α-syn PSer129 antibody. α-Syn was detected with anti-syn 131–140 antibody. The α-syn concentrations of Sarkosyl-insoluble fractions derived from human brains are shown in Additional file 1: Table S1A. **b** Quantification of immunoblot analyses shown in A. The results are expressed as means ± SEM ($n = 3$). $^*P < 0.05$. **c** SH-SY5Y cells into which synthetic human α-syn fibrils (2 μg) or sarkosyl-insoluble fractions from cerebellum of a MSA case and temporal cortex of a DLB case (2 μl) had been introduced were fixed and immunostained with PSer129 antibody EP1536Y. Scale bar, 100 μm. Cb: cerebellum, FC: frontal cortex, Pu: putamen, TC: temporal cortex

labeled α-syn aggregate formation in HEK 293 cells and earlier lethal CNS disorders in TgM83 hemizygous mice, whereas PD prions did not show similar infectivity [46, 66]. Next, we quantitated the prion-like seeding activities of MSA-syn and DLB-syn by using serially diluted samples (1/2, 1/5, 10^{-1}, 10^{-2} and 10^{-3}) of sarkosyl-insoluble fractions extracted from 3 cases of MSA (cerebellum, frontal cortex and putamen) and 1 case of DLB (frontal cortex). All MSA-syn exhibited high seeding activity at the concentration of 100 pg/ml, whereas DLB-syn exhibited much lower seeding activity at the same concentration (Fig. 4 and Additional file 3: Figure S2). Thus, these results indicated that MSA-syn possesses a strain-specific prion-like character distinct from that of DLB-syn. In addition, no significant differences in the seeding activity were detected among the different brain regions used in this study. MSA-syn has high seeding activity, similar to that of sonicated synthetic α-syn fibrils (Figs. 1c and 4).

Lewy-like α-syn pathology in WT mice inoculated with serial dilutions of synthetic α-syn fibrils

We characterized pathogenic α-syn in WT mice by means of the same approach as for SH-SY5Y cells. Series of diluted synthetic mouse α-syn fibrils were prepared and dilutions of 40, 10, 4, 2, 1, 10^{-1} to 10^{-5} μg were inoculated into striatum in the right hemisphere of C57BL6 mice. At 3 months after inoculation, phosphorylated α-syn pathology was examined by immunohistochemistry with phospho-α-syn antibody PS129. In mouse brains inoculated with more than 0.1 μg of synthetic mouse α-syn fibrils, Lewy-like pathologies were detected in striatum, frontal cortex, amygdala, substantia nigra and entorhinal

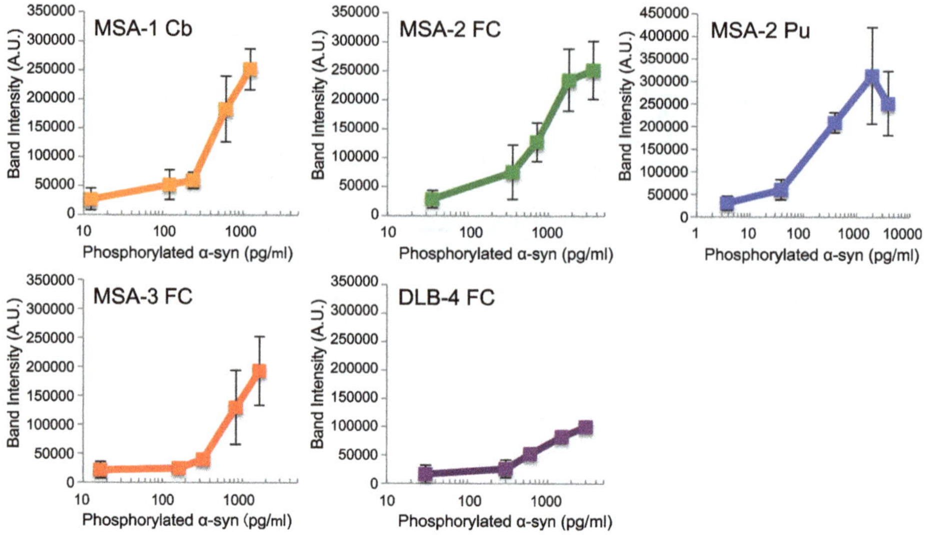

Fig. 4 Seed-dependent α-syn aggregation induced in SH-SY5Y cells by serial dilutions of insoluble fractions extracted from brains of patients with synucleinopathies. Serial dilutions of sarkosyl-insoluble fractions prepared from cerebellum, frontal cortex and putamen of 3 MSA cases and frontal cortex of a DLB case (2 μl) were introduced into SH-SY5Y cells transiently expressing human WT α-syn. Quantification of phosphorylated α-syn accumulated in SH-SY5Y cells induced by serial dilutions of pathogenic α-syn derived from brain samples. Band intensities of immunoblot analysis shown in Additional file 4: Figure S3 were measured. The results are expressed as means ± SEM ($n = 3$). Cb: cerebellum, FC: frontal cortex, Pu: putamen, TC: temporal cortex

cortex, as previously reported [35] (Fig. 5a), whereas inoculation of less than 0.01 μg α-syn fibrils did not induce α-syn pathology. To investigate the correlation between inoculum dose and spreading of α-syn pathology, we quantitated phosphorylated α-syn-positive cells and neurites in striatum, frontal cortex, amygdala and substantia nigra, where relatively abundant, conspicuous, broad-spectrum pathologies were observed in our previous study [58]. The numbers (areas) of phosphorylated α-syn-positive nerve cells and neurites were increased in parallel with the inoculated dose of α-syn fibrils (Fig. 5b). The increases were particularly marked in striatum and frontal cortex near the inoculation site. These results indicate that intracerebral inoculation of at least 0.1 μg of synthetic mouse α-syn fibrils per animal is required to induce Lewy-like pathology in WT mouse brain, in which the concentration of endogenous α-syn was determined to be 37.03 (± 6.71) μg/mL (Additional file 4: Figure S3).

MSA-syn induced PS129-positive α-syn pathology in WT mice

We next investigated whether these distinct pathogenic α-syn aggregates derived from MSA and DLB induce different types of pathology in WT mice. MSA-syn and DLB-syn were inoculated into the right striatum and α-syn pathology was evaluated by immunohistochemistry with PS129. Inoculation of MSA-syn derived from MSA-2 (putamen), which contained the highest concentration of phosphorylated α-syn, induced PS129-positive inclusions in striatum, frontal cortex, amygdala and substantia nigra at 3 months after inoculation (Fig. 6). α-Syn pathologies in MSA-syn-injected mouse brains did not resemble the GCIs-like pathology observed in MSA, but resembled the neuronal inclusions observed in PD and DLB. DLB-syn induced little α-syn pathology at 3 months after inoculation, and the pathology was mostly Lewy-neurite-like, even at 9 months after inoculation, as previously reported [36] (Fig. 6). No α-syn pathology was observed in mice inoculated with the control brain sample at 3 or 9 months after inoculation (Fig. 6). These results showed that α-syn aggregates derived from brains of patients with MSA and DLB induce distinct pathological forms of α-syn in WT mouse brains, supporting the view that MSA-syn and DLB-syn are distinct α-syn strains.

Thus, we determined the minimum amounts of synthetic α-syn and MSA-syn required for induction of seeded aggregation in SH-SY5Y cells and those of synthetic α-syn fibrils required for prion-like propagation of pathological α-syn in WT mice. In addition, we confirmed that MSA-syn and DLB-syn show distinct morphological and biochemical features and exhibit strain-specific prion-like properties in these models.

Degradation of synthetic α-syn fibrils by pre-vacuum steam sterilization and SDS

Having seen that small amounts of synthetic α-syn fibrils and MSA-syn can cause seeded aggregation of α-syn and induce α-syn pathology in vitro and in vivo, we next tested whether several procedures used to inactivate

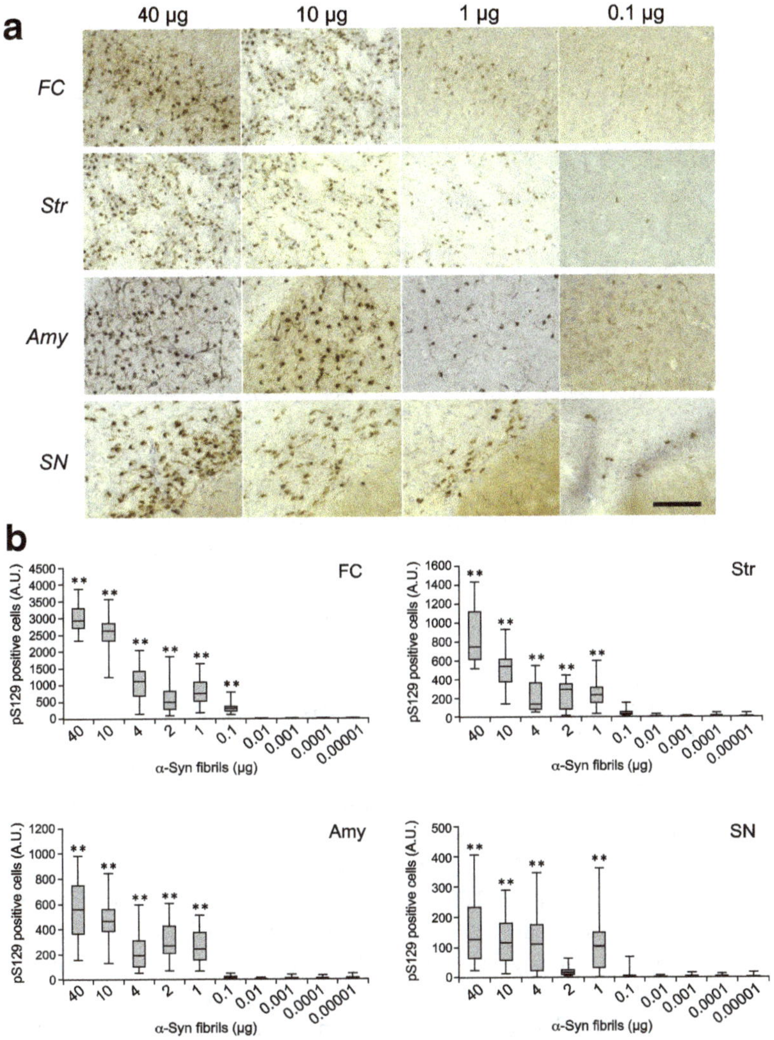

Fig. 5 Dose-dependent propagation following introduction of different amounts of synthetic α-syn fibrils in non-Tg mice. **a** Various amounts of mouse α-syn fibrils inoculated into WT mice dose-dependently induced α-syn pathology in frontal cortex, striatum, amygdala and substantia nigra. α-Syn pathology in mouse brains inoculated with 40, 10, 1, and 0.1 µg of α-syn fibrils into striatum at 3 months after inoculation is shown. The numbers of injected mice are shown in Additional file 5: Table S2A. Sections were evaluated by immunohistochemistry with PSer129 antibody EP1536Y. Scale bar, 100 µm. **b** Quantification of α-syn pathology in brains of mice inoculated with different amounts (40 µg to 10 pg) of mouse α-syn fibrils into striatum. The box plots show the number of pS129-positive cells in different regions. One-way ANOVA with Dunnett's post hoc test was used for multiple comparisons to 10 pg, $*P < 0.05$; $**P < 0.01$. FC: frontal cortex, Str: striatum, Amy: amygdala, SN: substantia nigra

PrP^{Sc} are also able to reduce the seeding activity of pathogenic α-syn. Synthetic α-syn fibrils and MSA-syn were subjected to general sterilization and inactivation procedures for PrP^{Sc}, and the residual seeding activities were examined using SH-SY5Y cells and WT mice. First, we tried SDS and autoclave treatments of synthetic α-syn fibrils. Synthetic human WT α-syn fibrils (2 mg/ml; 140 µM) were incubated for 1 h in the presence or absence of 0.1% or 1% SDS at room temperature or boiled at 100 °C for 3 min. Autoclave treatments of α-syn fibrils at 120 °C or 134 °C for 20 min were also conducted in the presence or absence of 0.1% and 1% SDS. The resulting samples were analyzed by immunoblotting with anti-α-syn antibodies. Some degradation bands of ~ 10 kDa were detected with the Syn102–116 antibody after autoclaving synthetic α-syn fibrils (Fig. 7a), suggesting that α-syn was hydrolysed by high-pressure and high-temperature treatments. Moreover, α-syn bands were hardly detectable with the anti-α-syn 131–140 antibody after autoclave treatment at 134 °C, indicating that the α-syn C-terminal region was mostly degraded after the higher-temperature autoclave treatment used in the inactivation of PrP^{Sc} (Fig. 7a). The proteinase K (ProK) resistance of these treated α-syn samples was also

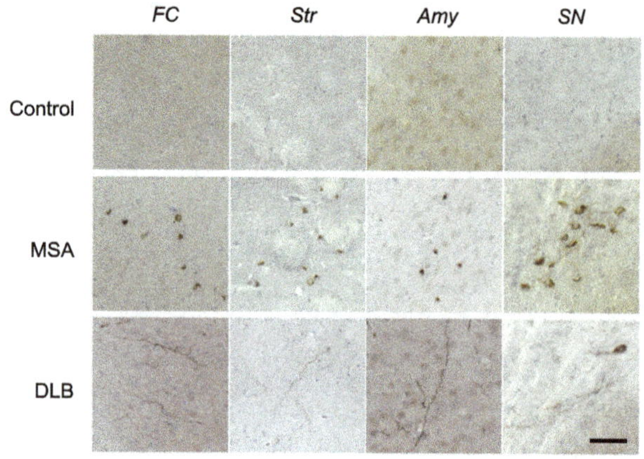

Fig. 6 α-Syn strain-specific pathology in non-Tg mice. Inoculation of sarkosyl-insoluble fractions extracted from MSA brain (MSA-2, putamen, 5 μl) into WT mice induced PS129-positive inclusions in frontal cortex, striatum, amygdala and substantia nigra at 3 months after inoculation (middle). Sarkosyl-insoluble fractions extracted from DLB brain (5 μl) induced Lewy-neurite-like α-syn pathology at 9 months after inoculation (lower). Control brain did not induce α-syn pathology (upper). Sections were evaluated by immunohistochemistry with PSer129 antibody EP1536Y. The α-syn concentrations of sarkosyl-insoluble fractions derived from human brains are shown in Additional file 2: Table S1B. The numbers of injected mice are shown in Additional file 5: Table S2C. FC: frontal cortex, Str: striatum, Amy: amygdala, SN: substantia nigra

examined to characterize the inactivation. ProK-resistant 10 and 15 kDa bands were detected with Syn102–116 in synthetic α-syn fibrils with or without boiling at 100 °C for 3 min, whereas no ProK-resistant band was detected in α-syn fibrils after autoclaving or 1% SDS treatment, although weak bands were observed after autoclaving at 120 °C in the presence and absence of 0.1% SDS (Fig. 7a).

Seeding properties of synthetic α-syn fibrils in SH-SY5Y cells after inactivation treatments

To test the effectiveness of the inactivation treatments, synthetic human α-syn fibrils after these treatments were introduced into SH-SY5Y cells and the intracellular accumulation of phosphorylated α-syn was examined by immunoblotting with PS129. Seeding activity of α-syn fibrils boiled at 100 °C for 3 min was almost equal to that of untreated fibrils (Fig. 7b and c). The single 1% SDS treatment and the autoclaving at 120 °C in the presence or absence of 0.1% SDS reduced the accumulation of α-syn but 50~ 80% of the seeding activity remained (Fig. 7b and c). On the other hand, the seeding activity was decreased by about 90% compared to that of untreated fibrils after autoclaving at 120 °C in the presence of 1% SDS, or 134 °C in the presence or absence of SDS (Fig. 7b, c and Table 1). In particular, combined treatments with 1% SDS and autoclaving resulted in almost complete abrogation of seeding activity (Fig. 7b, c and Table 1). Notably, the seeding activities of synthetic α-syn fibrils after various treatments corresponded well to the amounts of ProK-resistant bands detected with Syn102–116 and to the degree of degradation of α-syn fibrils (Fig. 7a).

To further investigate their inactivation, synthetic α-syn fibrils treated with 1% SDS at room temperature for 1 h, boiling at 100 °C for 3 min and autoclaving at 134 °C in the absence or presence of 1% SDS, then diluted serially from 10^{-1} to 10^{-6}, and introduced into SH-SY5Y cells. Synthetic α-syn fibrils after boiling at 100 °C for 3 min retained seeding activity equivalent to that of untreated fibrils, shown in Fig. 1c (Fig. 8 and Additional file 6: Figure S4). The single 1% SDS treatment reduced the seeding activity to about 1/100 (Fig. 8 and Additional file 6: Figure S4). The ID_{50} values per 2 μL of synthetic α-syn fibrils treated with 1% SDS and with boiling were calculated to be $10^{2.94}$ (± 0.67) and $10^{2.13}$ (± 0.48), respectively. On the other hand, α-syn fibrils after autoclaving at 134 °C in the absence or presence of 1% SDS showed little seeding activity (Fig. 8 and Additional file 6: Figure S4).

Inactivation of pathogenic α-syn derived from brains of MSA patients

We also investigated whether these inactivation treatments are effective for pathogenic α-syn derived from patients with MSA. Sarkosyl-insoluble fractions extracted from 2 cases of MSA (MSA-2, putamen and MSA-3) were treated with 1% SDS, boiling at 100 °C for 3 min, or autoclaving at 120 °C or 134 °C for 20 min in the presence or absence of 1% SDS. Immunoblotting with the Syn102–116 antibody showed marked degradation of insoluble α-syn after the autoclave treatments in the presence and absence of 1% SDS, in agreement with the results for synthetic α-syn fibrils shown in Fig. 7a (Fig. 9a). No apparent difference in the α-syn bands was detected between untreated MSA-syn and MSA-syn after single treatment with 1% SDS or boiling (Fig. 9a). When the treated MSA-syn was introduced into SH-SY5Y cells together with the untreated samples, we found that the seeding activity of MSA-syn from MSA-2 was dramatically reduced by about 90% after autoclaving at 121 °C or 134 °C in the presence of 1% SDS, compared to untreated MSA-syn (Fig. 9b, c and Table 1). Single autoclave treatment at 134 °C decreased the activity by about 80% (Fig. 9b, c and Table 1). The seeding activity was not completely lost after single 1% SDS treatment or autoclaving at 120 °C (Fig. 9b, c and Table 1). Boiling at 100 °C for 3 min had no effect (Fig. 9b, c and Table 1). Interestingly, MSA-syn derived from MSA-3 exhibited greater sensitivity to the inactivation treatments. The seeding activity was partially decreased after boiling at 100 °C for 3 min, and almost abolished after the other treatments (Fig. 9b, c and Table 1). These results suggest

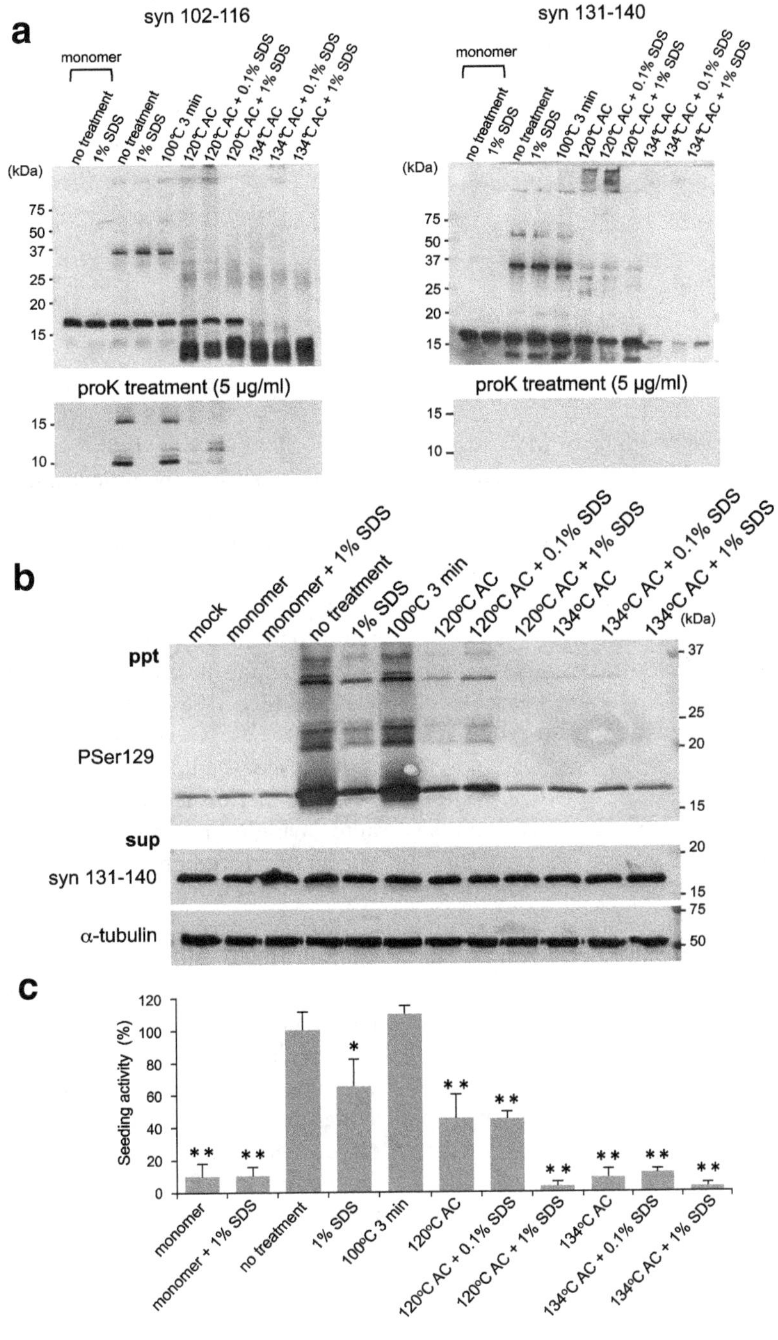

Fig. 7 Inactivation of synthetic α-syn fibrils by SDS treatment and autoclaving. **a** Synthetic α-syn fibrils were subjected to various inactivation treatments and analyzed by immunoblotting with Syn 102–116 and anti-syn 131–140 antibodies (upper). Treated α-syn samples were treated with protease K (5 μg/mL) and analyzed by immunoblotting (lower). **b** α-Syn fibrils were subjected to various inactivation treatments (2 μl) and introduced into SH-SY5Y cells transiently expressing human WT α-syn. Immunoblot analysis of sarkosyl-insoluble fractions (ppt) and sarkosyl-soluble fractions (sup) extracted from mock-transfected cells and cells transfected with α-syn monomer and fibrils, and treated with 1% SDS for 1 h at room temperature, or boiled, or autoclaved (AC) at 120 °C with or without 0.1%, 1% SDS, or autoclaved at 134 °C with or without 0.1% or 1% SDS are shown. Phosphorylated α-syn was detected with anti-phosphorylated α-syn PSer129 antibody. α-Syn was detected with anti-syn 131–140 antibody. **c** Quantification of immunoblot analysis shown in **b**. The results are expressed as means ± SEM ($n = 3$). "No treatment" was taken as 100%. One-way ANOVA with Dunnett's post hoc test were used for multiple comparisons to no treatment, *$P < 0.05$; **$P < 0.01$

Table 1 Inactivation effects of pathogenic α-syn derived from recombinant α-syn protein and MSA patients' brains in SH-SY5Y cells

Treatment	Synthetic α-syn fibrils	MSA-2 Pu	MSA-3 FC
No treatment	100 (± 11.22)	100 (± 3.38)	100 (± 11.49)
1% SDS	65.5 (± 16.48)	48.6 (± 18.66)	13.8 (± 2.96)
100 °C 3 min	109.7 (± 5.00)	114.2 (± 20.45)	29.5 (± 2.07)
120 °C 20 min	45.3 (± 14.75)	75.1 (± 13.45)	17.5 (± 2.37)
120 °C 20 min/0.1% SDS	44.9 (± 4.45)	not tested	not tested
120 °C 20 min/1% SDS	3.3 (± 2.94)	10.5 (± 2.91)	1.7 (± 1.23)
134 °C 20 min	8.7 (± 5.31)	19.0 (± 2.13)	6.3 (± 0.93)
134 °C 20 min/0.1% SDS	11.5 (± 2.31)	not tested	not tested
134 °C 20 min/1% SDS	2.8 (± 2.76)	3.5 (± 0.95)	6.8 (± 0.25)

that some varieties of pathogenic α-syn from MSA are resistant to inactivation, although differences in the concentration of pathological α-syn in the fractions may also affect the seeding activity. These results showed that the seeding activity of synthetic α-syn fibrils could be efficiently reduced by autoclaving treatment in presence of 1% SDS, and this procedure was also effective to inactivate pathogenic α-syn derived from MSA patients.

Seeding properties of inactivated pathogenic α-syn in WT mice

Finally, we investigated the effects of the inactivation procedures on seeding activity in vivo. Synthetic mouse α-syn fibrils after the inactivation treatments were inoculated into the right striatum of WT mouse brains. At 3 months after inoculation, α-syn pathology was evaluated by immunohistochemistry with PS129. Synthetic α-syn fibrils treated by boiling at 100 °C for 3 min induced Lewy-like pathology almost equivalent to that seen after inoculation of untreated fibrils, as had been found in the cellular model (Fig. 10a and b). Autoclaving of synthetic α-syn fibrils in the presence or absence of 0.1% SDS reduced the seeding activity, and the resulting α-syn pathologies were similar to those of mice inoculated with 0.1 μg of untreated synthetic fibrils, shown in Fig. 2a (Fig. 10a and b). The single autoclave treatment at 134 °C was the most effective treatment to reduce the seeding activity in mice (Fig. 10a and b). We also performed inoculation of synthetic fibrils after autoclaving in the presence or absence of 1% SDS, but the effects of treatments could not be compared because the mouse brains were partially lysed by SDS.

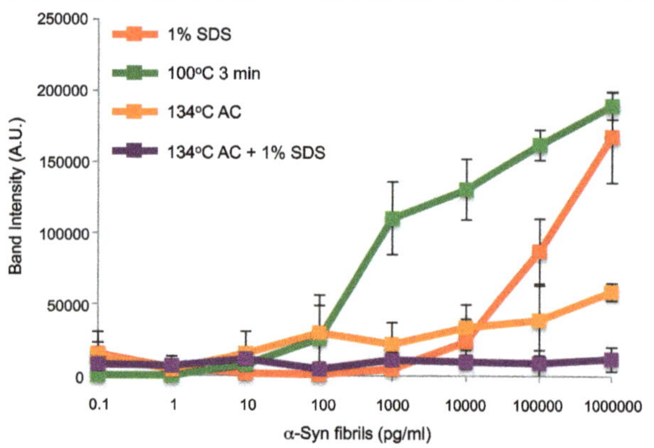

Fig. 8 Effects of inactivation treatments of synthetic α-syn fibrils on seeding activity in SH-SY5Y cells. Serial 10-fold dilutions of human α-syn fibrils treated with 1% SDS (red), boiling (green), autoclaving (AC) at 134 °C (orange) or autoclaving at 134 °C with 1% SDS (purple) were introduced into SH-SY5Y cells transiently expressing human WT α-syn. Phosphorylated α-syn accumulated in SH-SY5Y cells exposed to serial dilutions of synthetic human α-syn fibrils were quantified after each treatment. Band intensities from the immunoblot analyses shown in Additional file 6: Figure S4 were measured. The results are expressed as means ± SEM ($n = 3$)

MSA-syn derived from MSA-2 after boiling at 100 °C for 3 min and autoclaving at 134 °C was also inoculated into mouse brains. At 3 months after inoculation, PS129-positive inclusions were observed in mice injected with boiled MSA-syn, as shown in Fig. 5, whereas no pathology was detected in the mice injected with MSA-syn after autoclaving at 134 °C (Fig. 11). Thus, the autoclave treatment at 134 °C reduced the seeding activity of synthetic α-syn fibrils and MSA-syn sufficiently to block induction of α-syn pathology in WT mice.

Discussion

Many experimental studies on prion-like propagation of pathological proteins, such as α-syn, tau and TDP-43 strongly support the idea that cell-to-cell transmission of abnormal protein aggregates is a central mechanism in the pathogenesis and progression of many neurodegenerative diseases. Recent reports have also suggested that structurally different conformations of α-syn or tau exhibit strain-specific biochemical properties, including differences in the efficiency of propagation and in cellular toxicities. On the other hand, these findings raise the question of whether these pathogenic proteins can act as prions, i.e., infectious agents that may cause the onset and progression of neurodegenerative diseases, when

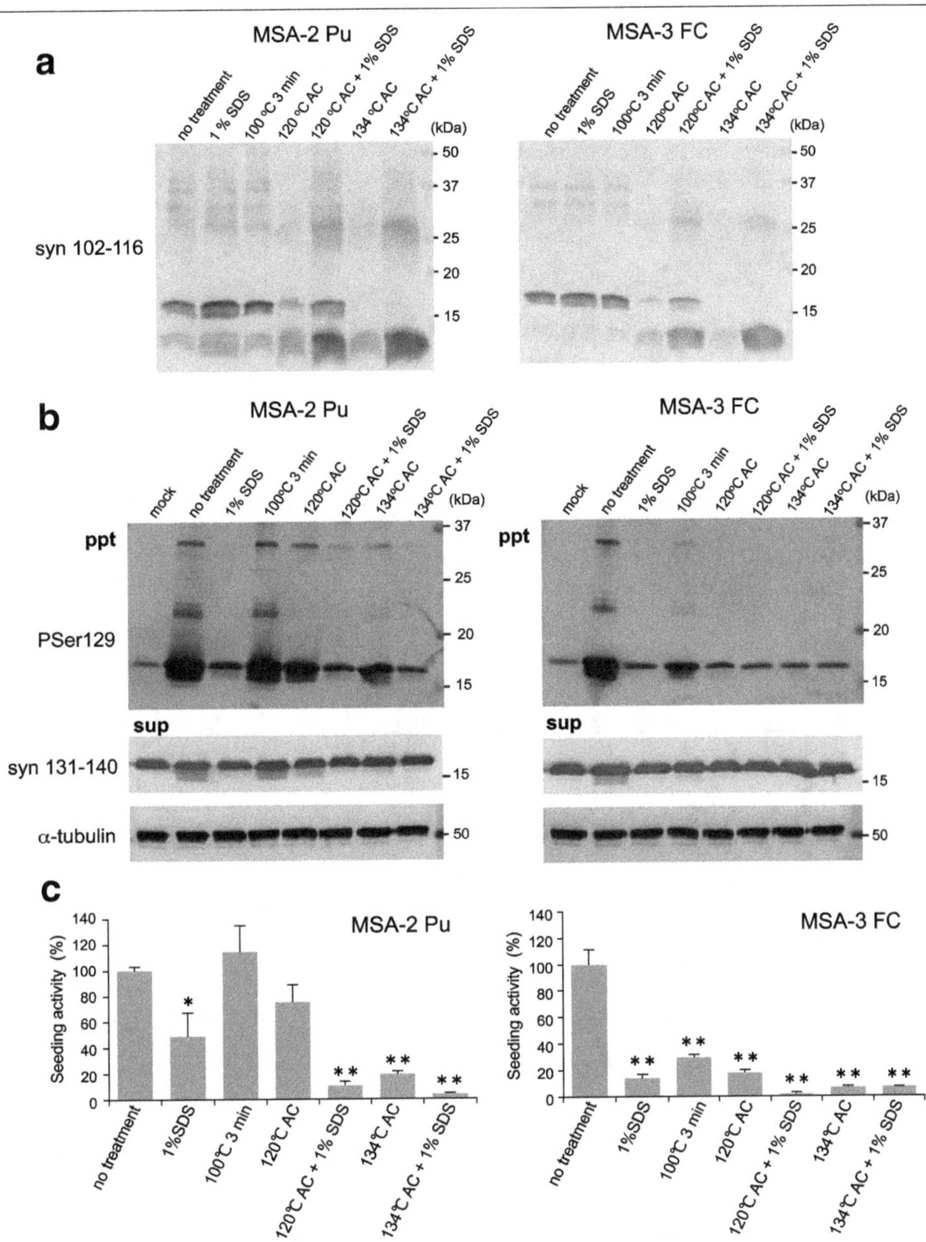

Fig. 9 Inactivation of pathogenic α-syn derived from brains of MSA patients. **a** Sarkosyl-insoluble fractions prepared from 2 MSA cases (MSA-2 Pu and MSA-3 FC) after various inactivation treatments were analyzed by immunoblotting with anti-syn 102–116 antibody. **b** Sarkosyl-insoluble fractions extracted from MSA brains after inactivation treatments (2 μl) were introduced into SH-SY5Y cells transiently expressing human WT α-syn. Immunoblot analyses of sarkosyl-insoluble fractions (ppt) and sarkosyl-soluble fractions (sup) extracted from mock-transfected cells or cells transfected with pathogenic α-syn derived from MSA brains and treated with 1% SDS for 1 h at room temperature, boiling, autoclaving (AC) at 120 °C with or without 1% SDS or AC at 134 °C with or without 1% SDS are shown. Phosphorylated α-syn was detected with anti-phosphorylated α-syn PSer129 antibody. α-Syn was detected with anti-syn 131–140 antibody. **c**, Quantification of immunoblot analyses shown in **b**. The results are expressed as means ± SEM ($n = 3$). "No treatment" was taken as 100%. One-way ANOVA with Dunnett's post hoc test were used for multiple comparisons to no treatment, $^*P < 0.05$; $^{**}P < 0.01$

humans are exposed to them. So far, there is no report of transmission of these pathogenic proteins between humans or from animals to humans, except in the case of PrP^{Sc}. However, considering the potential consequences of secondary infection to patients, clinicians and researchers, it is essential to establish whether there is actually a risk of iatrogenic or other infection. Therefore, in this study, we examined the ability of pathogenic α-syn proteins to induce prion-like seeded aggregation and to propagate in cellular and animal models. We also investigated the

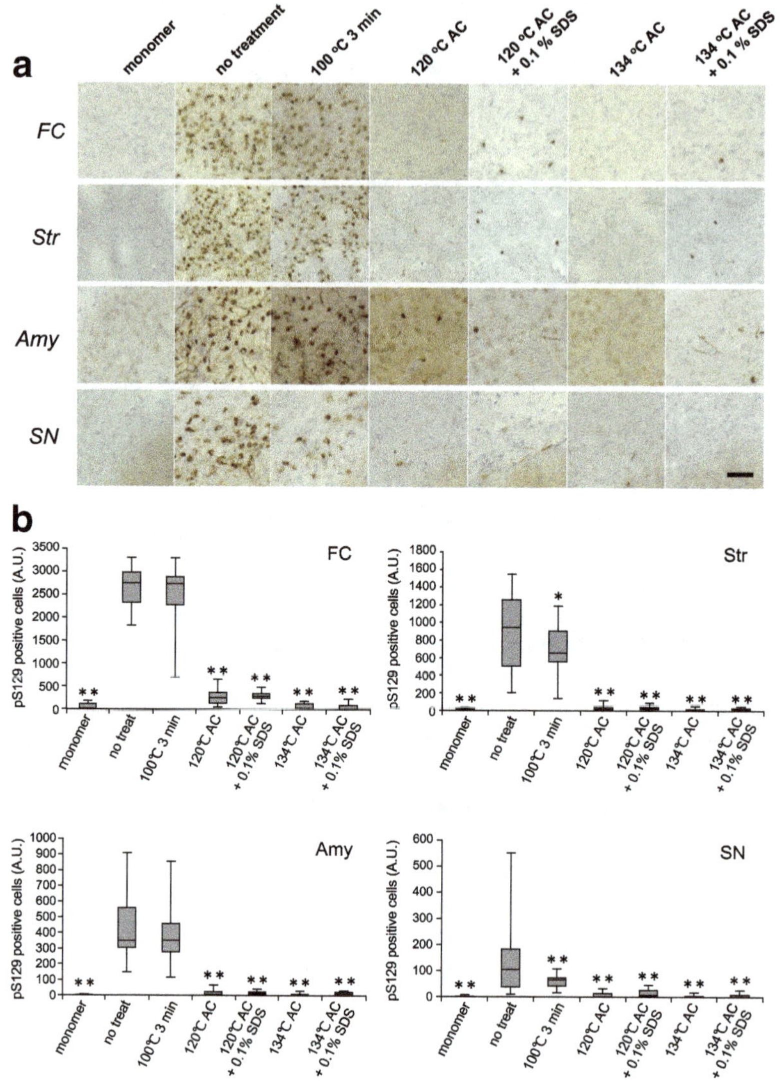

Fig. 10 Effects of inactivation treatments of synthetic α-syn fibrils on seeding activity in non-Tg mice. **a** 2 mg/ml mouse α-syn fibrils were exposed to various treatments (1% SDS for 1 h at room temperature, boiling, autoclaving (AC) at 120 °C with or without 0.1% SDS or autoclaving at 134 °C with or without 0.1% SDS), and 5 μl aliquots of the resulting samples were inoculated into WT mice. α-Syn pathologies in frontal cortex, striatum, amygdala and substantia nigra at 3 months after inoculation are shown. The numbers of injected mice are shown in Additional file 5: Table S2B. Sections were evaluated by immunohistochemistry with PSer129 antibody EP1536Y. Scale bar, 100 μm. **b** Quantification of α-syn pathology in mouse brains inoculated into striatum with α-syn fibrils exposed to various treatments. The box plots show the numbers of pS129-positive cells in different regions. One-way ANOVA with Dunnett's post hoc test were used for multiple comparisons to no treatment, *$P < 0.05$; **$P < 0.01$. FC: frontal cortex, Str: striatum, Amy: amygdala, SN: substantia nigra

efficacy of various inactivation methods for reducing the seeding activity of these pathogenic α-syn.

First, the seeding activities of serially diluted synthetic α-syn fibrils and α-syn aggregates derived from brains of synucleinopathy patients were characterized in SH-SY5Y cells transiently expressing human WT α-syn, in terms of formation of aggregated and phosphorylated α-syn. In this model, synthetic α-syn fibrils caused seeded aggregation of human α-syn at 7.14 pM and higher concentrations (Fig. 1c). The concentration of human soluble α-syn in the cells was estimated to be 2 μM, suggesting that the synthetic α-syn fibrils could function as seeds at 10^8 times lower concentration than that of normal α-syn. Further, MSA-syn showed similar seeding activity to the synthetic fibrils, although DLB-syn showed a lower seeding activity (Figs. 3b and 4). The concentration of pathogenic α-syn required for infection was similar to that reported by Prusiner's group, who detected seeded aggregation by fluorescence measurement in an HEK293 cell model [66]. In the present study, the synthetic fibrils were used after powerful sonication, which enhances their seeding activity, as shown in our previous report.

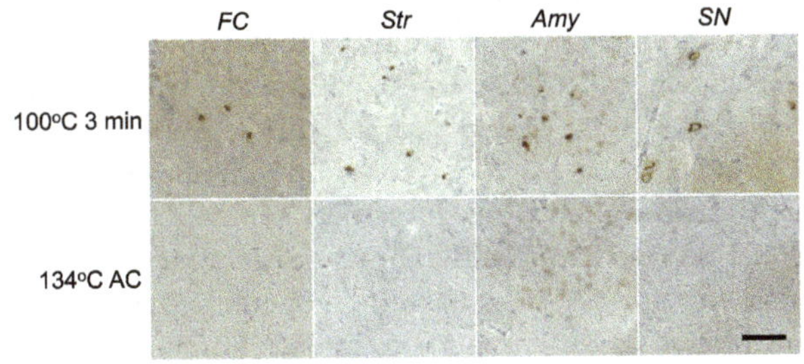

Fig. 11 Effects of inactivation treatments of pathogenic α-syn extracted from MSA patients' brains on seeding activity in non-Tg mice, α-Syn pathology in mouse brains inoculated into striatum with sarkosyl-insoluble fractions extracted from MSA brain (MSA-2, putamen) after boiling or autoclaving (AC) at 134 °C, at 3 months after injection. The numbers of injected mice are shown in Additional file 5: Table S2C. Sections were evaluated by immunohistochemistry with PSer129 antibody EP1536Y. Scale bar, 100 μm. FC: frontal cortex, Str: striatum, Amy: amygdala, SN: substantia nigra

However, MSA-syn showed high seeding activity even without this sonication. This may indicate that there are some structural differences between MSA-syn and the synthetic fibrils. We also found that MSA-syn is morphologically and biochemically distinct from DLB-syn (Fig. 2). It is plausible that these differences reflect the formation of the fibrils in different intracellular environments (oligodendrocytes in MSA and neuronal cells in PD and DLB). Further investigations will be required to understand the roles of different of α-syn strains in the clinical and pathological diversity of α-synucleinopathies.

We then used a WT mouse model to examine the minimum infectious amount, and found that as little as 0.1 μg of synthetic α-syn fibrils could induce Lewy-like pathology of endogenous mouse α-syn (Fig. 5). This is quite large compared to PrP^{Sc}, and thus the infectivity of α-syn fibrils as an environmentally acquired prion is expected to be considerably lower than that of PrP^{Sc}. The reason for this may be that normal prion protein is localized on the cell surface by a glycosylphosphatidylinositol (GPI) anchor, but the intracellular localization of α-syn requires that pathogens should first pass through the cell membrane to reach their target. Lewy-like pathologies in synthetic fibril-injected mice increased in proportion to the inoculation volume, especially around the injection site (Fig. 5). Similar dose-dependent induction of pathology was reported in the inoculation of synthetic tau fibrils into PS19 Tg mice overexpressing mutant human tau (P301S), in which MC1-positive tau pathology increased near the inoculation site when the inoculation volumes were increased [27].

For evaluation of prion-like properties, various methods are available, including RT-QuIC assay, prion-like propagation experimental models using cultured cells, primary cultures and animals, although they show different sensitivities. We analyzed the prion-like seeding activity by detecting formation of intracellular insoluble α-syn in SH-SY5Y cells transiently expressing α-syn or in WT mice expressing endogenous α-syn. In the cells, exposure to synthetic α-syn fibrils at 100 pg/mL or more induced seed-dependent aggregation. In WT mice, α-syn pathologies were detectable at 3 months after intracerebral inoculation of 0.1 μg synthetic mouse α-syn fibrils per animal. The concentration of endogenous α-syn in WT (C57BL6) mouse brain was quantitated and determined to be 37.03 (± 6.71) μg/mL. Previous studies using Tg mice, together with our study, indicate that sensitivity to pathogenic α-syn may vary depending upon the expression level of intracellular α-syn, although we did not use Tg mice in the present work. This is supported by the existence of copy number variations (duplication and triplication) in *SNCA* gene associated with early onset and rapid progression of PD [30]. Overall, these results show that both the amount of pathogenic protein and the concentration of intracellular normal soluble protein are key factors influencing the onset and progression of synucleinopathies. Thus, decreasing the expression level of intracellular soluble α-syn may contribute to suppression of aggregate formation, and inhibit intracerebral propagation.

It has been experimentally investigated whether exposure to pathological α-syn via peripheral routes can induce disease onset and pathology, as is the case for PrP^{Sc}. Several reports have shown that peripheral inoculation of synthetic α-syn fibrils or MSA brain homogenates into TgM83 mice can induce α-syn pathologies and lethal CNS disorders. Inoculations into the peritoneal cavity or hindlimb muscle resulted in disease onset with high infectivity compared with inoculation into the tongue [3, 10, 48]. On the other hand, α-syn pathology was not induced in WT mice by inoculation into hindlimb muscle or oral inoculation of even large amounts of synthetic α-syn fibrils [35]. These results may reflect the different expression levels of α-syn in the host animals, as noted above. Thus, the sensitivity to pathogenic proteins may depend strongly on the type of experimental model used. Surprisingly, implantation of stainless steel wires contaminated with MSA brain homogenates into TgM83 hemizygous mice resulted in the development of lethal CNS disorder [65]. In addition, PrP^{Sc} adhering to stainless steel wires has been reported to be more resistant to inactivation than PrP^{Sc} in brain homogenates [19, 44]. These findings imply that there may be a substantial risk of secondary infection from surgical instruments bearing pathogenic α-syn, such as instruments used in deep brain stimulation (DBS) surgery to restore motor function to PD patients. Similarly, stainless steel wires contaminated with amyloid-beta (Aβ) fraction caused amyloidosis in TgAPP23 mice [15]. Furthermore, Jaunmuktane et al. reported that transmission of Aβ seeds though surgical instruments might have occurred in patients who underwent neurosurgery in childhood [28]. Thus, to prevent iatrogenic infection, effective sterilization procedures seem mandatory.

Therefore, we next investigated the efficacy of various commonly used inactivation methods for PrP^{Sc} for abolishing the seeding activity of pathogenic α-syn. Autoclave treatments at 120 °C or 134 °C in the presence of 1% SDS dramatically reduced the seeding activity of pathogenic α-syn, including synthetic fibrils and MSA-syn, in the cultured cell model (Figs. 7c, 9c and Table 1). Further, pathogenic α-syn exposed to a single autoclave treatment at 134 °C did not induce α-syn pathology in WT mouse brain (Fig. 10b and 11). On the other hand, single autoclave treatment at 120 °C, which is commonly used as a general sterilization method, was insufficient to inactivate synthetic α-syn fibrils or MSA-syn (Figs. 7c and 9c). The seeding activity of pathogenic α-syn after boiling treatment for 3 min was almost the same as that of untreated pathogenic α-syn (Figs. 7c, 9c, 10b and 11). Similar heat resistance has been reported for Aβ aggregates and abnormal TDP-43 derived from ALS/frontotemporal lobar degeneration (FTLD) cases [15, 40].

Numerous studies on inactivation of PrP^{Sc} derived from various biological species and strains have been conducted, and have shown that various methods, including strong alkaline agents, protein-denaturing agents, proteolytic enzymes and autoclaving, are effective to abolish infectivity [20]. It has also been reported that the level of inactivation varies depending on the biological species and strain, but combinations of multiple treatments can reliably achieve complete inactivation [16, 59]. Thomzig and colleagues examined the removal of Aβ, tau, and α-syn adhering to medical devices by carrier assay using brain extracts of patients, and treatments with 1 M NaOH at room temperature for 1 h, combined treatments with 0.2% SDS or 0.3% NaOH and autoclaving at 134 °C for 5 min, and treatment with a commercial alkaline cleanser or a hydrogen peroxide solution containing Cu^{2+} were reported to be effective for removal of pathogenic α-syn [60]. On the other hand, formalin-fixed pathogenic Aβ, tau, and α-syn have been reported to retain high seeding activity in vitro and in vivo [17, 29, 50]. Surprisingly, an MSA patient's brain stored in formalin for over 20 years caused TgM83 hemizygous mice to develop lethal CNS disorder [65]. Thus, the suitability or unsuitability of various inactivation procedures for prion-like proteins is becoming clearer. Overall, PrP^{Sc} and other prion-like proteins seem to show similar responses to inactivation procedures, suggesting these pathogenic proteins have some common structural features. Regarding the handling of synthetic α-syn fibrils in laboratories, Bousset et al. reported that 1% SDS and the commercial cleanser Hellmanex can remove synthetic α-syn fibrils from surfaces of various materials, although they found differences in resistance to 1% SDS among distinct α-syn strains, fibrils and ribbons formed under different physiological conditions in vitro [7]. We also found differences of resistance to inactivation procedures between MSA-syn preparations derived from different cases (Fig. 9c). Thus, it remains important to manage pathogenic α-syn by using appropriate safety cabinets to avoid human exposure. Also, the use of a cup horn-type ultrasonicator is useful to avoid inhalation of aerosols containing fragmented pathogenic α-syn during sample preparation.

Conclusion

We investigated in detail the prion-like properties of pathogenic α-syn, including synthetic α-syn fibrils, MSA-syn and DLB-syn, using SH-SY5Y cells transiently expressing human WT α-syn and non-Tg mice. We found that synthetic α-syn fibrils and MSA-syn can induce both prion-like amplification of abnormal α-syn in cultured cells and spreading of phosphorylated α-syn pathologies in mouse brain. The seeding activity of MSA-syn is equivalent to or higher than that of synthetic α-syn fibrils, though DLB-syn showed much lower seeding activity. Various combinations of inactivation treatments were effective to abolish the seeding activity of these pathogenic α-syn. Our findings here provide further evidence of the prion-like properties of pathogenic α-syn and re-emphasize the importance of using appropriate inactivation treatments to prevent iatrogenic and secondary infections in the clinical and research fields.

Additional files

Additional file 1: Figure S1. Determination of protein concentration of phosphorylated α-syn in patients' brains. A, Sarkosyl-insoluble fractions prepared from patients' brains used in this study were analyzed by immunoblotting with anti-phosphorylated α-syn PSer129 antibody (upper) and anti-tau T46 antibody (lower). B, Standard curve of phosphorylated α-syn, generated by immunoblotting of phosphorylated monomer α-syn. Concentrations of phosphorylated α-syn were determined using this standard curve. Protein concentrations of sarkosyl-insoluble fractions extracted from patients' brains are shown in **Table S2**. (PDF 139 kb)

Additional file 2: Table S1. α-Syn concentrations in sarkosyl-insoluble fractions extracted from patients' brains, The α-syn concentrations of sarkosyl-insoluble fractions extracted from patients' brains used for experiments in the cultured cell model (A) and mouse model (B) are shown. (PDF 40 kb)

Additional file 3: Figure S2. Seeding activities of serial dilutions of sarkosyl-insoluble fractions from brains of α-synucleinopathy patients, Sarkosyl-insoluble fractions extracted from brains with synucleinopathy patients were diluted and introduced into SH-SY5Y cells transiently expressing human α-syn. Immunoblot analyses of sarkosyl-insoluble fractions (ppt) and sarkosyl-soluble fractions (sup) extracted from cells transfected with serial dilutions of MSA-1(Cb), MSA-2 (FC), MSA-2 (Pu), MSA-3 (FC) and DLB-4 (FC) are shown. Phosphorylated α-syn was detected with anti-phosphorylated α-syn PSer129 antibody. α-Syn was detected with anti-syn 131–140 antibody. Cb: cerebellum, FC: frontal cortex, Pu: putamen. (PDF 283 kb)

Additional file 4: Figure S3. Determination of protein concentration of α-syn in C57BL/6 mouse brain, Standard curve of mouse α-syn was generated by immunoblotting of serial dilutions of recombinant mouse α-syn protein. Protein concentrations of endogenous α-syn in mouse brains were determined by interpolation on a standard curve. A68 buffer-soluble fractions were extracted from C57BL/6 mouse brains ($n = 3$). Bands of recombinant proteins and A68 buffer-soluble fractions were detected with anti-mouse α-syn antibody. (PDF 78 kb)

Additional file 5: Table S2. Numbers of mice used in experiments. (PDF 52 kb)

Additional file 6: Figure S4. Seeding activities of serial dilutions of treated synthetic α-syn fibrils in SH-SY5Y cells, Serial dilutions of synthetic α-syn fibrils exposed to various inactivation treatments were introduced into SH-SY5Y cells. Immunoblot analysis of sarkosyl-insoluble fractions (ppt) and sarkosyl-soluble fractions (sup) extracted from cells transfected with serial dilutions of synthetic α-syn fibrils treated with 1% SDS for 1 h at room temperature, boiling, or autoclaving at 134 °C with or without 1% SDS are shown. Phosphorylated α-syn was detected with anti-phosphorylated α-syn PSer129 antibody. α-Syn was detected with anti-syn 131–140 antibody. (PDF 248 kb)

Acknowledgments

We are grateful to the patients and their families for making brains available for research. We thank Dr. Tetsuyuki Kitamoto and Dr. Shiro Mohri for useful comments on PrP prions. We also thank Dr. Masami Masuda-Suzukake for providing phosphorylated α-syn and Dr. Takashi Nonaka for helpful comments. This work was supported by Ministry of Education, Culture, Sports, Science, and Technology Grants-in-Aid for Scientific Research (KAKENHI) Grants JP26117005 (to M.H.), Japan Society for the Promotion of Science Grants-in-Aid for Scientific Research (KAKENHI) Grant JP23228004 (to M.H.), and a grant-in-aid for research on Brain Mapping by Integrated Neurotechnologies for Disease Studies (Brain/MINDS) from the Japan Agency for Medical Research and Development (AMED) JP14533254 (to M.H.).

Authors' contributions

MH and AT designed the research and wrote the manuscript. AT performed most of the experiments. TA and SM collected patients' brain samples and performed neuropathological diagnosis. SH, AT and MH analyzed the data. All authors read and approved the final manuscript.

Competing interests

The authors declare that they have no competing interests.

Author details

[1]Department of Dementia and Higher Brain Function, Tokyo Metropolitan Institute of Medical Science, 2-1-6 Kamikitazawa, Setagaya-ku, Tokyo 156-8506, Japan. [2]Department of Biological Science, Tokyo Metropolitan University, Minami-osawa, Hachioji, Tokyo 192-0397, Japan. [3]Department of Neuropsychiatry, Division of Clinical Medicine, Faculty of Medicine, University of Tsukuba, 1-1-1, Tennodai, Tsukuba, Ibaraki 305-8576, Japan. [4]Department of Neuropathology, Tokyo Metropolitan Geriatric Hospital and Institute of Gerontology, 35-2 Sakaecho, Itabashi-ku, Tokyo 173-0015, Japan.

References

1. Abeliovich A, Schmitz Y, Farinas I, Choi-Lundberg D, Ho WH, Castillo PE et al (2000) Mice lacking alpha-synuclein display functional deficits in the nigrostriatal dopamine system. Neuron 25:239–252
2. Anderson JP, Walker DE, Goldstein JM, de Laat R, Banducci K, Caccavello RJ et al (2006) Phosphorylation of Ser-129 is the dominant pathological modification of alpha-synuclein in familial and sporadic Lewy body disease. J Biol Chem 281:29739–29752
3. Ayers JI, Brooks MM, Rutherford NJ, Howard JK, Sorrentino ZA, Riffe CJ et al (2017) Robust central nervous system pathology in transgenic mice following peripheral injection of alpha-Synuclein fibrils. J Virol 91
4. Baba M, Nakajo S, Tu PH, Tomita T, Nakaya K, Lee VM et al (1998) Aggregation of alpha-synuclein in Lewy bodies of sporadic Parkinson's disease and dementia with Lewy bodies. Am J Pathol 152:879–884
5. Bernis ME, Babila JT, Breid S, Wusten KA, Wullner U, Tamguney G (2015) Prion-like propagation of human brain-derived alpha-synuclein in transgenic mice expressing human wild-type alpha-synuclein. Acta Neuropathol Commun 3:75
6. Bonini NM, Giasson BI (2005) Snaring the function of alpha-synuclein. Cell 123:359–361
7. Bousset L, Brundin P, Bockmann A, Meier B, Melki R (2016) An efficient procedure for removal and inactivation of alpha-Synuclein assemblies from laboratory materials. J Parkinsons Dis 6:143–151
8. Bousset L, Pieri L, Ruiz-Arlandis G, Gath J, Jensen PH, Habenstein B et al (2013) Structural and functional characterization of two alpha-synuclein strains. Nat Commun 4:2575
9. Braak H, Del Tredici K (2016) Potential pathways of abnormal tau and alpha-Synuclein dissemination in sporadic Alzheimer's and Parkinson's diseases. Cold Spring Harb Perspect Biol 8. https://doi.org/10.1101/cshperspect.a023630
10. Breid S, Bernis ME, Babila JT, Garza MC, Wille H, Tamguney G (2016) Neuroinvasion of alpha-Synuclein Prionoids after intraperitoneal and Intraglossal inoculation. J Virol 90:9182–9193
11. Brown P, Brandel JP, Sato T, Nakamura Y, MacKenzie J, Will RG et al (2012) Iatrogenic Creutzfeldt-Jakob disease, final assessment. Emerg Infect Dis 18:901–907
12. Burre J, Sharma M, Tsetsenis T, Buchman V, Etherton MR, Sudhof TC (2010) Alpha-synuclein promotes SNARE-complex assembly in vivo and in vitro. Science 329:1663–1667
13. Chandra S, Fornai F, Kwon HB, Yazdani U, Atasoy D, Liu X et al (2004) Double-knockout mice for alpha- and beta-synucleins: effect on synaptic functions. Proc Natl Acad Sci U S A 101:14966–14971
14. Crowther RA, Jakes R, Spillantini MG, Goedert M (1998) Synthetic filaments assembled from C-terminally truncated alpha-synuclein. FEBS Lett 436:309–312
15. Eisele YS, Bolmont T, Heikenwalder M, Langer F, Jacobson LH, Yan ZX et al (2009) Induction of cerebral beta-amyloidosis: intracerebral versus systemic Abeta inoculation. Proc Natl Acad Sci U S A 106:12926–12931
16. Fichet G, Comoy E, Duval C, Antloga K, Dehen C, Charbonnier A et al (2004) Novel methods for disinfection of prion-contaminated medical devices. Lancet 364:521–526
17. Fritschi SK, Langer F, Kaeser SA, Maia LF, Portelius E, Pinotsi D et al (2014) Highly potent soluble amyloid-beta seeds in human Alzheimer brain but not cerebrospinal fluid. Brain 137:2909–2915
18. Fujiwara H, Hasegawa M, Dohmae N, Kawashima A, Masliah E, Goldberg MS et al (2002) Alpha-Synuclein is phosphorylated in synucleinopathy lesions. Nat Cell Biol 4:160–164
19. Giles K, Glidden DV, Beckwith R, Seoanes R, Peretz D, DeArmond SJ et al (2008) Resistance of bovine spongiform encephalopathy (BSE) prions to inactivation. PLoS Pathog 4:e1000206
20. Giles K, Woerman AL, Berry DB, Prusiner SB (2017) Bioassays and inactivation of prions. Cold Spring Harb Perspect Biol 9. https://doi.org/10.1101/cshperspect.a023499
21. Goedert M (2015) NEURODEGENERATION. Alzheimer's and Parkinson's diseases: the prion concept in relation to assembled Abeta, tau, and alpha-synuclein. Science 349:1255555
22. Goedert M, Jakes R, Spillantini MG (2017) The Synucleinopathies: twenty years on. J Parkinsons Dis 7:S53–S71
23. Hasegawa M, Arai T, Nonaka T, Kametani F, Yoshida M, Hashizume Y et al (2008) Phosphorylated TDP-43 in frontotemporal lobar degeneration and amyotrophic lateral sclerosis. Ann Neurol 64:60–70
24. Hasegawa M, Fujiwara H, Nonaka T, Wakabayashi K, Takahashi H, Lee VM et al (2002) Phosphorylated alpha-synuclein is ubiquitinated in alpha-synucleinopathy lesions. J Biol Chem 277:49071–49076
25. Hasegawa M, Nonaka T, Masuda-Suzukake M (2016) Alpha-Synuclein: experimental pathology. Cold Spring Harb Perspect Med 6. https://doi.org/10.1101/cshperspect.a024273
26. Hughson AG, Race B, Kraus A, Sangare LR, Robins L, Groveman BR et al (2016) Inactivation of prions and amyloid seeds with Hypochlorous acid. PLoS Pathog 12:e1005914

27. Iba M, Guo JL, McBride JD, Zhang B, Trojanowski JQ, Lee VM (2013) Synthetic tau fibrils mediate transmission of neurofibrillary tangles in a transgenic mouse model of Alzheimer's-like tauopathy. J Neurosci 33:1024–1037
28. Jaunmuktane Z, Quaegebeur A, Taipa R, Viana-Baptista M, Barbosa R, Koriath C et al (2018) Evidence of amyloid-beta cerebral amyloid angiopathy transmission through neurosurgery. In: Acta Neuropathol
29. Kaufman SK, Thomas TL, Del Tredici K, Braak H, Diamond MI (2017) Characterization of tau prion seeding activity and strains from formaldehyde-fixed tissue. Acta Neuropathol Commun 5:41
30. Konno T, Ross OA, Puschmann A, Dickson DW, Wszolek ZK (2016) Autosomal dominant Parkinson's disease caused by SNCA duplications. Parkinsonism Relat Disord 22(Suppl 1):S1–S6
31. Luk KC, Kehm V, Carroll J, Zhang B, O'Brien P, Trojanowski JQ et al (2012) Pathological alpha-synuclein transmission initiates Parkinson-like neurodegeneration in nontransgenic mice. Science 338:949–953
32. Luk KC, Kehm VM, Zhang B, O'Brien P, Trojanowski JQ, Lee VM (2012) Intracerebral inoculation of pathological alpha-synuclein initiates a rapidly progressive neurodegenerative alpha-synucleinopathy in mice. J Exp Med 209:975–986
33. Maroteaux L, Campanelli JT, Scheller RH (1988) Synuclein: a neuron-specific protein localized to the nucleus and presynaptic nerve terminal. J Neurosci 8:2804–2815
34. Masuda M, Dohmae N, Nonaka T, Oikawa T, Hisanaga S, Goedert M et al (2006) Cysteine misincorporation in bacterially expressed human alpha-synuclein. FEBS Lett 580:1775–1779
35. Masuda-Suzukake M, Nonaka T, Hosokawa M, Kubo M, Shimozawa A, Akiyama H et al (2014) Pathological alpha-synuclein propagates through neural networks. Acta Neuropathol Commun 2:88
36. Masuda-Suzukake M, Nonaka T, Hosokawa M, Oikawa T, Arai T, Akiyama H et al (2013) Prion-like spreading of pathological alpha-synuclein in brain. Brain 136:1128–1138
37. Mougenot AL, Nicot S, Bencsik A, Morignat E, Verchere J, Lakhdar L et al (2012) Prion-like acceleration of a synucleinopathy in a transgenic mouse model. Neurobiol Aging 33:2225–2228
38. Neumann M, Kahle PJ, Giasson BI, Ozmen L, Borroni E, Spooren W et al (2002) Misfolded proteinase K-resistant hyperphosphorylated alpha-synuclein in aged transgenic mice with locomotor deterioration and in human alpha-synucleinopathies. J Clin Invest 110:1429–1439
39. Nonaka T, Iwatsubo T, Hasegawa M (2005) Ubiquitination of alpha-synuclein. Biochemistry 44:361–368
40. Nonaka T, Masuda-Suzukake M, Arai T, Hasegawa Y, Akatsu H, Obi T et al (2013) Prion-like properties of pathological TDP-43 aggregates from diseased brains. Cell Rep 4:124–134
41. Nonaka T, Watanabe ST, Iwatsubo T, Hasegawa M (2010) Seeded aggregation and toxicity of {alpha}-synuclein and tau: cellular models of neurodegenerative diseases. J Biol Chem 285:34885–34898
42. Nussbaum RL (2017) Genetics of Synucleinopathies. Cold Spring Harb Perspect Med. https://doi.org/10.1101/cshperspect.a024109
43. Peelaerts W, Bousset L, Van der Perren A, Moskalyuk A, Pulizzi R, Giugliano M et al (2015) Alpha-Synuclein strains cause distinct synucleinopathies after local and systemic administration. Nature 522:340–344
44. Peretz D, Supattapone S, Giles K, Vergara J, Freyman Y, Lessard P et al (2006) Inactivation of prions by acidic sodium dodecyl sulfate. J Virol 80:322–331
45. Prusiner SB (1998) Prions. Proc Natl Acad Sci U S A 95:13363–13383
46. Prusiner SB, Woerman AL, Mordes DA, Watts JC, Rampersaud R, Berry DB et al (2015) Evidence for alpha-synuclein prions causing multiple system atrophy in humans with parkinsonism. Proc Natl Acad Sci U S A 112:E5308–E5317
47. Recasens A, Dehay B, Bove J, Carballo-Carbajal I, Dovero S, Perez-Villalba A et al (2014) Lewy body extracts from Parkinson disease brains trigger alpha-synuclein pathology and neurodegeneration in mice and monkeys. Ann Neurol 75:351–362
48. Sacino AN, Brooks M, Thomas MA, McKinney AB, Lee S, Regenhardt RW et al (2014) Intramuscular injection of alpha-synuclein induces CNS alpha-synuclein pathology and a rapid-onset motor phenotype in transgenic mice. Proc Natl Acad Sci U S A 111:10732–10737
49. Saito Y, Kawashima A, Ruberu NN, Fujiwara H, Koyama S, Sawabe M et al (2003) Accumulation of phosphorylated alpha-synuclein in aging human brain. J Neuropathol Exp Neurol 62:644–654
50. Schweighauser M, Bacioglu M, Fritschi SK, Shimshek DR, Kahle PJ, Eisele YS et al (2015) Formaldehyde-fixed brain tissue from spontaneously ill alpha-synuclein transgenic mice induces fatal alpha-synucleinopathy in transgenic hosts. Acta Neuropathol 129:157–159
51. Serpell LC, Berriman J, Jakes R, Goedert M, Crowther RA (2000) Fiber diffraction of synthetic alpha-synuclein filaments shows amyloid-like cross-beta conformation. Proc Natl Acad Sci U S A 97:4897–4902
52. Shimonaka S, Nonaka T, Suzuki G, Hisanaga S, Hasegawa M (2016) Templated aggregation of TAR DNA-binding protein of 43 kDa (TDP-43) by seeding with TDP-43 peptide fibrils. J Biol Chem 291:8896–8907
53. Shimozawa A, Ono M, Takahara D, Tarutani A, Imura S, Masuda-Suzukake M et al (2017) Propagation of pathological alpha-synuclein in marmoset brain. Acta Neuropathol Commun 5:12
54. Spillantini MG, Crowther RA, Jakes R, Cairns NJ, Lantos PL, Goedert M (1998) Filamentous alpha-synuclein inclusions link multiple system atrophy with Parkinson's disease and dementia with Lewy bodies. Neurosci Lett 251:205–208
55. Spillantini MG, Crowther RA, Jakes R, Hasegawa M, Goedert M (1998) Alpha-Synuclein in filamentous inclusions of Lewy bodies from Parkinson's disease and dementia with lewy bodies. Proc Natl Acad Sci U S A 95:6469–6473
56. Spillantini MG, Schmidt ML, Lee VM, Trojanowski JQ, Jakes R, Goedert M (1997) Alpha-synuclein in Lewy bodies. Nature 388:839–840
57. Takahashi M, Miyata H, Kametani F, Nonaka T, Akiyama H, Hisanaga S et al (2015) Extracellular association of APP and tau fibrils induces intracellular aggregate formation of tau. Acta Neuropathol 129:895–907
58. Tarutani A, Suzuki G, Shimozawa A, Nonaka T, Akiyama H, Hisanaga S et al (2016) The effect of fragmented pathogenic alpha-Synuclein seeds on prion-like propagation. J Biol Chem 291:18675–18688
59. Tateishi J, Tashima T, Kitamoto T (1991) Practical methods for chemical inactivation of Creutzfeldt-Jakob disease pathogen. Microbiol Immunol 35:163–166
60. Thomzig A, Wagenfuhr K, Daus ML, Joncic M, Schulz-Schaeffer WJ, Thanheiser M et al (2014) Decontamination of medical devices from pathological amyloid-beta-, tau- and alpha-synuclein aggregates. Acta Neuropathol Commun 2:151
61. Wakabayashi K, Yoshimoto M, Tsuji S, Takahashi H (1998) Alpha-synuclein immunoreactivity in glial cytoplasmic inclusions in multiple system atrophy. Neurosci Lett 249:180–182
62. Walker LC, Jucker M (2015) Neurodegenerative diseases: expanding the prion concept. Annu Rev Neurosci 38:87–103
63. Watts JC, Giles K, Oehler A, Middleton L, Dexter DT, Gentleman SM et al (2013) Transmission of multiple system atrophy prions to transgenic mice. Proc Natl Acad Sci U S A 110:19555–19560
64. Wilham JM, Orru CD, Bessen RA, Atarashi R, Sano K, Race B et al (2010) Rapid end-point quantitation of prion seeding activity with sensitivity comparable to bioassays. PLoS Pathog 6:e1001217
65. Woerman AL, Kazmi SA, Patel S, Freyman Y, Oehler A, Aoyagi A et al (2017) MSA prions exhibit remarkable stability and resistance to inactivation. In: Acta Neuropathol
66. Woerman AL, Stohr J, Aoyagi A, Rampersaud R, Krejciova Z, Watts JC et al (2015) Propagation of prions causing synucleinopathies in cultured cells. Proc Natl Acad Sci U S A 112:E4949–E4958

13

Phosphorylated TDP-43 (pTDP-43) aggregates in the axial skeletal muscle of patients with sporadic and familial amyotrophic lateral sclerosis

Matthew D. Cykowski[1,2*], Suzanne Z. Powell[1,2,3], Joan W. Appel[3,4], Anithachristy S. Arumanayagam[1], Andreana L. Rivera[1,2,3] and Stanley H. Appel[2,3,4]

Abstract

Muscle atrophy with weakness is a core feature of amyotrophic lateral sclerosis (ALS) that has long been attributed to motor neuron loss alone. However, several studies in ALS patients, and more so in animal models, have challenged this assumption with the latter providing direct evidence that muscle can play an active role in the disease. Here, we examined the possible role of cell autonomous pathology in 148 skeletal muscle samples from 57 ALS patients, identifying phosphorylated TAR DNA-binding protein (pTDP-43) inclusions in the muscle fibers of 19 patients (33.3%) and 24 tissue samples (16.2% of specimens). A muscle group-specific difference was identified with pTDP-43 pathology being significantly more common in axial (paraspinous, diaphragm) than appendicular muscles ($P = 0.0087$). This pathology was not significantly associated with pertinent clinical, genetic (c9ALS) or nervous system pathologic data, suggesting it is not limited to any particular subgroup of ALS patients. Among 25 non-ALS muscle samples, pTDP-43 inclusions were seen only in the autophagy-related disorder inclusion body myositis (IBM) ($n = 4$), where they were more diffuse than in positive ALS samples ($P = 0.007$). As in IBM samples, pTDP-43 aggregates in ALS were p62/ sequestosome-1-positive, potentially indicating induction of autophagy. Phospho-TDP-43-positive ALS and IBM samples also showed significant up-regulation of *TARDBP* and *SQSTM1* expression. These findings implicate axial skeletal muscle as an additional site of pTDP-43 pathology in some ALS patients, including sporadic and familial cases, which is deserving of further investigation.

Keywords: Amyotrophic lateral sclerosis, Skeletal muscle, Inclusion body myositis, Paraspinous muscle, p62/ sequestosome-1, Autophagy, pTDP-43

Introduction

ALS is a progressive disorder characterized by motor neuron injury, muscle weakness, bulbar symptoms, such as dysarthria and dysphagia [1], and frontal-subcortical cognitive dysfunction in many patients [43, 44]. ALS has a lifetime risk of ~ 1 in 500 persons [51] and a prevalence in the United States reaching 17 per 100,000 individuals in the eighth decade [39]. Survival is generally poor and patients typically live only three to five years after diagnosis [49].

Pathologic studies of ALS nervous tissue have emphasized cell autonomous and non-cell autonomous pathologies in upper and lower motor neuron groups, and more recently, in non-motor brain regions [18, 38]. These include neuronal and glial inclusions comprising misfolded and phosphorylated TAR DNA-binding protein 43 kDA (pTDP-43) [10, 17, 35] and fused-in-sarcoma (FUS) protein [34], as well as dipeptide repeat pathology in C9ORF72 expansion-associated ALS (c9ALS) [54]. The critical role of glia and immune cells in disease progression is also recognized in human ALS and transgenic ALS models [26, 40, 58].

* Correspondence: mdcykowski@houstonmethodist.org
[1]Department of Pathology and Genomic Medicine, Houston Methodist Hospital, 6565 Fannin Street, Houston, TX 77030, USA
[2]Institute of Academic Medicine (IAM) in the Houston Methodist Research Institute (HMRI), Houston Methodist Hospital, 6565 Fannin Street, Houston, TX 77030, USA
Full list of author information is available at the end of the article

In contrast, since the original descriptions of ALS [16, 55], the secondary process of muscle atrophy following motor neuron loss and denervation has been emphasized. Indeed, electrophysiologic findings in ALS muscle are typically those of denervation atrophy [19, 29] and are accompanied by histopathologic changes of denervation, such as target fibers and fiber type grouping. At the same time, electrophysiological and functional studies of human ALS have supported an active and early role of skeletal muscle [48] and an early vulnerability of select muscle groups, such as paraspinous [29, 30]. Further, not all pathologies described in ALS muscle are those of denervation atrophy. Additional pathologies that have been described in some ALS muscle samples include myopathic features [28], fiber necrosis and inflammation [2], DNA fragmentation with expression of pro-apoptotic proteins [52], and reduced expression of mitochondrial proteins and mitochondrial DNA mutations/ deletions [4, 15, 56]. Studies of protein aggregates in human ALS muscle, that might indicate cell autonomous pathology, are much more limited. One study of 30 quadriceps biopsies did not identify pTDP-43 pathology in any samples [50]. Another recent study of deltoid samples found p62-positive, pTDP-43-negative inclusions [2] and p62-positive, pTDP-43-negative inclusions were recently described in the gastrocnemius of a single c9ALS patient [53].

Studies in ALS animal models have provided direct evidence that skeletal muscle can play a more active role in neurodegeneration. A variety of cell autonomous pathologies have been identified in the myofibers of transgenic (tg) mice expressing mutant Cu/Zn superoxide dismutase (mSOD1) [32]. These include increased endoplasmic reticulum stress response early in disease [12], reduction of heat shock protein expression [7], mitochondrial dysfunction [42], and pro-apoptotic signaling with increased cytosolic levels of calcium and calcium-binding proteins [13]. Aggregates of SOD1 protein have also been detected in the muscle of mSOD1 animals [6] and multiple studies have found an alteration in muscle expression of autophagy-related genes [14, 21]. The most compelling evidence to date for the active role of muscle in ALS is the finding that tg mice expressing G37R and G93A human SOD1 in skeletal muscle (hSOD1^{mus}), but not in nervous tissue, develop neurologic and pathologic ALS [57], with the wildtype motor neurons developing ubiquitinated aggregates. Other muscle-specific tg models have also shown muscular atrophy and reduced strength [22] and motor neuron degeneration [23].

To further examine whether cell autonomous pathology is present in the muscle of human ALS patients, we studied 148 muscle specimens from 57 patients to identify the prevalence and muscle group distribution of pTDP-43, a well-characterized marker of ALS pathology in motor neurons. To extend the work of prior studies, we included samples not only of appendicular muscle (quadriceps, deltoid), but also diaphragm and paraspinous muscle groups. We also studied pTDP-43-positive samples to determine whether the autophagy-related protein p62/ Sequestosome-1 was present in myofiber inclusions. To determine the specificity of these findings, we compared the ALS samples to an additional 25 non-ALS muscle samples with neurogenic atrophy, including four samples of clinical and pathologic inclusion body myositis (IBM). Finally, we examined whether pTDP-43 pathology in muscle was associated with salient disease characteristics, including age, site of onset, disease duration, familial or c9ALS status, and the burden of nervous system TDP-43 pathology.

Materials and methods

ALS muscle samples and clinical data

The 57 ALS patients with tissue examined in this study all underwent autopsy at our institution. The sample was representative of clinically diagnosed ALS patients seen at our institution with (1) pathologic confirmation and (2) skeletal muscle samples obtained at autopsy from one or multiple muscle groups. All pathologically confirmed ALS cases with skeletal muscle available for study were included. The majority of patients were evaluated in the clinic of two study authors (SHA, JWA). The study was conducted with the approval of the Institutional Review Board at Houston Methodist Hospital (IRB-(3 N)-0114–0013).

Clinical variables recorded included (a) disease duration, defined as the time between first symptoms and autopsy date, (b) age at death, (c) site of disease onset ("limb", "bulbar", or "multifocal/other"), and (d) whether the patient had familial (fALS) or sporadic ALS (sALS). As previously described [17], c9ALS status was identified (or confirmed) for the purposes of this retrospective study by the presence of TDP-43-negative, p62-positive inclusions on immunofluorescence (purified mouse anti-p62 Ick ligand, 1:50, BD Biosciences, San Jose, CA) in hippocampus and/or cerebellar granule cells. All c9ALS cases were confirmed using poly-GA (MABN889, EMD Millipore, 1:200, mouse monoclonal) and poly-GP (ABN455, EMD Millipore, 1:1000, rabbit polyclonal) antibodies. In 42 of the 57 patients in this study, the percentage of nervous system regions-of-interest (ROIs) with TDP-43 pathology, as previously reported [17], was also available.

Non-ALS muscle samples

Non-ALS patients ($n = 25$) included seventeen samples with neurogenic atrophy demonstrated on muscle biopsy.

These non-ALS patients comprised four cases of biopsy-proven inclusion body myositis (IBM), one case with neurogenic atrophy in a patient with myasthenic symptoms, one case of denervation atrophy in a patient with nerve plexus injury, one case of steroid myopathy, and 10 biopsies with a range of mild neurogenic changes (scattered nuclear clumps, esterase-positive angulated and atrophic fibers). Eleven of the non-ALS biopsies were from quadriceps and the remainder were obtained from biceps (2), gastrocnemius (2), or an unspecified site (2). An additional eight samples were included that contained fairly abundant paraspinous muscle among the various tissues obtained at laminectomy and submitted for routine pathologic examination. Two such specimens were from cervical spine with the remainder from lumbar spine and diagnoses included synovial cyst (2), radiculopathy (1), spinal stenosis (4), and spondylolisthesis (1).

Phospho(409/410)-TDP-43 immunohistochemistry

Phospho(409/410)-TDP43 antibody (1:500, rabbit polyclonal, 22309–1-AP, Proteintech, Rosemont, IL) was applied to all ALS samples, including paraspinous muscle (n = 44), deltoid (n = 34), diaphragm (n = 29), quadriceps (n = 26), skeletal muscle, NOS (n = 13), and one sample each of gastrocnemius and abdominal wall muscle. Immunostaining was performed on formalin-fixed, paraffin embedded (FFPE) tissue samples, sectioned at 4 μm, mounted on charged slides and dried for at least 2 h at 50–60 °C. Deparaffinization and rehydration were carried out using a series of xylenes, graded alcohols, and reagent grade water (ThermoFisher Scientific, Waltham, MA). Heat-based antigen retrieval was performed using a 1× antigen retrieval solution at pH 9 (Agilent Technologies, Santa Clara, CA) and was carried out for 1 h (30 min at 95 C^0, followed by 30 min on ice). Subsequent washing steps were carried out using a commercial Tris-buffered saline solution (1×) containing Tween 20, pH 7.6 (Agilent Technologies) with a 3% hydrogen peroxide solution (VWR International, Radnor, PA) used to block endogenous peroxidase. Primary antibody was applied for a minimum of 1 h following a one-hour blocking step at room temperature with 2.5% horse serum (Vector Laboratories, Burlingame, CA). Slides were thoroughly washed and a species appropriate ImmPress™ HRP IgG detection kit (Vector Laboratories) was applied for 1 h at room temperature. Following additional washing steps, target antigen was visualized using DAB chromogen in substrate buffer (Agilent Technologies). Hematoxylin counterstain was applied and slides were taken to xylene and mounted with Permount™ (ThermoFisher Scientific). Negative and positive controls were used with all staining reactions. Positive controls comprised ALS spinal cord or medulla and performed appropriately.

Evaluation of pTDP-43 inclusion pathology

Myofibers, adipose tissue, and neurovascular tissue were assessed for pTDP-43-reactive inclusions. For myofibers, only cases with unequivocal staining in the subsarcolemmal region or within sarcoplasm were recorded as positive (no intranuclear inclusions were identified). Semi-quantitation of pTDP43-positive samples was also performed. For pTDP-43 *density*, the number of involved fibers was quantitated in a single 100× low-power field (LPF). For pTDP-43 *extent*, the number of LPFs with pTDP-43 pathology per slide was expressed as a percentage of all LPFs with myofibers in the sample (e.g., 15 fields with pTDP-43 inclusion pathology of 25 total LPFs of muscle = 60% of fields with at least one pTDP-43 inclusion).

p62 and FUS immunohistochemistry

Using the procedures described above, skeletal muscle samples that were positive for pTDP-43 were screened for inclusions of p62 (purified mouse anti-p62 lck ligand, 1:100, BD Biosciences, San Jose, CA) and/or FUS/TLS (1:200, rabbit polyclonal, 11570–1-AP, Proteintech). Immunohistochemical procedures were identical to those described above. Negative and positive controls were used and performed appropriately. For p62, sections of spinal cord or medulla from ALS patients served as positive controls. For FUS, positive controls were sections of FTLD-FUS brain tissue.

Additional staining in a subset of cases

In a subset of ALS cases with pTDP-43 inclusions, double labeling immunofluorescence procedures were performed to assess co-expression of pTDP-43 (as above) with fast myosin (anti-mouse, 1:400, Sigma Aldrich, M4276), slow myosin (anti-mouse, 1:1000, Sigma Aldrich, M8421), or p62 (as above). Samples were incubated overnight with a mixture of primary antibodies at 4 °C following deparaffinization and rehydration steps, antigen retrieval procedures (10 mM citrate buffer), and a blocking step using 2.5% horse serum. After several washes with phosphate buffered saline, secondary antibodies (1:200) were applied for 1 h, including the secondary antibodies Alexa Fluor® 555 anti-rabbit IgG (Thermo Fisher, A-21429), Alexa Fluor® 555 anti-mouse IgG (Thermo Fisher, A32727), Alexa Fluor® 488 anti-mouse IgG (Thermo Fisher, A11001), and Alexa Fluor® 488 anti-rabbit IgG (Thermo Fisher, A-11034). Following further PBS washes, sections were mounted using Vectashield Antifade mounting media with DAPI (H-1200, Vector Laboratories, Burlingame, CA).

Additional staining for N-terminal TDP-43 antibody (1:1000, rabbit polyclonal, 10782-2-AP, Proteintech, Rosemont, IL), which stains both physiologic and pathologic TDP-43, was performed in three ALS samples with pTDP-43 inclusions (see Results), two ALS samples without pTDP-43 inclusions, and a control sample of frontotemporal lobar degeneration with TDP-43 inclusion pathology. 1% Thioflavin S staining was performed in the same five ALS samples undergoing N-terminal TDP-43 immunohistochemistry, as well as four samples of IBM, three samples of non-ALS, non-IBM neurogenic atrophy, and two control samples (Alzheimer's disease).

Evaluation of immunofluorescence studies

All immunofluorescence studies were reviewed within 24 h of staining and images were captured in cellSens software 1.13 (Olympus America, Inc., Center Valley, PA) on an Olympus BX-43 Microscope using a DP71 camera, a EGFP FITC/Cy2 filter cube (set number 49002, Olympus, Center Valley, PA) and a CY3/TRITC filter cube (set number 49004, Olympus, Center Valley, PA). Slides were examined separately under DAPI, TRITC, and FITC filters, to facilitate examination of antibody/ fluorophore-specific signal versus structures with autofluorescence (e.g., pigment). Images were captured in cellSens software, including merged images combining all three channels.

Electron microscopy of FFPE tissue

A protocol at our institution available for the ultrastructural study of specimens from FFPE blocks not fixed with glutaraldehyde was used to study four ALS muscle samples with comparatively extensive pTDP-43 inclusion pathology (see Results). A region of maximal pTDP-43 inclusion pathology was identified microscopically and marked on the tissue block face. A core of tissue was sampled from the corresponding tissue focus, deparaffinized and post fixed in buffered 2% osmium tetroxide. Tissues were dehydrated in a graded ethanol series, followed by resin infiltration with propylene oxide and EMbed 812 mixture (Electron Microscopy Sciences, Hatfield, PA). Samples were embedded overnight at 60 °C. Semi-thick and ultrathin sections were collected using a LEICA EM UC7 (Leica Microsystems, Buffalo Grove, IL). Stained thin sections were imaged with JEOL 1400 transmission electron microscope (JEOL Ltd., Tokyo, Japan) and AMT Imaging Software (Advanced Microscopy Techniques, Corp., Woburn, MA).

RNA isolation and real-time PCR

To examine *SQSTM1* (p62/ sequestosome-1) and *TARDBP* gene expression, RNA was isolated from four successive 10-μm sections of paraffin-embedded muscle tissue using an RNeasy® FFPE Kit (Qiagen, catalogue number 73504, Hilden, Germany) according to the manufacturer's protocol. RNA was isolated from five ALS samples (p62 and pTDP-43-positive), three IBM samples (p62 and pTDP-43-positive), and three samples of non-ALS, non-IBM neurogenic atrophy (p62 and pTDP-43-negative). Quantification of RNA was performed using a Nanodrop ND 100 spectrophotometer (Thermo Fisher Scientific).

Real-time PCR primer assays were performed using SYBR® Green dye-based chemistry (Bio-Rad, catalogue # 1725151, Hercules, CA, USA) with commercially available and experimentally validated PCR primer pairs for *SQSTM1* (Bio-Rad, catalogue # qHsaCED0045925) and *TARDBP* (Bio-Rad, catalogue # qHsaCED0043888). Housekeeping genes utilized for normalization of transcript levels included *GAPDH* (Bio-Rad, catalogue # qHsaCED0038674) and *RPS18* (Bio-Rad, catalogue # qHsaCED0037454). Each real-time PCR experiment included eleven ALS, IBM, and atrophy muscle RNA samples plus a no template control (12 experimental wells per primer × 4 primers). This experiment was duplicated in the other half of the 96-well plate and then repeated, again in duplicate, using a new 96-well plate. A one-step real-time PCR protocol was performed on a CFX96 Touch (Bio-Rad, Hercules, CA, USA), including a melt curve step to exclude non-specific amplification. Experiments were analyzed in CFX Maestro™ software for Mac (Bio-Rad, Hercules, CA, USA). *TARDBP* and *SQSTM1* expression were normalized to both reference genes (*GAPDH, RS18*) and relative normalized gene expression was compared between patient groups. Significance testing was performed using an unpaired t-test.

Descriptive statistics and statistical analyses

Fisher exact tests were used to determine the strength of association between pTDP-43 inclusion pathology in muscle fibers and individual muscle groups (deltoid, quadriceps, paraspinous, and diaphragm), as well as axial (diaphragm, paraspinous) versus appendicular (deltoid, quadriceps) musculature. Fisher exact tests were also used to examine the association between pTDP-43 inclusion pathology and c9ALS status, fALS status, and onset (limb versus bulbar). The strength of these associations was recorded by the *P*-value and odds ratio (OR).

Wilcoxon rank sum tests (Mann-Whitney U) were applied to examine the equality of medians in pTDP-43-positive and negative ALS patients with respect to age at death, disease duration, and percentage of central nervous system regions-of-interest (ROIs) positive for TDP-43 pathology [17]. As previously reported, the last of these measures was the percentage of 34 different brain regions positive for TDP-43 inclusions (using Proteintech 10782–2-AP) (ranging between 27.3 and 100%) and these data were available for 42 of the 57 patients studied here [17]. Similarly, Wilcoxon rank sum tests were applied to examine the equality of medians between IBM and ALS patients with respect to pTDP-43 density and pTDP-43 extent in positive skeletal muscle samples. Statistical testing was implemented in Matlab R2015b [37] and statistical significance was set at $P \leq 0.01$.

Results

Demographics and clinical characteristics

ALS patient characteristics are listed in Table 1. Briefly, the 57 patients in this study comprised 39 men and 18 women with a median age of 61 years at death (interquartile range, IQR 56–68 years). Ten patients had a history of fALS (17.5%) and the remaining cases were sporadic (n = 45, 79%), or family history was unknown (n = 2). c9ALS was present in 13 patients (22.8%), accounting for 90% of the clinically designated fALS patients in this study and 4 sALS patients (8.9% of sALS cases). Limb onset was seen in 38 patients (66.7%), bulbar onset in 12 (21.1%), and onset was other/ multifocal in six (10.5%). Onset site was not available in one patient. Median disease duration was 2.99 years (1090 days, IQR 781–1565 days).

Prevalence, distribution, and quantitation of pTDP-43 muscle pathology in ALS

pTDP-43 inclusion pathology was present in 24 of 148 ALS muscle specimens (16.2% of blocks) from 19 of 57 patients (33.3% of patients). pTDP-43 was identified in myofibers as cytoplasmic or subsarcolemmal aggregates, ranging from blocky, immunoreactive structures to dot- and dash-like and filamentous inclusions. Representative images of p62 and pTDP-43 pathology are shown in Fig. 1 for three IBM patients and three ALS patients. A subset of patients with and without pTDP-43 inclusions were studied and this showed N-terminal TDP-43 pathology in the same distribution as pTDP-43, with cytoplasmic staining and loss of normal nuclear staining (Fig. 2). Peripheral nerve elements were frequent components of the autopsy muscle specimens and no axonal or other neural pTDP-43 inclusions were identified in any samples, including those with pTDP-43 inclusions in muscle fibers (Fig. 3). Intranuclear inclusions were not identified.

Quantitatively, a range of inclusion density and spatial extent was seen across pTDP-43-positive ALS samples. The median number of pTDP-43 inclusions per 100× field was 2 (IQR, 2 to 14.3 inclusions, range of 1 to 64). The majority of positive samples had multiple LPFs of pTDP-43 pathology, with a median of 5 LPFs per case having pTDP-43 inclusions (IQR, 2–7 LPFs, range of 1 to 15). A median of 10% of all microscopic LPFs that included skeletal muscle had pTDP-43 pathology (range of 3%–60%), reflecting that the inclusion pathology was patchy and not typically diffuse.

Co-localization of pTDP-43 inclusion pathology was examined with respect to fast- and slow-myosin heavy chain expression in 5 ALS cases and 1 IBM sample. In ALS cases, a median of 2 pTDP-43-immunoreactive inclusions was seen in the positive high-power field studied (range of 1–14). Phospho-TDP-43 inclusions in both slow- and fast-myosin positive fibers were seen in two cases (one with 78.5% in fast-myosin expressing fibers, the other with 80% in slow-myosin expressing fibers). The remaining ALS cases had pTDP-43 positive inclusions only in slow fibers (2 cases) or fast fibers (1 case). The single IBM sample tested had 83.3% of pTDP-43-positive inclusions in myofibers expressing fast myosin.

Table 1 Demographic, clinical, and sample characteristics in 57 ALS patients

Characteristic	Entire cohort [a]
Age	61 years (IQR, 56–68), range 39–86 [b]
Duration	1090 days (IQR, 781–1565), range 315–4886
Men/ Women	39 men (68.4%)/ 18 women (31.6%)
fALS [c]/ sALS/ C9ALS	10 fALS (18.2%)/ 45 sALS (81.8%)/ 13 C9ALS
Onset site [c]	38 Limb (66.7%)/ 12 Bulbar (21.1%)/ 6 Multifocal (10.5%)
Axial muscle samples	44 Paraspinous (29.7%)/ 29 Diaphragm (19.6%)
Append. Muscle samples	34 Deltoid (22.9%)/ 26 Quadriceps (17.6%)
Other muscle samples	13 NOS [d] (8.8%)/ 1 gastrocnemius/ 1 abdominus rectus

[a]Data presented are medians with interquartile range (IQR) in parenthesis or number with percentage

[b]For the 17 non-ALS samples with atrophy studied, median age was 60 years (IQR, 51–62). For the 8 non-ALS paraspinous samples, median age was 62 years

[c]fALS/ sALS and c9ALS status were not available in 2 patients. One patient had an unknown onset site

[d]These samples were obtained without reference to anatomic site and simply labeled as "muscle" in the original autopsy report

p62 and FUS IHC in pTDP-43-positive ALS samples

All but one pTDP-43-positive ALS sample (23 of 24 samples) had pathologic inclusions of p62 in myofibers in the same distribution (Fig. 1). As in IBM cases, p62 was a more sensitive marker, revealing more extensive inclusion pathology than pTDP-43 alone. FUS immunohistochemistry was negative in all 24 ALS samples.

Muscle group distribution of pTDP-43 positive samples in ALS

Among the 24 pTDP-43-positive ALS muscle samples, 10 were obtained from paraspinous musculature (41.7% of positive samples), 7 from diaphragm (29.2%), three from deltoid (12.5%), and one from gastrocnemius (4.2%). Three positive samples were from a muscle group not specified in the original autopsy report (12.5%) and were simply designated as "muscle, NOS."

Axial muscle groups represented 17 of 24 positive samples (70.8%) (Fig. 4). Fisher's exact test revealed a

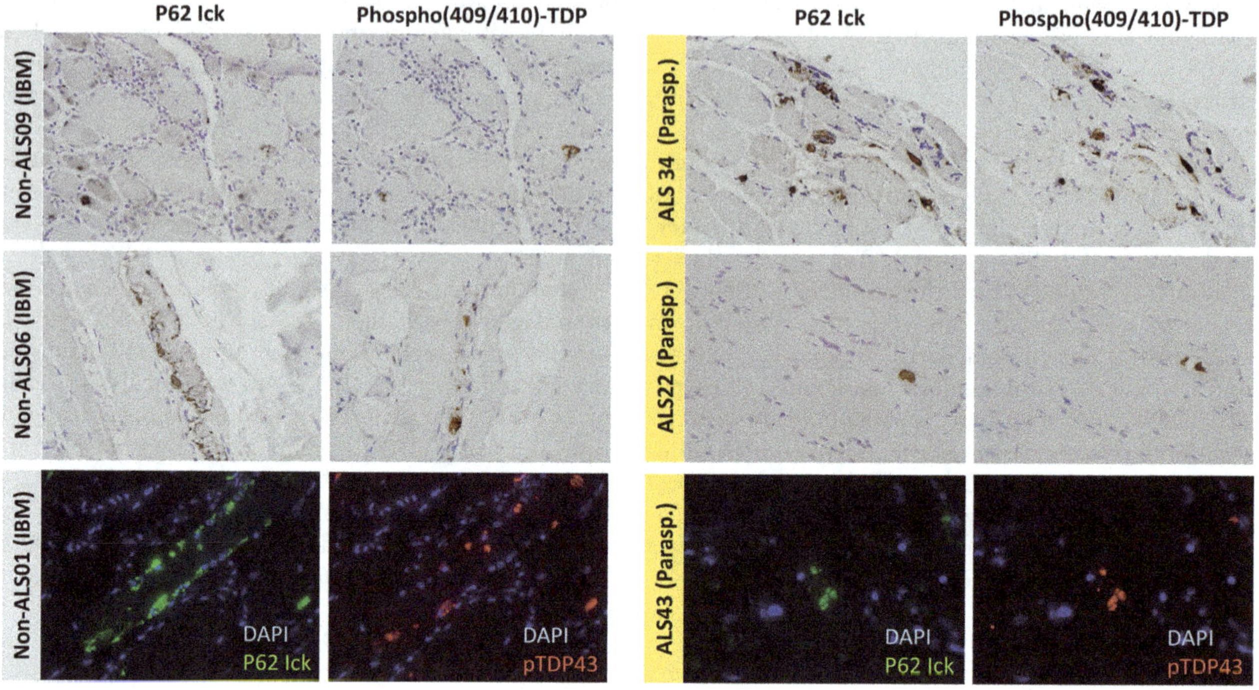

Fig. 1 p62 lck and pTDP-43 immunohistochemistry demonstrate p62-immunoreactive and pTDP-43-immunoreactive inclusions in three different IBM samples (left panels) and three different ALS samples (right panels; these examples all from paraspinous muscle). Immunofluorescence studies (bottom row) demonstrate co-localization of p62 lck and pTDP-43 in both IBM and ALS samples, although p62 is the more sensitive of the two in detecting subsarcolemmal/ sarcolemmal inclusion pathology. Top two rows (immunohistochemistry) photographed at 400× and bottom row (immunofluorescence) photographed at 600×

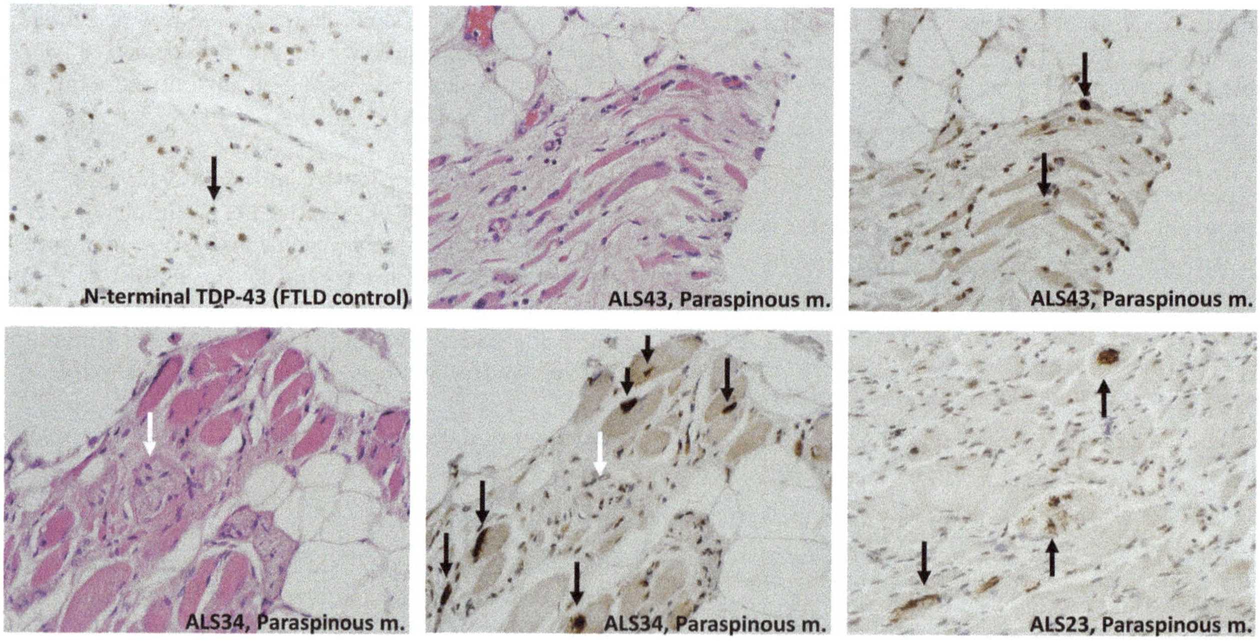

Fig. 2 N-terminal TDP-43 immunohistochemistry in a control brain (frontotemporal lobar degeneration) and three ALS muscle samples shown to have pTDP-43-reactive inclusions. N-terminal TDP-43 immunohistochemistry reveals cytoplasmic inclusions (black arrows), as demonstrated separately with pTDP-43 immunohistochemistry. There is a loss of normal nuclear staining in affected myofibers. In sample ALS34 (bottom left) a small nerve is present (white arrow), which does not show pathologic staining in the adjacent panel (white arrow). All images are photographed at 400×

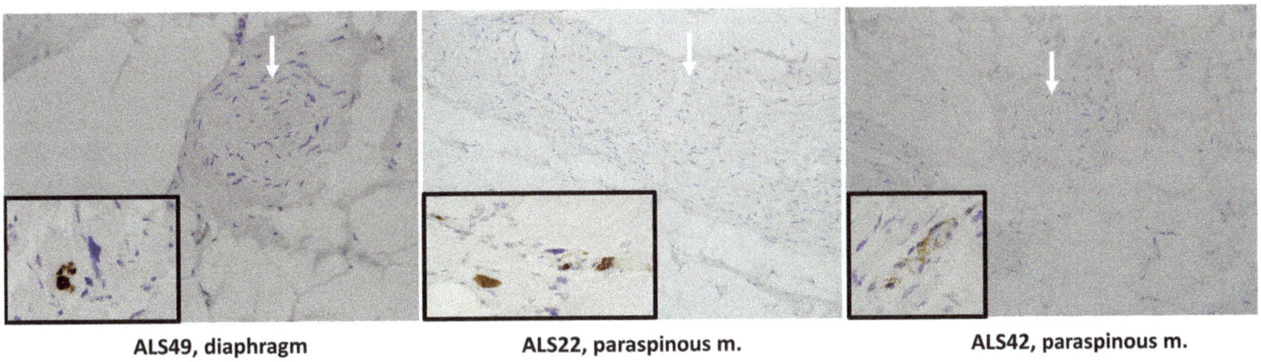

Fig. 3 Three additional ALS samples (ALS49, ALS22, and ALS42) with pTDP-43 inclusion pathology in muscle fibers, but not in adjacent nerve that was readily found and evaluated in autopsy-derived ALS muscle specimens. Main panels of pTDP-43-negative nerve (white arrows) photographed at 200×. Inset of each panel, showing pTDP-43-positive myofibers in the same slide, photographed at 400×

correspondingly strong and significant positive association between pTDP-43 pathology in ALS patients and axial musculature (paraspinous, diaphragm) versus appendicular muscle groups ($P = 0.0092$, OR = 4.25). No significant pTDP-43 and individual muscle group association (positive or negative) was seen for deltoid ($P = 0.2279$, OR = 0.44), quadriceps ($P = 0.07$, OR = 0.17), or for paraspinous ($P = 0.14$, OR = 2.1) or diaphragm ($P = 0.25$, OR = 2.04) considered separately (Fig. 4).

Among the 19 ALS patients with any pTDP-43-positive muscle sample, 4 patients had multiple pTDP-43-positive samples (7% of the cohort, 21% of positive samples). The combinations of pTDP-43-positive samples included: diaphragm and paraspinous (2 patients), diaphragm, paraspinous, and deltoid (1 patient), and diaphragm and deltoid (1 patient). Three of these patients had clinically-designated sALS (75%) and c9ALS was present in two of these four (50%).

Clinical and pathologic associations of pTDP-43 muscle pathology

The characteristics of ALS patients with and without pTDP-43-positive muscle samples are shown in Table 2. Briefly, patients with pTDP-43 skeletal muscle pathology ($n = 19$; 13 males, 6 females) had a median age of 64 years (IQR, 58.5–69.5 years), median disease duration of 1114 days (IQR, 840 to 2133.5 days), and included three fALS and four c9ALS patients. Patients had limb ($n = 11$), bulbar (5), and multifocal (3) sites of symptom onset. The group without pTDP-43 pathology had a median age of 59.5 years (IQR, 54.3–66.5 years), median disease duration of 1085 days (IQR, 723 to 1390 days),

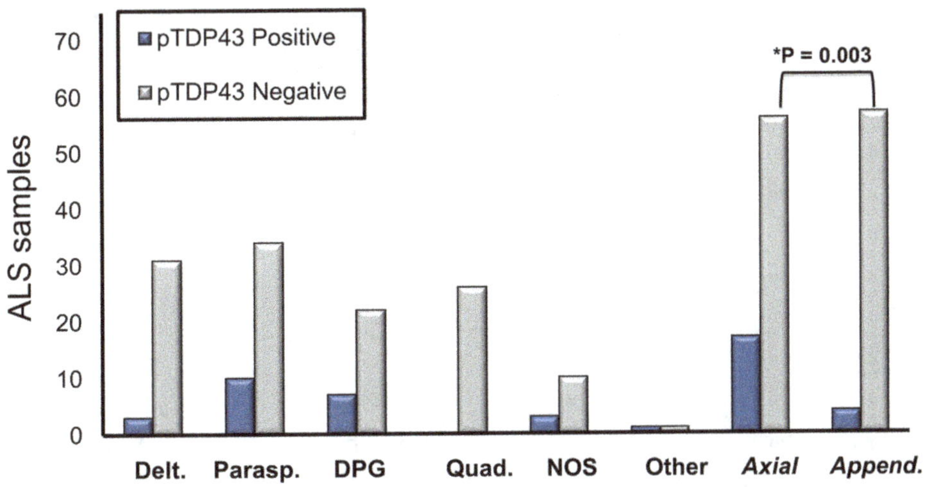

Fig. 4 Distribution of pTDP-43 pathology in 148 samples from ALS patients, including (from left to right) deltoid, paraspinous, diaphragm, and quadriceps. "NOS" represents muscles that were not specified by muscle group in the autopsy report and "Other" includes one positive gastrocnemius sample and one negative abdominal wall sample. The right-most bars show that pTDP-43 pathology was significantly more prevalent in axial (diaphragm, paraspinous) than appendicular (deltoid, quadriceps) samples

Table 2 Characteristics of muscle samples with and without pTDP-43 pathology

Variable	pTDP-43 Positive (n = 19)	pTDP-43 Negative (n = 38)	P-val [a]
Muscle group	17 Axial, 4 Appendicular [b]	56 Axial, 57 Appendicular [b]	*0.003*
Patient age	64 years (IQR, 58.5–69.5)	59.5 years (IQR, 54.3–66.5)	0.1
Disease duration	1114 days (IQR, 840–2134)	1085 days (IQR, 723–1390)	0.34
CNS TDP$^+$ ROI [c]	58.3% TDP+ (IQR, 45.5–79.4)	50.0% TDP+ (IQR, 42.3–76.5)	0.67
Men, Women	13 men, 6 women	26 men, 12 women	*NA*
fALS, sALS	3 fALS, 16 sALS	7 fALS, 29 sALS	0.78
C9ALS [d]	4 C9ALS	9 C9ALS	0.80
Onset site	11 Limb, 5 Bulb, 3 Multifocal	27 Limb, 7 Bulb, 3 Multifocal	0.49

[a]P-values represent differences using Fisher exact test or Mann-Whitney U test as appropriate (See Methods/ Results). [b] These numbers do not include three positive "NOS" samples, ten negative "NOS" samples, or negative abdominal wall muscle. [c] The percentage of brain and spinal cord ROIs positive for TDP-43 pathology as previously described in Cykowski et al., 2017 [17] (see Methods). [d] C9ALS status accounted for 9 of 10 fALS patients with one patient having an unknown genetic basis

and included 7 fALS and 9 c9ALS patients. These pTDP-43-negative patients had limb (n = 27), bulbar (7), and multifocal (3) sites of symptom onset.

No significant differences were identified between ALS patients with and without pTDP-43 muscle pathology with respect to age (z = 1.7, P = 0.1) or disease duration (z = 0.95, P = 0.34). Likewise, no significant association was seen between pTDP-43 status in muscle and fALS status (OR = 0.78), c9ALS status (OR = 0.8), or site of symptom onset (OR = 0.57). Utilizing data from an earlier study [17], ALS cases with pTDP-43 muscle pathology had a median of 58.3% and 50.0% of brain regions involved by TDP-43 inclusion pathology, respectively (z = 0.42, P = 0.67).

Inclusion pathology in IBM and non-IBM, non-ALS muscle

Non-ALS muscle biopsies with atrophy (n = 17) included 9 females and 8 males with a median age of 60 years (IQR, 51–62 years). Samples of non-ALS paraspinous muscle (n = 8) included 6 females and 2 males with a median age of 62 years (IQR, 58–66 years). Among non-ALS samples, only IBM cases showed pTDP-43-immunoreactive inclusions (see Figs. 1 and 5).

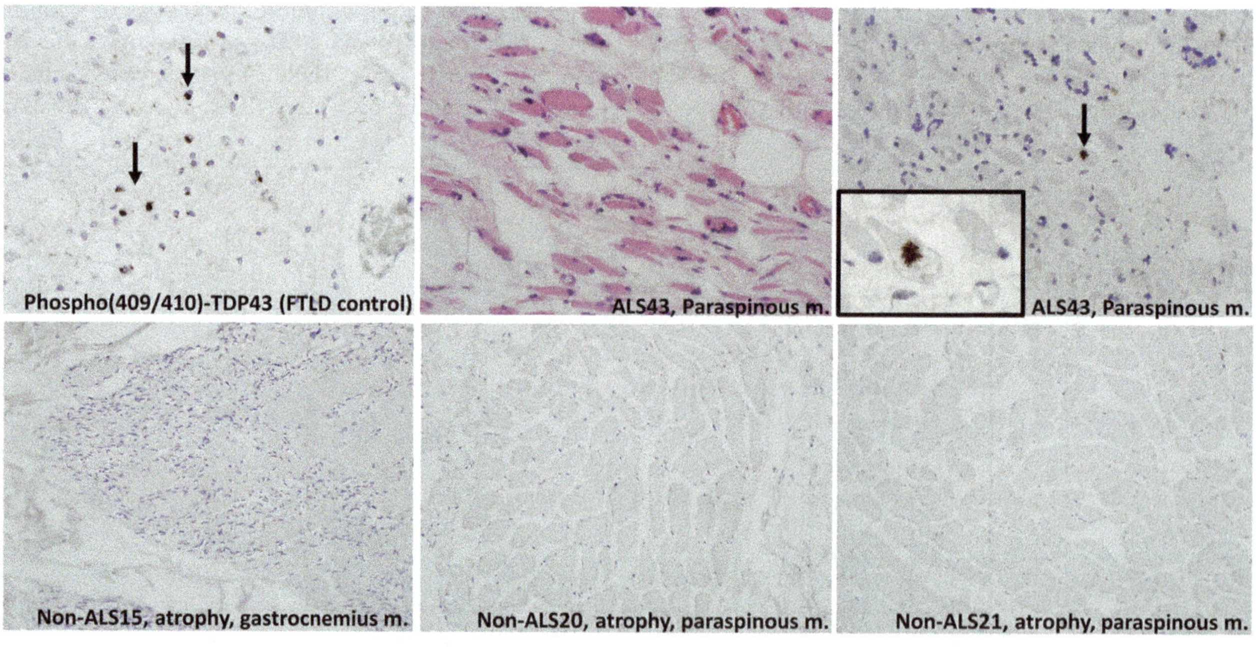

Fig. 5 Non-ALS, non-IBM samples were negative for pTDP-43 pathology. Representative brain section control from a patient with frontotemporal lobar degeneration (top left panel), stained for pTDP-43, followed by H&E-stained section and positive pTDP-43 myofiber in an ALS patient. Bottom panels show pTDP-43 negative results in a patient with long-term steroid use and profound fiber atrophy and two samples of pTDP-43-negative paraspinous muscle obtained in the course of laminectomy in non-ALS patients. Images in the top row all photographed at 400×, except for the inset of pTDP-43 staining at the top right (600×) for sample ALS43. Images in the bottom row all photographed at 200×

Four cases of IBM (clinically suspected and pathologically confirmed) were from three males and one female with a median age of 59 years. Among these samples, only IBM cases (100%) had pTDP-43 inclusions, which were also p62-immunoreactive (Fig. 1). Three non-ALS, non-IBM cases with mild neurogenic atrophy had granular, non-specific p62 immunoreactivity (pTDP-43 negative) that did not resemble that seen in either ALS or IBM patients. Likewise, in non-ALS paraspinous samples, p62 occasionally showed immunoreactive structures, but these were uniformly pTDP-43-negative and did not resemble those in ALS or IBM muscle. In IBM patients, within the focus of maximum pTDP-43 pathology (100× field), IBM cases had a median of 10 involved myofibers (IQR of 7–11.8), whereas for ALS cases the median was 2 (IQR of 2–14.3) ($z = -1.1$, $P = 0.26$). However, IBM and ALS patients with pTDP-43 inclusions did significantly differ in the spatial extent of pathology, with IBM patients having a median of 67% of LPFs involved ($z = -2.7$, $P = 0.007$).

pTDP-43 replication study in a subset of cases

A subset of 5 pTDP-43-positive muscle samples, two from patients with IBM and three from patients with ALS, were sent to an independent research laboratory for separate evaluation using their pTDP-43 immunohistochemistry protocol (phospho-TDP-43, 1D3 clone, 1: 500). Five unstained sections, cut at 4 μm and labeled "ALS1–3" and "IBM1–2", were shipped to the laboratory. Their results matched the spatial distribution and staining intensity of pTDP-43 in all IBM and ALS samples (see Online Resource Additional file 1: Figure S1).

Ultrastructural findings

A region of FFPE tissue, enriched for pTDP-43 pathology in ALS muscle samples, was prepared for electron microscopy (see Methods). Due to the nature of the specimen, autolytic changes and degradation of the sarcomere were present, as evidence by degeneration of myofibrils and Z-bands (Fig. 6). However, in each sample studied, sarcolemmal or subsarcolemmal filamentous material, ranging between 10 and 20 nm in width, was identified. This material was well demarcated from degenerating sarcomeres and is not identified in specimens with non-specific neurogenic atrophy or autolysis (personal experience of the authors). The structures resembled non-specific filamentous material that may be seen in muscle biopsy (filamentous bodies), although this material was more frequent in pTDP-43-positive ALS samples submitted for electron microscopy than we have observed for filamentous bodies in clinical muscle biopsy samples. Figure 6 shows the appearance of this material in sarcolemmal (top row), subsarcolemmal (middle row) and subsarcolemmal locations adjacent to a neuromuscular junction (bottom row), in three different patient samples. In this limited sample, no intranuclear inclusions, myelin-like figures, or lysosomal debris was identified. Mitochondria were too degenerated for evaluation.

Quantitative PCR

As shown in Fig. 7, real time PCR analyses revealed increased *TARDBP* and *SQSTM1* mRNA levels in both ALS and IBM patients relative to non-ALS, non-IBM control muscle. For ALS samples, relative to controls, there was a 4.21 fold increase (expression standard error of the mean (SEM) of 0.54) ($P = < 0.0001$) in *SQSTM1* and 1.67 fold increase in *TARDBP* (SEM = 0.31) ($P = 0.0128$). For IBM samples, relative to controls, there was a 1. 33 fold increase in *SQSTM1* expression (SEM of 0.26) ($P = 0.012$) and 1.31 fold increase in *TARDBP* expression (SEM of 0.29) ($P = 0.014$).

Discussion

This study demonstrates that aggregates of phosphorylated TDP-43 may be identified in the skeletal muscle of both sALS and fALS patients, including patients with and without c9ALS. This implicates axial skeletal muscle as an additional site of pTDP-43 pathology in ALS. A muscle group-specific difference in muscle pathology was also suggested by the finding that pTDP-43 inclusions were significantly more frequent in samples from axial muscle groups than appendicular groups (the absence of inclusion pathology in quadriceps samples is also consistent with the negative result of an earlier study [50] that did not assess axial muscle groups). Our finding that pTDP-43-positive (FUS-negative) aggregates in ALS samples are also positive for the autophagy pathway protein p62/ sequestosome-1 suggests the possibility of an engagement of endogenous autophagic mechanisms in ALS muscle, as in motor neurons. Indeed, this pattern resembled the co-localization of pTDP-43 and p62 inclusions in IBM [9, 31], an intrinsic myopathy in the differential diagnosis of ALS [33] with pathologic protein aggregates, progressive and asymmetrical weakness [46], and impairments in autophagy. Other characteristic features of IBM, however, were not identified in our ALS samples and there was significantly more extensive pTDP-43 inclusion pathology in IBM muscle than in ALS. Nonetheless, pTDP-43 aggregates in ALS and IBM muscle may arise through similar mechanisms, including impairments in autophagy and proteostasis.

To our knowledge this is the first study to systematically demonstrate the presence of pTDP-43 aggregates in the myofibers of ALS patients, particularly in axial muscle groups. This implicates ALS muscle as an additional site of pTDP-43 pathology, as previously demonstrated in motor neurons, non-motor neurons, and glia. The downstream effects of cytoplasmic pTDP-43 pathology in ALS muscle cells requires further study, though

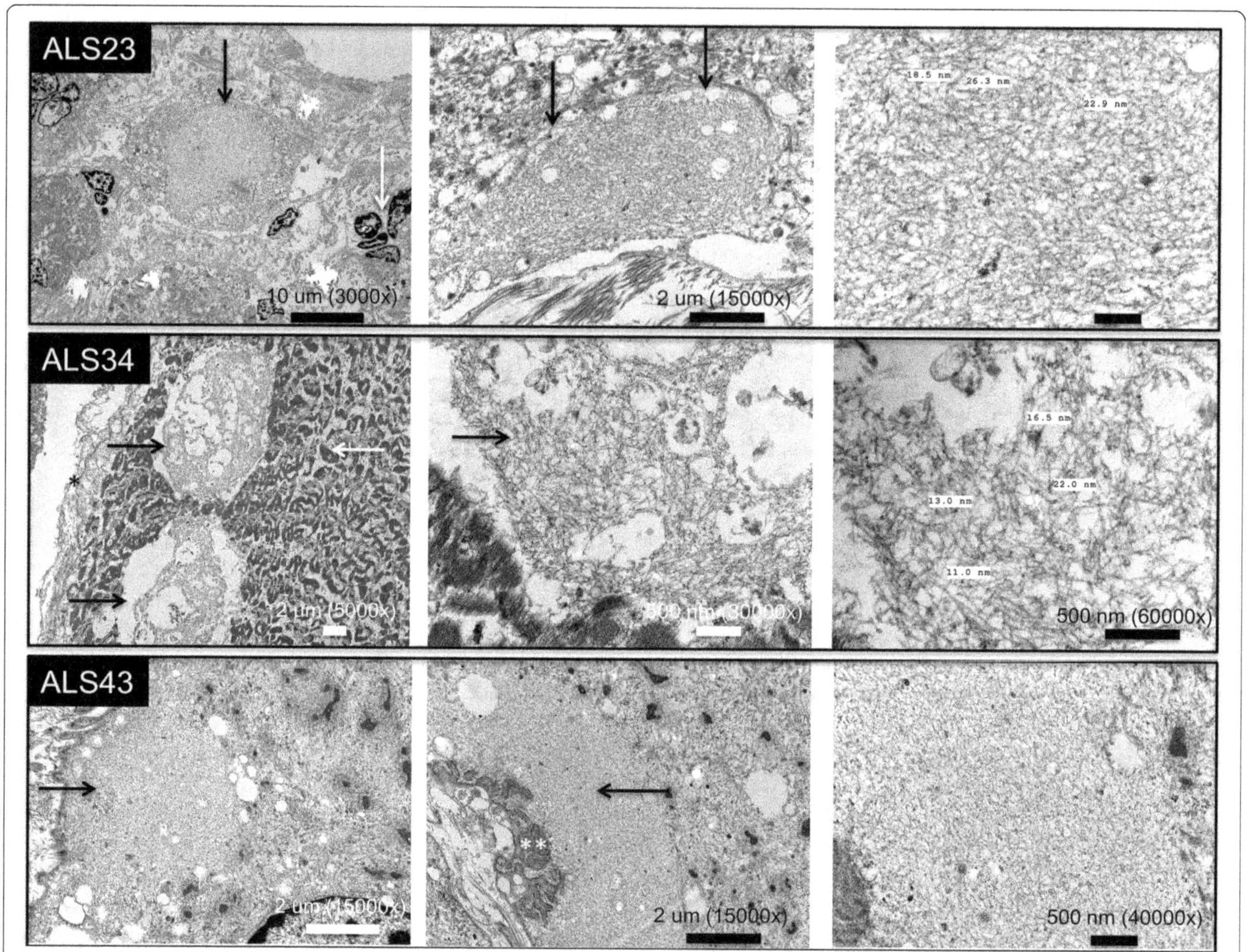

Fig. 6 Electron microscopy of three ALS muscle samples (study samples ALS23, ALS34, and ALS43). For each muscle sample, a region-of-interest was dissected out of the FFPE block in a region with maximal pTDP-43 and p62 inclusion pathology and subsequently processed for electron microscopy using a protocol for FFPE specimens (see Methods). Filamentous material (black arrows in all three rows) is present in these foci, entirely within myofibers and sharply demarcated from degenerating myofibrils (white arrow, middle row, left-most panel). Basement membrane (black asterisk, middle row, left panel) and nuclear clumps (white arrow, top row, left panel) are also identified, despite the degenerated nature of the specimen. The filamentous material identified predominantly measures between 10 and 20 nm in thickness (right panels of top and middle rows, which are enlargements of the middle panels in their respective rows). In the bottom row, the middle and right-most panels show accumulation of this material adjacent to invaginations of the cell membrane at an apparent neuromuscular junction (white asterisks). Scale bar and magnifications are shown for each panel

studies in transgenic animals expressing mutant human TDP-43 have identified a toxic gain-of-function from cytoplasmic aggregation, leading to transcriptional dysregulation, including within histone processing genes [3]. Several results of this study raise the question as to whether pTDP-43 in ALS muscle represents a cell autonomous pathology. First, the presence of pTDP-43 inclusions in muscle did not associate at all with disease duration or the burden of central nervous system TDP-43 pathology [17]. If cell-to-cell spread were the sole mechanisms explaining muscle pTDP-43 pathology, one would expect significant positive associations between muscle fiber inclusion pathology and either duration or the burden of nervous system TDP-43 pathology. Second, pTDP-43 co-localized with p62 in affected muscle fibers and a concomitant up-regulation of *TARDBP* and *SQSTM1* gene expression was seen by real-time PCR. Co-localization with an autophagy pathway protein (p62), and up-regulation in gene expression (for TDP-43 and p62), suggests this may be an endogenous pathology in muscle that engages the autophagy pathway. Increased expression of p62 has also been seen in non-ALS, non-IBM muscle diseases, including genetically driven forms of muscular dystrophy [20], so it may not implicate autophagy in all cases. Third, pTDP-43 co-localized with both fast- and slow-myosin expressing fibers in the same ALS sample (motor neurons innervating fibers of a single type) and was distributed within

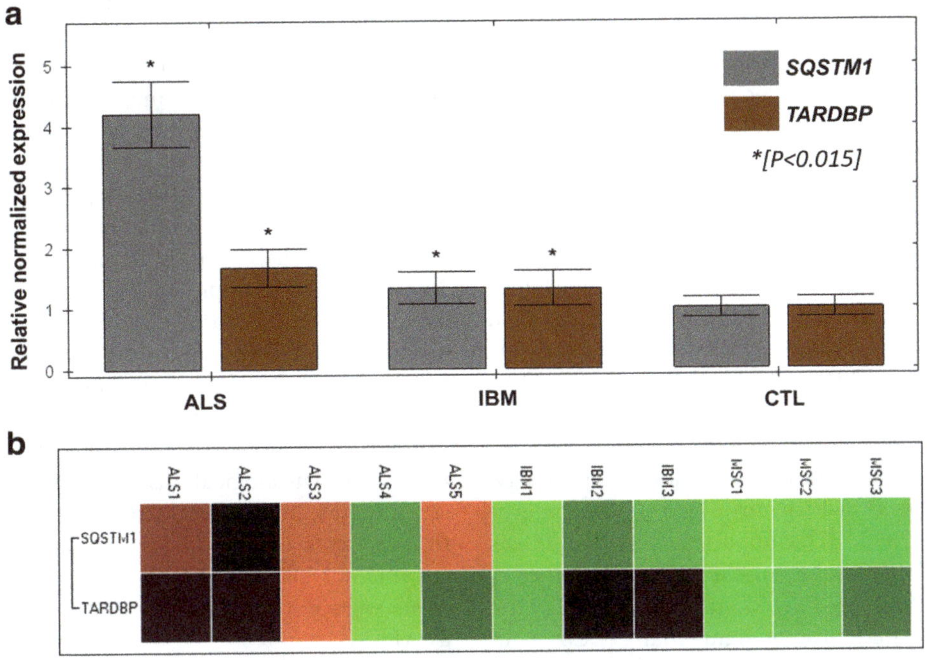

Fig. 7 qPCR analysis was performed in 5 ALS muscle samples ("ALS1–5") and 3 IBM muscle samples ("IBM1–3"), all containing p62 and pTDP-43 inclusions by immunohistochemical studies (see Results). Three non-ALS, non-IBM samples with mild neurogenic atrophy in the muscle biopsy were also studied ("MSC1–3"). *SQSTM1* and *TARDBP* were analyzed relative to the expression of two housekeeping genes (*18 s*, *GAPDH*) and data shown are combined from two 96-well plates (4 replicates per sample and primer). There was a significant increase in relative normalized gene expression for both ALS and IBM samples (**a**), relative to controls (right) and this was most significant for *SQSTM1* expression in ALS samples (> 4-fold expression relative to controls, $P < 0.0001$). Clustergram by gene target (**b**) shows heterogeneity across ALS and IBM samples with increase gene expression (red-brown) most conspicuous in ALS samples 1–3 and 5, as well as IBM samples 2 and 3

multiple fascicles rather than a single fascicle. However, it is also important to recognize that the majority of skeletal muscle samples were negative for pTDP-43. One reason for this may be that our study used single tissue samples obtained from between one and four muscle groups per patient. This approach is distinctly different from the postmortem examination of ALS nervous systems, where all anatomic regions (brain, spinal cord) are amenable to sampling and diagnostic pTDP-43 that may actually be quite limited in spatial extent. Recent autopsies at our institution, not included in this study, with paraspinous samples at multiple spinal levels, have indeed shown patchy, multifocal and segmental involvement of muscle (see Online Resource Additional file 1: Figure S2). This suggests that the true prevalence of pTDP-43 pathology in muscle cannot be ascertained from single biopsy-size samples and may be underestimated even in the present study.

An alternative mechanism explaining pTDP-43 aggregates in ALS muscle is a "prion-like" transfer of pTDP-43 protein, possibly through anterograde axonal transport. This model of neuron-to-neuron spread has been proposed to explain dissemination of pTDP-43 pathology in brain and spinal cord [8]. If trans-synaptic spread between neurons indeed takes place in ALS, then spread along the axons of motor neurons, across the neuromuscular junction, and into myofibers is plausible. A distance-dependent interaction between motor neurons and muscle, possibly acting in concert with muscle-specific pathology, may explain the enrichment of pTDP-43 inclusions in axial muscle. This question deserves further investigation, possibly through studies examining the density of spinal cord motor neuron pTDP-43 pathology in tandem with paraspinous muscle samples at the same spinal level.

Our study also identified co-localization of p62/sequestosome-1 in pTDP-43 inclusions of ALS muscle, which suggests the possibility that the autophagy pathway is activated. This recapitulates pathology well described in inclusion body myositis (IBM). Further comparison of ALS and IBM muscle samples may provide insight as to how pTDP-43 inclusions arise in vulnerable ALS muscle groups. To date, there have been few studies of pTDP-43 (or p62) pathology in ALS muscle. None of these, to our knowledge, have examined both axial and appendicular muscle groups or compared findings in ALS and IBM, and non-ALS, non-IBM samples with neurogenic atrophy. Previous studies do include a negative study of ALS quadriceps biopsies from 30 patients [50] (the 26 quadriceps samples studied here were also negative), a study of 31 deltoid biopsies finding p62-immunoreactive, pTDP-43-negative foci in 25.8% of samples [2], and a case report of a c9ALS patient with blocky p62 inclusions in gastrocnemius [53]. Inclusion pathologies have been much more extensively studied in IBM, where β-amyloid, α-synuclein, and p-tau inclusions have also been described [5]. IBM inclusions are also reported to be positive for Thioflavin S, a finding identified here in all four IBM samples studied and in three pTDP-43-positive ALS samples examined (see Online Resource Additional file 1: Figure S3). In IBM, p62 appears to be the most sensitive marker of inclusion pathology [27] and these additional inclusions have not been seen in all studies [9]. Nonetheless, these findings have led to the hypothesis that protein aggregates in IBM muscle result from impairments in autophagy, the cellular process by which misfolded protein aggregates are degraded [25, 31]. Supporting this hypothesis are the increased expression of the endosome marker clathrin, the autophagy-related protein ATG5, the microtubule-associated protein light chain (LC3), and beclin-1 [25] in IBM samples. IBM samples also demonstrate more frequent LC3-reactive fibers than in pTDP-43-negative, non-IBM inflammatory myopathy (e.g., polymyositis), which indicates that alterations in autophagy are critical in IBM and not linked to inflammation per se. For ALS, autophagy impairments in motor neurons, as in IBM muscle fibers, have been proposed as a mechanism leading to cell degeneration and toxic protein aggregates [11, 45]. Moreover, mutations in fALS have been reported in autophagy-related genes, including optineurin (*OPTN*) [36], ubiquilin 2 (*UBQLN2*), sequestosome 1 (*SQSTM1*) [24], and ubiquitin segregase (*VCP*) [51] (the last of these also being described in familial IBM). In ALS nervous systems, p62- and LC3-reactive inclusions have also been identified in spinal cord motor neurons [47], in addition to TDP-43 [41]. The findings of the current study, which extends the spectrum of pTDP-43 and p62 inclusion pathology to ALS skeletal muscle, particularly in axial muscles, suggests that impairments in autophagy may also involve ALS muscle. Future studies are needed to determine whether other autophagy-related proteins, such as LC3, beclin-1, and optineurin, are over- or under-expressed in ALS muscle.

An intriguing finding of this study was that pTDP-43 pathology was significantly enriched in axial muscle samples. It is known that physiologic abnormalities in paraspinous muscle by electromyography (EMG) are reliable in confirming the clinical diagnosis of ALS and help to distinguish the disease from its mimics [29]. Paraspinous abnormalities have also been described as being present early in the disease [30]. Denervation changes by EMG in paraspinous muscle are also associated with features of diaphragm denervation – an association possibly explained by the medial position of the relevant motor neurons in the ventral horn [19]. A recent study of multiple muscle groups, including thoracic (T10), lumbar (L3, L5), and sacral (S1) paraspinous muscle has also shown non-contiguous abnormalities by needle EMG (e.g., fibrillation potentials). This finding suggests the possibility of multifocal and discontinuous initiation of disease in different motor neuron pools. More extensive sampling of paraspinous muscle groups at autopsy will help to determine if pTDP-43 pathology is similarly multifocal and discontinuous. Further, a limitation of this study, to be addressed in future studies, is that autopsy-derived diaphragm and paraspinous muscle samples from non-ALS patients with other critical illnesses or neurological diseases were not available for study. Paraspinous muscle and muscle biopsy specimens from a range of non-ALS, non-IBM neurologic diagnoses did not show pTDP-43 pathology, but these specimens were not from patients with critical illnesses, such as ALS.

Studies in the mSOD1 mouse model of ALS have provided direct evidence that cell autonomous pathology in muscle can drive the development of the disease [32]. The muscle of mSOD1 animals has been reported to have alterations in the endoplasmic reticulum stress response [12] and heat shock protein expression [7], as well as mitochondrial dysfunction [42], pro-apoptotic signaling, and increased cytosolic levels of calcium and calcium-binding proteins [13]. Aggregates of SOD1 protein have also been detected in gastrocnemius, soleus, and flexor digitorum longus of the transgenic animal [6]. Further, as in IBM, increased gene expression of autophagy components LC3 and SQSTM1 is reported in mSOD1 muscle [14]. Most critically, studies of transgenic ALS mice have revealed that muscle-restricted and muscle-initiated pathologies may induce motor neuron degeneration. Specifically, expression of G37R and G93A human SOD1 in skeletal muscle (hSOD1^{mus}), but not nervous tissue, can lead to neurologic and pathologic ALS [57] with ubiquitinated aggregates in wild type neurons. Models with a muscle-restricted distribution of *SOD1* G93A mutation also show progressive muscular atrophy, mitochondrial dysfunction, and reduced muscle strength [22] and the atrophic muscles of these mice up-regulate autophagy genes, including *LC3*.

Conclusions

In summary, this study implicates axial skeletal muscle (diaphragm and paraspinous muscles) as an additional site of pTDP-43 pathology in ALS. Up-regulation of *TARDBP* and *SQSTM1* expression by real-time PCR supports this as a possible cell autonomous pathology in ALS, though future studies using unbiased techniques with a wide range of transcripts for normalization are needed (e.g., RNA-Seq). Additional studies utilizing tissue dedicated for electron microscopy study, with registration to histologic data, are required to clarify the ultrastructural features of the pTDP-43-positive material in ALS muscle. Nonetheless, our findings suggest that the impaired clearance of misfolded proteins in ALS, a well-recognized mechanism in motor neuron degeneration, may play an important role in pTDP-43 pathology in ALS muscle.

Additional file

Additional file 1: Figure S1. ALS muscle samples from three patients (top, middle, and bottom rows) with pTDP-43-immunoreactive inclusions. pTDP-43-stained sections (Proteintech clone 22309-1-AP) and H&E-stained sections from Houston Methodist (lab of MDC) are shown in the left three panels for each patient. The right-most panel of each patient shows repeat pTDP-43 staining at the University of Kentucky using the protocol of that laboratory and a different pTDP-43 antibody (1D3 clone, 1:500). All images are photographed at 400x without magnification except for five images photographed at 200x (top row, two right-most panels; middle row, H&E section; bottom row, two left-most panels). **Figure S2.** Four muscle samples from a recent autopsy of an ALS patient not included in this study. The patient had a clinical diagnosis of C9ALS and a positive family history of ALS (fALS). Examination of brain and spinal cord confirmed ALS and showed characteristic p62-immunoreactive and TDP-43-negative lesions in brain, consistent with C9ALS. Examination of seven muscle samples using p62 and pTDP-43 immunohistochemistry showed unequivocal pTDP-43-reactive lesions in muscle fibers of thoracic paraspinous and diaphragm muscle, an equivocal focus in sacral paraspinous muscle (not shown), but no pTDP-43-positive lesions in cervical paraspinous muscle (not shown). The inset of diaphragm shows the same focus on a deeper histologic section, also stained for pTDP-43, further revealing the thread- and dash-like inclusions in this sample. All images are photographed are 200x except for diaphragm, which is photographed at 400x. **Figure S3.** 1% Thioflavin S staining was performed in Alzheimer's disease (AD) control tissue from occipital cortex and hippocampus/ subiculum (top left panel, 200x, and top middle panel, 400x), IBM muscle (top right, Non-ALS09, photographed at 600x), pTDP-43-positive ALS muscle samples with electron microscopy data shown in Fig 6 (ALS43, ALS34, ALS23), all photographed at 600x magnification, and a pTDP-43-negative ALS muscle with atrophy and abundant lipofuscin pigment (ALS50) (600x). Green arrows highlight thioflavin S-reactive material in all samples, whereas white arrows indicate autofluorescent material, such as lipofuscin pigment (top left, bottom left, and bottom right panels), which appears yellow-orange in images combining FITC/ DAPI/ and TRITC filters (see Methods for detail on immunofluorescence microscopy). For ALS sample ALS43, the inset at lower left (600x) shows the similar shape of inclusions in this area by pTDP-43 immunohistochemistry. (PDF 1807 kb)

Acknowledgements
We appreciate the efforts of Ms. Claire Haueter of the Houston Methodist Hospital elecrtron microscopy core laboratory, who assisted in the preparation and ultrastructural examination of specimens. We appreciate the efforts of the neuropathology core at the University of Kentucky Alzheimer's Disease Center that assisted in external pTDP-43 staining in a subset of IBM and ALS samples, as well as the constructive feedback of core director Dr. Peter T. Nelson. We are grateful to the ALS patients and their family members for the donations that made this work possible.

Funding
Data collection, analysis, and interpretation, as well as writing of the manuscript, was supported by a Clinician-Scientist Research Award from the Institute of Academic Medicine in the Houston Methodist Research Institute (HMRI) of the Houston Methodist Hospital (to author MDC).

Authors' contributions
MDC conceived of the study, performed pathological and statistical analyses, and drafted the initial and final versions of the manuscript, tables, and figures, including supplementary material. SZP and ALR reviewed salient pathologic characteristics with MDC, assisted MDC in performing the primary autopsy examination in the patients studied herein, and reviewed the manuscript. ASA assisted MDC in the laboratory, including critical staining experiments, and critically evaluated the manuscript. SHA and JWA provided clinical data and expert clinical input and SHA provided critical feedback that improved study design. All authors read and approved the final manuscript.

Competing interests
The authors declare that they have no competing interests.

Author details
[1]Department of Pathology and Genomic Medicine, Houston Methodist Hospital, 6565 Fannin Street, Houston, TX 77030, USA. [2]Institute of Academic Medicine (IAM) in the Houston Methodist Research Institute (HMRI), Houston Methodist Hospital, 6565 Fannin Street, Houston, TX 77030, USA. [3]Houston Methodist Neurological Institute, Houston Methodist Hospital, 6565 Fannin Street, Houston, TX 77030, USA. [4]Department of Neurology, Houston Methodist Hospital, 6565 Fannin Street, Houston, TX 77030, USA.

References

1. Al-Chalabi A, Jones A, Troakes C, King A, Al-Sarraj S, van den Berg LH (2012) The genetics and neuropathology of amyotrophic lateral sclerosis. Acta Neuropathol 124:339–352. https://doi.org/10.1007/s00401-012-1022-4
2. Al-Sarraj S, King A, Cleveland M, Pradat PF, Corse A, Rothstein JD, Leigh PN, Abila B, Bates S, Wurthner J et al (2014) Mitochondrial abnormalities and low grade inflammation are present in the skeletal muscle of a minority of patients with amyotrophic lateral sclerosis; an observational myopathology study. Acta Neuropathol Commun 2:165. https://doi.org/10.1186/s40478-014-0165-z
3. Amlie-Wolf A, Ryvkin P, Tong R, Dragomir I, Suh E, Xu Y, Van Deerlin VM, Gregory BD, Kwong LK, Trojanowski JQ et al (2015) Transcriptomic changes due to cytoplasmic TDP-43 expression reveal dysregulation of histone transcripts and nuclear chromatin. PLoS One 10:e0141836. https://doi.org/10.1371/journal.pone.0141836
4. Artuso L, Zoccolella S, Favia P, Amati A, Capozzo R, Logroscino G, Serlenga L, Simone I, Gasparre G, Petruzzella V (2013) Mitochondrial genome aberrations in skeletal muscle of patients with motor neuron disease. Amyotroph Lateral Scler Frontotemp Degener 14:261–266. https://doi.org/10.3109/21678421.2012.735239
5. Askanas V, Engel WK (2007) Inclusion-body myositis, a multifactorial muscle disease associated with aging: current concepts of pathogenesis. Curr Opin Rheumatol 19:550–559. https://doi.org/10.1097/BOR.0b013e3282efdc7c
6. Atkin JD, Scott RL, West JM, Lopes E, Quah AK, Cheema SS (2005) Properties of slow- and fast-twitch muscle fibres in a mouse model of amyotrophic lateral sclerosis. Neuromuscul Disord 15:377–388. https://doi.org/10.1016/j.nmd.2005.02.005
7. Bhattacharya A, Wei R, Hamilton RT, Chaudhuri AR (2014) Neuronal cells but not muscle cells are resistant to oxidative stress mediated protein misfolding and cell death: role of molecular chaperones. Biochem Biophys Res Commun 446:1250–1254. https://doi.org/10.1016/j.bbrc.2014.03.097
8. Braak H, Brettschneider J, Ludolph AC, Lee VM, Trojanowski JQ, Del Tredici K (2013) Amyotrophic lateral sclerosis–a model of corticofugal axonal spread. Nat Rev Neurol 9:708–714. https://doi.org/10.1038/nrneurol.2013.221
9. Brady S, Squier W, Sewry C, Hanna M, Hilton-Jones D, Holton JL (2014) A retrospective cohort study identifying the principal pathological features useful in the diagnosis of inclusion body myositis. BMJ Open 4:e004552. https://doi.org/10.1136/bmjopen-2013-004552
10. Brettschneider J, Arai K, Del Tredici K, Toledo JB, Robinson JL, Lee EB, Kuwabara S, Shibuya K, Irwin DJ, Fang L et al (2014) TDP-43 pathology and neuronal loss in amyotrophic lateral sclerosis spinal cord. Acta Neuropathol 128:423–437. https://doi.org/10.1007/s00401-014-1299-6

11. Castillo K, Nassif M, Valenzuela V, Rojas F, Matus S, Mercado G, Court FA, van Zundert B, Hetz C (2013) Trehalose delays the progression of amyotrophic lateral sclerosis by enhancing autophagy in motoneurons. Autophagy 9: 1308–1320. https://doi.org/10.4161/auto.25188
12. Chen D, Wang Y, Chin ER (2015) Activation of the endoplasmic reticulum stress response in skeletal muscle of G93A*SOD1 amyotrophic lateral sclerosis mice. Front Cell Neurosci 9:170. https://doi.org/10.3389/fncel.2015.00170
13. Chin ER, Chen D, Bobyk KD, Mazala DA (2014) Perturbations in intracellular Ca2+ handling in skeletal muscle in the G93A*SOD1 mouse model of amyotrophic lateral sclerosis. Am J Physiol Cell Physiol 307:C1031–C1038. https://doi.org/10.1152/ajpcell.00237.2013
14. Crippa V, Boncoraglio A, Galbiati M, Aggarwal T, Rusmini P, Giorgetti E, Cristofani R, Carra S, Pennuto M, Poletti A (2013) Differential autophagy power in the spinal cord and muscle of transgenic ALS mice. Front Cell Neurosci 7:234. https://doi.org/10.3389/fncel.2013.00234
15. Crugnola V, Lamperti C, Lucchini V, Ronchi D, Peverelli L, Prelle A, Sciacco M, Bordoni A, Fassone E, Fortunato Fet al (2010) Mitochondrial respiratory chain dysfunction in muscle from patients with amyotrophic lateral sclerosis. Arch Neurol 67: 849–854 Doi https://doi.org/10.1001/archneurol.2010.128
16. Cruveilhier J (1853) Sur la paralysie musculaire progressive atrophique. Arch Gen Med I, 561
17. Cykowski MD, Powell SZ, Peterson LE, Appel JW, Rivera AL, Takei H, Chang E, Appel SH (2017) Clinical significance of TDP-43 neuropathology in amyotrophic lateral sclerosis. J Neuropathol Exp Neurol 76:402–413. https://doi.org/10.1093/jnen/nlx025
18. Cykowski MD, Takei H, Schulz PE, Appel SH, Powell SZ (2014) TDP-43 pathology in the basal forebrain and hypothalamus of patients with amyotrophic lateral sclerosis. Acta Neuropathol Commun 2:171. https://doi.org/10.1186/s40478 014 0171-1
19. de Carvalho M, Pinto S, Swash M (2010) Association of paraspinal and diaphragm denervation in ALS. Amyotroph Lateral Scler 11:63–66. https://doi.org/10.3109/17482960902730080
20. Dialynas G, Shrestha OK, Ponce JM, Zwerger M, Thiemann DA, Young GH, Moore SA, Yu L, Lammerding J, Wallrath LL (2015) Myopathic Lamin mutations cause reductive stress and activate the nrf2/keap-1 pathway. PLoS Genet 11:e1005231. https://doi.org/10.1371/journal.pgen.1005231
21. Dobrowolny G, Aucello M, Musaro A (2011) Muscle atrophy induced by SOD1G93A expression does not involve the activation of caspase in the absence of denervation. Skelet Muscle 1:3. https://doi.org/10.1186/2044-5040-1-3
22. Dobrowolny G, Aucello M, Rizzuto E, Beccafico S, Mammucari C, Boncompagni S, Belia S, Wannenes F, Nicoletti C, Del Prete Z et al (2008) Skeletal muscle is a primary target of SOD1G93A-mediated toxicity. Cell Metab 8:425–436. https://doi.org/10.1016/j.cmet.2008.09.002
23. Dupuis L, Gonzalez de Aguilar JL, Echaniz-Laguna A, Eschbach J, Rene F, Oudart H, Halter B, Huze C, Schaeffer L, Bouillaud F et al (2009) Muscle mitochondrial uncoupling dismantles neuromuscular junction and triggers distal degeneration of motor neurons. PLoS One 4:e5390. https://doi.org/10.1371/journal.pone.0005390
24. Fecto F, Yan J, Vemula SP, Liu E, Yang Y, Chen W, Zheng JG, Shi Y, Siddique N, Arrat H et al (2011) SQSTM1 mutations in familial and sporadic amyotrophic lateral sclerosis. Arch Neurol 68:1440–1446. https://doi.org/10.1001/archneurol.2011.250
25. Girolamo F, Lia A, Amati A, Strippoli M, Coppola C, Virgintino D, Roncali L, Toscano A, Serlenga L, Trojano M (2013) Overexpression of autophagic proteins in the skeletal muscle of sporadic inclusion body myositis. Neuropathol Appl Neurobiol 39:736–749. https://doi.org/10.1111/nan.12040
26. Graber DJ, Hickey WF, Harris BT (2010) Progressive changes in microglia and macrophages in spinal cord and peripheral nerve in the transgenic rat model of amyotrophic lateral sclerosis. J Neuroinflammation 7:8. https://doi.org/10.1186/1742-2094-7-8
27. Hiniker A, Daniels BH, Lee HS, Margeta M (2013) Comparative utility of LC3, p62 and TDP-43 immunohistochemistry in differentiation of inclusion body myositis from polymyositis and related inflammatory myopathies. Acta Neuropathol Commun 1:29. https://doi.org/10.1186/2051-5960-1-29
28. Iwasaki Y, Sugimoto H, Ikeda K, Takamiya K, Shiojima T, Kinoshita M (1991) Muscle morphometry in amyotrophic lateral sclerosis. Int J Neurosci 58:165–170
29. Kuncl RW, Cornblath DR, Griffin JW (1988) Assessment of thoracic paraspinal muscles in the diagnosis of ALS. Muscle Nerve 11:484–492. https://doi.org/10.1002/mus.880110512
30. Kyuno K, Ito H, Saito T, Kowa H, Tachibana S (1996) Needle electromyography in the thoracic paraspinal muscles of motor neuron disease. No To Shinkei 48:637–642
31. Lloyd TE (2010) Novel therapeutic approaches for inclusion body myositis. Curr Opin Rheumatol 22:658–664. https://doi.org/10.1097/BOR.0b013e32833f0f4a
32. Loeffler JP, Picchiarelli G, Dupuis L, Gonzalez De Aguilar JL (2016) The role of skeletal muscle in amyotrophic lateral sclerosis. Brain Pathol 26:227–236. https://doi.org/10.1111/bpa.12350
33. Ludolph AC, Knirsch U (1999) Problems and pitfalls in the diagnosis of ALS. J Neurol Sci 165(Suppl 1):S14–S20
34. Mackenzie IR, Ansorge O, Strong M, Bilbao J, Zinman L, Ang LC, Baker M, Stewart H, Eisen A, Rademakers R et al (2011) Pathological heterogeneity in amyotrophic lateral sclerosis with FUS mutations: two distinct patterns correlating with disease severity and mutation. Acta Neuropathol 122:87–98. https://doi.org/10.1007/s00401-011-0838-7
35. Mackenzie IR, Bigio EH, Ince PG, Geser F, Neumann M, Cairns NJ, Kwong LK, Forman MS, Ravits J, Stewart H et al (2007) Pathological TDP-43 distinguishes sporadic amyotrophic lateral sclerosis from amyotrophic lateral sclerosis with SOD1 mutations. Ann Neurol 61:427–434. https://doi.org/10.1002/ana.21147
36. Maruyama H, Morino H, Ito H, Izumi Y, Kato H, Watanabe Y, Kinoshita Y, Kamada M, Nodera H, Suzuki H et al (2010) Mutations of optineurin in amyotrophic lateral sclerosis. Nature 465:223–226. https://doi.org/10.1038/nature08971
37. MathWorks (2015) Matlab R2015b. City
38. McCluskey LF, Elman LB, Martinez-Lage M, Van Deerlin V, Yuan W, Clay D, Siderowf A, Trojanowski JQ (2009) Amyotrophic lateral sclerosis-plus syndrome with TAR DNA-binding protein-43 pathology. Arch Neurol 66: 121–124. https://doi.org/10.1001/archneur.66.1.121
39. Mehta P, Antao V, Kaye W, Sanchez M, Williamson D, Bryan L, Muravov O, Horton K (2014) Prevalance of amyotrophic lateral sclerosis - United States, 2010–2011. Morbidity and mortality weekly report (MMWR). Center for Disease Control and Prevention, City
40. Meyer K, Ferraiuolo L, Miranda CJ, Likhite S, McElroy S, Renusch S, Ditsworth D, Lagier-Tourenne C, Smith RA, Ravits J et al (2014) Direct conversion of patient fibroblasts demonstrates non-cell autonomous toxicity of astrocytes to motor neurons in familial and sporadic ALS. Proc Natl Acad Sci U S A 111:829–832. https://doi.org/10.1073/pnas.1314085111
41. Neumann M, Sampathu DM, Kwong LK, Truax AC, Micsenyi MC, Chou TT, Bruce J, Schuck T, Grossman M, Clark CM et al (2006) Ubiquitinated TDP-43 in frontotemporal lobar degeneration and amyotrophic lateral sclerosis. Science (New York, NY) 314:130–133
42. Palamiuc L, Schlagowski A, Ngo ST, Vernay A, Dirrig-Grosch S, Henriques A, Boutillier AL, Zoll J, Echaniz-Laguna A, Loeffler JP et al (2015) A metabolic switch toward lipid use in glycolytic muscle is an early pathologic event in a mouse model of amyotrophic lateral sclerosis. EMBO Mol Med 7:526–546. https://doi.org/10.15252/emmm.201404433
43. Ravits J, Appel S, Baloh RH, Barohn R, Brooks BR, Elman L, Floeter MK, Henderson C, Lomen-Hoerth C, Macklis JD et al (2013) Deciphering amyotrophic lateral sclerosis: what phenotype, neuropathology and genetics are telling us about pathogenesis. Amyotroph Lateral Scler Frontotemp Degener 14(Suppl 1):5–18. https://doi.org/10.3109/21678421.2013.778548
44. Ringholz GM, Appel SH, Bradshaw M, Cooke NA, Mosnik DM, Schulz PE (2005) Prevalence and patterns of cognitive impairment in sporadic ALS. Neurology 65:586–590. https://doi.org/10.1212/01.wnl.0000172911.39167.b6
45. Rudnick ND, Griffey CJ, Guarnieri P, Gerbino V, Wang X, Piersaint JA, Tapia JC, Rich MM, Maniatis T (2017) Distinct roles for motor neuron autophagy early and late in the SOD1G93A mouse model of ALS. Proc Natl Acad Sci U S A 114:E8294–E8303. https://doi.org/10.1073/pnas.1704294114
46. Sanmaneechai O, Swenson A, Gerke AK, Moore SA, Shy ME (2015) Inclusion body myositis and sarcoid myopathy: coincidental occurrence or associated diseases. Neuromuscul Disord 25:297–300. https://doi.org/10.1016/j.nmd.2014.12.005
47. Sasaki S (2011) Autophagy in spinal cord motor neurons in sporadic amyotrophic lateral sclerosis. J Neuropathol Exp Neurol 70:349–359. https://doi.org/10.1097/NEN.0b013e3182160690
48. Schiffman PL, Belsh JM (1993) Pulmonary function at diagnosis of amyotrophic lateral sclerosis. Rate Deteriorat Chest 103:508–513
49. Schmolck H, Mosnik D, Schulz P (2007) Rating the approachability of faces in ALS. Neurology 69:2232–2235. https://doi.org/10.1212/01.wnl.0000296001.16603.b3

50. Soraru G, Orsetti V, Buratti E, Baralle F, Cima V, Volpe M, D'Ascenzo C, Palmieri A, Koutsikos K, Pegoraro E et al (2010) TDP-43 in skeletal muscle of patients affected with amyotrophic lateral sclerosis. Amyotroph Lateral Scler 11:240–243. https://doi.org/10.3109/17482960902810890
51. Taylor JP, Brown RH Jr, Cleveland DW (2016) Decoding ALS: from genes to mechanism. Nature 539:197–206. https://doi.org/10.1038/nature20413
52. Tews DS, Goebel HH, Meinck HM (1997) DNA-fragmentation and apoptosis-related proteins of muscle cells in motor neuron disorders. Acta Neurol Scand 96:380–386
53. Turk M, Haaker G, Winter L, Just W, Nickel FT, Linker RA, Chevessier F, Schroder R (2014) C9ORF72-ALS: P62- and ubiquitin-aggregation pathology in skeletal muscle. Muscle Nerve 50:454–455. https://doi.org/10.1002/mus.24283
54. Vatsavayai SC, Yoon SJ, Gardner RC, Gendron TF, Vargas JN, Trujillo A, Pribadi M, Phillips JJ, Gaus SE, Hixson JD et al (2016) Timing and significance of pathological features in C9orf72 expansion-associated frontotemporal dementia. Brain. https://doi.org/10.1093/brain/aww250
55. Veltema AN (1975) The case of the saltimbanque prosper Lecomte. A contribution to the study of the history of progressive muscular atrophy (Aran-Duchenne) and amyotrophic lateral sclerosis (Charcot). Clin Neurol Neurosurg 78:204–209
56. Vielhaber S, Winkler K, Kirches E, Kunz D, Buchner M, Feistner H, Elger CE, Ludolph AC, Riepe MW, Kunz WS (1999) Visualization of defective mitochondrial function in skeletal muscle fibers of patients with sporadic amyotrophic lateral sclerosis. J Neurol Sci 169:133–139
57. Wong M, Martin LJ (2010) Skeletal muscle-restricted expression of human SOD1 causes motor neuron degeneration in transgenic mice. Hum Mol Genet 19:2284–2302. https://doi.org/10.1093/hmg/ddq106
58. Zhao W, Beers DR, Appel SH (2013) Immune-mediated mechanisms in the pathoprogression of amyotrophic lateral sclerosis. J NeuroImmune Pharmacol 8:888–899. https://doi.org/10.1007/s11481-013-9489-x

14

Preventing mutant huntingtin proteolysis and intermittent fasting promote autophagy in models of Huntington disease

Dagmar E. Ehrnhoefer[1,2*], Dale D. O. Martin[1], Mandi E. Schmidt[1], Xiaofan Qiu[1], Safia Ladha[1], Nicholas S. Caron[1], Niels H. Skotte[1], Yen T. N. Nguyen[1], Kuljeet Vaid[1], Amber L. Southwell[1], Sabine Engemann[1], Sonia Franciosi[1] and Michael R. Hayden[1*]

Abstract

Huntington disease (HD) is caused by the expression of mutant huntingtin (mHTT) bearing a polyglutamine expansion. In HD, mHTT accumulation is accompanied by a dysfunction in basal autophagy, which manifests as specific defects in cargo loading during selective autophagy. Here we show that the expression of mHTT resistant to proteolysis at the caspase cleavage site D586 (C6R mHTT) increases autophagy, which may be due to its increased binding to the autophagy adapter p62. This is accompanied by faster degradation of C6R mHTT in vitro and a lack of mHTT accumulation the C6R mouse model with age. These findings may explain the previously observed neuroprotective properties of C6R mHTT. As the C6R mutation cannot be easily translated into a therapeutic approach, we show that a scheduled feeding paradigm is sufficient to lower mHTT levels in YAC128 mice expressing cleavable mHTT. This is consistent with a previous model, where the presence of cleavable mHTT impairs basal autophagy, while fasting-induced autophagy remains functional. In HD, mHTT clearance and autophagy may become increasingly impaired as a function of age and disease stage, because of gradually increased activity of mHTT-processing enzymes. Our findings imply that mHTT clearance could be enhanced by a regulated dietary schedule that promotes autophagy.

Keywords: Huntington disease, Autophagy, Proteolysis, Caspase, Mutant huntingtin lowering

Introduction

Huntington disease (HD) is an autosomal dominant neurodegenerative disorder that is caused by an expansion of a polyglutamine tract in the huntingtin (HTT) protein [57]. Mutant HTT (mHTT) causes dysfunction in different cellular compartments and pathways [13] that are difficult to target individually. The removal of mHTT itself is therefore an attractive therapeutic strategy and is currently being pursued in both clinical and pre-clinical studies [61]. While most of these studies aim to lower HTT RNA, changes in mHTT protein levels through increased degradation have also been shown to ameliorate HD symptoms [31, 59]. Both soluble and aggregated forms of mHTT are thought to be cleared preferentially through autophagy [47, 49], and both mTOR-dependent and -independent autophagic pathways have been implicated in its degradation [31, 48]. Interestingly, a role for HTT in the regulation of autophagy has recently been discovered [2, 34, 35, 43, 50]. Both the HTT N- and C-termini play different but inter-dependent roles in autophagy [43], which may be promoted by the interaction of the two halves after proteolysis [18]. However, multiple proteolytic events may disrupt the interaction between the HTT N- and C-termini [18]. The cleavage of mHTT in HD increases with disease progression and age, and may prevent HTT from functioning as an autophagy-promoting factor [21, 35].

Here we use the C6R mouse model, which expresses full-length mHTT with a mutation preventing proteolysis at amino acid 586 by caspases 6 and 8 [23, 62], to investigate

* Correspondence: ehrnhoefer@bio.mx; mrh@cmmt.ubc.ca
[1]Centre for Molecular Medicine and Therapeutics (CMMT), CFRI, Department of Medical Genetics, University of British Columbia, 950 West 28th Avenue, Vancouver, BC V5Z 4H4, Canada
Full list of author information is available at the end of the article

the connection between mHTT cleavage and autophagy. We demonstrate a general increase in autophagy in cells and tissues from C6R mice compared to the YAC128 mouse model expressing fully cleavable full-length mHTT, and show that this is accompanied by reduced accumulation of mHTT protein.

HTT promotes autophagosome formation under basal, but not fasting conditions [50], suggesting that dietary interventions could circumvent mHTT-specific deficits in autophagy. In agreement with this hypothesis, we demonstrate that both fasting and scheduled feeding induce autophagy in the brains of HD mouse models, although only the longer scheduled feeding paradigm significantly reduces the levels of cleavable mHTT protein. These results provide a potential molecular mechanism for the beneficial effects of nutrient deprivation on neurodegenerative diseases [15, 31, 38, 54] and demonstrate that autophagy pathways that are not impacted by the HD pathology can be harnessed to lower mHTT protein levels in vivo.

Results

The expression of C6R mHTT promotes autophagy

HTT can act as a scaffold mediating cargo loading in basal autophagy [50], but as this function is dependent on the HTT C-terminus, it could be lost in HD due to proteolytic events [18, 35, 43]. To determine whether the expression of cleavable or C6R mHTT alters autophagy, we started by comparing mouse embryonic fibroblast (MEF) cultures derived from wt, YAC128 or C6R mice. The autophagy protein LC3-II decorates autophagosomes and is thus an indicator of autophagosome abundance, while the autophagy adapter protein p62 provides a link between LC3 and cargo proteins and is subsequently degraded together with the cargo [28]. Levels of these proteins are therefore commonly used to assess the autophagic state of cells [28].

We found that baseline levels of p62 and LC3-II were similar between MEFs of all three genotypes, while the non-lipidated LC3-I was not detectable (Fig. 1a, higher intensity blots shown in Additional file 1: Figure S1A). Using bafilomycin, an inhibitor of autophagic flux, both p62 and LC3-II levels increased, as expected, since their turnover was blocked (Fig. 1a). However, the levels of p62 after bafilomycin treatment were lower in YAC128 MEFs compared to wt, while C6R MEFs showed no such deficit (Fig. 1a). At the same time, no reduction in LC3-II turnover was observed in bafilomycin-treated YAC128 MEFs by Western blotting (Fig. 1a). To quantify the formation of autophagosomes in more detail, we next analyzed the formation of punctae immunopositive for p62 and LC3 by confocal microscopy. While no such punctae were observed under basal conditions (Additional file 1: Figure S1B), treatment with bafilomycin led to an increase in both p62- and LC3-positive structures (Fig. 1b). Quantitative image analysis revealed that both the density of p62- and LC3-punctae was increased in cultures derived from C6R mice, whereas MEFs expressing cleavable YAC128 mHTT showed a trend towards a decrease compared to wt cultures in these measures (Fig. 1b), and were significantly different from C6R cells. Interestingly, C6R MEFs show an increased number of LC3 punctae density but lower LC3 signal intensity within those punctae (Fig. 1b), indicating that the available LC3 is distributed over a larger number of autophagosomes. Accordingly, also the density of punctae with colocalization of p62 and LC3 was increased in C6R MEFs, confirming their identity as autophagosomes (Fig. 1b).

In addition to its role as a cargo-binding protein in basal and starvation-induced autophagy, p62 also associates with misfolded proteins upon proteasomal inhibition and proteotoxic stress [14, 32]. In this context, we found that treatment with the proteasomal inhibitor MG132 led to a dramatic increase in p62-positive structures, which was again exacerbated in MEFs expressing C6R but not cleavable mHTT (Fig. 1c). Proteasomal inhibition leads to an accumulation of ubiquitinated proteins, which are then bound by p62 [29]. This can lead to a feedback loop of transcriptional upregulation of p62 through Nrf2 [14]. Indeed, we observed a strong upregulation of p62 mRNA expression after MG132 treatment (Fig. 1d), which was dampened in MEFs derived from YAC128 mice. Taken together, our data therefore suggest that cells derived from C6R mice upregulate autophagic pathways more efficiently than YAC128 cells, both at baseline and under conditions of proteotoxic stress, a situation most relevant to neurodegenerative diseases such as HD.

Interestingly, none of these measures were altered in MEFs derived from YAC18 mice overexpressing wild-type human HTT [24], suggesting that the changes in autophagosome formation are related to the C6R mutation in the mHTT protein, and not merely overexpression of a non-pathogenic variant of HTT (Additional file 2: Figure S2A + B).

Reduced interaction between mHTT and p62 is normalized with the C6R mutation

To further investigate the role of mHTT in autophagy, we next assessed its interaction with p62, and found that the presence of the expanded polyglutamine tract significantly reduced the binding efficiency of HTT_{1-1212} to p62 in co-transfected cells (Fig. 2a). As p62-interaction domains have only been described for the HTT C-terminus [43, 50] which is absent in our expression construct, we next decided to map this novel binding site. Using a series of truncation mutants, we determined that HTT interacts with p62 between amino acids 800-1004 (Fig. 2b), which is an area known to harbour an ULK1 binding domain and may therefore be involved in binding the ULK1/p62 complex during autophagosome formation [50].

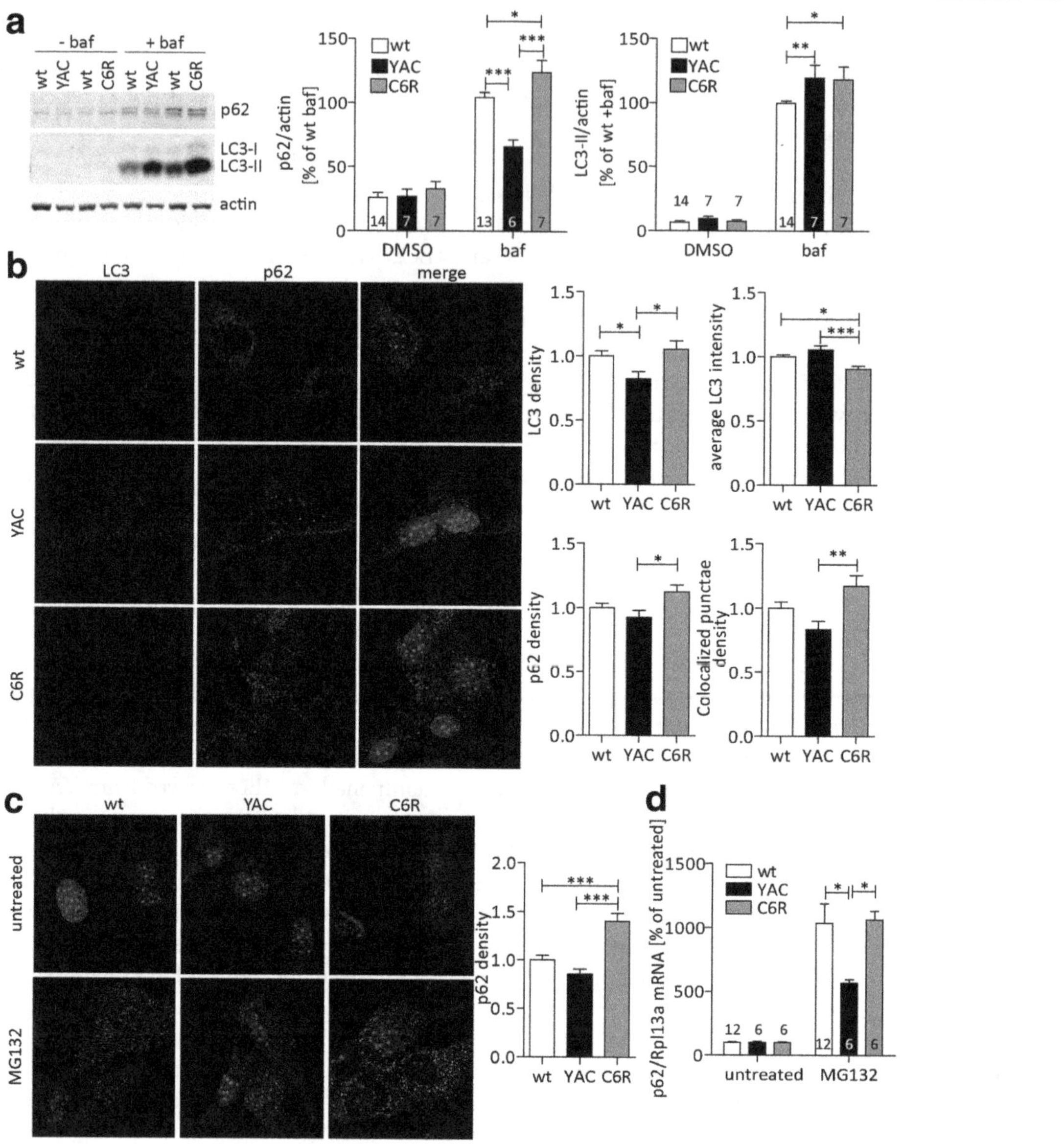

Fig. 1 The expression of C6R mHTT promotes autophagy. **a** Primary MEF cultures from YAC128, C6R or wt littermate embryos were treated with bafilomycin or DMSO as a control. Levels of p62 and LC3-II were analyzed by Western blot. p62: 2way-ANOVA genotype $p < 0.0001$, bafilomycin $p < 0.0001$, LC3-II: 2way-ANOVA genotype $p = 0.0239$, bafilomycin $p < 0.0001$. **b** Primary MEF cultures from YAC128, C6R or wt littermate embryos were seeded onto coverslips and treated with bafilomycin. Cells were fixed and stained for p62 and LC3, Hoechst dye was used for nuclear counterstaining. Samples were imaged on a confocal microscope and the density of punctae, staining intensity as well as the co-localization of LC3 and p62 staining were analyzed. p62 density: 1way-ANOVA $p = 0.0167$, LC3 density: 1way-ANOVA $p = 0.0116$, LC3 staining intensity: 1way-ANOVA $p = 0.0003$, colocalization: 1way-ANOVA $p = 0.0051$. **c** Primary MEF cultures from YAC128, C6R or wt littermate embryos were seeded onto coverslips and treated with MG132 or DMSO as a control. Cells were fixed and stained for p62, Hoechst dye was used for nuclear counterstaining. Samples were imaged on a confocal microscope and the density of punctae was analyzed. 1way-ANOVA $p < 0.0001$. **d** Primary MEF cultures from YAC128, C6R or wt littermate embryos were seeded onto coverslips and treated with MG132 or DMSO as a control. RNA levels of p62 were determined by quantitative RT-PCR (qPCR), normalized to the expression level of Rpl13a. 2way-ANOVA: genotype $p = 0.0461$, treatment $p < 0.0001$. Representative blots/images and pooled quantification data with S.E.M. are shown, 3-5 independent cultures were analyzed. Number of replicates is shown as insets for Western blot and qPCR experiments, for imaging experiments 24-30 cells per condition were analyzed. Statistical significance was determined 2way-ANOVA with post-hoc Bonferroni correction. *: $p < 0.05$, **: $p < 0.01$, ***: $p < 0.001$

Furthermore, we found that C6R $mHTT_{1-1212}$ interacts approximately twice as strongly with p62 compared to cleavable mHTT (Fig. 2c), which was confirmed with co-immunoprecipitation of HTT with p62 (Additional file 3: Figure S3A). Consistent with our findings for wt HTT (Fig. 2b), the interaction between p62 and a $mHTT_{1-586}$ fragment was also barely detectable, confirming that also for mHTT the p62 interaction domain is located C-

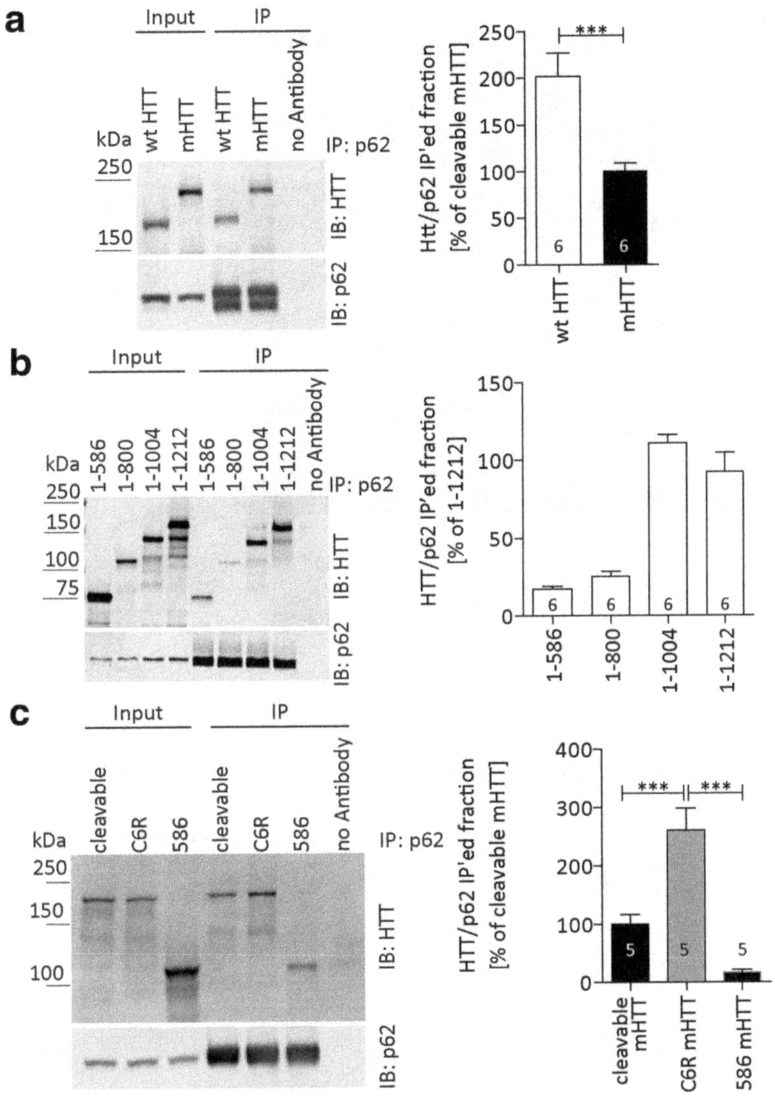

Fig. 2 The C6R mutation improves the binding of mHTT to the autophagy adapter p62. **a** COS-7 cells were cotransfected with wt or mHTT aa1-1212 and p62 as indicated and treated with bafilomycin to block autophagic flux. After immunoprecipitation of p62, the ratio of co-immunoprecipitated HTT was quantified (normalized to input to control for transfection efficiency). **b** COS-7 cells were cotransfected with wt HTT fragments of different lengths and p62 as indicated and treated with bafilomycin to block autophagic flux. After immunoprecipitation of p62, the ratio of co-immunoprecipitated HTT was quantified (normalized to input to control for transfection efficiency). **c** COS-7 cells were cotransfected with cleavable mHTT$_{1-1212}$, C6R mHTT$_{1-1212}$ or mHTT$_{1-586}$ and p62 as indicated and treated with bafilomycin to block autophagic flux. After immunoprecipitation of p62, the ratio of co-immunoprecipitated HTT was quantified (normalized to input to control for transfection efficiency). 1way-ANOVA $p < 0.0001$. Blots and quantification data with S.E.M. from a representative of 3 independent experiments are shown, number of technical replicates is shown as insets. Statistical significance was determined by Student's t-test (**a**) or 1way-ANOVA with Tukey's post-hoc correction (**c**). *: $p < 0.05$, **: $p < 0.01$, ***: $p < 0.001$

terminal of the D586 caspase cleavage site (Fig. 2c). However, as the interaction is not completely abolished for the mHTT-586aa fragment, HTT may have additional p62 binding sites or multiple interaction domains that can be separated by proteolysis.

Immunofluorescence staining confirmed the preferential localization of C6R mHTT to p62-positive areas (Fig. 3a), which was much reduced for cleavable mHTT or the mHTT-586aa fragment. This colocalization may relate to the role of HTT in autophagosome formation [43, 50], but may also influence the autophagic clearance of HTT itself. We therefore performed cycloheximide-chase experiments in COS cells co-transfected with cleavable or C6R mHTT$_{1-1212}$ and p62. In the absence of p62 overexpression, cleavable mHTT is degraded more slowly than C6R mHTT (Fig. 3b) within the first 4 h of chase time. However, when p62 is overexpressed, the degradation of cleavable mHTT is accelerated and rendered indistinguishable

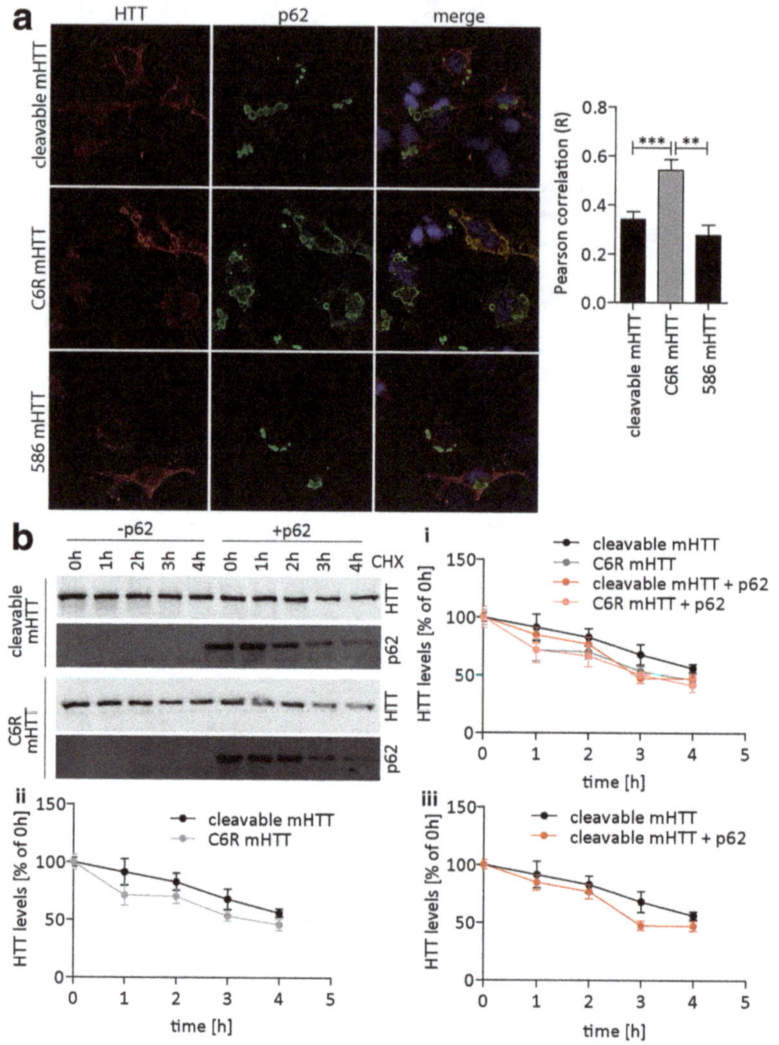

Fig. 3 C6R mHTT preferentially colocalizes with p62 and is degraded faster than cleavable mHTT. **a** COS-7 cells were seeded onto coverslips, cotransfected with cleavable $mHTT_{1-1212}$, C6R $mHTT_{1-1212}$ or $mHTT_{1-586}$ and p62 as indicated and treated with bafilomycin to block autophagic flux. Cells were fixed and stained for p62 and HTT, Hoechst dye was used for nuclear counterstaining. Samples were imaged on a confocal microscope and the colocalization of HTT and p62 signals was analyzed. 1way-ANOVA $p < 0.0001$. **b** COS-7 cells were cotransfected with cleavable $mHTT_{1-1212}$, C6R $mHTT_{1-1212}$ and p62 as indicated and treated with MG132 to enforce autophagic degradation. Cycloheximide was added for the indicated periods of time and samples were analyzed by Western blot. Data are graphed in three different versions to better visualize differences between groups: (i) all four conditions, (ii) cleavable mHTT vs. C6R mHTT, 2way-ANOVA mHTT construct $p = 0.0146$, time $p < 0.0001$, (iii) cleavable mHTT without/with p62, 2way-ANOVA p62 $p = 0.0436$, time $p < 0.0001$. Representative blots/images and pooled quantification data with S.E.M. are shown, for imaging experiments 14-21 cells per condition were analyzed, for Western blotting 3 independent experiments were performed with 3 technical replicates each. Statistical significance was determined by 1way-ANOVA with Tukey's post-hoc correction for A and 2way-ANOVA with Bonferroni's post-hoc correction for B. *: $p < 0.05$, **: $p < 0.01$, ***: $p < 0.001$

from C6R mHTT (Fig. 3b), suggesting that a sufficiently large supply of p62 can overcome degradation deficits of cleavable mHTT. Overexpressed p62 was almost completely degraded within the 4 h timeframe of the experiment (Fig. 3b, quantified in Additional file 3: Figure S3B). We furthermore confirmed that the decrease in full-length HTT and p62 levels are not due to proteolysis, since no accumulation of degradation products was observed on the full Western blots (shown in Additional file 4: Figure S4C).

p62 interacts with ubiquitinated substrates, and preferentially those that are linked to ubiquitin through lysine 63 (K63), promoting their autophagic degradation [4, 53]. HTT can be ubiquitinated by K63 or K48 linkages, and both types of ubiquitinated mHTT accumulate in cell and mouse models of HD, which has been attributed to impaired clearance by both autophagy and the proteasome [6, 7]. Co-transfection of cleavable or C6R $mHTT_{1-122}$ with either wt ubiquitin, or ubiquitin mutants that can only bind their target proteins through lysine 48 (K48 ubiquitin) or lysine 63 (K63 ubiquitin), revealed that C6R mHTT co-immunoprecipitated with significantly more ubiquitin in general (wt ubiquitin, Additional file 3: Figure S3C). Interestingly, the interaction with K48 ubiquitin was equal between cleavable and C6R mHTT, but K63 ubiquitin preferentially co-immunoprecipitated with C6R mHTT, indicating that the K63 linkage is preferred in the presence of the C6R mutation (Additional file 3: Figure S3C). Increased K63-ubiquitination of C6R mHTT would thus be expected to mediate increased p62 binding and may therefore account for its preferential autophagic clearance.

Fasting-induced autophagy is functional in the presence of mHTT

As a next step, we decided to investigate autophagy pathways in vivo. Since the liver heavily relies on autophagy to maintain its basal function [33], and HD-specific dysfunction in autophagic and metabolic pathways has been found in livers from HD mouse models and human patients [9, 36, 58, 59], we decided to focus on both brain and liver tissues from YAC128 and C6R mice.

We first compared baseline levels of autophagy with a food deprivation paradigm, which is expected to activate autophagy [12]. A fasting period of 24 h was sufficient to observe significant changes in hepatic levels of key autophagy proteins in wt, YAC128 and C6R mice: fasting decreased p62 levels, in agreement with its increased autophagic turnover following food deprivation (Fig. 4a) [28]. Furthermore, LC3-II levels were increased by fasting (Fig. 4b), indicating enhanced autophagosome formation. Interestingly, LC3-I levels were strikingly elevated in C6R mice under fed conditions (Fig. 4b). Fasting eliminated this increase (Fig. 4b), suggesting that fasting leads to a rapid conversion of available LC3-I pools into LC3-II. This was further analyzed by qRT-PCR, which showed similar expression levels of LC3 for mice of all three genotypes at baseline (Additional file 5: Figure S5A), demonstrating that the differences observed by Western blotting are post-transcriptional.

To determine whether alterations in autophagy had an impact on the degradation of mHTT, we next assessed HTT protein levels in the liver of YAC128 and C6R mice. We found a strong age-dependent increase in wt and mHTT protein that reached statistical significance at 12 months in YAC128 animals (Fig. 4c). On the other hand, C6R mice showed no age-dependent alterations in wt or mHTT levels, suggesting that this change is specific to the expression of cleavable mHTT (Fig. 4c). To confirm that the changes are post-transcriptional, we performed qRT-PCR analyses on liver tissues from 12 month old mice. Interestingly, mHTT mRNA levels are higher in C6R compared to YAC128 liver tissues (Additional file 5: Figure S5B), confirming that the lack of mHTT accumulation observed by Western blot are not due to decreased expression, but rather due to post-transcriptional effects such as increased protein degradation.

Fasting-induced autophagy in the liver was paralleled by a significant reduction of mHTT protein in YAC128 mice (Fig. 4d), while the levels of wt HTT remained unchanged (Additional file 5: Figure S5C). mRNA levels of the mHTT transgene were also not affected by fasting, confirming that this intervention likely reduced mHTT protein through autophagic degradation (Additional file 5: Figure S5D). Fasting also had an impact on hepatic mHTT protein levels in C6R mice, although the reduction was more subtle in this genotype (Additional file 5: Figure S5E). This is not surprising, given the already low levels of mHTT protein in C6R compared to YAC128 mice. Nevertheless, the trend towards a further decrease suggests that fasting-induced autophagy can still lower mHTT even in C6R mice.

Taken together, these findings demonstrate that basal autophagy is altered in the liver of C6R mice and may be responsible for the lack of age-dependent mHTT accumulation in this mouse model. Fasting-induced autophagy mechanisms on the other hand are intact and can be activated in the liver of both YAC128 and C6R mice. Furthermore, our data suggest that the age-dependent accumulation of mHTT can be reversed by activating such protein degradation pathways simply through dietary changes.

Prolonged regulation of food intake induces mHTT clearance in the brain

Recent studies have demonstrated that acute fasting also induces autophagy in the CNS [1, 10]. We therefore examined LC3 and p62 levels in cortical tissues from fasted as well as mice fed ad libitum, and found that a 24 h fasting period increased LC3-I, LC3-II and p62 protein levels in the cortex of both wt and YAC128 animals (Additional file 6: Figure S6A). While both the increased cortical p62 and LC3-I levels differ from our findings in the liver (Fig. 4a and b), this may suggest different timing of autophagy induction in the two organs. These differences not only manifest on the protein level, but are also observed transcriptionally: While YAC128 mice show a trend towards reduced p62 expression in both the liver and the cortex at baseline (Additional file 6: Figure S6B + C), fasting induces a reduction in p62 mRNA in the liver but not the cortex of wt animals (Additional file 6: Figure S6B + C). Furthermore, unlike hepatic mHTT (Fig. 4d), cortical mHTT levels remained unaffected by a 24 h fasting period (Additional file 6: Figure S6D). We therefore hypothesized that the lack of mHTT degradation after acute fasting may be due to the delayed induction of autophagy in the brain compared to the liver, and designed a fasting schedule that could be maintained for a longer period of time.

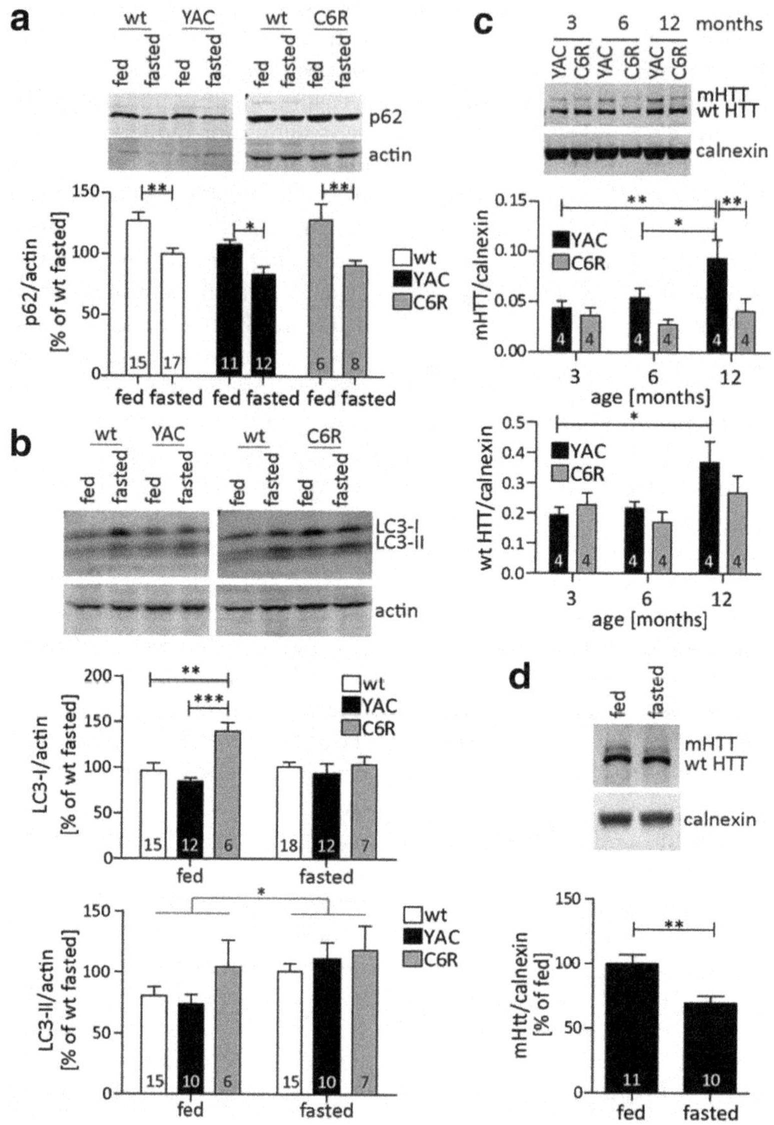

Fig. 4 mHTT levels increase in aging YAC128 liver and can be reduced by fasting-induced autophagy. **a**, **b** + **d** 12 month old YAC128 and C6R mice, as well as their wt littermates, were subjected to a 24 h fasting period, sacrificed immediately and liver samples were compared to littermates with ad libitum access to food. p62 (**a**) and LC3 (**b**) protein levels were analyzed by Western blot. p62: 2way-ANOVA genotype $p = 0.0103$, fasting $p < 0.0001$, LC3-I: 2way-ANOVA genotype $p = 0.0043$, fasting $p = 0.3161$, LC3-II: 2way-ANOVA genotype $p = 0.2012$, fasting $p = 0.0151$. **c** Liver tissues from YAC128 and C6R mice at different ages were analyzed for HTT expression using the MAB2166 antibody. mHTT 2way-ANOVA genotype $p = 0.0047$, age $p = 0.0342$; wt HTT 2way-ANOVA genotype $p = 0.3168$, age $p = 0.0232$. **d** HTT protein levels in YAC128 liver were analysed by Western blot using the MAB2166 antibody. Representative blots and pooled quantification data with S.E.M. are shown, number of replicates is shown as insets. Statistical significance was determined by 2way-ANOVA with Bonferroni's post-hoc correction for **a** - **c**, or two-tailed Student's t-test for **d**. *: $p < 0.05$, **: $p < 0.01$, ***: $p < 0.001$

In our paradigm, mice were fasted for 18 h and allowed full access to food for 6 h periods. We hypothesized that this schedule would induce autophagy in vivo daily, without necessarily reducing caloric intake. Long-term caloric restriction has beneficial effects on aging and neurodegenerative phenotypes [11, 42], and previous studies have implicated both mTOR inhibition and SIRT1 activation in these phenomena [11, 20, 25, 26]. Consistent with these reports, we observed that our scheduled feeding diet decreased phosphorylated mTOR (Fig. 5a), an indication of mTOR inhibition similar to the effect of nutrient deprivation [64]. In addition, RNA levels of SIRT1 were increased in mice subjected to scheduled feeding (Fig. 5b), which can further contribute to the downregulation of mTOR signaling [20] and thus induce autophagy.

While the steady-state cortical p62 protein levels were not altered by scheduled feeding (Additional file 7: Figure S7A), we observed a significant induction of p62 expression at the RNA level (Fig. 5c). This is consistent with the

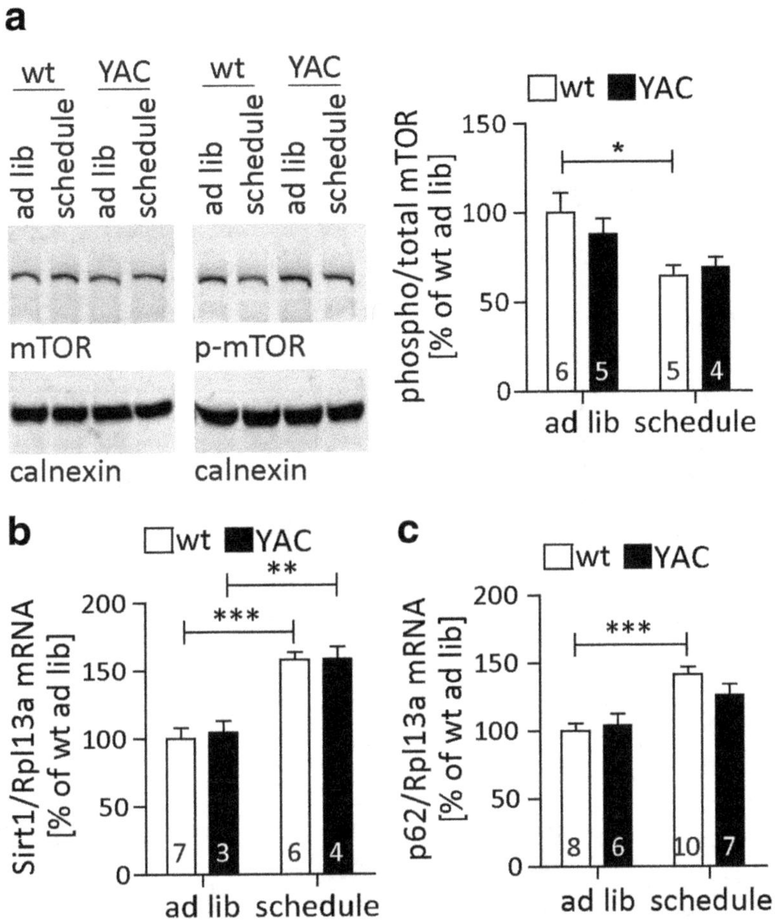

Fig. 5 Scheduled feeding alters nutrient-sensing pathways in the brain. **a - c** YAC128 mice and their wt littermates were subjected to 1 week of scheduled feeding and compared to littermates with ad libitum access to food. **a** Levels of total and phosphorylated mTOR were analyzed by Western blot. 2way-ANOVA genotype $p = 0.6796$, feeding $p = 0.0082$. **b + c** mRNA levels of SIRT1 (**b**) and p62 (**c**) were analyzed by qRT-PCR. SIRT1: 2way-ANOVA genotype $p = 0.7651$, feeding $p < 0.0001$, p62: 2way-ANOVA genotype $p = 0.4121$, feeding $p < 0.0001$. Representative blots and pooled quantification data with S.E.M. are shown. Statistical significance was determined by 2way-ANOVA with Bonferroni's post-hoc correction, number of replicates is shown as insets. *: $p < 0.05$, **: $p < 0.01$, ***: $p < 0.001$

previously demonstrated replenishing of p62 protein levels through increased expression during long-term fasting [5, 51]. Although LC3-I levels were not altered by scheduled feeding (Additional file 7: Figure S7B), C6R mice responded to the paradigm with significantly lower levels of LC3-II compared to wt or YAC128 animals (Fig. 6a). Furthermore, confocal microscopy demonstrated a strong reduction in LC3 punctae in C6R mice at baseline, with levels that are only reached after scheduled feeding in wt and YAC128 mice (Fig. 6b). Taken together, these data point towards higher autophagic flux in the CNS of C6R mice, but also suggest that it is possible to reach similar autophagy levels in YAC128 animals through scheduled feeding.

Next, EM analysis was performed to quantify the formation of autophagosomes and autophagolysosomes in the cortex of scheduled-fed mice. In this experiment we observed predominantly autolysosomes with electron-dense content with some remaining ultrastructure [28], which are the most abundant form of autophagic vesicles (AVs) in neurons [8]. We found that the overall number of AVs per cell significantly increased after scheduled feeding, confirming that autophagosomes are successfully transported to the neuronal soma and cargo degradation increased (Fig. 6c). Consistent with this data we found that the scheduled feeding paradigm also significantly reduced the levels of cortical mHTT protein in YAC128 mice (Fig. 6d), similar to the effect of short-term fasting on mHTT the liver (Fig. 4d). No changes were observed for wt HTT protein (Additional file 7: Figure S7C) or mHTT mRNA (Additional file 7: Figure S7D). Taken together our data therefore suggests that scheduled feeding increases mHTT clearance in the brain through the upregulation of autophagy, and that this mechanism is functional in a mouse model expressing cleavable mHTT.

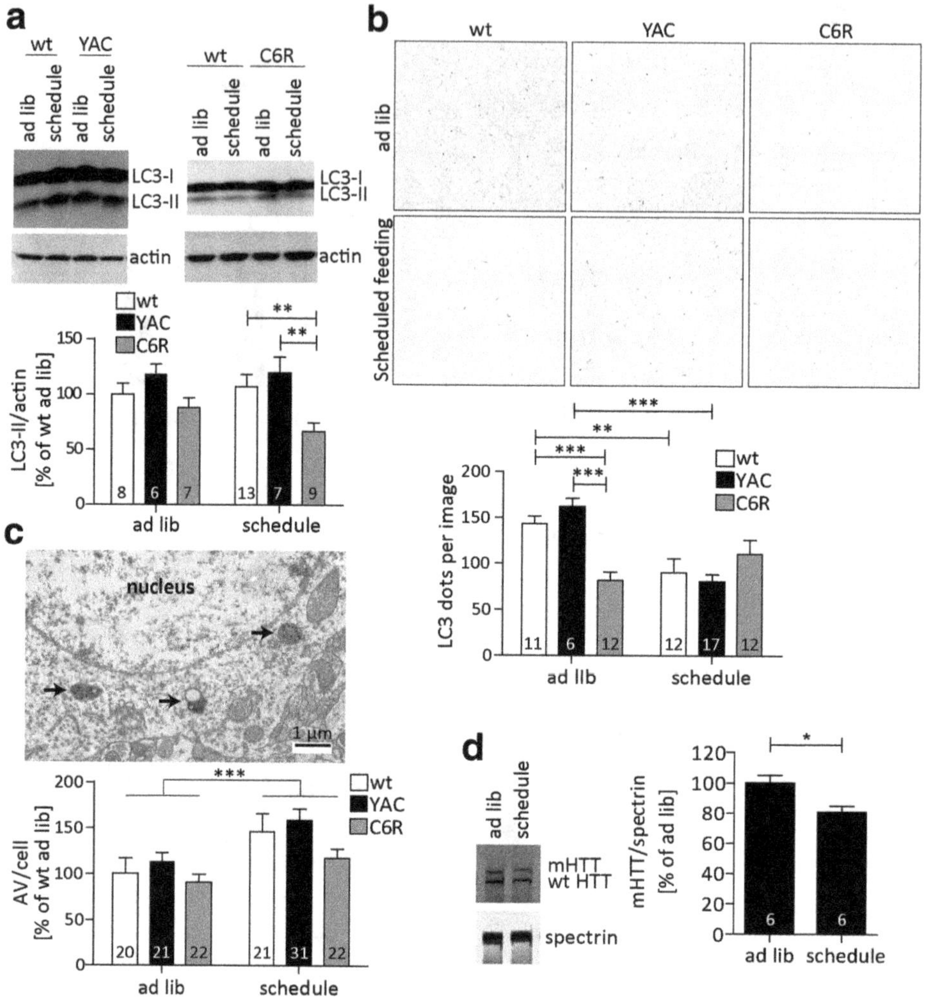

Fig. 6 Scheduled feeding induces autophagy and lowers mHTT protein in the brain. **a - d** YAC128 and C6R mice as well as their wt littermates were subjected to 1 week of scheduled feeding and cortical tissue was compared to littermates with ad libitum access to food. **a** LC3-II levels in cortical lysates were determined by Western blotting. 2way-ANOVA genotype $p = 0.0034$, feeding $p = 0.6776$. **b** Cortical brain sections were stained for LC3 and confocal images were analyzed. 2way-ANOVA genotype $p = 0.0815$, feeding $p = 0.0006$. **c** Brain sections of the motor cortex were analyzed by EM, and autophagic vesicles (AV) surrounding the nuclei were counted in a blinded fashion. 2way-ANOVA genotype $p = 0.0636$, feeding $p = 0.0006$. **d** mHTT protein levels in cortical tissues were analyzed by Western blotting using antibody MAB2166. Representative images/ blots and pooled quantification data with S.E.M. are shown, number of replicates is shown as insets. Statistical significance in **a** - **c** was determined by 2way-ANOVA with Bonferroni's post-hoc correction, in D by two-tailed Student's t-test. *: $p < 0.05$, **: $p < 0.01$, ***: $p < 0.001$

Discussion

The expansion of the CAG tract in HTT is the single cause for HD. Recent efforts in therapeutic development have therefore focused on different strategies to lower the levels of mHTT [61]. While a major focus of these efforts lies on the reduction of mHTT expression, there is strong evidence for dysfunction of mHTT clearance pathways in HD [30]. In particular, impaired autophagy has been linked to the well-documented accumulation of mHTT in the CNS [30, 39].

Here, we show that the expression of mHTT resistant to proteolytic cleavage at D586 (C6R mHTT) leads to increased basal and proteotoxicity-induced autophagy in primary MEFs. Together with the finding that autophagy is normal in MEFs derived from mice overexpressing wt HTT (YAC18), our data therefore suggest that the C6R mutation in particular causes the observed alterations in autophagy pathways. This may be due to an altered structure of C6R compared to cleavable mHTT, since we also find that C6R mHTT preferentially interacts with p62 compared to the full-length form of cleavable mHTT. As this interaction site localizes to an area also bound by ULK1 [50], the aa800-1004 region of HTT may form an ULK1/p62/HTT complex that can initiate autophagosome formation [34, 35, 50]. At the same time, the increased interaction may promote the autophagic degradation of C6R mHTT itself. This mechanism may explain why C6R mice fail to accumulate mHTT in the liver with age, despite sufficient expression levels and in contrast to YAC128 animals. C6R mice are thus better protected from the accumulation of toxic, aggregated forms of mHTT compared to YAC128 animals, which may shed light on the remarkable lack of HD phenotypes in the former mouse model [21, 23, 40, 45].

We only observe very subtle and specific deficits in autophagy in MEFs derived from YAC128 mice: Western blotting revealed a decrease in p62 turnover, with no deficit in LC3, while defects in autophagosome formation monitored by immunofluorescence were also less pronounced. However, the cargo recognition failure and specific defects in selective, but not bulk autophagy reported previously for HD model systems [36, 50] may be related to the decreased ability of mHTT to bind p62. This defect may not only prevent the degradation of mHTT, but through impaired formation of p62/ULK1/HTT complexes could impact selective autophagy in general. Recent studies have shown that the C-terminus of the HTT protein can act as a scaffold similar to Atg11, and promote autophagosome formation [43]. This function is regulated by an interaction between the HTT N- and C-termini [43], which is disrupted in the case of multiple proteolytic events within the HTT protein [18]. We therefore propose a model in which the negative effects of mHTT N-terminal fragments on autophagosome formation, transport and fusion are repaired in C6R mice since mHTT cleavage at D586 is prevented (Fig. 7). This furthermore boosts the normal function of the intact HTT C-terminus in promoting autophagosome formation and more efficient degradation of mHTT itself (Fig. 7). Supporting this hypothesis, increased autophagy and reduced mHTT levels have been demonstrated previously in HD mouse models crossed to a $C6^{-/-}$ line, an intervention that reduces (but does not completely abolish) mHTT cleavage at D586 [19, 62].

Although the C6R mutation is beneficial, it is not directly translatable to human HD patients. We therefore set out to test a therapeutic intervention that has the potential to alter autophagy pathways in vivo and to monitor its effects in the presence of cleavable mHTT. Caloric restriction can slow aging in a large variety of animal models [37] and upregulate key transcription factors such as *SIRT1* that are beneficial in different neurodegenerative conditions including HD [11, 25, 26]. However, such an intervention is not advisable for human patients, since HD already leads to a significant reduction in body weight [3] which may be exacerbated by further caloric reduction. We show here that scheduled feeding is sufficient to upregulate *SIRT1* expression and activate the mTOR pathway in a mouse model of HD. Importantly, intermittent fasting can still trigger starvation-induced autophagy and mHTT clearance in the YAC128 mouse model of HD, even though the overall calorie intake was not restricted. Furthermore, subtle deficits in autophagic pathways caused by the expression of cleavable mHTT did not prevent autophagy induction, suggesting that any such defects can be overcome by strong autophagy-inducing stimuli.

Circadian rhythms are disrupted in HD patients as well as in animal models of the disease, and this phenotype can be ameliorated by forcing a circadian pattern of food intake in mice, even at late stages of the disease [38]. Since

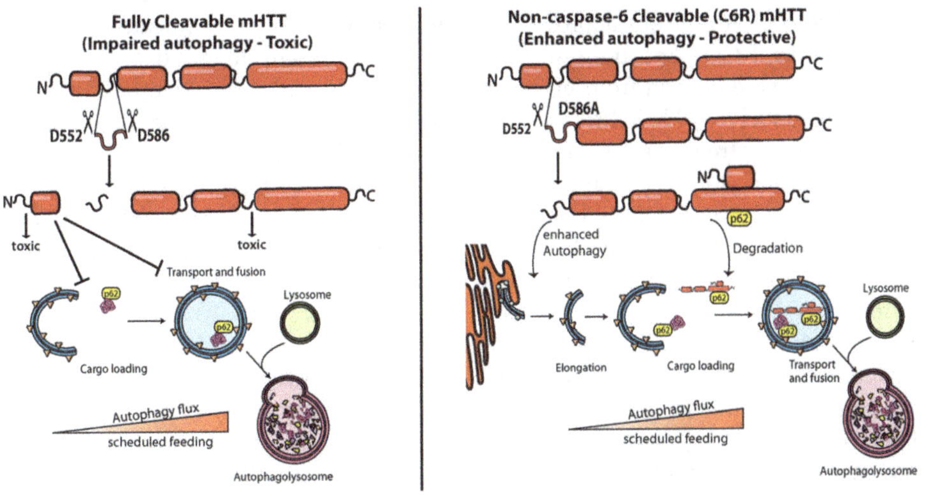

Fig. 7 Schematic representation of the effects of cleavable or C6R mHTT on autophagy. mHTT is subject to proteolysis by different proteases, with a number of cleavage sites clustering in the PEST2 domain [17]. Cleavage at D552 and D586 liberate a small fragment that is myristoylated at G553 [34] and induces autophagosome formation. However, both the N-terminal and C-terminal fragments resulting from mHTT double cleavage are toxic and interfere with autophagic cargo loading and autophagosome transport and fusion [18, 36, 43, 63]. In the C6R mice, cleavage at D586 is prevented, and we observed enhanced autophagy as well as improved degradation of C6R mHTT. In both YAC128 and C6R mice, autophagic flux and mHTT degradation can be enhanced in peripheral tissues by fasting and in the CNS by scheduled feeding

autophagy follows a circadian pattern in the brain [1], it is possible that the disruption of circadian rhythms in neurodegenerative disease may cause autophagic dysfunction and contribute to the accumulation of autophagy substrates such as mHTT. Furthermore, treating disruptions in circadian rhythm through lifestyle changes may ameliorate symptoms such as depression, anxiety and cognitive dysfunction in human HD patients [41], and our data suggest that such an intervention has the potential to lower mHTT protein levels through increased autophagy.

Conclusions

In this study, we provide evidence that not only prolonged fasting but also scheduled feeding without forcibly reducing calorie intake alters nutrient-sensing pathways and activates autophagy in mouse brain. This intervention furthermore reduces the amounts of mHTT protein, and may thus contribute to its clearance. As mHTT levels are closely correlated with pathology, these findings therefore correlate environmental influences with disease in a mouse model of HD.

In addition, we show that dysregulation of autophagy caused by the expression of mHTT is not observed when the protein is rendered resistant to cleavage at D586 (C6R mHTT). Age-dependent accumulation of mHTT is curtailed in C6R mice, and increased autophagy observed in cells derived from this mouse model may be responsible for the puzzling lack of HD phenotypes in these animals [21, 23, 40, 45].

Materials and methods

Animal models and statistics

All mouse experiments were carried out in accordance with protocols (Animal protocol A07-0106) approved by the UBC Committee on Animal Care and the Canadian Council on Animal Care. Mice are derived from in-house breeding pairs, maintained under a 12 h light:12 h dark cycle in a clean facility and given free access to food and water except otherwise indicated (for fasting and scheduled feeding protocols). YAC128 (line HD53 [56]) and C6R (line W13 [23]) mice are on a FVB/N background, mixed sexes were analyzed. Cortex and liver tissue was dissected and snap-frozen on dry ice for protein analyses.

Sample sizes were chosen based on extensive experience with biochemical differences between YAC128 mice and their WT littermates for experiments using mouse tissues [21–23, 44, 46, 58, 62]. Cell culture experiments were repeated independently at least three times to ensure reproducibility. Samples were only excluded if technical issues were apparent (i.e. bubble on a Western blot) or if determined statistical outliers using Grubb's outlier test (α = 0.05, no more than one sample per group was excluded).

For randomization, mice were assigned numbers not related to genotype. Scientists performing experiments were blinded for genotypes, unless it was necessary to ensure the appropriate order of samples on a gel. Data analyses was performed by a separate person in possession of the genotype information. For image analysis of electron microscopy and confocal microscopy data, unblinding was performed after all quantitation was complete.

Statistical significance was assessed using Student's t-test for comparison of two groups, one-way ANOVA with post-hoc Tukey's correction for the comparison of one variable between more than two groups, and two-way ANOVA with post-hoc Bonferroni correction for the comparison of two variables between groups. Variances between groups were similar. All analyses were performed using the GraphPad Prism 5.01 software package.

Generation of primary cell cultures

Primary MEF and neuronal cultures from YAC128 (line 53, [56]), YAC18 (line 212 [24]) and C6R (line W13, [23]) embryos, as well as their wt littermates were set up as described previously [16, 55]. In brief, embryos were collected on day 15.5–16.5 of gestation for neuronal cultures and at day 12.5 for MEF cultures. Tissues were extracted and transferred to Hibernate E (Invitrogen) for up to 24 h, during which time samples from the remaining embryonic tissues were genotyped [55]. For MEFs, the body without head, limbs, liver, lung and heart was minced, digested with 0.25% trypsin-EDTA and taken up in MEF medium (Dulbeccos's modified Eagle medium with high glucose, 10% fetal calf serum, 2 mM L-Glutamine, 100 μM non-essential amino acids, 1 mM sodium pyruvate, 1 μ M β-mercaptoethanol). Cells were triturated with a pipette tip, digested with DNAse I and a single cell suspension without clumps was seeded. When indicated, cells were treated with 20 nM bafilomycin A1 (Cayman Chemicals) or DMSO for 16 h. Cells were harvested by scraping and lysed for Western blot analysis as described [16] or fixed for immunofluorescence.

For neuronal cultures, cortices were micro-dissected in ice-cold Hank's balanced salt solution (HBSS+; Gibco), then diced and pooled for each genotype. Cells were dissociated with 0.05% trypsin-EDTA (Gibco), followed by neutralization with 10% fetal calf serum in neuro basal medium (NBM+) and DNAse I treatment (153 U/mL). Tissue was triturated with a pipette five to six times. Cells were plated on poly-D-lysine coated 6-well plates with 2 ml of Neurobasal media (Gibco #21103-049), B27 (Gibco #17504-044), 100 U/mLpenicillin-streptomycin (PS) (Gibco), 0.5 mM L-glutamine and maintained at 37° C, 5% CO2 with humidity. Cells were fed with 200 mL fresh medium every fifth day. On day 9-11 in culture, cells were treated with 10 nM bafilomycin A1 (Cayman Chemicals) or DMSO for 2 h. Cells were harvested by scraping and lysed for Western blot analysis as described [16].

Western blotting

Western blots were performed on samples lysed in SDP lysis buffer (50 mM Tris pH 8, 150 mM NaCl, 1% Igepal with 'Complete' protease inhibitor cocktail (Roche)). Protein concentration was measured using the DC protein assay kit (Bio Rad, USA) and equal amounts were separated on 7% Bis-Tris gels for the detection of HTT, or 4-12% gradient gels (Invitrogen, USA) for the detection of LC3 and p62. Protein was transferred to PVDF Immobilon-FL membranes by electroblotting and membranes were developed with primary antibodies in 5% bovine serum albumin/phosphate buffered saline. The following antibodies were used for immunoblotting: anti-HTT BKP1 (1:100) generated in-house [27], anti-HTT 2166 (1:1000) from Millipore (MAB2166), anti-polyglutamine expansion antibody (1C2, MAB1574) from Millipore (1:2000), anti-p62 (1:1000) from ENZO (BML-PW9860), anti-LC3b (1:1000) from Cell Signaling Technologies (2775), anti-mTOR (1:1000) from Cell Signaling Technologies (2983), anti-phospho-mTOR (1:1000) from Cell Signaling Technologies (5536), anti-HA (1:1000) from COVANCE (MMS-101R), anti-Actin (1:10,000) from Sigma (A2103), anti-calnexin (1:5000) from Sigma (C4731), anti-spectrin (1:4000) from ENZO (bm-FG6090). Fluorescently labelled secondary antibodies conjugated to either 700 or 800 IR dye (1:5000; Rockland, USA) and the LiCor Odyssey Infrared Imaging system were used for detection. The following antibodies were used for immunocytochemistry experiments: anti-p62 from R&D Systems (MAB8028; 1:200), anti-LC3β from Cell Signaling (2775S; 1:200), anti-polyglutamine expansion antibody (1C2, MAB1574;1:1000) from Millipore, Alexa Fluor 488 goat anti-mouse IgG from Invitrogen (A11001; 1:500), and Alexa Fluor 568 goat anti-rabbit IgG from Invitrogen (A11011; 1:500).

Immunocytochemistry

Cells (MEFs or COS-7) were cultured on coverslips in 24-well plates and treated with bafilomycin (16 h; 20 nM), MG132 (4 h; 10 μM), or DMSO followed by fixation with 4% paraformaldehyde in PBS for 15 min at room temperature (RT). Cells were treated with ice-cold methanol for 5 min at – 20 °C, washed 3× in PBS, permeabilized in 0.03% Triton-X/PBS for 5 min at RT, washed 3× in PBS, and incubated in blocking buffer (0.2% gelatin/PBS) at RT for 30 min. Coverslips were transferred to primary antibody solution made up in blocking buffer and incubated overnight at 4 °C, followed by 3xPBS washes and incubation with secondary antibody in blocking buffer at RT for 1.5 h. Coverslips were washed and mounted on slides with ProLong Gold antifade reagent with DAPI (Molecular Probes).

Confocal imaging and image analysis

Single z-plane images were acquired on a Leica TCS SP8 confocal laser scanning microscope at 63X objective magnification. Images were imported into Image J, background subtracted using a rolling ball radius of 15 pixels, and de-speckled. 1-3 cells per image were analysed by selecting 3 random regions of interest (ROIs) within the cytosol of each cell, manually thresholding punctae from each channel, and evaluating punctae size, density, and overlap using the Image J Colocalization plugin and the Analyse Particles function. All data were normalized to the mean of the appropriate wild-type littermate control values.

For COS cell analysis, punctae analysis was not possible due to the diffuse staining pattern of transfected HTT. Instead, 1-3 cells per image were outlined to generate ROIs, and the Coloc2 plugin was utilized to calculate a Pearson correlation coefficient as measures of colocalization between channels.

COS-7 cell transfection and immunoprecipitation

COS-7 cells were maintained in DMEM with 10% FBS, 1% L-glutamine, 100 U/mL penicillin and 0.1 mg/mL streptomycin at 37 °C and 5% CO2 in a humidified incubator. HTT expression constructs aa1-1212 and 1-586 were described previously [60], fragments aa1-800 and aa1-1004 were generated from HTT_{1-1212} 15Q using the Q5 site-directed mutagenesis kit (NEB) with the following primers:

HTT 800 For: 5′ - AACCCTCACATGAAATACATTTTCTTTG - 3'
HTT 800 Rev.: 5′ - CTAATGGTGCCCATCCAATC - 3'
HTT 1004 For: 5′ - AAATAACCTTTGAAGAGTTAT TGCAG - 3'
HTT 1004 Rev.: 5′ - TCCATAGTGACGTCTGTTATG - 3'

Correct insertion of the stop codons was verified by sequencing.

Cells were transiently cotransfected with the aa1-1212 15Q, aa1-586 15Q, aa1-800 15Q, aa1-1004 15Q, aa1-1212 128Q (cleavable), aa1-1212 138Q-C6R or aa1-586 Q128 HTT constructs (11) together with RFP-p62 (obtained from Addgene (12)) or HA-ubiquitin wt, K63 or K48 (obtained from Addgene (13)). The Xtreme gene 9 transfection reagent (Roche Applied Science, Quebec, Canada) was used according to the manufacturer's protocol.

The day after transfection, cells were treated with 100 nM bafilomycin for 4 h to prevent HTT-p62 and HTT-ubiquitin complexes from degradation. Cell lysates were prepared in SDP buffer and immunoprecipitated over night at 4 °C using anti-p62 (MBL PM045) or anti-HTT 2166 antibodies (Millipore MAB2166). Immunoprecipitates and cell lysates were subjected to SDS-PAGE and Western blot as described above.

Cycloheximide chase assay

COS-7 cells were transfected as above. 6 h after transfection, 10 μM MG132 were added to prevent proteasomal degradation and enforce autophagic clearance of mHTT. 16 h later, 0 h timepoints were harvested and 100 μg/ml cycloheximide were added for the indicated timepoints. Samples were lysed and analyzed by Western blotting as described above.

qRT-PCR

RNA was extracted using the PureLink mini RNA extraction kit (Life Technologies). RNA was treated with DNase I (Invitrogen) and 500 ng of RNA were reverse transcribed using SuperScript III (Invitrogen) and oligo-dT primers according to manufacturer's instructions to generate cDNA for qRT-PCR. The PCR was run with SYBR Green Power master mix (Applied Biosystems) on the ABI Prism 7500 Sequence Detection System.

Each sample was run in triplicate. Relative gene expression was determined by using the $\Delta\Delta C_T$ method, normalizing to *Rpl13a* mRNA levels in cortical tissues and MEF cells and to *Pgk1* mRNA levels in liver. The following primers were used:

Human *Htt* forward: 5′-
GAAAGTCAGTCCGGGTAGAAC -3'
Human *Htt* reverse: 5′-
CAGATACCCGCTCCATAGCAA -3′
mouse *Rpl13a* forward: 5'-
GGAGGAGAAACGGAAGGAAAAG-3′
mouse *Rpl13a* reverse: 5′-
CCGTAACCTCAAGATCTGCTTCTT-3′
mouse *Pgk1* forward: 5′ -
ACCTGCTGGCTGGATGG - 3′
mouse *Pgk1* reverse: 5′ -
CACAGCCTCGGCATATTTCT - 3′
mouse *Sirt1* forward: 5′-
CAGTGTCATGGTTCCTTTGC -3′
mouse *Sirt1* reverse: 5′–
CACCGAGGAACTACCTGAT -3′
mouse *p62* forward: 5′-
CTCAGCCCTCTAGGCATTG – 3′
mouse *p62* reverse: 5′-
TCCTTCCTGTGAGGGGTCT – 3′
mouse *LC3b1* forward: 5′ -
CTCACTCGTGGTCTGAGGACTTC - 3′
mouse *LC3b1* reverse: 5′ -
GGTGGCTATGCTGGCTTCA - 3′

Transmission electron microscopy (TEM)

Mice were anesthetized with avertin and injected with 15 μL of heparin intracardially. Mice were perfused with 4% paraformaldehyde and 0.125% glutaraldehyde for 20 min at a rate of 6 mL/min. Brains were dissected and left overnight in fixative at room temperature. 400 μm sections were cut on a vibratome and 1 mm^2 tissue blocks of motor cortex were dissected. Postfixing, embedding, sectioning and staining were performed at the University of British Columbia BioImaging facility. Briefly, samples were rinsed in 0.1 M sodium cacodylate buffer and secondary fixed in 1% osmium tetroxide with 1.5% potassium ferricyanide in 0.1 M sodium cacodylate for 2 h. Tissue was washed two times in distilled water and dehydrated in a series of ethanol dilutions, followed by graded resin infiltration and embedding. Ultrathin sections were prepared on a Leica Ultracut 7 using 45 degree diamond histoknife. Thin sections were counterstained with Sato's lead. Images were taken using a Hitachi H7600 Transmission Electron Microscope and analyzed using Image J. 10-15 cells per mouse were identified and pictures taken systematically around the nucleus, covering all visible cytoplasm. 4-5 mice per genotype from 2 to 4 separate litters of YAC and wt mice were analyzed in a randomized and blinded fashion. AV were identified as either autophagosomes with a double membrane and visible cytoplasmic content such as mitochondria, or autolysosomes (vesicles with electron-dense content and some remaining ultrastructure) [28] and counted manually. The number of AV/cell was calculated and normalized to wt littermates. Imaging and counting were performed by separate blinded investigators.

Immunohistochemistry and image analysis

Samples from the same mouse brains as used in electron microscopy were mounted on slides and stained with anti-LC3b (1:1000) from Cell Signaling Technologies (2775). Slides were imaged on a Leica SP5 laser-scanning confocal microscope with a 63X immersion plan-apochromat objective. Fixed and stained mouse cortices were imaged at 100 Hz with a 1024 × 1024 pixel scan format, a zoom factor of 1 and a pinhole size of 75 μm. LC3 staining was imaged using the 543 laser at 15% laser power (50% intensity and 100% gain) and DAPI was imaged using the UV laser at full laser power (25% intensity and 10% gain).

Background subtraction on the LC3 image stack was performed using the rolling ball method using a radius of 10 pixels. A threshold mask was then applied to the image stack based on intensities ranging from 100 to 255 to generate binary images. Subsequently, ImageJ [52] automated particle analysis was performed on the image stack and particle counts, size and area were measured for all images.

Additional files

Additional file 1: Figure S1. LC3 and p62 are barely detectable at baseline in MEF cultures. **A** Higher exposure of blots shown in Fig. 1a demonstrates low baseline levels of p62 and LC3 in MEF cells. **B** Immunofluorescent staining for LC3 and p62 is barely detectable in MEFs in the absence of bafilomycin. (TIFF 2834 kb)

Additional file 2: Figure S2. Autophagy pathways are not altered in MEFs derived from YAC18 mice. **A** Primary MEF cultures from YAC18 or wt littermate embryos were seeded onto coverslips and treated with bafilomycin. Cells were fixed and stained for p62 and LC3, Hoechst dye was used for nuclear counterstaining. Samples were imaged on a confocal microscope and the density of punctae as well as the co-localization of LC3 and p62 staining were analyzed. **B** Primary MEF cultures from YAC18 or wt littermate embryos were seeded onto coverslips and treated with MG132 or DMSO as a control. Cells were fixed and stained for p62, Hoechst dye was used for nuclear counterstaining. Samples were imaged on a confocal microscope and the density of punctae were analyzed. Representative images and pooled quantification data with S.E.M. are shown, 3 independent cultures were analyzed. Number of replicates is shown as insets for Western blot experiments, for imaging experiments 24-30 cells per condition were analyzed. Statistical significance was determined by Student's t-test. No statistically significant differences were found. (TIFF 5239 kb)

Additional file 3: Figure S3. Increased association of p62 and K63 ubiquitin with C6R mHTT. **A** COS-7 cells were cotransfected with mHTT aa 1-1212 (cleavable or C6R) or mHTT aa 1-586 and p62 as indicated. After immunoprecipitation of HTT, the ratio of co-immunoprecipitated p62 was quantified (normalized to input to control for transfection efficiency). **B** COS-7 cells were cotransfected with cleavable $mHTT_{1-1212}$, C6R $mHTT_{1-1212}$ and p62 as indicated and treated with MG132 to enforce autophagic degradation. Cycloheximide was added for the indicated periods of time and samples were analyzed by Western blot. Representative blots are shown as part of Fig. 3b. 2way-ANOVA HTT construct p=0.1451, time $p<0.0001$. **C** COS-7 cells were cotransfected with mHTT aa1-1212 (cleavable or C6R) and HA-tagged wt, K63 or K48 ubiquitin (allowing all, only K63 or only K48 linkage to target proteins) as indicated. After immunoprecipitation of HTT, the ratio of co-immunoprecipitated ubiquitin/HTT was quantified (normalized to input to control for transfection efficiency). Blots and quantification data with S.E.M. from a representative of 3 independent experiments are shown, number of technical replicates is shown as insets. Statistical significance was determined by 1way ANOVA with Tukey's post-hoc correction (A), 2way-ANOVA with Bonferroni's post-hoc correction (B) or Student's t-test (D). *: $p<0.05$, **: $p<0.01$, ***: $p<0.001$. (TIFF 2089 kb)

Additional file 4: Figure S4. Full blots corresponding to Fig. 3b. (TIFF 4590 kb)

Additional file 5: Figure S5. 24h fasting does not alter wt HTT protein or mHTT RNA levels while it reduces C6R mHTT in the liver. **A** Liver tissue from 12 month old YAC128 and C6R mice as well as their wt littermates was analyzed for mRNA expression of *LC3b* by qRT-PCR. Data were normalized to the expression of *Pgk1*. 1way-ANOVA $p=0.6552$. **B** Liver tissue from 12 month old YAC128 and C6R mice was analyzed for mRNA expression of *mHTT* by qRT-PCR. Data were normalized to the expression of *Pgk1*. **C - E** 12 month old YAC128 and C6R mice as well as their wt littermates were subjected to a 24h fasting period, sacrificed immediately and liver samples were compared to littermates with ad libitum access to food. **C** Protein levels for wt HTT were analyzed by Western blotting with antibody MAB2166 in liver tissues derived from YAC128 mice. **D** mRNA levels for transgenic human mHTT were analyzed by qRT-PCR in liver tissues derived from YAC128 mice. **E** Protein levels for mHTT were analyzed by Western blotting with antibody MAB2166 in liver tissues derived from C6R mice. Representative blots and pooled quantification data with S.E.M. are shown, the blot matching panel C is shown in Fig. 5d. Statistical significance was determined by 1way-ANOVA (A) or two-tailed Student's t-test (B-E), number of replicates is shown as insets. (TIFF 1130 kb)

Additional file 6: Figure S6. 24h fasting increases autophagy but does not cause mHTT degradation in the brain. **A + B** 3 month old YAC128 and C6R mice as well as their wt littermates were subjected to a 24h fasting period, sacrificed immediately and cortical samples were compared to littermates with ad libitum access to food. **A** Protein levels of p62, LC3-I and LC3-II were analyzed by Western blotting in cortical tissues of wt and YAC128 mice. p62: 2way-ANOVA genotype $p=0.2568$, feeding $p=0.0002$, LC3-I: 2way-ANOVA genotype $p=0.7914$, feeding $p<0.0001$, LC3-II: 2way-ANOVA genotype $p=0.5499$, feeding $p=0.0039$. **B** Protein levels of mHTT were analyzed by Western blotting with antibody MAB2166 in cortical tissues of YAC128 mice. Representative blots and pooled quantification data with S.E.M. are shown, number of replicates is shown as insets. Statistical significance was determined by 2way-ANOVA with Bonferroni's post-hoc correction for A, or two-tailed Student's t-test for B. *: $p<0.05$, **: $p<0.01$, ***: $p<0.001$. (TIFF 1574 kb)

Additional file 7: Figure S7. Cortical p62, LC3-I and wt HTT protein levels as well as mHTT mRNA are not altered by scheduled feeding. **A** YAC128 and C6R mice as well as their wt littermates were subjected to one week of scheduled feeding and compared to littermates with ad libitum access to food. Protein levels of p62 were analyzed by Western blotting in cortical tissues. 2way-ANOVA, genotype $p=0.2138$, feeding $p=0.5807$. **B** YAC128 and C6R mice as well as their wt littermates were subjected to one week of scheduled feeding and compared to littermates with ad libitum access to food. Protein levels of LC3-I were analyzed by Western blotting in cortical tissues. 2way-ANOVA, genotype $p=0.5798$, feeding $p=0.2548$. **C + D** YAC128 mice and their wt littermates were subjected to one week of scheduled feeding and compared to littermates with ad libitum access to food. **C** Protein levels of wt HTT were analyzed by Western blotting with antibody MAB2166 in cortical tissues. 2way-ANOVA genotype $p=0.6115$, feeding $p=0.1818$. **D** mRNA levels for transgenic human mHTT were analyzed by qRT-PCR in cortical tissues derived from YAC128 mice. Representative blots and pooled quantification data with S.E.M. are shown, number of replicates is shown as insets. The blot corresponding to panel B is shown in Fig. 6a, the blot corresponding to panel C is shown in Fig. 6d. Statistical significance was determined by 2way ANOVA (A-C) or Student's t-test (D). (TIFF 1304 kb)

Acknowledgements

The authors thank Dr. Ana-Maria Cuervo for assistance in the identification of AVs and Mandi Schmidt for assistance with image analysis. We thank Piers Ruddle, Mahsa Amirabbasi, Sheng Yu, Mark Wang, Yun Ko, Yuanyun Xie and Qingwen Xia for their technical support. DDOM and NHS were supported by postdoctoral fellowships from CIHR. DDOM was also supported by Michael Smith Foundation for Health Research and the Bluma Tischler Fellowship from UBC. MS was supported by a Vanier Canada Graduate Scholarship. SL was supported by a doctoral scholarship from CIHR. NSC was supported by postdoctoral fellowships from CIHR and the James Family. This work was supported by the Canadian Institutes of Health Research (CIHR 20R90174) and a sponsored research agreement with Teva Pharmaceuticals.

Authors' contributions

DEE designed and performed experiments, coordinated author contributions and wrote the manuscript. DDOM designed and performed experiments, provided intellectual input and edited the manuscript. MS, XQ, SL, NSC, NHS, YTNN, KV, ALS, SE and SF performed experiments. MRH supervised the project and edited the manuscript. All authors read and approved the final manuscript.

Competing interests

M.R.H. was an employee of Teva Pharmaceuticals, Inc. Teva did not play a role in the design, analysis or interpretation of this study. All other authors declare no competing financial interests.

Author details

[1]Centre for Molecular Medicine and Therapeutics (CMMT), CFRI, Department of Medical Genetics, University of British Columbia, 950 West 28th Avenue, Vancouver, BC V5Z 4H4, Canada. [2]Present address: BioMed X Innovation Center, Im Neuenheimer Feld 515, 69120 Heidelberg, Germany.

References

1. Alirezaei M, Kemball CC, Flynn CT, Wood MR, Whitton JL, Kiosses WB (2010) Short-term fasting induces profound neuronal autophagy. Autophagy 6:702–710
2. Atwal RS, Xia J, Pinchev D, Taylor J, Epand RM, Truant R (2007) Huntingtin has a membrane association signal that can modulate huntingtin aggregation, nuclear entry and toxicity. Hum Mol Genet 16: 2600–2615. https://doi.org/10.1093/hmg/ddm217
3. Aziz NA, van der Burg JM, Landwehrmeyer GB, Brundin P, Stijnen T, Group ES, Roos RA (2008) Weight loss in Huntington disease increases with higher

CAG repeat number. Neurology 71:1506–1513. https://doi.org/10.1212/01.wnl.0000334276.09729.0e
4. Babu JR, Seibenhener ML, Peng J, Strom AL, Kemppainen R, Cox N, Zhu H, Wooten MC, Diaz-Meco MT, Moscat J et al (2008) Genetic inactivation of p62 leads to accumulation of hyperphosphorylated tau and neurodegeneration. J Neurochem 106:107–120. https://doi.org/10.1111/j.1471-4159.2008.05340.x
5. Bae SH, Sung SH, Oh SY, Lim JM, Lee SK, Park YN, Lee HE, Kang D, Rhee SG (2013) Sestrins activate Nrf2 by promoting p62-dependent autophagic degradation of Keap1 and prevent oxidative liver damage. Cell Metab 17: 73–84. https://doi.org/10.1016/j.cmet.2012.12.002
6. Bennett EJ, Shaler TA, Woodman B, Ryu KY, Zaitseva TS, Becker CH, Bates GP, Schulman H, Kopito RR (2007) Global changes to the ubiquitin system in Huntington's disease. Nature 448:704–708. https://doi.org/10.1038/nature06022
7. Bhat KP, Yan S, Wang CE, Li S, Li XJ (2014) Differential ubiquitination and degradation of huntingtin fragments modulated by ubiquitin-protein ligase E3A. Proc Natl Acad Sci U S A 111:5706–5711. https://doi.org/10.1073/pnas.1402215111
8. Boland B, Kumar A, Lee S, Platt FM, Wegiel J, Yu WH, Nixon RA (2008) Autophagy induction and autophagosome clearance in neurons: relationship to autophagic pathology in Alzheimer's disease. J Neurosci 28:6926–6937. https://doi.org/10.1523/JNEUROSCI.0800-08.2008
9. Carroll JB, Bates GP, Steffan J, Saft C, Tabrizi SJ (2015) Treating the whole body in Huntington's disease. Lancet Neurol 14:1135–1142. https://doi.org/10.1016/S1474-4422(15)00177-5
10. Chen X, Kondo K, Motoki K, Homma H, Okazawa H (2015) Fasting activates macroautophagy in neurons of Alzheimer's disease mouse model but is insufficient to degrade amyloid-beta. Sci Rep 5:12115. https://doi.org/10.1038/srep12115
11. Cunha-Santos J, Duarte-Neves J, Carmona V, Guarente L, Pereira de Almeida L, Cavadas C (2016) Caloric restriction blocks neuropathology and motor deficits in Machado-Joseph disease mouse models through SIRT1 pathway. Nat Commun 7:11445. https://doi.org/10.1038/ncomms11445
12. Czaja MJ, Ding WX, Donohue TM Jr, Friedman SL, Kim JS, Komatsu M, Lemasters JJ, Lemoine A, Lin JD, Ou JH et al (2013) Functions of autophagy in normal and diseased liver. Autophagy 9:1131–1158. https://doi.org/10.4161/auto.25063
13. De Souza RA, Leavitt BR (2015) Neurobiology of Huntington's disease. Curr Top Behav Neurosci 22:81–100. https://doi.org/10.1007/7854_2014_353
14. Dikic I (2017) Proteasomal and Autophagic degradation systems. Annu Rev Biochem 86:193–224. https://doi.org/10.1146/annurev-biochem-061516-044908
15. Duan W, Guo Z, Jiang H, Ware M, Li XJ, Mattson MP (2003) Dietary restriction normalizes glucose metabolism and BDNF levels, slows disease progression, and increases survival in huntingtin mutant mice. Proc Natl Acad Sci U S A 100:2911–2916. https://doi.org/10.1073/pnas.0536856100
16. Ehrnhoefer DE, Skotte NH, Savill J, Nguyen YT, Ladha S, Cao LP, Dullaghan E, Hayden MR (2011) A quantitative method for the specific assessment of caspase-6 activity in cell culture. PLoS One 6: e27680. https://doi.org/10.1371/journal.pone.0027680
17. Ehrnhoefer DE, Sutton L, Hayden MR (2011) Small changes, big impact: posttranslational modifications and function of huntingtin in Huntington disease. Neuroscientist 17:475–492. https://doi.org/10.1177/1073858410390378
18. El-Daher MT, Hangen E, Bruyere J, Poizat G, Al-Ramahi I, Pardo R, Bourg N, Souquere S, Mayet C, Pierron G et al (2015) Huntingtin proteolysis releases non-polyQ fragments that cause toxicity through dynamin 1 dysregulation. EMBO J 34:2255–2271. https://doi.org/10.15252/embj.201490808
19. Gafni J, Papanikolaou T, Degiacomo F, Holcomb J, Chen S, Menalled L, Kudwa A, Fitzpatrick J, Miller S, Ramboz S et al (2012) Caspase-6 activity in a BACHD mouse modulates steady-state levels of mutant huntingtin protein but is not necessary for production of a 586 amino acid proteolytic fragment. J Neurosci 32:7454–7465. https://doi.org/10.1523/JNEUROSCI.6379-11.2012
20. Ghosh HS, McBurney M, Robbins PD (2010) SIRT1 negatively regulates the mammalian target of rapamycin. PLoS One 5:e9199. https://doi.org/10.1371/journal.pone.0009199
21. Graham RK, Deng Y, Carroll J, Vaid K, Cowan C, Pouladi MA, Metzler M, Bissada N, Wang L, Faull RL et al (2010) Cleavage at the 586 amino acid caspase-6 site in mutant huntingtin influences caspase-6 activation in vivo. J Neurosci 30:15019–15029. https://doi.org/10.1523/JNEUROSCI.2071-10.2010
22. Graham RK, Deng Y, Pouladi MA, Vaid K, Ehrnhoefer DE, Southwell AL, Bissada N, Franciosi S, Hayden MR (2012) Caspase-6-resistant mutant huntingtin does not rescue the toxic effects of caspase-cleavable mutant huntingtin in vivo. J Huntington's Dis 1:243–260
23. Graham RK, Deng Y, Slow EJ, Haigh B, Bissada N, Lu G, Pearson J, Shehadeh J, Bertram L, Murphy Z et al (2006) Cleavage at the caspase-6 site is required for neuronal dysfunction and degeneration due to mutant huntingtin. Cell 125: 1179–1191. https://doi.org/10.1016/j.cell.2006.04.026
24. Hodgson JG, Smith DJ, McCutcheon K, Koide HB, Nishiyama K, Dinulos MB, Stevens ME, Bissada N, Nasir J, Kanazawa I et al (1996) Human huntingtin derived from YAC transgenes compensates for loss of murine huntingtin by rescue of the embryonic lethal phenotype. Hum Mol Genet 5:1875–1885
25. Jeong H, Cohen DE, Cui L, Supinski A, Savas JN, Mazzulli JR, Yates JR 3rd, Bordone L, Guarente L, Krainc D (2011) Sirt1 mediates neuroprotection from mutant huntingtin by activation of the TORC1 and CREB transcriptional pathway. Nat Med 18:159–165. https://doi.org/10.1038/nm.2559
26. Jiang M, Wang J, Fu J, Du L, Jeong H, West T, Xiang L, Peng Q, Hou Z, Cai H et al (2011) Neuroprotective role of Sirt1 in mammalian models of Huntington's disease through activation of multiple Sirt1 targets. Nat Med 18:153–158. https://doi.org/10.1038/nm.2558
27. Kalchman MA, Graham RK, Xia G, Koide HB, Hodgson JG, Graham KC, Goldberg YP, Gietz RD, Pickart CM, Hayden MR (1996) Huntingtin is ubiquitinated and interacts with a specific ubiquitin-conjugating enzyme. J Biol Chem 271:19385–19394
28. Klionsky DJ, Abdelmohsen K, Abe A, Abedin MJ, Abeliovich H, Acevedo Arozena A, Adachi H, Adams CM, Adams PD, Adeli K et al (2016) Guidelines for the use and interpretation of assays for monitoring autophagy (3rd edition). Autophagy 12:1–222. https://doi.org/10.1080/15548627.2015.1100356
29. Korolchuk VI, Mansilla A, Menzies FM, Rubinsztein DC (2009) Autophagy inhibition compromises degradation of ubiquitin-proteasome pathway substrates. Mol Cell 33:517–527. https://doi.org/10.1016/j.molcel.2009.01.021
30. Krainc D (2010) Clearance of mutant proteins as a therapeutic target in neurodegenerative diseases. Arch Neurol 67:388–392. https://doi.org/10.1001/archneurol.2010.40
31. Lee JH, Tecedor L, Chen YH, Monteys AM, Sowada MJ, Thompson LM, Davidson BL (2015) Reinstating aberrant mTORC1 activity in Huntington's disease mice improves disease phenotypes. Neuron 85: 303–315. https://doi.org/10.1016/j.neuron.2014.12.019
32. Lim J, Lachenmayer ML, Wu S, Liu W, Kundu M, Wang R, Komatsu M, Oh YJ, Zhao Y, Yue Z (2015) Proteotoxic stress induces phosphorylation of p62/SQSTM1 by ULK1 to regulate selective autophagic clearance of protein aggregates. PLoS Genet 11:e1004987. https://doi.org/10.1371/journal.pgen.1004987
33. Ma D, Panda S, Lin JD (2011) Temporal orchestration of circadian autophagy rhythm by C/EBPbeta. EMBO J 30:4642–4651. https://doi.org/10.1038/emboj.2011.322
34. Martin DD, Heit RJ, Yap MC, Davidson MW, Hayden MR, Berthiaume LG (2014) Identification of a post-translationally myristoylated autophagy-inducing domain released by caspase cleavage of huntingtin. Hum Mol Genet 23:3166–3179. https://doi.org/10.1093/hmg/ddu027
35. Martin DD, Ladha S, Ehrnhoefer DE, Hayden MR (2015) Autophagy in Huntington disease and huntingtin in autophagy. Trends Neurosci 38:26–35. https://doi.org/10.1016/j.tins.2014.09.003
36. Martinez-Vicente M, Talloczy Z, Wong E, Tang G, Koga H, Kaushik S, de Vries R, Arias E, Harris S, Sulzer D et al (2010) Cargo recognition failure is responsible for inefficient autophagy in Huntington's disease. Nat Neurosci 13:567–576. https://doi.org/10.1038/nn.2528
37. Mattison JA, Colman RJ, Beasley TM, Allison DB, Kemnitz JW, Roth GS, Ingram DK, Weindruch R, de Cabo R, Anderson RM (2017) Caloric restriction improves health and survival of rhesus monkeys. Nat Commun 8:14063. https://doi.org/10.1038/ncomms14063
38. Maywood ES, Fraenkel E, McAllister CJ, Wood N, Reddy AB, Hastings MH, Morton AJ (2010) Disruption of peripheral circadian timekeeping in a mouse model of Huntington's disease and its restoration by temporally scheduled feeding. J Neurosci 30:10199–10204. https://doi.org/10.1523/JNEUROSCI.1694-10.2010
39. Menzies FM, Fleming A, Rubinsztein DC (2015) Compromised autophagy and neurodegenerative diseases. Nat Rev Neurosci 16:345–357. https://doi.org/10.1038/nrn3961
40. Metzler M, Gan L, Mazarei G, Graham RK, Liu L, Bissada N, Lu G, Leavitt BR, Hayden MR (2010) Phosphorylation of huntingtin at Ser421 in YAC128 neurons is associated with protection of YAC128 neurons from NMDA-mediated excitotoxicity and is modulated by PP1 and PP2A. J Neurosci 30: 14318–14329. https://doi.org/10.1523/JNEUROSCI.1589-10.2010
41. Morton AJ (2013) Circadian and sleep disorder in Huntington's disease. Exp Neurol 243:34–44. https://doi.org/10.1016/j.expneurol.2012.10.014

42. Ntsapi C, Loos B (2016) Caloric restriction and the precision-control of autophagy: a strategy for delaying neurodegenerative disease progression. Exp Gerontol 83:97–111. https://doi.org/10.1016/j.exger.2016.07.014
43. Ochaba J, Lukacsovich T, Csikos G, Zheng S, Margulis J, Salazar L, Mao K, Lau AL, Yeung SY, Humbert S et al (2014) Potential function for the huntingtin protein as a scaffold for selective autophagy. Proc Natl Acad Sci U S A 111: 16889–16894. https://doi.org/10.1073/pnas.1420103111
44. Okamoto S, Pouladi MA, Talantova M, Yao D, Xia P, Ehrnhoefer DE, Zaidi R, Clemente A, Kaul M, Graham RK et al (2009) Balance between synaptic versus extrasynaptic NMDA receptor activity influences inclusions and neurotoxicity of mutant huntingtin. Nat Med 15:1407–1413. https://doi.org/10.1038/nm.2056
45. Pouladi MA, Graham RK, Karasinska JM, Xie Y, Santos RD, Petersen A, Hayden MR (2009) Prevention of depressive behaviour in the YAC128 mouse model of Huntington disease by mutation at residue 586 of huntingtin. Brain 132:919–932. https://doi.org/10.1093/brain/awp006
46. Pouladi MA, Xie Y, Skotte NH, Ehrnhoefer DE, Graham RK, Kim JE, Bissada N, Yang XW, Paganetti P, Friedlander RM et al (2010) Full-length huntingtin levels modulate body weight by influencing insulin-like growth factor 1 expression. Hum Mol Genet 19:1528–1538. https://doi.org/10.1093/hmg/ddq026
47. Ravikumar B, Duden R, Rubinsztein DC (2002) Aggregate-prone proteins with polyglutamine and polyalanine expansions are degraded by autophagy. Hum Mol Genet 11:1107–1117
48. Rose C, Menzies FM, Renna M, Acevedo-Arozena A, Corrochano S, Sadiq O, Brown SD, Rubinsztein DC (2010) Rilmenidine attenuates toxicity of polyglutamine expansions in a mouse model of Huntington's disease. Hum Mol Genet 19:2144–2153. https://doi.org/10.1093/hmg/ddq093
49. Rubinsztein DC (2006) The roles of intracellular protein-degradation pathways in neurodegeneration. Nature 443:780–786. https://doi.org/10.1038/nature05291
50. Rui YN, Xu Z, Patel B, Chen Z, Chen D, Tito A, David G, Sun Y, Stimming EF, Bellen HJ et al (2015) Huntingtin functions as a scaffold for selective macroautophagy. Nat Cell Biol 17:262–275. https://doi.org/10.1038/ncb3101
51. Sahani MH, Itakura E, Mizushima N (2014) Expression of the autophagy substrate SQSTM1/p62 is restored during prolonged starvation depending on transcriptional upregulation and autophagy-derived amino acids. Autophagy 10:431–441. https://doi.org/10.4161/auto.27344
52. Schneider CA, Rasband WS, Eliceiri KW (2012) NIH image to ImageJ: 25 years of image analysis. Nat Methods 9:671–675
53. Seibenhener ML, Babu JR, Geetha T, Wong HC, Krishna NR, Wooten MW (2004) Sequestosome 1/p62 is a polyubiquitin chain binding protein involved in ubiquitin proteasome degradation. Mol Cell Biol 24:8055–8068. https://doi.org/10.1128/MCB.24.18.8055-8068.2004
54. Skillings EA, Wood NI, Morton AJ (2014) Beneficial effects of environmental enrichment and food entrainment in the R6/2 mouse model of Huntington's disease. Brain Behav 4:675–686. https://doi.org/10.1002/brb3.235
55. Skotte NH, Southwell AL, Ostergaard ME, Carroll JB, Warby SC, Doty CN, Petoukhov E, Vaid K, Kordasiewicz H, Watt AT et al (2014) Allele-specific suppression of mutant huntingtin using antisense oligonucleotides: providing a therapeutic option for all Huntington disease patients. PLoS One 9:e107434. https://doi.org/10.1371/journal.pone.0107434
56. Slow EJ, van Raamsdonk J, Rogers D, Coleman SH, Graham RK, Deng Y, Oh R, Bissada N, Hossain SM, Yang YZ et al (2003) Selective striatal neuronal loss in a YAC128 mouse model of Huntington disease. Hum Mol Genet 12:1555–1567
57. The Huntington's disease Collaborative Research Group (1993) A novel gene containing a trinucleotide repeat that is expanded and unstable on Huntington's disease chromosomes. Huntington's Dis Collab Res Group Cell 72:971–983
58. Van Raamsdonk JM, Gibson WT, Pearson J, Murphy Z, Lu G, Leavitt BR, Hayden MR (2006) Body weight is modulated by levels of full-length huntingtin. Hum Mol Genet 15:1513–1523. https://doi.org/10.1093/hmg/ddl072
59. Walter C, Clemens LE, Muller AJ, Fallier-Becker P, Proikas-Cezanne T, Riess O, Metzger S, Nguyen HP (2016) Activation of AMPK-induced autophagy ameliorates Huntington disease pathology in vitro. Neuropharmacology. https://doi.org/10.1016/j.neuropharm.2016.04.041
60. Warby SC, Doty CN, Graham RK, Carroll JB, Yang YZ, Singaraja RR, Overall CM, Hayden MR (2008) Activated caspase-6 and caspase-6-cleaved fragments of huntingtin specifically colocalize in the nucleus. Hum Mol Genet 17:2390–2404. https://doi.org/10.1093/hmg/ddn139
61. Wild EJ, Tabrizi SJ (2014) Targets for future clinical trials in Huntington's disease: what's in the pipeline? Movement Disord 29: 1434–1445. https://doi.org/10.1002/mds.26007
62. Wong BK, Ehrnhoefer DE, Graham RK, Martin DD, Ladha S, Uribe V, Stanek LM, Franciosi S, Qiu X, Deng Y et al (2015) Partial rescue of some features of Huntington disease in the genetic absence of caspase-6 in YAC128 mice. Neurobiol Dis 76:24–36. https://doi.org/10.1016/j.nbd.2014.12.030
63. Wong YC, Holzbaur EL (2014) The regulation of autophagosome dynamics by huntingtin and HAP1 is disrupted by expression of mutant huntingtin, leading to defective cargo degradation. J Neurosci 34:1293–1305. https://doi.org/10.1523/JNEUROSCI.1870-13.2014
64. Young JE, Martinez RA, La Spada AR (2009) Nutrient deprivation induces neuronal autophagy and implicates reduced insulin signaling in neuroprotective autophagy activation. J Biol Chem 284:2363–2373. https://doi.org/10.1074/jbc.M806088200

15

White matter changes in Alzheimer's disease: a focus on myelin and oligodendrocytes

Sara E. Nasrabady[1*], Batool Rizvi[4], James E. Goldman[2,4] and Adam M. Brickman[3,4]

Abstract

Alzheimer's disease (AD) is conceptualized as a progressive consequence of two hallmark pathological changes in grey matter: extracellular amyloid plaques and neurofibrillary tangles. However, over the past several years, neuroimaging studies have implicated micro- and macrostructural abnormalities in white matter in the risk and progression of AD, suggesting that in addition to the neuronal pathology characteristic of the disease, white matter degeneration and demyelination may be also important pathophysiological features. Here we review the evidence for white matter abnormalities in AD with a focus on myelin and oligodendrocytes, the only source of myelination in the central nervous system, and discuss the relationship between white matter changes and the hallmarks of Alzheimer's disease. We review several mechanisms such as ischemia, oxidative stress, excitotoxicity, iron overload, Aβ toxicity and tauopathy, which could affect oligodendrocytes. We conclude that white matter abnormalities, and in particular myelin and oligodendrocytes, could be mechanistically important in AD pathology and could be potential treatment targets.

Keywords: Alzheimer's disease, White matter, Myelin, Oligodendrocyte, Neurodegeneration, Oxidative stress

Introduction

Alzheimer's disease (AD) is conceptualized as a progressive consequence of two hallmark pathological changes: extracellular neuritic plaques, which are composed of amyloid-beta (Aβ) surrounded by dystrophic neuritic processes, and neurofibrillary tangles, which are intraneuronal aggregates of insoluble cytoskeletal elements, composed mainly of phosphorylated tau protein. These pathological changes are believed to result in neurodegeneration, which can be appreciated with structural neuroimaging as regional and global atrophy [73]. Because of the distribution of this pathology and its associated neurodegeneration, AD is typically considered a disease of the brain's grey matter. However, over the past several years, neuroimaging studies have implicated micro- and macrostructural abnormalities in white matter in the risk and progression of AD, suggesting that in addition to the neuronal loss characteristic of the disease, white matter degeneration and demyelination may be important pathophysiological features. Myelin loss and the inability of the oligodendrocytes, the cells responsible for the production and maintenance of myelin, to repair myelin damage may be additional central features of AD [5, 53, 55, 60]. Because of the essential role of oligodendrocyte cell lineage in myelin production and remyelination processes, changes in the number of oligodendrocytes or their precursor cells and/or their dysfunction can affect myelin integrity and therefore be potentially implicated in AD pathogenesis.

The purpose of this review is to discuss the evidence for white matter abnormalities in AD with a focus on myelin damage and oligodendrocyte lineage cells and to review the relationship between white matter changes and the pathological hallmarks of AD. In addition, we discuss whether white matter changes are a secondary result of cortical AD pathology or whether they contribute directly or indirectly to the pathogenesis and clinical manifestation of AD.

* Correspondence: se2351@columbia.edu
[1]Department of Psychiatry, Columbia University, New York, NY, USA
Full list of author information is available at the end of the article

Evidence of white matter abnormalities from imaging studies

The observation that neuroimaging-defined white matter abnormalities are characteristic of AD is relatively new. Work from our laboratory, for example, demonstrated that the burden of white matter hyperintensities (WMH), distributed signal abnormalities visualized on T2-weighted magnetic resonance imaging (MRI), predicts incident AD [18, 19, 21], the rate of cognitive decline among individuals with prevalent AD [78], and is associated with genetic risk factors for late onset AD [20]. We recently showed in the Dominantly Inherited Alzheimer's Network that WMH volume is elevated among individuals with autosomal dominant, fully penetrant mutations for AD up to 20 years before the expected onset of symptoms, demonstrating that white matter abnormalities are indeed a core feature of AD. Furthermore, the appearance of WMH in these patients emerges contemporaneously with AD-related cerebrospinal fluid (CSF) amyloid and tau abnormalities [49]. WMH severity also correlates with CSF levels of Aβ1–42 in preclinical AD [49] and predicts increasing CSF tau levels in individuals with mild cognitive impairment [79]. White matter hyperintensity severity is associated with cerebrospinal fluid (CSF) amyloid levels independent of vascular risk factors [71].

The important role of vascular disease in the development of white matter damage should be emphasized. White matter hyperintensities tend to be distributed in brain areas with relatively low perfusion levels, particularly in the deep, periventricular white matter. The density of vessels in these areas decreases both with normal aging and in AD [23], consistent with reports of decreased blood flow to white matter [69], which could cause hypoxic/ischemic damage in these areas. White matter hyperintensities are related to small vessel disease, and inflammation [26, 61, 64], but comprehensive analysis of postmortem tissue in areas known to be affected by WMH, including evaluation of possible hypoxic damage to oligodendrocyte lineage cells, has not been completed. A recent study reported that parietal WMH pathogenesis in AD is related to axonal loss, through Wallerian-like degeneration, which corresponds to cortical phosphorylated tau burden, and demyelination in patients with AD but to vasculopathy and ischemia (by sclerotic index as a marker of small vessel disease and myelin associated glycoprotein to proteolipid protein ratio as a measure of hypoperfusion) in individuals without AD, suggesting that some degree of WMH is secondary to neurodegeneration in the context of AD [57]. However, neuroimaging studies showed that white matter networks are defective in preclinical AD, at a time when neurodegenerative changes, cortical atrophy, or cortical glucose reduction were not apparent [33]. Vascular and blood brain barrier (BBB) impairments, small hemorrhagic lesions and buildup of iron have been reported in the brains of AD patients even in the preclinical stages of the disease [86].

Histopathological evidence of white matter abnormalities

The neuroimaging studies establish that there is some degree of white matter abnormality in the context of AD, which may be radiological manifestations of more widespread white matter pathological abnormalities. White matter hyperintensities have been associated histopathologically with myelin pallor, myelin loss [31, 38] (as shown in Fig. 1) and the loss of myelinated axons, as well as changes in arterial adventitia in deep white matter [68]. In our aim to review the widespread white matter abnormalities, we focus on the changes in the myelin sheath and oligodendrocyte lineage cells.

Myelin damage

In the normal development of the central nervous system (CNS), different brain regions are myelinated at different times. Myelination begins in the fourth month of human embryonic development and continues until the third or fourth decade of life [22, 47] . In general, the spinal cord and brain stem myelinate earlier, while other areas, such as the telencephalon, the entorhinal cortex, hippocampus and the amygdala myelinate later [17, 30]. Diffusion tensor imaging studies show the development of association tracts in post-adolescent subjects [47]. In addition, there is a particular susceptibility for demyelination in areas that are myelinated at older ages, a phenomenon referred to as "neuropathologic retrogenesis" [8, 12, 17, 66, 76]. Myelin loss has been observed consistently in AD and the later-myelinated areas are also most vulnerable [13, 36, 65]. They demonstrate significantly greater myelin loss compared with areas that myelinate earlier [6]. Analysis of postmortem brain tissue of AD patients has revealed that the white matter is altered chemically, compared with that of patients without dementia: the amounts of total protein, myelin basic protein (MBP), myelin proteolipid protein (PLP), Cyclic nucleotide phosphohydrolase (CNPase), and cholesterol is significantly decreased, indicating a loss of myelin. White matter fatty acid ratios are also altered in AD [67].

White matter and myelin changes in AD need to be taken with respect to changes during aging. For example, the overall hemispheric white matter volume decreases with age [50]. How much of this is due to changes in water content or water infusibility is not completely clear [42]. However, a decrease in the total length of myelinated fibers, reaching a 45% decrease from 20 to 80 year-old individuals and the appearance of thinner axons has been reported [50]. Thus, a number of investigations conclude that with age, myelin production by oligodendrocytes continues but leads to thinner myelin sheaths and shorter internodes [50]. Axon caliber decreases in experimental models of demyelination and remyelination [52]. Thinner

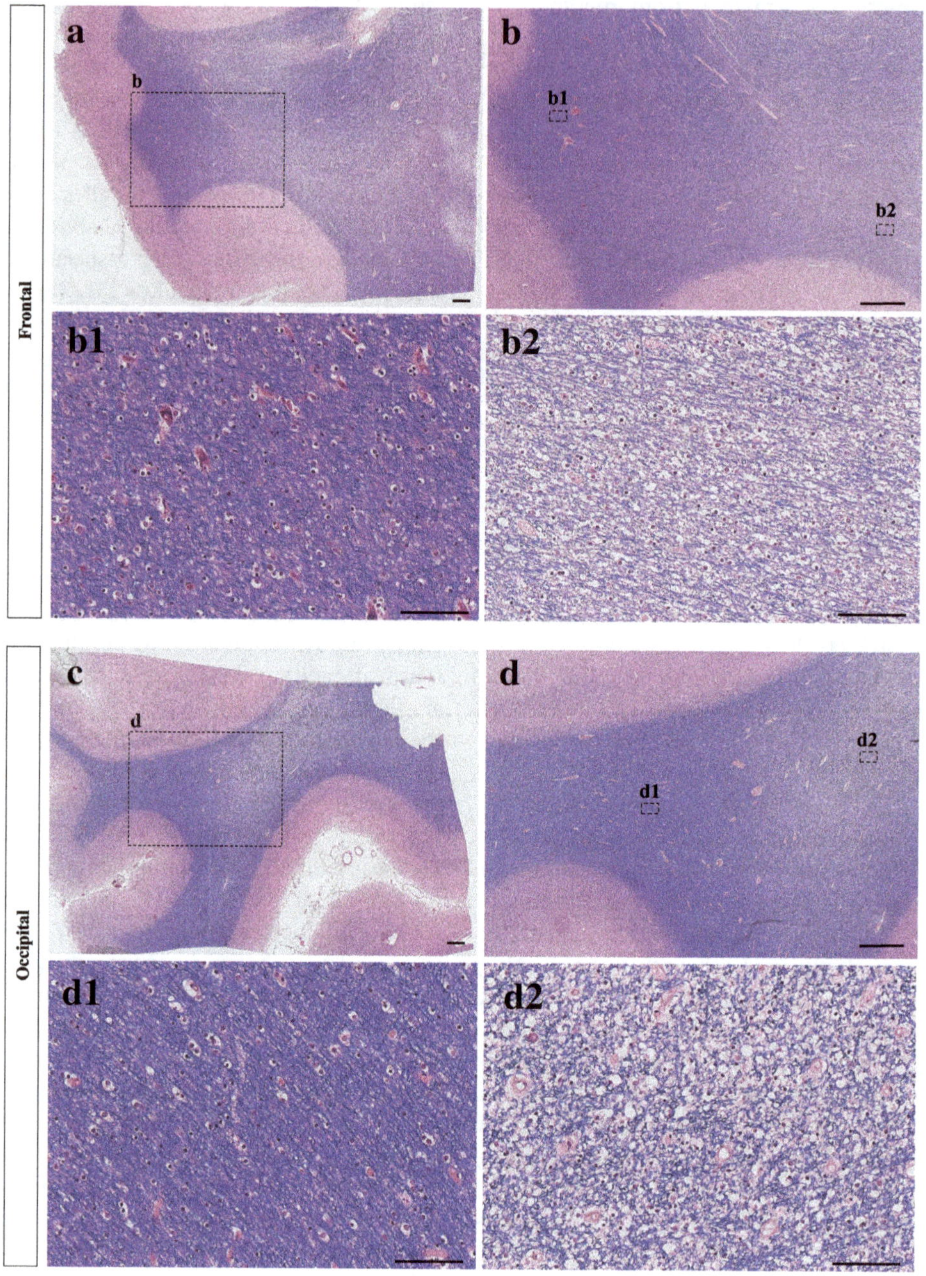

Fig. 1 This figure demonstrates examples of white matter myelin loss in brain sections from a patient with Alzheimer's disease. Tissues from frontal and occipital areas are stained with Luxol fast blue-hematoxylin and eosin (LHE). b2 and b1 represent the regions with and without myelin pallor in the frontal area, respectively. d2 and d1 represent the regions with and without myelin pallor in the occipital area, respectively. The scale bars in images **a**, **b**, **c** and **d** are 1000 μm. The scale bars in images *b1*, *b2*, *d1* and *d2* are 100 μm

myelin sheaths and smaller axons can lead to functional white matter deficits due to conduction failure and by a greater vulnerability to trauma, oxidative stress, or Aβ toxicity [5]. Axonal loss and demyelination are both associated with white matter abnormalities in AD and are predictors of severity of white matter abnormalities [57]. Future studies with the aim of preventing or repairing myelin damage could elucidate the impact of white matter changes as one of the core pathologies of AD.

Abnormalities of oligodendrocyte lineage cells in AD

The primary role of oligodendrocytes is to produce myelin, but they also play a supportive, modulatory and regulatory role for neurons, including the production of neurotrophic factors, inhibition of neurite growth, and stabilization of neuronal connectivity [44, 70]. The adult central nervous system contains both precursor cells for oligodendrocytes in addition to mature, myelinating cells [10]. Oligodendrocyte precursor cells (OPCs) in the adult central nervous system are capable of proliferating and migrating and effecting new myelination after demyelinating insults. Animal studies have shown that during adulthood, oligodendrocytes are generated from ventricular-subventricular zone and the new oligodendrocytes progenitors migrate to white matter tracks from there [59]. Mature human oligodendrocytes in the condition of being deprived from their myelin sheath may return into their previous subtype capacity and change their phenotype and their myelination program [37]. The different oligodendrocyte lineage cells express changes in morphology during their development and maturation [10]. Figure 2 shows an example of oligodendrocyte distribution throughout white matter areas in an adult postmortem human brain. In mammals, OPCs, by presence of intrinsic hypoxia-inducible factor (HIF) signaling, control white matter angiogenesis, axonal integrity, and the onset of myelination at postnatal stages [85]. Oligodendrocytes are able to modulate ion homeostasis in the axon environment [60]. OPCs are the specific glial cells that directly make synapses with neurons; they build synapses with glutamatergic neurons in the hippocampus (rat) [15], cortex (mouse) [24], white matter tracks (rat) [46] and other areas. However, they only make postsynaptic connection with neurons. The behavior of OPCs can be controlled by neurotransmitters and by surrounding neuronal demands. For example, in the presence of higher neural activity, oligodendrocytes change the amounts of myelin sheaths, which affects the

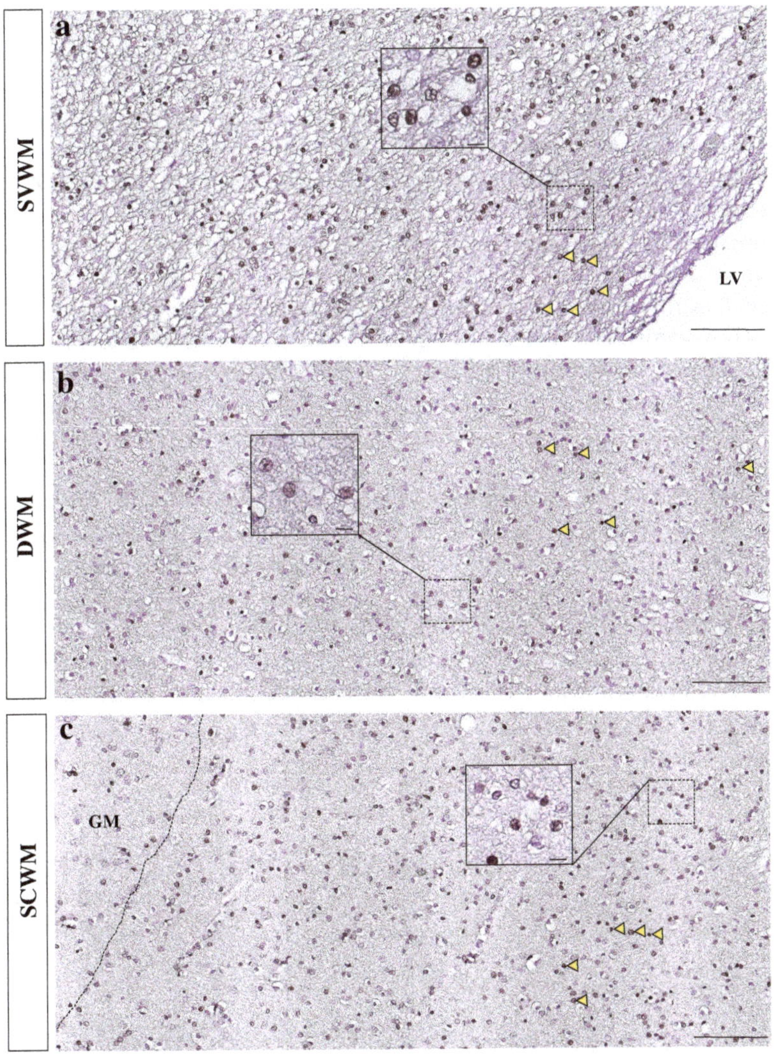

Fig. 2 An example of Olig2+ oligodendrocyte distribution throughout the white matter from a neurologically-healthy adult, postmortem brain. The insets show Olig2+ nuclei at higher magnification. H&E counterstaining. Arrowheads: Olig2+ nuclei (brown). Dashed line: the border of white and grey matter. LV: lateral ventricle; SVWM: subventricular white matter; DWM: deep white matter; SCWM: subcortical white matter; GM: grey matter. The scale bars in **a**, **b** and **c** are 100 μm and the scale bars in the insets are 10 μm

electrical transmission in the neuronal network [32]. We could speculate that neuronal AD pathology, which is characterized by neuronal and axonal dysfunction, could alter the amounts of myelin produced by oligodendrocytes. This dynamicity of myelin and oligodendrocytes thus could ultimately affect behavior [58].

A number of human and animal studies investigated oligodendrocyte changes in AD. In one study, 6–8-month-old APPPS1 mice showed an increase in the numbers of OPCs, while the number of Olig2+ cells in postmortem tissues of AD patients was decreased [11]. Another study reported a higher number of MAP-2 positive remyelinating oligodendrocytes in the areas adjacent to periventricular white matter lesions and a higher number of PDGFR-α positive OPCs in white matter lesions [74]. In a PS1 knock-in mouse model, increased vulnerability and death of oligodendrocytes due to glutamate and Aβ were demonstrated and these cells showed a deficit in calcium regulation [60]. This study suggests that the abnormalities of oligodendrocytes in the presence of a PS1 mutation could be an early event in the disease course. Another study demonstrated that MBP and the number of myelinating oligodendrocytes were decreased in 6-month old triple transgenic mice (3xTg-AD), the number of immature oligodendrocytes remained unchanged and mature non-myelinating cells were increased [29]. The authors reported that myelinating oligodendrocytes are highly sensitive to oxidative stress due to their higher metabolic demand, higher iron, and lipid content. Reduction of the diameter of oligodendrocyte nuclei in AD patients in parahippocampal white matter was also reported [35] while the mean nuclear diameter of neurons remained unchanged. Alzheimer's-related changes in oligodendrocytes for human studies and animal models are summarized in Table 1.

One of the frequently accepted themes related to oligodendrocyte damage in AD is that these cells suffer from *oxidative stress*, which can be produced by a wide range of factors. The adult CNS contains oligodendrocyte precursor cells, which can be mobilized to differentiate into myelinating oligodendrocytes [10]. Oxidative stress impairs the differentiation of OPCs, in part by decreasing the levels of expression of genes that promote oligodendrocytes differentiation, such as Shh, Sox10 and HDAC3 [34]. In cell culture, pre-oligodendrocytes show a sensitivity to oxidative stress and glutathione depletion [2]. In rat cell cultures, low antioxidant content and high iron capacity, in addition to excitotoxicity through metabotropic glutamate receptors, makes oligodendrocytes more vulnerable to oxidative stress [27, 77]. Other factors affecting oligodendrocytes are listed below.

Aβ and tau: Several studies suggest that Aβ is toxic to oligodendrocytes [28, 29, 41, 48, 84]. For example, a cell culture study of rat oligodendrocytes demonstrated that Aβ-induced oxidative stress can drive oligodendrocyte death and dysfunction [84]. This study also showed that mitochondrial DNA damage and the consequent NF-kB and AP-1 activation are other possible mechanisms of Aβ toxicity for oligodendrocytes [84]. Note that although amyloid plaques are exceedingly rare in AD white matter, the levels of soluble Aβ are elevated in the white matter [25]. Thus, a direct exposure of white matter oligodendrocytes to increased amounts of Aβ is likely. Although there are toxic effects of Aβ on oligodendrocytes, clinical trials that have aimed to remove the Aβ plaque in symptomatic AD patients, did not prevent the progressive neurodegeneration and cognitive decline in AD patients [39, 72]. These findings suggest that this toxic effect needs to be targeted earlier or it could not be the only pathology leading to cell death and atrophy in symptomatic patients. In addition to the effects of amyloid pathology, the impact of tau pathology on white matter needs to be considered. Tau can affect the normal function of neurons through a toxic gain of function or a loss of its normal function in stabilizing microtubules. Although severe neocortical tauopathy occurs in later stages of AD and mostly affects grey matter, phosphorylated tau transforms into neurofibrillary tangles in neurons as well as glial tangles in astrocytes

Table 1 This table summarizes the studies, the specimen that was used, and oligodendrocyte alterations in AD animal models and human

The model and specimen	Oligodendrocyte changes			Source
PS1 knock-in mouse	Vulnerability and death of OLs			Pak et al. 2003
Postmortem AD	Increased MAP-2 positive remyelinating OLs adjacent to WM lesions	Increased PDGFR- α positive OPCs in WM lesions	No change in Myelinating OLs in deep white matter	Simpson et al. 2007
3xTg-AD mouse	Decreased myelinating OLs	No change in immature OLs	Increased mature non-myelinating OLs	Desai et al. 2010
Postmortem AD	Reduced OLs nuclear diameter in parahippocampal white matter			Gagyi et al. 2011
APPPS1 mouse	Increased OPCs number			Behrendt et al. 2013
Postmortem AD	Decreased Olig2+			Behrendt et al. 2013

It depicts the verity of the results in different animal models and human studies. *PS1* Presenelin-1, *OL* oligodendrocyte, *MAP* microtubule associated protein, *PDGFR* platelet-derived growth factor receptor, *OPCs* oligodendrocyte progenitor cells, *WM* white matter, *3xTg-AD* triple transgenic AD mouse model. *APPPS1 mouse* mouse with both APP and PS1 transgenes

or oligodendroglia [4]. Furthermore, phosphorylated tau in grey matter is associated with white matter abnormalities and demyelination in AD patients [56, 57]. The increased levels of calpain2 in the AD white matter, an indicator of axonal loss, was shown to be associated with increased cortical phosphorylated tau and amyloid [57] and the phosphorylated tau showed to be a predictor for white matter hyperintensities [56].

Iron: During myelination, oligodendrocytes require 2–3 fold higher energy levels than other cell types in the CNS to produce such an extensive amount of membrane. Oligodendrocytes synthesize cholesterol, a process that is highly metabolically demanding, making them vulnerable to hypoperfusion, excitotoxicity, heavy metals, and free radicals that induce oxidative stress. Oligodendrocytes have the highest iron content of all cell types, which increases with age and even further in AD [5]. Oligodendrocytes at all stages of their differentiation, compared with other glial cells contain smaller amounts of antioxidant agents (e.g. glutathione peroxidase) and only half of the glutathione reductase activity [43]. Thus, a high iron content and a low antioxidant content make oligodendrocytes one of the most vulnerable cell classes to oxidative stress in the CNS. If oxidative stress is exacerbated by age, it may lead to increased cell damage [81]. Bartzokis by comparing a map of cortical myelination with maps of Aβ deposition hypothesized that age-associated myelin breakdown leads to iron release from oligodendrocytes and that this iron release promotes Aβ oligomerization in the parenchyma [7].

Hypoxia/Ischemia: Deep white matter areas lie at the ends of the CNS arterial circulation, making them susceptible to decreases in blood flow and oxygenation. Some anterior and posterior white matter lies in watershed zones between the anterior cerebral and middle cerebral arteries and middle cerebral and posterior cerebral arteries respectively. Vascular pathology in these regions is greater in patients with AD than in individuals without dementia [23, 69]. Late-stage oligodendrocyte progenitors are more sensitive to hypoxic or ischemic damage than early-stage progenitors and more mature oligodendrocytes [3]. A recent rodent study, using single cell RNA sequencing, identified a population of oligodendrocyte precursors as vascular and leptomeningeal cells. These OPCs are located along vessels and they show similarities with pericyte lineage cells [51]. In addition, to emphasize the importance of relationship between vascular system and oligodendrocyte lineage cells Tsai showed that those OPCs require the physical infrastructure provided by the vascular system to facilitate their migration during development [80].

Excitotoxicity: In general, oligodendrocytes show a great vulnerability to excessive ATP and/or activation of glutamate receptors [55]. Oligodendrocytes express a wide variety of receptors and membrane channels (e.g. ionotropic glutamate and ATP receptors, ligand gated Ca^{2+} channels and P2x7 receptors). Because of the lack of the GluR2 subunit in oligodendrocyte AMPA receptors, there is a higher permeability to Ca^{2+} ions compared with neurons [54]. Another example is the sustained activation of p2x7 receptors in oligodendrocytes due to excitotoxicity or to high levels of ATP/ADP/AMP, which leads to excessive Ca^{2+} in the cytosol and the activation of apoptosis through caspase-3 activation. Extensive activation of these receptors can result in oligodendrocyte damage and subsequently myelin destruction. Back and colleagues showed maturation-dependent vulnerability of oligodendrocytes caused by intracellular glutathione depletion [2]. In addition, as we mentioned, oligodendrocytes and myelin damage due to excitotoxicity and calcium dysregulation could be an early pathological feature of AD [45, 60].

DNA damage: Age related DNA damage in myelinating oligodendrocytes may contribute to myelin loss [81, 82]. Postmortem analysis of white matter lesions obtained from aging individuals shows the presence of oxidative damage (8-OHdG immunoreactivity) in oligodendrocyte nuclear DNA. These cells are also positive for senescence markers such as SA-β-gal [1]. In older adults, excessive DNA damage occurs in vulnerable oligodendrocytes and the DNA repair mechanism becomes overwhelmed. Studies of changes in genomic integrity and genomic instability of oligodendrocytes in the white matter of patients and animal models could illuminate the role of oligodendrocyte in white matter damage and pathology of AD [81, 82]. In addition, oligodendrocyte lineage transcription factor 2 (Olig2) is located on chromosome 21 which is 6.8 Mb telomeric of the amyloid precursor protein (APP) gene. The possibility of these two genes interacting in a context of the disease needs to be studied [75].

Discussion

A variety of structural, histopathological and biochemical pathologies take place in the white matter of AD patients (summarized in Fig. 3). In this review, we have tried to answer two questions:

> *What changes occur in white matter in the course of AD and what is the relationship between these changes and the pathological hallmarks of the disease?*

Radiological, pathological, and molecular changes occur in the white matter of AD patients. Radiological markers of white matter damage occur as early as 22 years before the estimated age of symptom onset in humans who carry AD mutations [49]. These white matter changes are believed to reflect demyelination and axon damage [63]. It is possible that the oligodendrocytes or the precursors responsible for remyelination of these areas are altered in number and in DNA stability or are functionally less efficient in the presence of genetic changes, oxidative stress, increased iron

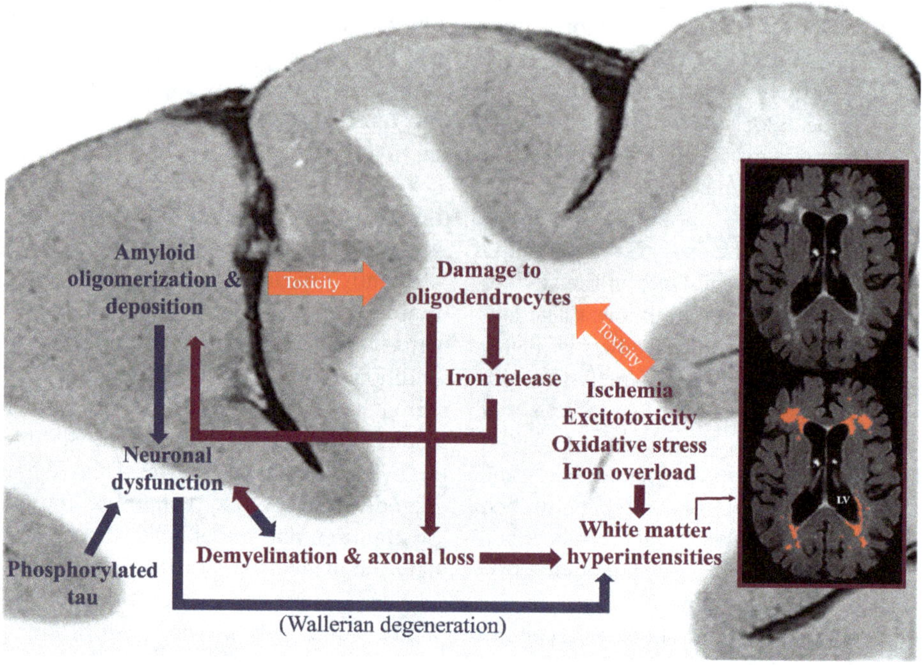

Fig. 3 This figure summarizes the pathological cascades, and their relation with each other, occurring during the development of Alzheimer's disease in white matter and cortex. While ischemia, excitotoxicity, oxidative stress, and iron overload in white matter damage oligodendrocytes, on one hand, and amyloid toxicity affects them, on the other hand, the iron released from damaged oligodendrocytes promotes amyloid polymerization and deposition in grey matter. The consequent demyelination and axonal loss result in further white matter damage and neuronal dysfunction. Neuronal dysfunction is also a result of amyloid deposition in cortex and a proposed cause for white matter abnormalities in AD patients. White matter hyperintensities are labelled with red in the MRI (FLAIR) scan of an AD patient. Blue arrows: direction of the damages originating in grey matter. Maroon arrows: direction of the damages originating in white matter. LV lateral ventricle

levels, and vascular pathology [5, 81]. In addition to gross white matter damage in AD, there are chemical alterations marked by loss of proteins and cholesterol. The decreases in the levels of myelin proteins, such as myelin basic protein (MBP), myelin proteolipid protein (PLP) and CNPase, in white matter reflects the changes in oligodendrocytes and myelin sheaths. In animal models of AD, the white matter disruption and changes in myelin marker expression are among the earliest pathological changes [16, 30]. Although white matter changes are believed to be partly related to neuronal degeneration in the cortex [57], there is also evidence that oligodendrocyte and myelin pathology, which are detected in AD mouse models, are affected prior to appearance of amyloid and cortical pathology. It is not clear if these changes are independent of cortical pathology or the cortical structural damages are beyond the detection limits of methods at early stages of the disease [29, 30, 40] and subtle neurodegenerative changes could precede or promote white matter changes even if they are not detectable with conventional methods. In terms of therapeutic implications, contemporary clinical trials have focused on the removal of fibrillar forms of amyloid protein as a primary target, motivated by the "amyloid hypothesis" that has dominated the field's conceptualization of the disease for many years [73]. Accordingly, interventions that target the removal of amyloid would arrest the progression of disease and improve cognitive outcomes. However, to date, clinical trials aimed to clear Aβ plaques in AD have not resulted in clinical improvement or reduction in the rates of disease progression. New strategies for disease treatment and prevention are therefore necessary. The consistent observations that implicate white matter abnormalities in AD pathogenesis and progression point to opportunities to target potential novel mechanisms implicated in the disease.

Are the clinical changes in AD secondary only to the cortical hallmarks of the disease or do white matter abnormalities contribute directly or indirectly to the disease?

Beside amyloid hypothesis as the cause of AD, it is crucial to note that there is a weak association between amyloid plaques and AD symptoms [5]. Further, senile plaques can be found in about 20–40% of older adults without symptoms of dementia and cognitive impairment [14, 62]. As discussed above, myelin loss contributes to cognitive decline in humans [67, 83] and in AD animal models, early changes in white matter are followed by the first cognitive impairment detected after intracellular accumulation of Aβ but before Aβ plaques appear [29]. Altering axonal conduction by demyelination or axonal damage could directly and/or indirectly affect cognition. Future studies with the aim of repairing myelin loss could clarify the impact of white matter changes on AD pathogenesis and may have therapeutic benefit. In addition, dysfunctional oligodendrocytes early in the course of the disease may not be able to play a protective role for neurons and their axons. Hence, the process of remyelination and myelin repair will be affected. Signal conductivity, and synchronicity of impulses, which are required for information processing between neurons, depend on the amount of myelin produced by oligodendrocytes and therefore will be affected [10]. In general, a number of animal AD model studies suggest that white matter pathology emerges prior to appearance of cortical plaques and tangles [29, 30, 40]. Human studies with autosomal dominant forms of AD suggest that Aβ levels begin to change as early as 25–30 years prior to symptom onset, followed by tau pathology about 15 years prior to symptom onset, cerebral hypometabolism, brain atrophy, and cognitive and functional deficits [9, 29]. As noted above white matter abnormalities are also early findings in these patients [49], but causal relationships among AD biomarkers in humans are difficult to infer even from observed temporally-ordered observations; white matter changes appear to emerge contemporaneously with other AD pathology, but it is unclear if one is causing the other. Studies of 3xTg-AD triple transgenic AD mice show that the first pathological features start to appear in 2 to 6-month old mice as white matter disruption and changes in myelin marker expression in the hippocampus and entorhinal cortex. At this age, the mice do not show learning or memory deficits [16, 30]. Cognitive impairment emerges after at around 3 to 6-months of age [29]. The studies discussed regarding vascular insufficiency in white matter suggest that the white matter pathology is not caused by cortical pathology. On the other hand, neuronal accumulation of tangles and neuronal death will lead to axonal loss in white matter [57]. It is not clear how this would produce white matter hyperintensities in deep white matter, however, it could well contribute to a more widespread decrease in axons and myelin.

In conclusion, the various observations suggest that white matter abnormalities and in particular impaired myelin and oligodendrocytes could promote cognitive impairment and AD pathology and could be the important targets for studying and early treatments of AD. Future studies with the aim of repairing myelin damage, beside other efforts focused on the hallmark of Alzheimer's disease, could elucidate the impact of white matter changes as one of the core pathologies of AD.

Abbreviations

3xTg-AD: triple transgenic AD mice model; AD: Alzheimer's disease; AP-1: activator protein 1; ATP: adenosine triphosphate; Aβ: amyloid-beta; BBB: blood brain barrier; CNPase: cyclic nucleotide phosphohydrolase; CNS: central nervous system; CSF: cerebrospinal fluid; HDAC3: histone deacetylase 3; HIF: hypoxia-inducible factor; MBP: myelin basic protein; MRI: magnetic resonance imaging; NF-kB: nuclear factor kappa-light-chain-enhancer of activated B cells; OPC: oligodendrocyte precursor cell; P2x7 receptors: P2X purinoceptor 7; PLP: myelin proteolipid protein; Shh: sonic hedgehog; Sox-10: SRY-related HMG-box; WMH: white matter hyperintensity

Acknowledgements

This work was supported by grants from the Alzheimer's Association, the Taub Institute at Columbia University, the Mary E. Groff Surgical Medical Research and Education Charitable Trust Groff Foundation, and NIH (P50 AG008702). Dr. Nasrabady is supported by NIH T32 grant (MH 20004-19), Division of Late-Life NeuroPsychiatric Disorders, Department of Psychiatry.

Authors' contributions

SEN, JEG and AMB conceptualized the review, drafted the manuscript, read and approved the final manuscript. BR contributed towards the creation of the figures, read and approved the final manuscript.

Competing interests

The authors declare that they have no competing interests.

Author details

[1]Department of Psychiatry, Columbia University, New York, NY, USA. [2]Department of Pathology and Cell Biology, Columbia University, New York, NY, USA. [3]Department of Neurology, Columbia University, New York, NY, USA. [4]The Taub Institute for Research in Alzheimer's Disease and the Aging Brain, Columbia University, New York, NY, USA.

References

1. Al-Mashhadi S, Simpson JE, Heath PR, Dickman M, Forster G, Matthews FE, Brayne C, Ince PG, Wharton SB (2015) Oxidative glial cell damage associated with white matter lesions in the aging human brain. Brain pathology (Zurich, Switzerland) 25:565–574. https://doi.org/10.1111/bpa.12216
2. Back SA, Gan X, Li Y, Rosenberg PA, Volpe JJ (1998) Maturation-dependent vulnerability of oligodendrocytes to oxidative stress-induced death caused by glutathione depletion. J Neurosci 18:6241–6253
3. Back SA, Han BH, Luo NL, Chricton CA, Xanthoudakis S, Tam J, Arvin KL, Holtzman DM (2002) Selective vulnerability of late oligodendrocyte progenitors to hypoxia-ischemia. J Neurosci 22:455–463
4. Ballatore C, Lee VM, Trojanowski JQ (2007) Tau-mediated neurodegeneration in Alzheimer's disease and related disorders. Nat Rev Neurosci 8:663–672. https://doi.org/10.1038/nrn2194
5. Bartzokis G (2011) Alzheimer's disease as homeostatic responses to age-related myelin breakdown. Neurobiol Aging 32: 1341-1371 Doi 0.1016/j.Neurobiolaging.2009.08.007
6. Bartzokis G, Cummings JL, Sultzer D, Henderson VW, Nuechterlein KH, Mintz J (2003) White matter structural integrity in healthy aging adults and patients with Alzheimer disease: a magnetic resonance imaging study. Arch Neurol 60:393–398
7. Bartzokis G, Lu PH, Mintz J (2007) Human brain myelination and amyloid beta deposition in Alzheimer's disease. Alzheimers Dement 3:122–125. https://doi.org/10.1016/j.jalz.2007.01.019
8. Bartzokis G, Sultzer D, Lu PH, Nuechterlein KH, Mintz J, Cummings JL (2004) Heterogeneous age-related breakdown of white matter structural integrity: implications for cortical "disconnection" in aging and Alzheimer's disease. Neurobiol Aging 25:843–851. https://doi.org/10.1016/j.neurobiolaging.2003.09.005
9. Bateman RJ, Xiong C, Benzinger TL, Fagan AM, Goate A, Fox NC, Marcus DS, Cairns NJ, Xie X, Blazey TMet al (2012) Clinical and biomarker changes in

dominantly inherited Alzheimer's disease. N Engl J Med 367: 795–804 Doi https://doi.org/10.1056/NEJMoa1202753
10. Baumann N, Pham-Dinh D (2001) Biology of oligodendrocyte and myelin in the mammalian central nervous system. Physiol Rev 81:871–927
11. Behrendt G, Baer K, Buffo A, Curtis MA, Faull RL, Rees MI, Gotz M, Dimou L (2013) Dynamic changes in myelin aberrations and oligodendrocyte generation in chronic amyloidosis in mice and men. Glia 61:273–286. https://doi.org/10.1002/glia.22432
12. Bender AR, Volkle MC, Raz N (2016) Differential aging of cerebral white matter in middle-aged and older adults: a seven-year follow-up. NeuroImage 125:74–83. https://doi.org/10.1016/j.neuroimage.2015.10.030
13. Benitez A, Fieremans E, Jensen JH, Falangola MF, Tabesh A, Ferris SH, Helpern JA (2014) White matter tract integrity metrics reflect the vulnerability of late-myelinating tracts in Alzheimer's disease. NeuroImage Clinical 4:64–71. https://doi.org/10.1016/j.nicl.2013.11.001
14. Bennett DA, Schneider JA, Arvanitakis Z, Kelly JF, Aggarwal NT, Shah RC, Wilson RS (2006) Neuropathology of older persons without cognitive impairment from two community-based studies. Neurology 66:1837–1844. https://doi.org/10.1212/01.wnl.0000219668.47116.e6
15. Bergles DE, Roberts JD, Somogyi P, Jahr CE (2000) Glutamatergic synapses on oligodendrocyte precursor cells in the hippocampus. Nature 405:187–191. https://doi.org/10.1038/35012083
16. Billings LM, Oddo S, Green KN, McGaugh JL, LaFerla FM (2005) Intraneuronal Abeta causes the onset of early Alzheimer's disease-related cognitive deficits in transgenic mice. Neuron 45:675–688. https://doi.org/10.1016/j.neuron.2005.01.040
17. Braak H, Braak E (1996) Development of Alzheimer-related neurofibrillary changes in the neocortex inversely recapitulates cortical myelogenesis. Acta Neuropathol 92:197–201
18. Brickman AM (2013) Contemplating Alzheimer's disease and the contribution of white matter hyperintensities. Curr Neurol Neurosci Rep 13: 415. https://doi.org/10.1007/s11910-013-0415-7
19. Brickman AM, Provenzano FA, Muraskin J, Manly JJ, Blum S, Apa Z, Stern Y, Brown TR, Luchsinger JA, Mayeux R (2012) Regional white matter hyperintensity volume, not hippocampal atrophy, predicts incident Alzheimer disease in the community. Arch Neurol 69:1621–1627. https://doi.org/10.1001/archneurol.2012.1527
20. Brickman AM, Schupf N, Manly JJ, Stern Y, Luchsinger JA, Provenzano FA, Narkhede A, Razlighi Q, Collins-Praino L, Artero S et al (2014) APOE epsilon4 and risk for Alzheimer's disease: do regionally distributed white matter hyperintensities play a role? Alzheimers Dement 10:619–629. https://doi.org/10.1016/j.jalz.2014.07.155
21. Brickman AM, Zahodne LB, Guzman VA, Narkhede A, Meier IB, Griffith EY, Provenzano FA, Schupf N, Manly JJ, Stern Y et al (2015) Reconsidering harbingers of dementia: progression of parietal lobe white matter hyperintensities predicts Alzheimer's disease incidence. Neurobiol Aging 36: 27–32. https://doi.org/10.1016/j.neurobiolaging.2014.07.019
22. Brody BA, Kinney HC, Kloman AS, Gilles FH (1987) Sequence of central nervous system myelination in human infancy. I. An autopsy study of myelination. J Neuropathol Exp Neurol 46:283–301
23. Brown WR, Thore CR (2011) Review: cerebral microvascular pathology in ageing and neurodegeneration. Neuropathol Appl Neurobiol 37:56–74. https://doi.org/10.1111/j.1365-2990.2010.01139.x
24. Chittajallu R, Aguirre A, Gallo V (2004) NG2-positive cells in the mouse white and grey matter display distinct physiological properties. J Physiol 561:109–122. https://doi.org/10.1113/jphysiol.2004.074252
25. Collins-Praino LE, Francis YI, Griffith EY, Wiegman AF, Urbach J, Lawton A, Honig LS, Cortes E, Vonsattel JP, Canoll PD et al (2014) Soluble amyloid beta levels are elevated in the white matter of Alzheimer's patients, independent of cortical plaque severity. Acta Neuropathol Commun 2:83. https://doi.org/10.1186/s40478-014-0083-0 10.1186/preaccept-3091772881321882
26. De Leeuw FE, Barkhof F, Scheltens P (2004) Alzheimer's disease–one clinical syndrome, two radiological expressions: a study on blood pressure. J Neurol Neurosurg Psychiatry 75:1270–1274. https://doi.org/10.1136/jnnp.2003.030189
27. Deng W, Wang H, Rosenberg PA, Volpe JJ, Jensen FE (2004) Role of metabotropic glutamate receptors in oligodendrocyte excitotoxicity and oxidative stress. Proc Natl Acad Sci U S A 101:7751–7756. https://doi.org/10.1073/pnas.0307850101
28. Desai MK, Guercio BJ, Narrow WC, Bowers WJ (2011) An Alzheimer's disease-relevant presenilin-1 mutation augments amyloid-beta-induced oligodendrocyte dysfunction. Glia 59:627–640. https://doi.org/10.1002/glia.21131
29. Desai MK, Mastrangelo MA, Ryan DA, Sudol KL, Narrow WC, Bowers WJ (2010) Early oligodendrocyte/myelin pathology in Alzheimer's disease mice constitutes a novel therapeutic target. Am J Pathol 177:1422–1435. https://doi.org/10.2353/ajpath.2010.100087
30. Desai MK, Sudol KL, Janelsins MC, Mastrangelo MA, Frazer ME, Bowers WJ (2009) Triple-transgenic Alzheimer's disease mice exhibit region-specific abnormalities in brain myelination patterns prior to appearance of amyloid and tau pathology. Glia 57:54–65. https://doi.org/10.1002/glia.20734
31. Erten-Lyons D, Woltjer R, Kaye J, Mattek N, Dodge HH, Green S, Tran H, Howieson DB, Wild K, Silbert LC (2013) Neuropathologic basis of white matter hyperintensity accumulation with advanced age. Neurology 81:977–983. https://doi.org/10.1212/WNL.0b013e3182a43e45
32. Fields RD (2015) A new mechanism of nervous system plasticity: activity-dependent myelination. Nat Rev Neurosci 16:756–767. https://doi.org/10.1038/nrn4023
33. Fischer FU, Wolf D, Scheurich A, Fellgiebel A (2015) Altered whole-brain white matter networks in preclinical Alzheimer's disease. NeuroImage Clinical 8:660–666. https://doi.org/10.1016/j.nicl.2015.06.007
34. French HM, Reid M, Mamontov P, Simmons RA, Grinspan JB (2009) Oxidative stress disrupts oligodendrocyte maturation. J Neurosci Res 87: 3076–3087. https://doi.org/10.1002/jnr.22139
35. Gagyi E, Kormos B, Castellanos KJ, Valyi-Nagy K, Korneff D, LoPresti P, Woltjer R, Valyi-Nagy T (2012) Decreased oligodendrocyte nuclear diameter in Alzheimer's disease and Lewy body dementia. Brain pathology (Zurich, Switzerland) 22:803–810. https://doi.org/10.1111/j.1750-3639.2012.00595.x
36. Gao J, Cheung RT, Lee TM, Chu LW, Chan YS, Mak HK, Zhang JX, Qiu D, Fung G, Cheung C (2011) Possible retrogenesis observed with fiber tracking: an anteroposterior pattern of white matter disintegrity in normal aging and Alzheimer's disease. Journal of Alzheimer's disease : JAD 26:47–58. https://doi.org/10.3233/jad-2011-101788
37. Gogate N, Verma L, Zhou JM, Milward E, Rusten R, O'Connor M, Kufta C, Kim J, Hudson L, Dubois-Dalcq M (1994) Plasticity in the adult human oligodendrocyte lineage. The Journal of neuroscience : the official journal of the Society for Neuroscience 14:4571–4587
38. Gouw AA, Seewann A, Vrenken H, van der Flier WM, Rozemuller JM, Barkhof F, Scheltens P, Geurts JJ (2008) Heterogeneity of white matter hyperintensities in Alzheimer's disease: post-mortem quantitative MRI and neuropathology. Brain : a journal of neurology 131:3286–3298. https://doi.org/10.1093/brain/awn265
39. Holmes C, Boche D, Wilkinson D, Yadegarfar G, Hopkins V, Bayer A, Jones RW, Bullock R, Love S, Neal JWet al (2008) Long-term effects of Abeta42 immunisation in Alzheimer's disease: follow-up of a randomised, placebo-controlled phase I trial. Lancet (London, England) 372: 216-223 Doi https://doi.org/10.1016/s0140-6736(08)61075-2
40. Horiuchi M, Maezawa I, Itoh A, Wakayama K, Jin LW, Itoh T, Decarli C (2012) Amyloid beta1-42 oligomer inhibits myelin sheet formation in vitro. Neurobiol Aging 33:499–509. https://doi.org/10.1016/j.neurobiolaging.2010.05.007
41. Jantaratnotai N, Ryu JK, Kim SU, McLarnon JG (2003) Amyloid beta peptide-induced corpus callosum damage and glial activation in vivo. Neuroreport 14:1429–1433. https://doi.org/10.1097/01.wnr.0000086097.47480.a0
42. Jorgensen AM, Marner L, Pakkenberg B (2008) No change in total length of white matter fibers in Alzheimer's disease. Neuroscience 157:878–883. https://doi.org/10.1016/j.neuroscience.2008.06.075
43. Juurlink BH, Thorburne SK, Hertz L (1998) Peroxide-scavenging deficit underlies oligodendrocyte susceptibility to oxidative stress. Glia 22:371–378
44. Kapfhammer JP, Schwab ME (1994) Inverse patterns of myelination and GAP-43 expression in the adult CNS: neurite growth inhibitors as regulators of neuronal plasticity? J Comp Neurol 340:194–206. https://doi.org/10.1002/cne.903400206
45. Kelleher RJ 3rd, Shen J (2017) Presenilin-1 mutations and Alzheimer's disease. Proc Natl Acad Sci U S A 114:629–631. https://doi.org/10.1073/pnas.1619574114
46. Kukley M, Capetillo-Zarate E, Dietrich D (2007) Vesicular glutamate release from axons in white matter. Nat Neurosci 10:311–320. https://doi.org/10.1038/nn1850
47. Lebel C, Beaulieu C (2011) Longitudinal development of human brain wiring continues from childhood into adulthood. J Neurosci 31:10937–10947. https://doi.org/10.1523/jneurosci.5302-10.2011
48. Lee JT, Xu J, Lee JM, Ku G, Han X, Yang DI, Chen S, Hsu CY (2004) Amyloid-beta peptide induces oligodendrocyte death by activating the neutral sphingomyelinase-ceramide pathway. J Cell Biol 164:123–131. https://doi.org/10.1083/jcb.200307017

49. Lee S, Viqar F, Zimmerman ME, Narkhede A, Tosto G, Benzinger TL, Marcus DS, Fagan AM, Goate A, Fox NC et al (2016) White matter hyperintensities are a core feature of Alzheimer's disease: evidence from the dominantly inherited Alzheimer network. Ann Neurol 79:929–939. https://doi.org/10.1002/ana.24647
50. Marner L, Nyengaard JR, Tang Y, Pakkenberg B (2003) Marked loss of myelinated nerve fibers in the human brain with age. J Comp Neurol 462: 144–152. https://doi.org/10.1002/cne.10714
51. Marques S, Zeisel A, Codeluppi S, van Bruggen D, Mendanha Falcao A, Xiao L, Li H, Haring M, Hochgerner H, Romanov RAet al (2016) Oligodendrocyte heterogeneity in the mouse juvenile and adult central nervous system. Science (New York, NY) 352: 1326-1329 Doi https://doi.org/10.1126/science.aaf6463
52. Mason JL, Langaman C, Morell P, Suzuki K, Matsushima GK (2001) Episodic demyelination and subsequent remyelination within the murine central nervous system: changes in axonal calibre. Neuropathol Appl Neurobiol 27: 50–58
53. Matute C (2010) Calcium dyshomeostasis in white matter pathology. Cell Calcium 47:150–157. https://doi.org/10.1016/j.ceca.2009.12.004
54. Matute C (2006) Oligodendrocyte NMDA receptors: a novel therapeutic target. Trends Mol Med 12:289–292. https://doi.org/10.1016/j.molmed.2006.05.004
55. Matute C, Alberdi E, Domercq M, Sanchez-Gomez MV, Perez-Samartin A, Rodriguez-Antiguedad A, Perez-Cerda F (2007) Excitotoxic damage to white matter. J Anat 210:693–702. https://doi.org/10.1111/j.1469-7580.2007.00733.x
56. McAleese KE, Firbank M, Dey M, Colloby SJ, Walker L, Johnson M, Beverley JR, Taylor JP, Thomas AJ, O'Brien JT et al (2015) Cortical tau load is associated with white matter hyperintensities. Acta neuropathologica communications 3:60. https://doi.org/10.1186/s40478-015-0240-0
57. McAleese KE, Walker L, Graham S, Moya ELJ, Johnson M, Erskine D, Colloby SJ, Dey M, Martin-Ruiz C, Taylor JP et al (2017) Parietal white matter lesions in Alzheimer's disease are associated with cortical neurodegenerative pathology, but not with small vessel disease. Acta neuropathologica. https://doi.org/10.1007/s00401-017-1738-2
58. McKenzie IA, Ohayon D, Li H, de Faria JP, Emery B, Tohyama K, Richardson WD (2014) Motor skill learning requires active central myelination. Science (New York, NY) 346:318–322. https://doi.org/10.1126/science.1254960
59. Menn B, Garcia-Verdugo JM, Yaschine C, Gonzalez-Perez O, Rowitch D, Alvarez-Buylla A (2006) Origin of oligodendrocytes in the subventricular zone of the adult brain. J Neurosci 26:7907–7918. https://doi.org/10.1523/jneurosci.1299-06.2006
60. Pak K, Chan SL, Mattson MP (2003) Presenilin-1 mutation sensitizes oligodendrocytes to glutamate and amyloid toxicities, and exacerbates white matter damage and memory impairment in mice. NeuroMolecular Med 3:53–64. https://doi.org/10.1385/nmm:3:1:53
61. Pantoni L, Garcia JH (1997) Cognitive impairment and cellular/vascular changes in the cerebral white matter. Ann N Y Acad Sci 826:92–102
62. Price JL, McKeel DW Jr, Buckles VD, Roe CM, Xiong C, Grundman M, Hansen LA, Petersen RC, Parisi JE, Dickson DW et al (2009) Neuropathology of nondemented aging: presumptive evidence for preclinical Alzheimer disease. Neurobiol Aging 30:1026–1036. https://doi.org/10.1016/j.neurobiolaging.2009.04.002
63. Prins ND, Scheltens P (2015) White matter hyperintensities, cognitive impairment and dementia: an update. Nat Rev Neurol 11:157–165. https://doi.org/10.1038/nrneurol.2015.10
64. Raz N, Yang Y, Dahle CL, Land S (2012) Volume of white matter hyperintensities in healthy adults: contribution of age, vascular risk factors, and inflammation-related genetic variants. Biochim Biophys Acta 1822:361–369. https://doi.org/10.1016/j.bbadis.2011.08.007
65. Reisberg B, Franssen EH, Hasan SM, Monteiro I, Boksay I, Souren LE, Kenowsky S, Auer SR, Elahi S, Kluger A (1999) Retrogenesis: clinical, physiologic, and pathologic mechanisms in brain aging, Alzheimer's and other dementing processes. Eur Arch Psychiatry Clin Neurosci 249(Suppl 3):28–36
66. Reisberg B, Franssen EH, Souren LE, Auer SR, Akram I, Kenowsky S (2002) Evidence and mechanisms of retrogenesis in Alzheimer's and other dementias: management and treatment import. Am J Alzheimers Dis Other Demen 17:202–212. https://doi.org/10.1177/153331750201700411
67. Roher AE, Weiss N, Kokjohn TA, Kuo YM, Kalback W, Anthony J, Watson D, Luehrs DC, Sue L, al WD (2002) Increased a beta peptides and reduced cholesterol and myelin proteins characterize white matter degeneration in Alzheimer's disease. Biochemistry 41:11080–11090
68. Scheltens P, Barkhof F, Leys D, Wolters EC, Ravid R, Kamphorst W (1995) Histopathologic correlates of white matter changes on MRI in Alzheimer's disease and normal aging. Neurology 45:883–888
69. Schuff N, Matsumoto S, Kmiecik J, Studholme C, Du A, Ezekiel F, Miller BL, Kramer JH, Jagust WJ, Chui HC et al (2009) Cerebral blood flow in ischemic vascular dementia and Alzheimer's disease, measured by arterial spin-labeling magnetic resonance imaging. Alzheimers Dement 5:454–462. https://doi.org/10.1016/j.jalz.2009.04.1233
70. Schwab ME (1990) Myelin-associated inhibitors of neurite growth and regeneration in the CNS. Trends Neurosci 13:452–456
71. Scott JA, Braskie MN, Tosun D, Thompson PM, Weiner M, DeCarli C, Carmichael OT (2015) Cerebral amyloid and hypertension are independently associated with white matter lesions in elderly. Front Aging Neurosci 7:221. https://doi.org/10.3389/fnagi.2015.00221
72. Selkoe DJ (2011) Resolving controversies on the path to Alzheimer's therapeutics. Nat Med 17:1060–1065. https://doi.org/10.1038/nm.2460
73. Selkoe DJ, Hardy J (2016) The amyloid hypothesis of Alzheimer's disease at 25 years. EMBO Mol Med 8:595–608. https://doi.org/10.15252/emmm.201606210
74. Simpson JE, Fernando MS, Clark L, Ince PG, Matthews F, Forster G, O'Brien JT, Barber R, Kalaria RN, Brayne C et al (2007) White matter lesions in an unselected cohort of the elderly: astrocytic, microglial and oligodendrocyte precursor cell responses. Neuropathol Appl Neurobiol 33:410–419. https://doi.org/10.1111/j.1365-2990.2007.00828.x
75. Sims R, Hollingworth P, Moskvina V, Dowzell K, O'Donovan MC, Powell J, Lovestone S, Brayne C, Rubinsztein D, Owen MJ et al (2009) Evidence that variation in the oligodendrocyte lineage transcription factor 2 (OLIG2) gene is associated with psychosis in Alzheimer's disease. Neurosci Lett 461:54–59. https://doi.org/10.1016/j.neulet.2009.05.051
76. Stricker NH, Schweinsburg BC, Delano-Wood L, Wierenga CE, Bangen KJ, Haaland KY, Frank LR, Salmon DP, Bondi MW (2009) Decreased white matter integrity in late-myelinating fiber pathways in Alzheimer's disease supports retrogenesis. NeuroImage 45:10–16. https://doi.org/10.1016/j.neuroimage.2008.11.027
77. Thorburne SK, Juurlink BH (1996) Low glutathione and high iron govern the susceptibility of oligodendroglial precursors to oxidative stress. J Neurochem 67:1014–1022
78. Tosto G, Zimmerman ME, Carmichael OT, Brickman AM (2014) Predicting aggressive decline in mild cognitive impairment: the importance of white matter hyperintensities. JAMA neurology 71:872–877. https://doi.org/10.1001/jamaneurol.2014.667
79. Tosto G, Zimmerman ME, Hamilton JL, Carmichael OT, Brickman AM (2015) The effect of white matter hyperintensities on neurodegeneration in mild cognitive impairment. Alzheimers Dement 11:1510–1519. https://doi.org/10.1016/j.jalz.2015.05.014
80. Tsai HH, Niu J, Munji R, Davalos D, Chang J, Zhang H, Tien AC, Kuo CJ, Chan JR, Daneman R et al (2016) Oligodendrocyte precursors migrate along vasculature in the developing nervous system. Science (New York, NY) 351: 379–384. https://doi.org/10.1126/science.aad3839
81. Tse KH, Herrup K (2017) DNA damage in the oligodendrocyte lineage and its role in brain aging. Mech Ageing Dev 161:37–50. https://doi.org/10.1016/j.mad.2016.05.006
82. Tse KH, Herrup K (2017) Re-imagining Alzheimer's disease - the diminishing importance of amyloid and a glimpse of what lies ahead. J neurochemistry. https://doi.org/10.1111/jnc.14079
83. Vlkolinsky R, Cairns N, Fountoulakis M, Lubec G (2001) Decreased brain levels of 2',3'-cyclic nucleotide-3'-phosphodiesterase in down syndrome and Alzheimer's disease. Neurobiol Aging 22:547–553
84. Xu J, Chen S, Ahmed SH, Chen H, Ku G, Goldberg MP, Hsu CY (2001) Amyloid-beta peptides are cytotoxic to oligodendrocytes. The journal of neuroscience : the official journal of the Society for Neuroscience 21: Rc118
85. Yuen TJ, Silbereis JC, Griveau A, Chang SM, Daneman R, Fancy SP, Zahed H, Maltepe E, Rowitch DH (2014) Oligodendrocyte-encoded HIF function couples postnatal myelination and white matter angiogenesis. Cell 158:383–396. https://doi.org/10.1016/j.cell.2014.04.052
86. Zhao Z, Nelson AR, Betsholtz C, Zlokovic BV (2015) Establishment and dysfunction of the blood-brain barrier. Cell 163:1064–1078. https://doi.org/10.1016/j.cell.2015.10.067

Permissions

All chapters in this book were first published in ANC, by BioMed Central; hereby published with permission under the Creative Commons Attribution License or equivalent. Every chapter published in this book has been scrutinized by our experts. Their significance has been extensively debated. The topics covered herein carry significant findings which will fuel the growth of the discipline. They may even be implemented as practical applications or may be referred to as a beginning point for another development.

The contributors of this book come from diverse backgrounds, making this book a truly international effort. This book will bring forth new frontiers with its revolutionizing research information and detailed analysis of the nascent developments around the world.

We would like to thank all the contributing authors for lending their expertise to make the book truly unique. They have played a crucial role in the development of this book. Without their invaluable contributions this book wouldn't have been possible. They have made vital efforts to compile up to date information on the varied aspects of this subject to make this book a valuable addition to the collection of many professionals and students.

This book was conceptualized with the vision of imparting up-to-date information and advanced data in this field. To ensure the same, a matchless editorial board was set up. Every individual on the board went through rigorous rounds of assessment to prove their worth. After which they invested a large part of their time researching and compiling the most relevant data for our readers.

The editorial board has been involved in producing this book since its inception. They have spent rigorous hours researching and exploring the diverse topics which have resulted in the successful publishing of this book. They have passed on their knowledge of decades through this book. To expedite this challenging task, the publisher supported the team at every step. A small team of assistant editors was also appointed to further simplify the editing procedure and attain best results for the readers.

Apart from the editorial board, the designing team has also invested a significant amount of their time in understanding the subject and creating the most relevant covers. They scrutinized every image to scout for the most suitable representation of the subject and create an appropriate cover for the book.

The publishing team has been an ardent support to the editorial, designing and production team. Their endless efforts to recruit the best for this project, has resulted in the accomplishment of this book. They are a veteran in the field of academics and their pool of knowledge is as vast as their experience in printing. Their expertise and guidance has proved useful at every step. Their uncompromising quality standards have made this book an exceptional effort. Their encouragement from time to time has been an inspiration for everyone.

The publisher and the editorial board hope that this book will prove to be a valuable piece of knowledge for researchers, students, practitioners and scholars across the globe.

List of Contributors

Jordan R. Warford, Anna-Claire Lamport, Derek R. Clements, Alicia Malone, Barry E. Kennedy, Youra Kim, Shashi A. Gujar, David W. Hoskin and Alexander S. Easton
Department of Pathology, Dalhousie University, Sir Charles Tupper Medical Building, 5850 College Street, Halifax, NS B3H 4R2, Canada

David W. Hoskin
Department of Microbiology and Immunology, Dalhousie University, Sir Charles Tupper Medical Building, 5850 College Street, Halifax, NS B3H 4R2, Canada

Melissa L. Cooper, John W. Collyer and David J. Calkins
Department of Ophthalmology and Visual Sciences, The Vanderbilt Eye Institute, Vanderbilt University Medical Center, 1105 Medical Research Building IV, Nashville, TN 37232-0654, USA

Daniel A. Mordes, Joseph R. Klim, Rob Moccia, Francesco Limone, Olli Pietilainen, Kaitavjeet Chowdhary and Kevin Eggan
Department of Stem Cell and Regenerative Biology, Harvard University, Cambridge, MA 02138, USA
Harvard Stem Cell Institute, Harvard University, Cambridge, MA 02138, USA

Daniel A. Mordes, Joseph R. Klim, Rob Moccia, Francesco Limone, Olli Pietilainen Petrucelli and Kevin Eggan
Stanley Center for Psychiatric Research, Broad Institute of MIT and Harvard, Cambridge, MA 02142, USA

Daniel A. Mordes
Department of Pathology, Massachusetts General Hospital, Boston, MA 02114, USA

Dennis W. Dickson, Rosa Rademakers, Leonard Petrucelli and Mercedes Prudencio
Department of Neuroscience, Mayo Clinic, Jacksonville, FL 32224, USA

Nancy M. Bonini and Lindsey D. Goodman
Department of Biology, University of Pennsylvania, Philadelphia, PA 19104, USA

Rob Moccia
Pfizer, Cambridge, MA 02139, USA

Asad Jan
Aarhus Institute of Advanced Studies, Department of Biomedicine, Aarhus University, Høegh-Guldbergs Gade 6B, DK-8000 Aarhus, Denmark

Alberto Delaidelli, Gian Luca Negri, Poul H. Sorensen and Ian R. Mackenzie
Department of Pathology and Laboratory Medicine, University of British Columbia, Vancouver, Canada

Brandon Jansonius and Poul H. Sorensen
British Columbia Cancer Research Centre, 675 West 10th Avenue, Vancouver, BC V5Z 1L3, Canada

Forum Bhanshali, Yi Andy An and Stefan Taubert
Centre for Molecular Medicine and Therapeutics, BC Children's Hospital Research Institute, Department of Medical Genetics, University of British Columbia, Vancouver, BC V5Z 4H4, Canada

Nelson Ferreira and Poul H. Jensen
Danish Research Institute of Translational Neuroscience, Department of Biomedicine, Aarhus University, Ole Worms Allé 3, DK-8000 Aarhus, Denmark

Lisa M. Smits and Jens C. Schwamborn
Developmental and Cellular Biology, Luxembourg Centre for Systems Biomedicine (LCSB), University of Luxembourg, 7, avenue des Hauts-Fourneaux, 4362 Esch-sur-Alzette, Luxembourg

Leah C. Beauchamp, Jacky Chan, Lin W. Hung, Laura J. Vella, Xiang M. Liu, Ashley I. Bush, Laura Jacobson and Kevin J. Barnham
The Florey Institute of Neuroscience and Mental Health, The University of Melbourne, Parkville, VIC 3010, Australia

Leah C. Beauchamp, Laura Jacobson and Kevin J. Barnham
The Department of Pharmacology and Therapeutics, The University of Melbourne, Parkville, VIC 3010, Australia

Benjamin S. Padman
Monash Biomedicine Discovery Institute, Monash University, Clayton, VIC 3800, Australia

Bradley Coleman and Andrew F. Hill
The Department of Biochemistry and Molecular Biology, Bio21 Institute, The University of Melbourne, Parkville, VIC 3010, Australia

Andrew F. Hill
The Department of Biochemistry and Genetics, La Trobe Institute for Molecular Science, La Trobe University, Bundoora, VIC 3083, Australia

Christina E. Murray, Priya Gami-Patel, Janice L. Holton, Tamas Revesz and Tammaryn Lashley
The Queen Square Brain Bank for Neurological Disorders, Department of Molecular Neuroscience, UCL Institute of Neurology, London WC1N 3BG, UK

Eleni Gkanatsiou, Gunnar Brinkmalm, Erik Portelius and Henrik Zetterberg
Institute of Neuroscience and Physiology, Department of Psychiatry and Neurochemistry, The Sahlgrenska Academy at the University of Gothenburg, Mölndal, Sweden

Erik Portelius, Kaj Blennow and Henrik Zetterberg
Clinical Neurochemistry Laboratory, Sahlgrenska University Hospital, Mölndal, Sweden

Oliver Wirths
Department of Psychiatry and Psychotherapy, University Medical Center (UMG), Georg-August-University, Goettingen, Germany

Wendy Heywood and Kevin Mills
Centre for Translational Omics, Great Ormond Street Institute of Child health, UCL, London, UK

Jorge Ghiso
New York University, New York, NY, USA

Christina E. Murray and Henrik Zetterberg
Dementia Research Institute, UCL, London, UK

Joan Y. W. Liu, Mar Matarin, Cheryl Reeves, Andrew W. McEvoy, Pamela Thompson, Sanjay M. Sisodiya and Maria Thom
Department of Clinical and Experimental Epilepsy, UCL Institute of Neurology, Queen Square, London WCN1BG, UK

Joan Y. W. Liu, Cheryl Reeves and Maria Thom
Department of Neuropathology, National Hospital for Neurology and Neurosurgery, UCL Institute of Neurology, Queen Square, London WC1N 3BG, UK

Sanjay M. Sisodiya
Department of Neurology, National Hospital for Neurology and Neurosurgery, London, UK

Pamela Thompson
Department of Neuropsychology, National Hospital for Neurology and Neurosurgery, London, UK

Andrew W. McEvoy
Department of Neurosurgery, National Hospital for Neurology and Neurosurgery, London, UK

Pamela Thompson, Anna Miserocchi and Sanjay M. Sisodiya
Chalfont Centre for Epilepsy, Chesham Lane, Chalfont St Peter, Buckinghamshire SL9 0RJ, UK

Joan Y. W. Liu
Department of Biomedical Sciences, University of Westminster, W1W6UW, London, UK

Karin M. E. Forsberg
Department of Medical Biosciences & Pathology, Umeå Universitet, Umeå, Sweden

Yingshuang Zhang
Department of Neurology, Peking University Third Hospital, Beijing, China

Johanna Reiners, Martina Ander, Alexandra Niedermayer, Lubin Fang, Kelly Del Tredici, Heiko Braak and Deniz Yilmazer-Hanke
Clinical Neuroanatomy Section, Neurology, School of Medicine, Ulm University, Helmholtzstr. 8/1, 89081 Ulm, Germany

Hermann Neugebauer, Jan Kassubek and Albert C. Ludolph
Department of Neurology, Ulm University Hospital, Ulm University, Ulm, Germany

Istvan Katona and Joachim Weis
Institute of Neuropathology, School of Medicine, RTWH Aachen University Hospital, Aachen, Aachen, Germany

Satish Kumar Nemani, Silvio Notari, Ignazio Cali, Mark Cohen and Pierluigi Gambetti
Department of Pathology, Case Western Reserve University, School of Medicine, Cleveland, OH 44106, USA

Victor E Alvarez and Ann McKee
VA Boston Healthcare System, Boston, MA 02130, USA

Victor E Alvarez and Ann McKee
Department of Neurology and Pathology, Boston University School of Medicine, Boston, MA 02118, USA

Victor E Alvarez, Robert A. Stern and Ann McKee
Alzheimer's Disease Center and CTE Program, Boston University School of Medicine, Boston, MA 02118, USA

Diane Kofskey, Mark Cohen and Brian Appleby
National Prion Disease Pathology Surveillance Center, Case Western Reserve University, Cleveland, OH 44106, USA

Robert A. Stern
Departments of Neurology,Neurosurgery, and Anatomy and Neurobiology, Boston University School ofMedicine, Boston, MA 02118, USA

Brian Appleby
Departments of Neurology and Psychiatry, Case Western Reserve University, School of Medicine, Cleveland, OH 44106, USA

Joseph Abrams and Lawrence Schonberger
Division of High-Consequence Pathogens and Pathology, National Center for Emerging and Zoonotic Infectious Diseases, Center for Disease Control and Prevention, Atlanta, GA 30333, USA

Jurre den Haan, Philip Scheltens and Femke H. Bouwman
Department of Neurology, Alzheimer Center Amsterdam, Amsterdam Neuroscience, Vrije Universiteit Amsterdam, Amsterdam UMC, Mailbox 7057, Amsterdam 1007 MB, The Netherlands

Tjado H. J. Morrema, Jeroen J. Hoozemans and Annemieke J. Rozemuller
Department of Pathology, Amsterdam Neuroscience, Amsterdam UMC, Vrije Universiteit Amsterdam, Amsterdam, The Netherlands

Frank D. Verbraak
Ophthalmology Department, VU University Medical Center, Amsterdam, The Netherlands

Johannes F. de Boer
Department of Physics, Bio Laser Lab Amsterdam, VU University, Amsterdam, The Netherlands

Arthur A. B. Bergen
Departments of Clinical genetics and Ophthalmology, Amsterdam UMC, Academic Medical Center, University of Amsterdam, Amsterdam, The Netherlands
The Netherlands Institute for Neuroscience (NIN-KNAW), Amsterdam, The Netherlands

Iliana Michailidou, Theodosia Georgakopoulou, Marit B. de Wissel, Ruud A. Wolterman, Patrick Ruizendaal and Valeria Ramaglia
Department of Genome Analysis, Academic Medical Center, Amsterdam, The Netherlands

Iliana Michailidou, Jeroen P. Vreijling, Kees Fluiter and Frank Baas
Department of Clinical Genetics, Leiden University Medical Center, Einthovenweg 20, 2333, ZC, Leiden, The Netherlands

Aldo Jongejan
Department of Bioinformatics, Academic Medical Center, Amsterdam, The Netherlands

Ngaisah Klar-Mohamad and Cees van Kooten
Department of Nephrology, Leiden University Medical Center, Leiden, The Netherlands

Anita E. Grootemaat, Daisy I. Picavet and Nicole N. van der Wel
Electron Microscopy Centre Amsterdam, Department of Medical Biology, Academic Medical Center, Amsterdam, The Netherlands

Vinod Kumar and Trent M. Woodruff
School of Biomedical Sciences, The University of Queensland, Brisbane, Australia

B. Paul Morgan
Systems Immunity University Research Institute, School of Medicine, Cardiff University, Cardiff, UK

Valeria Ramaglia
Department of Immunology, University of Toronto, Toronto, Canada

Airi Tarutani and Masato Hasegawa
Department of Dementia and Higher Brain Function, Tokyo Metropolitan Institute of Medical Science, 2-1-6 Kamikitazawa, Setagaya-ku, Tokyo 156-8506, Japan

Airi Tarutani and Shin-ichi Hisanaga
Department of Biological Science, Tokyo Metropolitan University, Minami-osawa, Hachioji, Tokyo 192-0397, Japan

Tetsuaki Arai
Department of Neuropsychiatry, Division of Clinical Medicine, Faculty of Medicine, University of Tsukuba, 1-1-1, Tennodai, Tsukuba, Ibaraki 305-8576, Japan

Shigeo Murayama
Department of Neuropathology, Tokyo Metropolitan Geriatric Hospital and Institute of Gerontology, 35-2 Sakaecho, Itabashi-ku, Tokyo 173-0015, Japan

Matthew D. Cykowski, Suzanne Z. Powell, Anithachristy S. Arumanayagam and Andreana L. Rivera
Department of Pathology and Genomic Medicine, Houston Methodist Hospital, 6565 Fannin Street, Houston, TX 77030, USA

Matthew D. Cykowski, Suzanne Z. Powell, Andreana L. Rivera and Stanley H. Appel
Institute of Academic Medicine (IAM) in the Houston Methodist Research Institute (HMRI), Houston Methodist Hospital, 6565 Fannin Street, Houston, TX 77030, USA

Suzanne Z. Powell and Joan W. Appel
Houston Methodist Neurological Institute, Houston Methodist Hospital, 6565 Fannin Street, Houston, TX 77030, USA

Joan W. Appel and Stanley H. Appel
Department of Neurology, Houston Methodist Hospital, 6565 Fannin Street, Houston, TX 77030, USA

Dagmar E. Ehrnhoefer, Dale D. O. Martin, Mandi E. Schmidt, Xiaofan Qiu, Safia Ladha, Nicholas S. Caron, Niels H. Skotte, Yen T. N. Nguyen, Kuljeet Vaid, Amber L. Southwell, Sabine Engemann, Sonia Franciosi and Michael R. Hayden
Centre for Molecular Medicine and Therapeutics (CMMT), CFRI, Department of Medical Genetics, University of British Columbia, 950 West 28th Avenue, Vancouver, BC V5Z 4H4, Canada

Dagmar E. Ehrnhoefer
BioMed X Innovation Center, Im Neuenheimer Feld 515, 69120 Heidelberg, Germany

Sara E. Nasrabady
Department of Psychiatry, Columbia University, New York, NY, USA

James E. Goldman
Department of Pathology and Cell Biology, Columbia University, New York, NY, USA

Adam M. Brickman
Department of Neurology, Columbia University, New York, NY, USA

Batool Rizvi, James E. Goldman and Adam M. Brickman
The Taub Institute for Research in Alzheimer's Disease and the Aging Brain, Columbia University, New York, NY, USA

Index

www.ingramcontent.com/pod-product-compliance
Lightning Source LLC
LaVergne TN
LVHW080719210926
848485LV00003B/490